Intrauterine Growth Restriction: Aetiology and Management

Intrauterine Growth Restriction: Aetiology and Management

Editor: Timmy Glass

FOSTER ACADEMICS

www.fosteracademics.com

www.fosteracademics.com

FOSTER ACADEMICS

Cataloging-in-Publication Data

Intrauterine growth restriction : aetiology and management / edited by Timmy Glass.
p. cm.
Includes bibliographical references and index.
ISBN 978-1-64646-598-9
1. Fetal growth retardation. 2. Fetal growth retardation--Etiology. 3. Fetal growth retardation--Treatment.
4. Fetus--Growth. 5. Pregnancy--Complications. 6. Fetus--Diseases--Etiology. 7. Fetus--Abnormalities. I. Glass, Timmy.
RG629.G76 I58 2023
618.32--dc23

Foster Academics,
118-35 Queens Blvd., Suite 400,
Forest Hills, NY 11375, USA

ISBN 978-1-64646-598-9 (Hardback)

Contents

Preface

Intrauterine growth restriction (IUGR) or fetal growth restriction is a condition in which the fetus does not grow normally in the womb during pregnancy. This condition may be caused due to maternal, fetal, or placental complications. Certain important causes include placenta abnormalities, high blood pressure in mother, infections, smoking or alcohol abuse, cardiovascular disease, hypertension, blood clotting disorder, etc. One of the major consequences of IUGR is that a baby is born weighing less than 90 percent of other babies at the same gestational age. IUGR is broadly classified into asymmetrical IUGR and symmetrical IUGR. A decreased oxygen or nutrient supply to the fetus during the third trimester of pregnancy due to placental insufficiency is called asymmetrical IUGR. Symmetrical IUGR, also known as global growth restriction, shows that the fetus has grown slowly during the pregnancy, and has been affected from the start. This book is compiled in such a manner, that it will provide in-depth knowledge about intrauterine growth restriction. It outlines the aetiology and management of this medical condition in detail. Those in search of information to further their knowledge will be greatly assisted by this book.

This book has been the outcome of endless efforts put in by authors and researchers on various issues and topics within the field. The book is a comprehensive collection of significant researches that are addressed in a variety of chapters. It will surely enhance the knowledge of the field among readers across the globe.

It gives us an immense pleasure to thank our researchers and authors for their efforts to submit their piece of writing before the deadlines. Finally in the end, I would like to thank my family and colleagues who have been a great source of inspiration and support.

Editor

1

Influence of Low Protein Diet-Induced Fetal Growth Restriction on the Neuroplacental Corticosterone Axis in the Rat

Marius Schmidt[1], Manfred Rauh[1], Matthias C. Schmid[2], Hanna Huebner[3], Matthias Ruebner[3], Rainer Wachtveitl[1], Nada Cordasic[1], Wolfgang Rascher[1], Carlos Menendez-Castro[1], Andrea Hartner[1] and Fabian B. Fahlbusch[1]*

[1] Department of Pediatrics and Adolescent Medicine, Friedrich-Alexander University Erlangen-Nuremberg, Erlangen, Germany, [2] Institute of Medical Biometry, Informatics and Epidemiology, Faculty of Medicine, Rheinische Friedrich-Wilhelms-University, Bonn, Germany, [3] Department of Gynaecology and Obstetrics/ Comprehensive Cancer Center Erlangen-EMN, Friedrich-Alexander University Erlangen-Nuremberg, Erlangen, Germany

***Correspondence:**
Fabian B. Fahlbusch
fabian.fahlbusch@uk-erlangen.de

Objectives: Placental steroid metabolism is linked to the fetal hypothalamus-pituitary-adrenal axis. Intrauterine growth restriction (IUGR) might alter this cross-talk and lead to maternal stress, in turn contributing to the pathogenesis of anxiety-related disorders of the offspring, which might be mediated by fetal overexposure to, or a reduced local enzymatic protection against maternal glucocorticoids. So far, direct evidence of altered levels of circulating/local glucocorticoids is scarce. Liquid chromatography tandem-mass spectrometry (LC-MS/MS) allows quantitative endocrine assessment of blood and tissue. Using a rat model of maternal protein restriction (low protein [LP] vs. normal protein [NP]) to induce IUGR, we analyzed fetal and maternal steroid levels via LC-MS/MS along with the local expression of 11beta-hydroxysteroid-dehydrogenase (*Hsd11b*).

Methods: Pregnant Wistar dams were fed a low protein (8%, LP; IUGR) or an isocaloric normal protein diet (17%, NP; controls). At E18.5, the expression of *Hsd11b1* and *2* was determined by RT-PCR in fetal placenta and brain. Steroid profiling of maternal and fetal whole blood, fetal brain, and placenta was performed via LC-MS/MS.

Results: In animals with LP-induced reduced body ($p < 0.001$) and placental weights ($p < 0.05$) we did not observe any difference in the expressional *Hsd11b1/2*-ratio in brain or placenta. Moreover, LP diet did not alter corticosterone (Cort) or 11-dehydrocorticosterone (DH-Cort) levels in dams, while fetal whole blood levels of Cort were significantly lower in the LP group ($p < 0.001$) and concomitantly in LP brain ($p = 0.003$) and LP placenta ($p = 0.002$). Maternal and fetal progesterone levels (whole blood and tissue) were not influenced by LP diet.

Conclusion: Various rat models of intrauterine stress show profound alterations in placental Hsd11b2 gatekeeper function and fetal overexposure to corticosterone. In contrast, LP diet in our model induced IUGR without altering maternal steroid levels or placental enzymatic glucocorticoid barrier function. In fact, IUGR offspring showed significantly reduced levels of circulating and local corticosterone. Thus, our LP model might not represent a genuine model of intrauterine stress. Hypothetically, the observed changes might reflect a fetal attempt to maintain anabolic conditions in the light of protein restriction to sustain regular brain development. This may contribute to fetal origins of later neurodevelopmental sequelae.

Keywords: IUGR intrauterine growth restriction, steroids, brain, placenta, Hsd11b2, rat model, low protein, neuroplacentology

INTRODUCTION

The association of intrauterine growth restriction (IUGR) with the development of metabolic disorders [i.e., type 2 diabetes, hyperlipidemia (1)] and cardiac disease [i.e., arterial hypertension, cardiovascular disease (2)] in later life is well-recognized based on several animal (3, 4) and human (5) studies. Barker introduced the hypothesis of "fetal programming," postulating that an adverse intrauterine environment affects growth and differentiation of the fetus and subsequently contributes to the development of the above sequelae later in life (6).

The mechanistic basis of "developmental origins of health and disease" (DOHaD) are subject of ongoing research (7). A possible mechanism that links maternal gestational adversity to long-term health outcomes in offspring is the diaplacental transfer of glucocorticoids (8): during pregnancy the placental enzyme 11beta-hydroxysteroid dehydrogenase 2 (Hsd11b2) catalyses the oxidation of cortisol to cortisone [predominant in humans (9)] and of corticosterone (Cort) to 11-dehydrocorticosterone [DH-Cort, predominant in rats (9)], thereby inactivating these glucocorticoids. There is evidence that low birth weight might be associated with a reduced placental HSD11b2 activity in both humans (10) and rodents (11–13) contributing to fetal hypercortisolism and programming of hypertension and metabolic syndrome in adult rat offspring.

Beyond these major schemes of fetal programming, a potential negative influence of poor fetal growth on brain development with anxiety-related sequelae is being critically discussed (14). In human pregnancy, heightened maternal anxiety with endogenous elevation of glucocorticoids might predispose the offspring for schizophrenia (15), hyperactive disorder (16) and/or impaired emotional and cognitive development (17). It has been shown that maternal anxiety is negatively correlated with placental *HSD11b2* mRNA expression (18). Additionally, a reduction of placental HSD11b2 seems to be associated with IUGR (19). We have also found that the *HSD11b2* mRNA expression is negatively correlated with postnatal catch-up growth in IUGR (10).

There is evidence that iatrogenic administration of exogenous glucocorticoids for lung maturation might exert negative fetal effects: A single course of antenatal betamethasone (not metabolized by HSD11b2) treatment before 34 + 0 weeks of gestation seems to be associated with an impairment of cognitive ability in treated infants (20, 21) and a reduced head circumference in females (22) at term. Moreover, betamethasone treatment (23) and inhibition of HSD11b2 activity (24) was associated with a certain impairment of hypothalamic-pituitary-adrenal (HPA)-axis function in humans.

Similar to humans, fetal exposure of rats to gestational stress (e.g., via inhibition of Hsd11b2 or treatment with glucocorticoids) seemed to induce low birth weight and trigger processes in the HPA-axis with negative effects on postnatal neurodevelopment. Affected rats showed increased stress responsivity, anxiety-like behavior and altered social interaction postnatally (25–28). Experiments with Hsd11b2 null mice are indicative of direct fetal programming effects on animal behavior via endogenous glucocorticoids (29).

Various non-surgical rat models for the induction of gestational maternal adversity exist (28). In general, maternal stress is either directly [e.g., chronic restraint stress (30)] or indirectly [e.g., nutritional restriction (13, 31)], induced during various stages of gestation. Maternal glucocorticoids are deemed to be among the main effectors of fetal programming in these animals (32), as prenatal effects can be averted via adrenalectomy of the dams (33). Noteworthy, the glucocorticoid system is known to be tightly interlinked with other essential regulators of fetal neurodevelopment, such as the neuroplacental serotonin (5-hydroxytryptamine; 5-HT) axis (34, 35). Perturbations of the fetal serotonin system during early development by prenatal maternal stress have been linked to processes of fetal programming of psychiatric disorders in later life (35).

In our study we investigated the maternal and fetal (E18.5) HPA-axis in an established nutritionally-induced IUGR model (36), using a novel methodological approach. So far, endocrine changes in such models were mainly studied using multiple ELISA measurements of single hormones in serum or RT-PCR of *Hsd11b2* in target tissues (i.e., placenta and brain) (11, 12, 22, 37–40). We have recently established a liquid chromatography tandem mass-spectrometry method (LC-MS/MS) that allows for the detection of multiple glucocorticoids in a single tissue/serum probe (9, 41), minimizing tissue-matrix interactions (42, 43). The combination of LC-MS/MS with volumetric adhesive microsampling devices enables individual sampling without the need for pooling of fetal samples (44). We set out to determine the steroid profile in maternal and fetal circulation, along with placental and brain steroid profiles, in IUGR vs. control rats and to compare these findings to *Hsd11b2* mRNA expression in these tissues. We were especially interested to identify steroid profiles characteristic for IUGR. In the face of potential IUGR-related neurologic sequelae and the role of placental Hsd11b2, we aimed to provide evidence of a neuroplacental cross-talk on the glucocorticoid level in these animals.

METHODS

Animals and Diets

Animal procedures were carried out as previously described (36). This study was carried out in accordance with the recommendations of the NIH *Guide for the Care and Use of Laboratory Animals* and the *EU Directive 2010/63/EU.* All procedures and protocols were governmentally approved by the corresponding board (Regierung von Mittelfranken, AZ #54-2531.31-31/09). Wistar rats were ordered from Charles River (Sulzfeld, Germany). Virgin female rats (240–260 g) were housed individually and maintained at 22°C on a 12 h light–dark cycle. After mating, pregnancy was confirmed via vaginal plug formation (day 1 of gestation). The use of our alimentary IUGR model for the analysis of postnatal sequelae of fetal programming has been previously described by us (3, 36, 45, 46). In short, 12 dams were randomly assigned to two groups receiving semi-purified diets (Altromin Spezialfutter GmbH & Co. KG, Lage, Germany) of either low protein diet (LP group, 25 g/d of Altromin C1003, 8.1% protein, 13% fat, 78% carbohydrates [2% monosaccharides, 18% disaccharides, 49% polysaccharides] or an isocaloric diet of normal protein content (NP group, 25 g/d of Altromin C1000, 17.3% protein, 13% fat, 67% carbohydrates [10% disaccharides, 47% polysaccharides], and were weighed daily. Animal characteristics are displayed in **Table 1**.

Additionally, a second set of four dams (conversion set) was mated and received NP diet *ad libitum*. Blood samples of these animals and the respective fetuses were used to establish a conversion factor for volumetric adhesive microsampling (VAMS) to EDTA-blood in order to improve comparability of data with findings from the literature (**Supplementary Table S1**). Moreover, LC-MS/MS pretesting of placental tissue and brain in these animals helped to optimize run settings for steroid and CRH detection.

Sample and Data Collection

At E18.5 fetuses were obtained via cesarean section under isoflurane anesthesia. Starting out with six dams per group, one dam of the NP group (NP) had to be excluded as litter size (<10 fetuses) was extremely low. Additionally, two dams (one NP and LP, each) did not follow their expected growth trajectories and were subsequently excluded by the veterinarian due to suspected health issues. For our final analysis six fetuses ($n = 3$ females, $n = 3$ males each) per dam ($n = 4$ NP, $n = 5$ LP) were chosen based on their matching positions in the proximal uterine horns. Fetuses were sacrificed via decapitation, followed by individual Mitra™ (Neoteryx, LLC, Torrance, CA, USA) VAMS of mixed arterio-venous blood from the trunk's cutting surface, as described (44). Brain and placenta samples were instantly snap-frozen in liquid nitrogen and stored at −80°C. Fetal tail-tip biopsies were used for sex determination. We did not perform fetal saline-perfusion prior to tissue collection, as this procedure has been shown to interfere with cerebral tissue steroid detection (47). Subsequently, dams were sacrificed via aortic transection. Arterial blood was drawn via syringe and collected in K3 EDTA blood collection tubes (Sarstedt, Nümbrecht, Germany). Additionally, whole blood samples were collected via VAMS.

In the conversion set of animals (see above), trunk blood of fetuses from one litter was pooled in EDTA-tubes to facilitate the measurement of a maximum number of steroids for the purpose of converting VAMS steroid measurements into EDTA standard values (**Supplementary Table S1**).

TABLE 1 | Rat auxologic data.

Weight (g)	NP	LP	*p*-value
Litter (*n*)	4	5	
Fetus	1.38 ± 0.09	0.84 ± 0.06	<0.001#
Brain	0.08 ± 0.01	0.08 ± 0.05	ns§
Placenta	0.34 ± 0.04	0.29 ± 0.02	<0.050#
Placenta/Fetus	0.25 ± 0.02	0.35 ± 0.03	<0.001#
Litter size	12.75 ± 2.22	14.20 ± 2.59	ns#

(#) Welch's t-test, (§) Mann–Whitney U-test.

RNA Extraction, RT-PCR, and Real-Time Quantitative PCR

For measurement of *Hsd11b1* and *2*, RNA was extracted from fetal placenta and brain using peqGOLD TriFast™, according to the manufacturer's instruction (VWR International GmbH, Darmstadt, Germany). RNA concentration was quantified via NanoDrop ND1000 spectrophotometry (Peqlab) and adjusted to 1 ng/ml. After DNase treatment, RNA was transcribed into cDNA using the QuantiTect Reverse Transcription Kit (Qiagen, Hilden, Germany) and random hexamers as primers. Reactions without Quantiscript Reverse Transcriptase served as negative controls. Quantitative real-time PCR was performed with SYBR Green (Applied Biosystems, Darmstadt, Germany; ThermoFisher Scientific) using the StepOnePlus Real-Time PCR System (Applied Biosystems). Samples were run in duplicates and mRNA levels were normalized to the housekeeping gene *18S* rRNA. SYBR-Green based real-time PCR results were compared between groups using the $2^{-\Delta\Delta CT}$-method. Primers sequences were as following (5′-3′): *r18s* forward (fw) TTGATTAAGTCC CTGCCCTTTGT, *r18s* reverse (rev) CGATCCGAGGGCCTC ACTA; *Hsd11b1* fw TAGACACAGAAACAGCTTTG, *Hsd11b1* rev AATTCCATGATCCTCCTTCC; *Hsd11b2* fw CAGGAGACA TGCCATACC, *Hsd11b2* rev GATGATGCTGACCTTGATAC.

Sex verification was carried out via sex-determining region Y (*Sry*) gene PCR (45). DNA from tail-tip biopsies was extracted using the MyTaq™ Extract-PCR Kit (Bioline, London, UK). Sex determination was performed via commercially available PCR *Sry* assay (Rn04224592; ThermoScientific, Waltham, USA) with *18S* rRNA as housekeeping gene. PCR conditions were adopted from the manufacturer's protocol (ThermoFisher). For male gender a cut-off <23 cycles was chosen, while the threshold for female sex was >29 cycles. When verification was needed, we repeated the measurement with corresponding liver samples.

Liquid Chromatography—Tandem Mass Spectrometry (LC-MS/MS)

We have previously established and validated LC-MS/MS methods for the determination of steroids in human placenta (41) and amniotic fluid (48), as well as in rat placenta and brain (9). We determined corticosterone (Cort), 11-dehydrocorticosterone (DH-Cort), 11-deoxycorticosterone (DOC), progesterone, androstenedione, and testosterone in maternal and fetal whole blood, fetal brain, and placenta. While others were able to detect testosterone in pooled fetal plasma on E19 by RIA (49), androstenedione and testosterone were below the detection limit in whole blood (data not shown), due to individual sampling. LC-MS/MS allows for the combined quantification of corticotropin-releasing hormone (CRH) and steroids. As CRH is not present in rat placenta (9), our study involves its determination in fetal brain only. The following adjustments were made to the methods above: We used 1 ml of ethanol solvent containing protease inhibitor cocktail (Aprotinin 2.0 μl/ml, Pepstatin 6.7 μl/ml and Leupeptin 10.0 μl/ml, all from Carl Roth, Karlsruhe, Germany) per 150 mg tissue for homogenization and waived ultrasonification based on tissue softness. The reduced fetal organ size allowed for the reduction of the amount of resuspended tissue homogenate to 1/10th. Thus, 30 μl of homogenized supernatant were added to 90 μl methanol (MeOH) containing 1% formic acid (FA) for LC-MS/MS sample preparation. Thereby, we could maintain our established sample to solution ratio of 1:3. For steroid profiling, sample protein precipitation was adjusted to the initial reduction of homogenate quantity, such that 50 μl of the above methanol/FA supernatant was added to 50 μl MeOH/zinc sulfate (50 g/L, 1/1 v/v), while the addition of 100 μl internal standard remained unmodified (41). The concentration of standards dilution series encompassed a range of 1.0–250.0 ng/ml. CRH quantification was performed with the remaining homogenate *in toto*. We added MeOH/FA (99/1 v/v) containing 0.24 μg/ml bovine CRH as internal standard (IS, Bachem AG, Bubendorf, Switzerland) relative to 1/3rd of the homogenate volume. Serial standard dilutions of CRH with equivalent IS-ratio covered a detection range of 0.1–20.0 ng/ml. LC-MS/MS measurements of steroids in VAMS of fetal whole blood via MITRA capillary blood collection device (Neoteryx LLC, Torrance, CA, USA) has been previously established and validated by us (44). The final fetal and maternal conversion factors from VAMS whole blood to EDTA blood are given in **Supplementary Table S1**.

Statistical Analysis

Data processing and imaging was performed with Microsoft Office 2016 (Microsoft, Redmond, WA, USA) and Adobe Photoshop CS6 (Adobe Systems, San José, CA, USA). For statistical analysis we used GraphPad PRISM Version 7.0 (GraphPad Software, La Jolla, CA, USA). For every litter, the mean levels of the respective individual fetal hormones in tissue and blood were calculated. Outliers of all laboratory parameters and respective ratios within litters and groups were corrected by using the PRISM "robust regression and outlier removal" (ROUT) method (Q = 1%, equivalent to a false discovery rate of 1%), as described by Motulsky and Brown (50) and Hughes and Hekimi (51). Excluded data points ($n = 6$) are given in **Supplementary Table S2** and were not included in the calculation of the mean per litter. Subsequently, the means per litter ($n = 4$ for the NP group, $n = 5$ for the LP group) were subjected to further statistical analysis. Before performing groupwise comparisons, we checked the normality assumption of the mean values by carrying out a Shapiro Wilk test in each experimental group, followed by a Bonferroni correction of the resulting p-values (one per experimental group). The null hypothesis of normality in both groups was rejected if at least one Bonferroni-corrected Shapiro Wilk $p < 0.05$. When normal distribution was present, Welch's t-test was performed, otherwise a Mann–Whitney U-test was executed. For sex-specific subgroup comparison between NP and LP groups, we used two-way analysis of variance (two-way ANOVA with Sidak's multiple comparison analysis). The normality assumption for the ANOVA residuals was verified using normal quantile-quantile (QQ) plots. All data in this manuscript represent mean ± standard deviation (SD) regardless of their normality, facilitating comparative overview. A $p < 0.05$ was considered statistically significant.

RESULTS

Auxologic Data

We did not observe significant differences in litter size in our LP group secondary to their dietary restriction (**Table 1**). The fetal and placental weights were both significantly lower in the LP group compared to the NP group ($p < 0.001$ and $p < 0.05$, respectively, **Table 1**), while brain weight did not differ (**Table 1**). The ratio of placenta-to-body weight was significantly increased in the LP group ($p < 0.001$, **Table 1**). Thus, while LP diet negatively affected both body and placental weight, its influence on fetal body weight appeared to be more prominent (**Table 1**).

Quantitative Real-Time PCR (qRT-PCR)

The results of our qRT-PCR of fetal brain and placental tissue are listed in **Table 2**. We did not detect significant differences in *Hsd11b1* and *2* mRNA expressions between the NP and LP groups in both brain and placenta. Moreover, the ratio of *Hsd11b1* to *Hsd11b2* was not significantly influenced by LP diet in brain (**Figure 1A**) and placenta (**Figure 1B**). Sex-specific analysis of *Hsd11b1/2*-ratio between NP and LP groups did not reveal significant differences (data not shown).

Steroid Analysis via LC-MS/MS in Maternal and Fetal Whole Blood

Steroid profiles of maternal, as well as of fetal whole blood can be found in **Tables 3, 4**, respectively. NP and LP dams showed

TABLE 2 | qRT-PCR results.

		NP	LP	p-value
Brain	*n*	4	5	
	Fold change (*Hsd11b1*)	1.00 ± 0.69	0.89 ± 0.94	ns[#]
	Fold change (*Hsd11b2*)	1.00 ± 0.51	1.11 ± 0.53	ns[#]
	Ratio	0.98 ± 0.33	0.88 ± 0.77	ns[#]
Placenta	Fold change (*Hsd11b1*)	1.00 ± 0.92	1.96 ± 0.84	ns[#]
	Fold change (*Hsd11b2*)	1.00 ± 0.82	1.84 ± 0.55	ns[#]
	Ratio	1.40 ± 1.24	1.15 ± 0.60	ns[#]

(#) Welch's t-test.

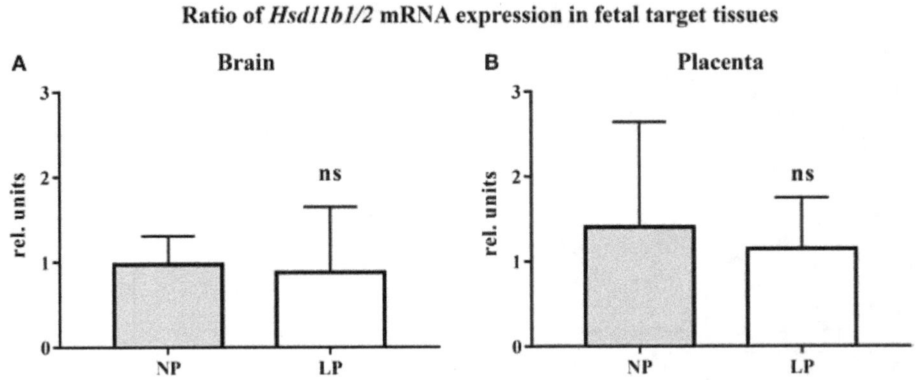

FIGURE 1 | Ratio of *Hsd11b1/2* mRNA expression (qRT-PCR, relative units) in fetal target tissues. **(A)** Fetal rat brain, **(B)** Rat placenta. Legend: Gray column represents NP group ($n = 4$), white column represents LP group ($n = 5$). Legend: rel. units, relative units; ns, not significant.

TABLE 3 | Steroid analysis of maternal whole blood.

Steroids in maternal whole blood (nmol/l)	NP	LP	*p*-value
n	4	5	
Corticosterone (Cort)	1333.00 ± 343.30	1191.00 ± 289.20	ns[§]
Dehydrocorticosterone (DH-Cort)	91.21 ± 25.23	89.12 ± 34.19	ns[#]
Ratio (Cort/DH-Cort)	15.32 ± 5.51	14.37 ± 3.71	ns[#]
Deoxycorticosterone (DOC)	27.63 ± 17.12	14.63 ± 6.49	ns[#]
Progesterone	761.40 ± 466.50	430.00 ± 177.90	ns[§]
Testosterone	1.68 ± 0.89	2.21 ± 0.47	ns[#]

(#)Welch's t-test, (§) Mann–Whitney U-test.

TABLE 4 | Steroid analysis of fetal whole blood.

Steroids in fetal whole blood (nmol/l)	NP	LP	*p*-value
n	4	5	
Corticosterone (Cort)	1740.00 ± 209.90	856.50 ± 177.10	<0.001[#]
Dehydrocorticosterone (DH-Cort)	218.80 ± 47.30	246.10 ± 46.12	ns[#]
Ratio (Cort/DH-Cort)	8.10 ± 1.20	3.54 ± 0.73	0.001[#]
Deoxycorticosterone (DOC)	72.23 ± 16.56	42.54 ± 9.41	0.028[#]
Progesterone	31.52 ± 4.94	29.38 ± 7.09	ns[#]

(#) Welch's t-test.

similar profiles of circulating steroids and Cort/DH-Cort-ratios (**Table 3**). In LP fetuses circulating levels of corticosterone were significantly reduced by 50.78% ($p < 0.001$, **Figure 2A**), while significant group differences regarding circulating levels of 11-dehydrocorticosterone were not detected (**Table 4**, **Figure 2A**). The ratio of Cort/DH-Cort was significantly reduced in LP rat fetuses ($p = 0.001$, **Table 4**, **Figure 2B**). As the pools of fetal and maternal glucocorticoids are diaplacentally linked (52, 53), we determined the feto-maternal Cort/DH-Cort-ratio (i.e., normalization of fetal to maternal steroid levels). No significant alteration of fetal Cort/DH-Cort-ratio was found in the LP group compared to NP fetuses (data not shown). Moreover, we found a significant reduction in circulating DOC levels in the LP group ($p = 0.028$, **Table 4**), while progesterone levels were not significantly different.

Subsequently, we examined fetal steroid profiles with regard to sex (**Table 5**). This subgroup analysis revealed no sex-specific differences between NP and LP groups, with regard to circulating steroids.

Steroid Analysis via LC-MS/MS in Fetal Tissue

Brain and placental tissue steroid profiles are listed in **Tables 6**, **7**, respectively. LP diet significantly lowered local corticosterone levels of both brain and placenta by 45.75% ($p = 0.003$, **Figure 3A**) and 45.56% ($p = 0.002$, **Figure 3C**), respectively. In both brain and placenta, levels of 11-dehydrocorticosterone were not significantly altered compared to the NP groups (**Table 6**, **Figure 3A**; **Table 7**, **Figure 3C**, respectively). In the LP group the local Cort/DH-Cort-ratio was significantly lower in fetal brain ($p = 0.016$; **Figure 3B**; **Table 6**) and placenta ($p = 0.014$; **Figure 3D**; **Table 7**) when compared to NP. Furthermore, local DOC levels were significantly reduced in brain ($p = 0.029$, **Table 6**) and placenta ($p = 0.036$, **Table 7**) of LP fetuses. No significant differences of local progesterone in brain and placenta were observed.

In the brain, LP diet significantly reduced local levels of androstenedione and testosterone in males only ($p = 0.011$, $p = 0.025$, respectively; **Supplementary Table S3a**). In contrast to humans (54), the rat placenta synthesizes significant amounts of androgens (androstenedione and testosterone) (55). In our model, local androgen levels of placenta did not significantly differ between NP and LP groups (**Table 7**), even when sex was regarded (**Supplementary Table S3b**). CRH levels were at the detection limit in fetal brain. Subsequently, we were only able to observe a trend to lower CRH in the brain of LP rats ($p = 0.156$, **Table 6**, **Figure 4**). CRH levels in the fetal brain did not show sex-specific differences between NP and LP groups (**Supplementary Table S3a**).

Further examining sex-specific local tissue steroid profiles of brain and placenta between NP and LP

LC-MS/MS analysis of glucocorticoids in fetal whole blood

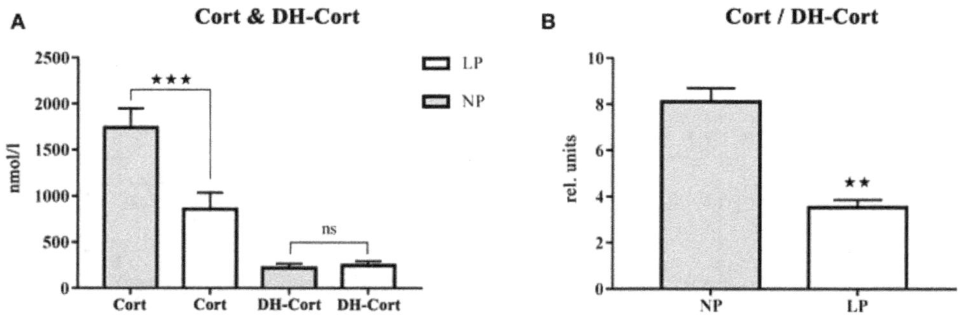

FIGURE 2 | LC-MS/MS analysis of circulating glucocorticoid levels in fetal whole blood. **(A)** Differences of circulating corticosterone (Cort) and 11-dehydrocorticosterone (DH-Cort) levels of fetal NP ($n = 4$) and LP ($n = 5$) whole blood (pmol/g). **(B)** Differences of Cort/DH-Cort -ratio in whole blood. Legend: Gray column represents NP group ($n = 4$), white column represents LP group ($n = 5$), rel. units, relative units; ns, not significant; $^{**}p < 0.01$ and $^{***}p < 0.001$.

TABLE 5 | Sex-specific steroid analysis of fetal whole blood.

	Steroids in fetal whole blood (nmol/l)	**NP**	**LP**	***p*-value**
	n	4	5	
Male	Corticosterone (Cort)	1803.00 ± 191.20	838.50 ± 152.30	<0.001‡
	Dehydrocorticosterone (DH-Cort)	210.40 ± 56.29	238.50 ± 67.45	ns‡
	Ratio (Cort/DH-Cort)	8.95 ± 2.22	3.71 ± 1.07	<0.001‡
	Deoxycorticosterone (DOC)	73.71 ± 17.00	42.06 ± 14.24	0.014‡
	Progesterone	33.02 ± 4.31	27.27 ± 13.01	ns‡
Female	Corticosterone (Cort)	1677.00 ± 239.00	874.40 ± 218.40	<0.001‡
	Dehydrocorticosterone (DH-Cort)	227.20 ± 47.31	253.70 ± 41.84	ns‡
	Ratio (Cort/DH-Cort)	7.48 ± 0.78	3.49 ± 0.90	0.001‡
	Deoxycorticosterone (DOC)	70.75 ± 16.61	43.02 ± 12.40	0.030‡
	Progesterone	30.01 ± 7.05	31.49 ± 17.89	ns‡

(‡) Two-way Anova.

TABLE 6 | Steroid and CRH analysis of fetal brain.

Steroids and CRH in fetal brain (pmol/g)	**NP**	**LP**	***p*-value**
n	4	5	
Corticosterone (Cort)	98.86 ± 12.77	53.63 ± 6.09	0.003#
Dehydrocorticosterone (DH-Cort)	104.50 ± 25.86	122.10 ± 37.66	ns#
Ratio (Cort/DH-Cort)	0.99 ± 0.13	0.48 ± 0.10	0.016§
Deoxycorticosterone (DOC)	13.05 ± 2.67	7.68 ± 3.19	0.029#
Progesterone	47.64 ± 7.81	37.86 ± 12.29	ns#
Androstenedione	3.21 ± 0.48	2.35 ± 0.70	ns#
Testosterone	1.87 ± 0.49	1.02 ± 0.81	ns#
CRH (ng/g)	1.50 ± 0.87	0.68 ± 0.31	ns (0.156)#

(#) Welch's t-test, (§) Mann–Whitney U-test.

TABLE 7 | Steroid analysis of placenta.

Steroids in fetal placenta (pmol/g)	**NP**	**LP**	***p*-value**
n	4	5	
Corticosterone (Cort)	272.80 ± 19.63	148.50 ± 45.76	0.002#
Dehydrocorticosterone (DH-Cort)	309.80 ± 52.00	236.20 ± 43.48	ns#
Ratio (Cort/DH-Cort)	0.93 ± 0.14	0.58 ± 0.18	0.014#
Deoxycorticosterone (DOC)	17.56 ± 4.33	10.17 ± 1.65	0.036#
Progesterone	44.29 ± 12.86	45.89 ± 8.83	ns#
Androstenedione	7.94 ± 1.65	8.58 ± 2.24	ns#
Testosterone	1.09 ± 0.43	0.83 ± 0.25	ns#

(#) Welch's t-test.

groups (**Supplementary Table S2**), we found that local levels of corticosterone in fetal brain and placenta were significantly diminished in both male and female LP rats (**Supplementary Tables S3a,b**, respectively). Furthermore, the sex-specific Cort/DH-Cort-ratio in these organs remained significantly reduced (**Supplementary Table S3**). However, the influence of LP diet on the Cort/DH-Cort-ratio reduction in the female placenta was only a trend ($p = 0.086$, **Supplementary Table S3b**). In the male brain, no difference between NP and LP groups was observed for DOC, while DOC was significantly reduced in female brain ($p = 0.032$, **Supplementary Table S3a**) and in the placenta of both sexes.

Normalization of Tissue LC-MS/MS Results to Body Size

Glucocorticoids and mineralocorticoids are known to significantly influence brain and body weight in rats, respectively (56). As the LP group is characterized by a significant reduction of both body and placental weight (**Table 1**), we normalized local corticosterone, 11-dehydrocorticosterone and deoxycorticosterone levels of brain and placenta in both groups to their respective organ-to-body weight ratio (i.e., steroid x organ weight/body weight, data not shown). Cort/DH-Cort-ratio in brain and placenta of LP fetuses remained

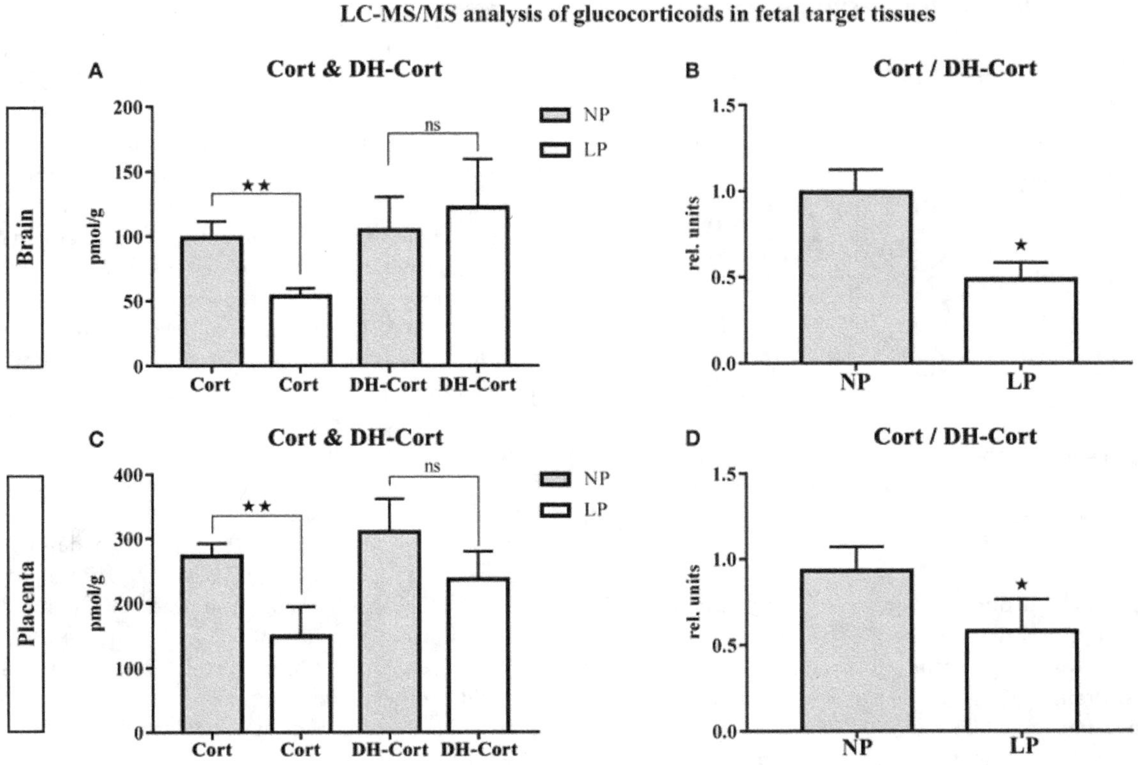

FIGURE 3 | LC-MS/MS analysis of local glucocorticoid levels in fetal target tissues. Results of fetal brain are shown in **(A,B)**, results of placenta are shown in **(C,D)**. **(A)** Differences of corticosterone (Cort) and 11-dehydrocorticosterone (DH-Cort) levels in fetal brains of NP ($n = 4$) and LP ($n = 5$) groups (pmol/g). **(B)** Differences of Cort/DH-Cort -ratio in fetal brain (relative units). **(C)** Differences of corticosterone (Cort) and 11-dehydrocorticosterone (DH-Cort) levels in placenta of NP ($n = 4$) and LP ($n = 5$) groups (pmol/g). **(D)** Differences of Cort/DH-Cort-ratio in placenta of NP ($n = 4$) and LP ($n = 5$) groups (relative units). Legend: Gray column represents NP group ($n = 4$), white column represents LP ($n = 5$) group, rel. units, relative units; ns, not significant; $^{*}p < 0.05$, $^{**}p < 0.01$.

unaffected, i.e., significantly reduced ($p = 0.016$ and $p = 0.014$, respectively). Moreover, levels of placental corticosterone were significantly reduced ($p = 0.043$). No significance was obtained for deoxycorticosterone. While these results seemed largely independent of sex, the reduction of Cort/DH-Cort-ratio of female placenta remained a trend ($p = 0.086$, data not shown).

Analysis of Steroid Levels Relative to Progesterone

In the rat, progesterone serves as a precursor for mineralocorticoids (DOC) and glucocorticoids (57). Thus, we analyzed the ratio of progesterone to DOC and corticosterone. The results are given in **Supplementary Table S4**. In general, ratios of progesterone to DOC and to corticosterone were increased in all LP specimens tested. However, significance was only reached for progesterone/corticosterone-ratio in whole blood ($p = 0.026$, **Supplementary Table S4**) and progesterone/DOC-ratio in placenta ($p = 0.003$, respectively; **Supplementary Table S4**).

DISCUSSION

Our study analyzed steroid profiles via LC-MS/MS in fetal and maternal whole blood and the corresponding fetal placentas and brains in an established rat model of IUGR by maternal protein restriction. We found that LP nutrition did not alter maternal steroid profiles at E18.5. Furthermore, LP diet did not induce fetal hypercortisolism in our model. Instead, levels of circulating corticosterone were lower in LP litters along with a significant reduction in Cort/DH-Cort-ratio. Circulating DOC levels were reduced in the LP group, while progesterone levels remained constant. These results were independent of sex. Similar to our observation in whole blood, we also found a reduction of fetal corticosterone and Cort/DH-Cort-ratio in our analysis of LP brain and placental steroid profiles.

Effects of Low Protein Diet on Steroid Profiles and CRH of the Fetal Brain

The Cort/DH-Cort-ratio in the brain was largely independent of sex in NP and LP groups. While normalization to organ-to-body weight ratio did not affect Cort/DH-Cort-ratio, the observed reduction in DOC tissue levels seemed secondary to the reduced LP weight development (56). It has been shown by others (56) that levels of corticosterone inversely correlate with brain mass in the rat. Also, there is evidence that administration of antenatal betamethasone might be associated with a reduction in head circumference (22) at term and subsequent impairment of cognitive function in treated infants (20, 21). Thus, a reduced

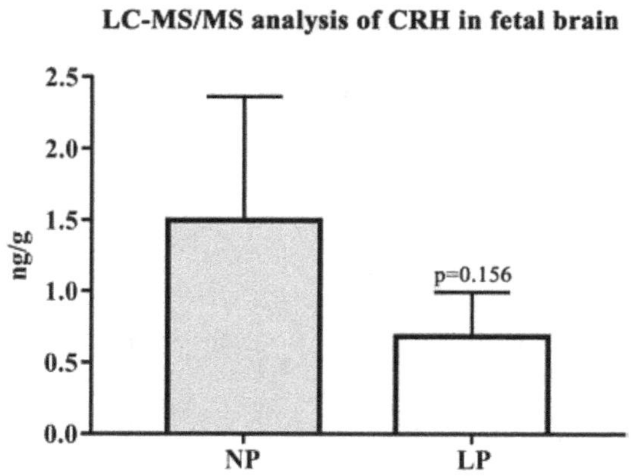

FIGURE 4 | LC-MS/MS analysis of local CRH levels in fetal brain. Differences of CRH of NP ($n = 4$) and LP ($n = 5$) group in brain given in ng/g. Legend: Gray column represents NP ($n = 4$) group, white column represents LP ($n = 5$) group.

Cort/DH-Cort-ratio in our model might argue for a brain sparing effect [reviewed by Miller et al. (58)] in our LP group, as brain weight was not significantly different when compared to NP animals. Brain sparing is associated with asymmetric fetal growth due to increased allocation of nutrients, oxygen, as well as fetal cardiac output to the brain in comparison to other organ systems (58). While this effect promotes survival, it is now apparent that brain sparing might negatively affect brain development in IUGR fetuses (58, 59). Fetal adaptations to adverse intrauterine environment may contribute to an increased postnatal vulnerability for neurodevelopmental and behavioral problems (58, 59). While most animal studies [reviewed by Miller et al. (58)] examined brain sparing effects in rat models of hypoxia or ligation of the uterine artery, García-Contreras et al. (60) examined brain sparing in a malnourished piglet model. They were able to show that nutritional shortage was able to induce local changes in neurotransmitter levels (catecholamines and indoleamines) in swine fetuses, dependent of their sex (60). These transmitters are thought to be related to important cognitive functions (e.g., learning, memory, reward-motivated behavior and stress) (61). To our knowledge, such postnatal behavioral sequelae and neuroendocrine effects have not been studied in our rat model so far. Thus, the potential presence of brain sparing in our LP animals requires future investigation. In line with the observation of sex-specific influences of IUGR on neurotransmitters in swine fetuses (60), we observed differences in brain androgen metabolism (significant reduction of androstenedione and testosterone levels) in our LP male rat fetuses only. These effects might point to brain-specific alterations in local *de novo* synthesis (62) of androgens, as placental androgen levels were not altered by LP diet. It is well-recognized that androgens are important neurodevelopmental factors (63). Androstenedione significantly alters the free fatty acid composition of the fetal brain (64). Excessive levels of androstenedione may induce cellular energy deficits and oxidative stress, potentially driving apoptosis (64). Thus, it might be hypothesized that the reduced androgen levels in the brain of LP males might serve to protect these animals from these adverse effects of IUGR [reviewed by Miller et al. (58)]. Brain compositional changes in free fatty acids warrant further research in our model. The stable androgen levels in the brain of female LP rats could be associated with their ability to metabolize androgens as precursors for estradiol (not determined in this study) (65). Beyond its impact on neurodevelopment, estradiol is known to exert anti-apoptotic effects (66). However, Fernandez-Twinn et al. (39) could only detect an end-gestational rise in circulating estradiol in LP dams of their protein restriction rat model, while no such effect was evident in the fetuses.

Fetal brain CRH levels were close to the lower limit of quantification via LC-MS/MS. Our finding that LP whole brains showed a trend to lower levels of CRH might, however, indicate alterations of superordinate control centers of the HPA-axis. As further targeted histomorphological assessment of these centers (67) is pending in our animal model, we hypothesize that the reduced levels of circulating corticosterone in LP whole blood are associated with reduced CRH in LP brain, despite the lack of significance. A study by Li et al. regarding HPA-axis function in nutritional IUGR of the baboon showed that CRH was the major releasing hormone driving ACTH and cortisol secretion in their model (68). In contrast to our results in the LP rat, the baboon (68), alike other models of maternal nutritional restriction (discussed below), showed an up-regulation of HPA-axis activity. We are currently unaware of other studies examining fetal CRH in the brain of LP rats.

Effects of Low Protein Diet on Placental Hsd11b2 Expression and Function

LP diet led to a significantly reduced placental Cort/DH-Cort-ratio. The reduction of placental corticosterone levels appeared to be independent of organ-to-body weight ratio, similarly to whole blood. While Cort/DH-Cort-reduction did not reach significance in female LP placentas, the Cort/DH-Cort-ratio in whole blood of female LP rats was significantly reduced, alike in male littermates. The lack of significance in female LP placentas might be associated with the small group size. Thus, we concluded that LP diet did not induce fetal hypercortisolism in both sexes in our model.

There is a controversy (39) as to whether intrauterine glucocorticoid exposure is responsible for the reduction of birth weights in the LP model beyond the prevalent deprivation of amino acids (39, 69–71). Our own data does not support this notion. Steroid measurements of whole blood and tissue, via LC-MS/MS, might help to clarify this issue as direct evidence of altered levels of circulating glucocorticoids in the protein restriction model is scarce [ELISA, (39)] and largely based on reports on reduced mRNA expression levels of *Hsd11b2* as a surrogate for enzymatic activity (11, 12, 37, 38).

Jensen Peña et al. recently showed that chronic maternal restraint stress during gestational days 14–20 induced IUGR in Long Evans rats. They observed a significant decrease in placental *Hsd11b2* mRNA expression, associated with an increase in local *Hsd11b2* DNA methylation (40). Accordingly, fetal overexposure to maternal corticosterone was assumed to be involved in the pathogenesis of IUGR. However, no local or circulating glucocorticoid levels were determined in this study. Interestingly, while *Hsd11b2* mRNA levels in the brain remained unaffected (40), the DNA methylation patterns within the *Hsd11b2* promoter were similar to the ones determined in placenta, indicating a certain neuroplacental correlation (40).

In our model, we did not detect significant expressional changes of *Hsd11b1* and *2* mRNA in placenta. Our tissue LC-MS/MS method allows for the direct analysis of local steroid metabolism. Based on the observed dichotomy between our qRT-PCR and LC-MS/MS, we hypothesize that the latter method might be superior regarding the detection sensitivity of alterations in glucocorticoid metabolism. Interestingly, others have just recently found great variability in multiple mRNA species associated with cortisol production, metabolism, and action (72).

Rat Models of Intrauterine Malnutrition and the Role of Glucocorticoids

The role of fetal overexposure to glucocorticoids in IUGR animal models of nutritional restriction remains somewhat unclear, partly due to the differences in feeding, and analytical methods used: employing a rat model where dams were kept on a restricted diet in late gestation (50% of their daily *ad libitum* intake), Blondeau et al. found increased maternal and fetal levels of corticosterone using radio-immunoassays (73). Fetuses had low birth weight and significantly reduced pancreatic insulin content. Thus, an inverse correlation of circulating maternal glucocorticoid levels with fetal β-cell mass was hypothesized (73). Similarly, other studies involving maternal undernutrition (either 50% or protein restriction) showed an increase in maternal levels of corticosterone and a reduction of placental *Hsd11b2* in rats (11, 13).

In contrast, Fernandez-Twinn et al. found serum corticosterone (ELISA detection) in both maternal and fetal circulation (39) to be unaffected by maternal protein restriction using a Wistar rat model of isoenergetic protein restriction throughout gestation]80 g protein/kg vs. 200 g protein/kg (74), *ad libitum*]. However, they were able to identify endocrine changes in their dams (hyperglycemia with concomitant hyperinsulinism, increased levels of prolactin and decreased progesterone levels in early pregnancy; compensatory elevated oestradiol levels and reduced leptin levels in late pregnancy), that might contribute to the programming of poor glucose tolerance, insulin resistance, and the metabolic syndrome in their animals (39). By then, glucocorticoid levels had not been studied in the rat protein restriction model. Hence, based on these findings, Fernandez-Twinn et al. concluded that glucocorticoid levels may not have played a major role in direct programming of eventual adult disease in the developing fetus of their model of protein restriction (39).

Our model of protein restriction has not been characterized to develop postnatal disturbance of glucose tolerance or diabetes in young animals (75) and we have found a significant reduction of corticosterone in our LP rats. Thus, we hypothesize, that the hyperglycemic metabolic state of their dams (39) might have masked potentially reduced glucocorticoid levels so that corticosterone levels presumably matched those found in their NP controls. Exaggerated glucocorticoid secretion has been described to be present in diabetic animals and patients (76). Etiopathologically, the observed maternal hyperglycemia might have been due to the fact that their protein restriction model (74) mainly used monosaccharides to achieve isocaloric energy supplementation (39) and that *ad libitum* fed LP dams further showed an increased daily food intake (39). In contrast, such an effect did not occur in our model (daily food intake 25 g) and isocaloric conditions were fostered by increased substitution of polysaccharides and fat. Also, we observed an increase of the placenta-to-body weight ratio at E18.5, while Fernandez-Twinn et al. observed the ratio to be unchanged (E18), or rather reduced (E21) (39). This might suggest a higher placental capacity for the compensation of maternal protein restriction in our model.

In light of the presented results, one might hypothesize that the maternal food restriction model (i.e., 50% total intake restriction) might more closely resemble models of intrauterine stress than our model of protein restriction, as it leads to increased fetal glucocorticoids. Conclusions drawn from comparison of our study with the only other protein restriction model that examined fetal corticosterone levels (39) seem limited by the above-mentioned maternal metabolic differences. However, corticosterone levels of LP fetuses never exceeded NP levels in both studies. In line with this finding, our previous work (77) indicates that adult male LP rats did not show changes in their circulating glucocorticoid levels, postnatally.

Potential Role of Progesterone in Energy Homeostasis

Progesterone is an essential neuroactive steroid during gestation (78). It is synthesized in maternal tissue, placenta, and the fetal brain, the latter of which is the major target of the steroid (79). Increased local biosynthesis of progesterone and its derivatives may contribute to adaptive processes in maternal and fetal brain during pregnancy (80). Progesterone also exerts neuroprotective functions (78).

While others found progesterone levels of protein restricted dams to be temporarily reduced, we did not detect an influence of LP diet on maternal and fetal progesterone levels at E18.5, despite a reduction in corticosterone and Cort/DH-Cort-ratio in placenta, fetal whole blood, and fetal brain. Thus, it might be speculated that the observed reduction of active glucocorticoids in our LP animals could have resulted, in part, from an organismal effort to maintain constant progesterone levels. Based on our findings, it can be hypothesized that glucocorticoid metabolism is reduced in favor of progesterone maintenance in our LP rats. Interestingly, progesterone is also known to enhance amino acid utilization by the liver (81, 82), which could be of relevance for energy homeostasis in our LP rats.

Limitations

The presented results are limited by the small power of our study. Thus, some of our findings, especially of sex-related differences, represent trends and have to be interpreted with care. The expression of *Hsd11b 1* and *2* was determined on the mRNA level only, however, it remains elusive how mRNA expression translates to protein levels and enzymatic activity in target tissues. While LC-MS/MS has already served as a valid tool for the investigation of glucocorticoid turnover rates in tissue (9), we lacked sufficient amounts of material to perform microsomal enzymatic activity analyses in our study. Furthermore, as only a single time-point of gestation was examined, so far, dynamics in steroid metabolism during pregnancy remain undetermined. It needs to be noted, that the displayed results of our work are only focused on the analysis of fetuses from the proximal uterine horn, which represents the site with the highest maternal blood supply (13). Methodologically, we have avoided brain perfusion prior to LC-MS/MS tissue analysis, as blood contamination has been shown to have little effect on brain steroid levels and saline perfusion may significantly alter local steroid levels (47). Furthermore, we used anesthesia by isoflurane before sacrifice in all animals. While this technique avoids induction of glucocorticoids caused by the injection of anesthetic compounds (83), Bekhbat et al. have recently shown that the use of isoflurane might sex-specifically alter corticosterone levels as determined via ELISA (84). As we currently cannot rule out artifacts in response to collection paradigms, caution has to be used when transferring the presented data to models with different anesthesia.

CONCLUSION

LP diet induced IUGR in our rats, yet it did not impair placental Hsd11b2 gatekeeping function in our study. We did not observe fetal hypercortisolism, as described by other rat models of IUGR (especially general undernutrition and stress models). In contrast, fetal corticosterone levels were significantly reduced in the LP group. This finding seemed independent of sex and was evident in whole blood, placenta and fetal brain. We hypothesize that our LP model does not represent a genuine model of intrauterine stress. Accordingly, our model might not be appropriate to study mechanisms involved in modulating fetal exposure to maternal steroids in IUGR. Thus, while the above-mentioned IUGR models imply that alterations of neuroplacental glucocorticoid cross-talk predispose for neurodevelopmental sequelae, this mechanism might not be present in our LP model. Our maternal protein restriction model may be seen as an equivalent to maternal protein malnutrition in developing countries (85) and might aid in understanding of mechanisms involved in fetal development under protein restriction conditions and the associated postnatal sequelae [especially reno-vascular and cardiac (3, 4, 46, 86)]. However, these may not be significant to and/or representative of mechanisms involved in intrauterine stress in general. At this time we cannot exclude that fetal hypercortisolism was preexistent at earlier gestational stages and that our analysis only determined a certain fatigue of HPA-axis function at the end of pregnancy. Nevertheless, the observed endocrine traits could suggest fetal efforts to achieve anabolic conditions, e.g., brain sparing, in the state of amino acid shortage. If such an effect was present in LP fetuses, it might negatively affect neurodevelopment. Our future studies will, therefore, include additional analysis of postnatal behavior, glucocorticoid levels, tissue metabolomics, and longitudinal steroid profiling beyond corticosterone, e.g., of progesterone derivatives.

AUTHOR CONTRIBUTIONS

AH and FF designed the experiments and supervised the study. MS, RW, NC, and FF conducted and interpreted the experiments. MS, MCS, FF, and MRa performed the data analysis. MS, FF, and MRa wrote the manuscript. FF, MCS, and MS participated in the statistical analysis. WR, CM-C, AH, HH, MCS, and MRu critically revised the manuscript. All authors read and approved the final version of the manuscript.

ACKNOWLEDGMENTS

We gratefully acknowledge the technical assistance of I. Allabauer and K. Heussner at the research facility of the Department of Pediatrics and Adolescent Medicine, Friedrich-Alexander University Erlangen-Nuremberg, Erlangen, Germany. Animal procedures, endocrine analysis and respective data acquisition were performed by MS in fulfillment of the requirements for obtaining the degree Dr. med. at the Friedrich-Alexander-University of Erlangen-Nuremberg, Department of Pediatrics and Adolescent Medicine, Germany. The authors kindly thank S. Fahlbusch, Kirkland, USA for proofreading and language editing. We acknowledge support by Deutsche Forschungsgemeinschaft and Friedrich-Alexander-University Erlangen-Nürnberg (FAU) within the funding programme Open Access Publishing.

REFERENCES

1. McMillen IC, Robinson JS. Developmental origins of the metabolic syndrome: prediction, plasticity, and programming. *Physiol Rev.* (2005) 85:571–633. doi: 10.1152/physrev.00053.2003
2. Barker DJ. *In utero* programming of cardiovascular disease. *Theriogenology.* (2000) 53:555–74. doi: 10.1016/S0093-691X(99)00258-7
3. Menendez-Castro C, Fahlbusch F, Cordasic N, Amann K, Munzel K, Plank C, et al. Early and late postnatal myocardial and vascular changes in a protein restriction rat model of intrauterine growth restriction. *PLoS ONE.* (2011) 6:e20369. doi: 10.1371/journal.pone.0020369
4. Menendez-Castro C, Rascher W, Hartner A. Intrauterine growth restriction - impact on cardiovascular diseases later in life. *Mol Cell Pediatr.* (2018) 5:4. doi: 10.1186/s40348-018-0082-5
5. Crispi F, Miranda J, Gratacos E. Long-term cardiovascular consequences of fetal growth restriction: biology, clinical implications, and opportunities for prevention of adult disease. *Am J Obstet Gynecol.* (2018) 218:S869–79. doi: 10.1016/j.ajog.2017.12.012

6. Barker DJ. *In utero* programming of chronic disease. *Clin Sci.* (1998) 95:115–28.
7. Gluckman PD, Hanson MA, Buklijas T. A conceptual framework for the developmental origins of health and disease. *J Dev Orig Health Dis.* (2010) 1:6–18. doi: 10.1017/S2040174409990171
8. Seckl JR, Holmes MC. Mechanisms of disease: glucocorticoids, their placental metabolism and fetal 'programming' of adult pathophysiology. *Nat Clin Pract Endocrinol Metab.* (2007) 3:479–88. doi: 10.1038/ncpendmet0515
9. Heussner K, Ruebner M, Huebner H, Rascher W, Menendez-Castro C, Hartner A, et al. Species differences of 11beta-hydroxysteroid dehydrogenase type 2 function in human and rat term placenta determined via LC-MS/MS. *Placenta.* (2016) 37:79–84. doi: 10.1016/j.placenta.2015.11.009
10. Tzschoppe A, Struwe E, Blessing H, Fahlbusch F, Liebhaber G, Dorr HG, et al. Placental 11beta-HSD2 gene expression at birth is inversely correlated with growth velocity in the first year of life after intrauterine growth restriction. *Pediatr Res.* (2009) 65:647–53. doi: 10.1203/PDR.0b013e31819e7337
11. Langley-Evans SC, Phillips GJ, Benediktsson R, Gardner DS, Edwards CR, Jackson AA, et al. Protein intake in pregnancy, placental glucocorticoid metabolism and the programming of hypertension in the rat. *Placenta.* (1996) 17:169–72.
12. Seckl JR. Glucocorticoids, feto-placental 11 beta-hydroxysteroid dehydrogenase type 2, and the early life origins of adult disease. *Steroids.* (1997) 62:89–94.
13. Belkacemi L, Jelks A, Chen CH, Ross MG, Desai M. Altered placental development in undernourished rats: role of maternal glucocorticoids. *Reprod Biol Endocrinol.* (2011) 9:105. doi: 10.1186/1477-7827-9-105
14. Jaekel J, Baumann N, Bartmann P, Wolke D. Mood and anxiety disorders in very preterm/very low-birth weight individuals from 6 to 26 years. *J Child Psychol Psychiatry.* (2018) 59:88–95. doi: 10.1111/jcpp.12787
15. Khashan AS, Abel KM, McNamee R, Pedersen MG, Webb RT, Baker PN, et al. Higher risk of offspring schizophrenia following antenatal maternal exposure to severe adverse life events. *Arch Gen Psychiatry.* (2008) 65:146–52. doi: 10.1001/archgenpsychiatry.2007.20
16. Rodriguez A, Bohlin G. Are maternal smoking and stress during pregnancy related to ADHD symptoms in children? *J Child Psychol Psychiatry.* (2005) 46:246–54. doi: 10.1111/j.1469-7610.2004.00359.x
17. Roberts G, Anderson PJ, Davis N, De Luca C, Cheong J, Doyle LW, et al. Developmental coordination disorder in geographic cohorts of 8-year-old children born extremely preterm or extremely low birthweight in the 1990s. *Dev Med Child Neurol.* (2011) 53:55–60. doi: 10.1111/j.1469-8749.2010.03779.x
18. O'Donnell KJ, Bugge Jensen A, Freeman L, Khalife N, O'Connor TG, Glover V. Maternal prenatal anxiety and downregulation of placental 11beta-HSD2. *Psychoneuroendocrinology.* (2012) 37:818–26. doi: 10.1016/j.psyneuen.2011.09.014
19. Shams M, Kilby MD, Somerset DA, Howie AJ, Gupta A, Wood PJ, et al. 11Beta-hydroxysteroid dehydrogenase type 2 in human pregnancy and reduced expression in intrauterine growth restriction. *Hum Reprod.* (1998) 13:799–804.
20. French NP, Hagan R, Evans SF, Godfrey M, Newnham JP. Repeated antenatal corticosteroids: size at birth and subsequent development. *Am J Obstet Gynecol.* (1999) 180:114–21.
21. Jensen RB, Juul A, Larsen T, Mortensen EL, Greisen G. Cognitive ability in adolescents born small for gestational age: associations with fetal growth velocity, head circumference and postnatal growth. *Early Hum Dev.* (2015) 91:755–60. doi: 10.1016/j.earlhumdev.2015.08.014
22. Braun F, Hardt A, Ehrlich L, Sloboda DM, Challis JRG, Plagemann A, et al. Sex-specific and lasting effects of a single course of antenatal betamethasone treatment on human placental 11β-HSD2. *Placenta.* (2018) 69:9–19. doi: 10.1016/j.placenta.2018.07.007
23. Davis EP, Townsend EL, Gunnar MR, Guiang SF, Lussky RC, Cifuentes RF, et al. Antenatal betamethasone treatment has a persisting influence on infant HPA axis regulation. *J Perinatol.* (2006) 26:147–53. doi: 10.1038/sj.jp.7211447
24. Raikkonen K, Seckl JR, Heinonen K, Pyhala R, Feldt K, Jones A, et al. Maternal prenatal licorice consumption alters hypothalamic-pituitary-adrenocortical axis function in children. *Psychoneuroendocrinology.* (2010) 35:1587–93. doi: 10.1016/j.psyneuen.2010.04.010
25. Welberg LA, Seckl JR, Holmes MC. Inhibition of 11beta-hydroxysteroid dehydrogenase, the foeto-placental barrier to maternal glucocorticoids, permanently programs amygdala GR mRNA expression and anxiety-like behaviour in the offspring. *Eur J Neurosci.* (2000) 12:1047–54. doi: 10.1046/j.1460-9568.2000.00958.x
26. Patin V, Lordi B, Vincent A, Caston J. Effects of prenatal stress on anxiety and social interactions in adult rats. *Brain Res Dev Brain Res.* (2005) 160:265–74. doi: 10.1016/j.devbrainres.2005.09.010
27. Shoener JA, Baig R, Page KC. Prenatal exposure to dexamethasone alters hippocampal drive on hypothalamic-pituitary-adrenal axis activity in adult male rats. *Am J Physiol Regul Integr Comp Physiol.* (2006) 290:R1366–73. doi: 10.1152/ajpregu.00757.2004
28. Weinstock M. The long-term behavioural consequences of prenatal stress. *Neurosci Biobehav Rev.* (2008) 32:1073–86. doi: 10.1016/j.neubiorev.2008.03.002
29. Holmes MC, Abrahamsen CT, French KL, Paterson JM, Mullins JJ, Seckl JR. The mother or the fetus? 11beta-hydroxysteroid dehydrogenase type 2 null mice provide evidence for direct fetal programming of behavior by endogenous glucocorticoids. *J Neurosci.* (2006) 26:3840–4. doi: 10.1523/JNEUROSCI.4464-05.2006
30. Mairesse J, Lesage J, Breton C, Breant B, Hahn T, Darnaudery M, et al. Maternal stress alters endocrine function of the feto-placental unit in rats. *Am J Physiol Endocrinol Metab.* (2007) 292:E1526–33. doi: 10.1152/ajpendo.00574.2006
31. Lesage J, Blondeau B, Grino M, Breant B, Dupouy JP. Maternal undernutrition during late gestation induces fetal overexposure to glucocorticoids and intrauterine growth retardation, and disturbs the hypothalamo-pituitary adrenal axis in the newborn rat. *Endocrinology.* (2001) 142:1692–702. doi: 10.1210/endo.142.5.8139
32. Cottrell EC, Seckl JR. Prenatal stress, glucocorticoids and the programming of adult disease. *Front Behav Neurosci.* (2009) 3:19. doi: 10.3389/neuro.08.019.2009
33. Barbazanges A, Piazza PV, Le Moal M, Maccari S. Maternal glucocorticoid secretion mediates long-term effects of prenatal stress. *J Neurosci.* (1996) 16:3943–9.
34. Bonnin A, Goeden N, Chen K, Wilson ML, King J, Shih JC, et al. A transient placental source of serotonin for the fetal forebrain. *Nature.* (2011) 472:347–50. doi: 10.1038/nature09972
35. St-Pierre J, Laurent L, King S, Vaillancourt C. Effects of prenatal maternal stress on serotonin and fetal development. *Placenta.* (2016) 48 (Suppl. 1):S66–71. doi: 10.1016/j.placenta.2015.11.013
36. Beinder L, Faehrmann N, Wachtveitl R, Winterfeld I, Hartner A, Menendez-Castro C, et al. Detection of expressional changes induced by intrauterine growth restriction in the developing rat mammary gland via exploratory pathways analysis. *PLoS ONE.* (2014) 9:e100504. doi: 10.1371/journal.pone.0100504
37. Langley-Evans SC. Maternal carbenoxolone treatment lowers birthweight and induces hypertension in the offspring of rats fed a protein-replete diet. *Clin Sci.* (1997) 93:423–9
38. Lesage J, Hahn D, Leonhardt M, Blondeau B, Breant B, Dupouy JP. Maternal undernutrition during late gestation-induced intrauterine growth restriction in the rat is associated with impaired placental GLUT3 expression, but does not correlate with endogenous corticosterone levels. *J Endocrinol.* (2002) 174:37–43. doi: 10.1677/joe.0.1740037
39. Fernandez-Twinn DS, Ozanne SE, Ekizoglou S, Doherty C, James L, Gusterson B, et al. The maternal endocrine environment in the low-protein model of intra-uterine growth restriction. *Br J Nutr.* (2003) 90:815–22. doi: 10.1079/BJN2003967
40. Jensen Pena C, Monk C, Champagne FA. Epigenetic effects of prenatal stress on 11beta-hydroxysteroid dehydrogenase-2 in the placenta and fetal brain. *PLoS ONE.* (2012) 7:e39791. doi: 10.1371/journal.pone.0039791
41. Fahlbusch FB, Ruebner M, Rascher W, Rauh M. Combined quantification of corticotropin-releasing hormone, cortisol-to-cortisone ratio and progesterone by liquid chromatography-Tandem mass spectrometry in placental tissue. *Steroids.* (2013) 78:888–95. doi: 10.1016/j.steroids.2013.04.015

42. Rauh M. Steroid measurement with LC-MS/MS in pediatric endocrinology. *Mol Cell Endocrinol.* (2009) 301:272–81. doi: 10.1016/j.mce.2008.10.007
43. Taves MD, Ma C, Heimovics SA, Saldanha CJ, Soma KK. Measurement of steroid concentrations in brain tissue: methodological considerations. *Front Endocrinol.* (2011) 2:39. doi: 10.3389/fendo.2011.00039
44. Heussner K, Rauh M, Cordasic N, Menendez-Castro C, Huebner H, Ruebner M, et al. Adhesive blood microsampling systems for steroid measurement via LC-MS/MS in the rat. *Steroids.* (2017) 120:1–6. doi: 10.1016/j.steroids.2017.01.006
45. Nusken KD, Schneider H, Plank C, Trollmann R, Nusken E, Rascher W, et al. Fetal programming of gene expression in growth-restricted rats depends on the cause of low birth weight. *Endocrinology.* (2011) 152:1327–35. doi: 10.1210/en.2010-1116
46. Menendez-Castro C, Toka O, Fahlbusch F, Cordasic N, Wachtveitl R, Hilgers KF, et al. Impaired myocardial performance in a normotensive rat model of intrauterine growth restriction. *Pediatr Res.* (2014) 75:697–706. doi: 10.1038/pr.2014.27
47. Taves MD, Schmidt KL, Ruhr IM, Kapusta K, Prior NH, Soma KK. Steroid concentrations in plasma, whole blood and brain: effects of saline perfusion to remove blood contamination from brain. *PLoS ONE.* (2010) 5:e15727. doi: 10.1371/journal.pone.0015727
48. Fahlbusch FB, Heussner K, Schmid M, Schild R, Ruebner M, Huebner H, et al. Measurement of amniotic fluid steroids of midgestation via LC-MS/MS. *J Steroid Biochem Mol Biol.* (2015) 152:155–60. doi: 10.1016/j.jsbmb.2015.05.014
49. Houtsmuller EJ, de Jong FH, Rowland DL, Slob AK. Plasma testosterone in fetal rats and their mothers on day 19 of gestation. *Physiol Behav.* (1995) 57:495–9.
50. Motulsky HJ, Brown RE. Detecting outliers when fitting data with nonlinear regression - a new method based on robust nonlinear regression and the false discovery rate. *BMC Bioinformatics.* (2006) 7:123. doi: 10.1186/1471-2105-7-123
51. Hughes BG, Hekimi S. Different mechanisms of longevity in long-lived mouse and caenorhabditis elegans mutants revealed by statistical analysis of mortality rates. *Genetics.* (2016) 204:905–20. doi: 10.1534/genetics.116.192369
52. Dupouy JP, Coffigny H, Magre S. Maternal and foetal corticosterone levels during late pregnancy in rats. *J Endocrinol.* (1975) 65:347–52.
53. Benediktsson R, Calder AA, Edwards CR, Seckl JR. Placental 11 beta-hydroxysteroid dehydrogenase: a key regulator of fetal glucocorticoid exposure. *Clin Endocrinol.* (1997) 46:161–6
54. Conley AJ, Mason JI. Placental steroid hormones. *Baill Clin Endocrinol Metab.* (1990) 4:249–72.
55. Warshaw ML, Johnson DC, Khan I, Eckstein B, Gibori G. Placental secretion of androgens in the rat. *Endocrinology.* (1986) 119:2642–8. doi: 10.1210/endo-119-6-2642
56. Devenport LD, Devenport JA. Adrenocortical hormones and brain growth: reversibility and differential sensitivity during development. *Exp Neurol.* (1985) 90:44–52.
57. Kostadinova F, Schwaderer J, Sebeo V, Brunner T. Why does the gut synthesize glucocorticoids? *Ann Med.* (2014) 46:490–7. doi: 10.3109/07853890.2014.932920
58. Miller SL, Huppi PS, Mallard C. The consequences of fetal growth restriction on brain structure and neurodevelopmental outcome. *J Physiol.* (2016) 594:807–23. doi: 10.1113/JP271402
59. Roza SJ, Steegers EA, Verburg BO, Jaddoe VW, Moll HA, Hofman A, et al. What is spared by fetal brain-sparing? Fetal circulatory redistribution and behavioral problems in the general population. *Am J Epidemiol.* (2008) 168:1145–52. doi: 10.1093/aje/kwn233
60. Garcia-Contreras C, Valent D, Vazquez-Gomez M, Arroyo L, Isabel B, Astiz S, et al. Fetal growth-retardation and brain-sparing by malnutrition are associated to changes in neurotransmitters profile. *Int J Dev Neurosci.* (2017) 57:72–6. doi: 10.1016/j.ijdevneu.2017.01.005
61. Vazquez-Gomez M, Valent D, Garcia-Contreras C, Arroyo L, Ovilo C, Isabel B, et al. Sex and intrauterine growth restriction modify brain neurotransmitters profile of newborn piglets. *Int J Dev Neurosci.* (2016) 55:9–14. doi: 10.1016/j.ijdevneu.2016.09.004
62. Konkle AT, McCarthy MM. Developmental time course of estradiol, testosterone, and dihydrotestosterone levels in discrete regions of male and female rat brain. *Endocrinology.* (2011) 152:223–35. doi: 10.1210/en.2010-0607
63. Hiort O. The differential role of androgens in early human sex development. *BMC Med.* (2013) 11:152. doi: 10.1186/1741-7015-11-152
64. Kim CS, Ross IA, Sprando RL, Johnson WD, Sahu SC, Flynn TJ, et al. Distribution of androstenedione and its effects on total free fatty acids in pregnant rats. *Toxicol Ind Health.* (2007) 23:65–74. doi: 10.1177/0748233707076774
65. Jackson JA, Albrecht ED. The development of placental androstenedione and testosterone production and their utilization by the ovary for aromatization to estrogen during rat pregnancy. *Biol Reprod.* (1985) 33:451–7.
66. McCarthy MM. Estradiol and the developing brain. *Physiol Rev.* (2008) 88:91–124. doi: 10.1152/physrev.00010.2007
67. Zohar I, Weinstock M. Differential effect of prenatal stress on the expression of corticotrophin-releasing hormone and its receptors in the hypothalamus and amygdala in male and female rats. *J Neuroendocrinol.* (2011) 23:320–8. doi: 10.1111/j.1365-2826.2011.02117.x
68. Li C, Ramahi E, Nijland MJ, Choi J, Myers DA, Nathanielsz PW, et al. Up-regulation of the fetal baboon hypothalamo-pituitary-adrenal axis in intrauterine growth restriction: coincidence with hypothalamic glucocorticoid receptor insensitivity and leptin receptor down-regulation. *Endocrinology.* (2013) 154:2365–73. doi: 10.1210/en.2012-2111
69. Malandro MS, Beveridge MJ, Kilberg MS, Novak DA. Effect of low-protein diet-induced intrauterine growth retardation on rat placental amino acid transport. *Am J Physiol.* (1996) 271(1 Pt 1):C295–303. doi: 10.1152/ajpcell.1996.271.1.C295
70. Jansson N, Pettersson J, Haafiz A, Ericsson A, Palmberg I, Tranberg M, et al. Down-regulation of placental transport of amino acids precedes the development of intrauterine growth restriction in rats fed a low protein diet. *J Physiol.* (2006) 576:935–46. doi: 10.1113/jphysiol.2006.116509
71. Vaughan OR, Sferruzzi-Perri AN, Fowden AL. Maternal corticosterone regulates nutrient allocation to fetal growth in mice. *J Physiol.* (2012) 590:5529–40. doi: 10.1113/jphysiol.2012.239426
72. Sheehan PM, Bousman C, Komiti A, Judd F, Newman L, Tonge B, et al. Assessment of placental cortisol pathway gene expression in term pregnant women with anxiety. *Neuropsychobiology.* (2018) 77:1–7. doi: 10.1159/000490428
73. Blondeau B, Lesage J, Czernichow P, Dupouy JP, Breant B. Glucocorticoids impair fetal beta-cell development in rats. *Am J Physiol Endocrinol Metab.* (2001) 281:E592–9. doi: 10.1152/ajpendo.2001.281.3.E592
74. Snoeck A, Remacle C, Reusens B, Hoet JJ. Effect of a low protein diet during pregnancy on the fetal rat endocrine pancreas. *Biol Neonate.* (1990) 57:107–18. doi: 10.1159/000243170
75. Bertram CE, Hanson MA. Animal models and programming of the metabolic syndrome. *Br Med Bull.* (2001) 60:103–21 doi: 10.1093/bmb/60.1.103
76. Repetto EM, Sanchez R, Cipelli J, Astort F, Calejman CM, Piroli GG, et al. Dysregulation of corticosterone secretion in streptozotocin-diabetic rats: modulatory role of the adrenocortical nitrergic system. *Endocrinology.* (2010) 151:203–10. doi: 10.1210/en.2009-0592
77. Plank C, Meissner U, Rauh M, Wollmann H, Dorr HG, Rascher W, et al. Cortisol-cortisone ratios in small for gestational age (SGA) children without postnatal catch-up growth. *Clin Endocrinol.* (2007) 67:304–9. doi: 10.1111/j.1365-2265.2007.02884.x
78. Pluchino N, Russo M, Genazzani AR. The fetal brain: role of progesterone and allopregnanolone. *Horm Mol Biol Clin Investig.* (2016) 27:29–34X. doi: 10.1515/hmbci-2016-0020
79. Schumacher M, Guennoun R, Stein DG, De Nicola AF. Progesterone: therapeutic opportunities for neuroprotection and myelin repair. *Pharmacol Ther.* (2007) 116:77–106. doi: 10.1016/j.pharmthera.2007.06.001
80. Hirst JJ, Kelleher MA, Walker DW, Palliser HK. Neuroactive steroids in pregnancy: key regulatory and protective roles in the foetal brain. *J Steroid Biochem Mol Biol.* (2014) 139:144–53. doi: 10.1016/j.jsbmb.2013.04.002
81. Landau RL, Lugibihl K. The effect of progesterone on amino acid metabolism. *J Clin Endocrinol Metab.* (1961) 21:1355–63. doi: 10.1210/jcem-21-11-1355
82. Landau RL, Lugibihl K. The effect of progesterone on the concentration of plasma amino acids in man. *Metabolism.* (1967) 16:1114–22.

83. Wu XY, Hu YT, Guo L, Lu J, Zhu QB, Yu E, et al. Effect of pentobarbital and isoflurane on acute stress response in rat. *Physiol Behav.* (2015) 145:118–21. doi: 10.1016/j.physbeh.2015.04.003
84. Bekhbat M, Merrill L, Kelly SD, Lee VK, Neigh GN. Brief anesthesia by isoflurane alters plasma corticosterone levels distinctly in male and female rats: implications for tissue collection methods. *Behav Brain Res.* (2016) 305:122–5. doi: 10.1016/j.bbr.2016.03.003
85. Vehaskari VM, Woods LL. Prenatal programming of hypertension: lessons from experimental models. *J Am Soc Nephrol.* (2005) 16:2545–56. doi: 10.1681/ASN.2005030300
86. Menendez-Castro C, Hilgers KF, Amann K, Daniel C, Cordasic N, Wachtveitl R, et al. Intrauterine growth restriction leads to a dysregulation of Wilms' tumour supressor gene 1 (WT1) and to early podocyte alterations. *Nephrol Dial Transplant.* (2013) 28:1407–17. doi: 10.1093/ndt/gfs517

2

Hormonal Changes Associated with Intra-Uterine Growth Restriction: Impact on the Developing Brain and Future Neurodevelopment

Olivier Baud [1,2]* *and Nadia Berkane* [3]

[1] *Division of Neonatology and Pediatric Intensive Care, Department of Women-Children-Teenagers, University Hospitals Geneva, Geneva, Switzerland,* [2] *Inserm U1141, Sorbonne, Paris Diderot University, Paris, France,* [3] *Division of Obstetrics and Gynecology, Department of Women-Children-Teenagers, University Hospitals Geneva, Geneva, Switzerland*

Correspondence:
Olivier Baud
olivier.baud@hcuge.ch

The environment in which a fetus develops is not only important for its growth and maturation but also for its long-term postnatal health and neurodevelopment. Several hormones including glucocorticosteroids, estrogens and progesterone, insulin growth factor and thyroid hormones, carefully regulate the growth of the fetus and its metabolism during pregnancy by controlling the supply of nutrients crossing the placenta. In addition to fetal synthesis, hormones regulating fetal growth are also expressed and regulated in the placenta, and they play a key role in the vulnerability of the developing brain and its maturation. This review summarizes the current understanding and evidence regarding the involvement of hormonal dysregulation associated with intra-uterine growth restriction and its consequences on brain development.

Keywords: intra-uterine growth restriction, brain development, glucocorticoids, neurosteroids, insulin growth factor, thyroid hormones

FETAL GROWTH RESTRICTION, BRAIN DEVELOPMENT, AND HORMONES

Fetal growth depends on several factors of maternal, fetal and placental origin, in particular genetic background, nutrients and oxygen supply to the fetus, maternal nutrition and various growth factors and hormones (1). Suboptimal fetal growth is likely to be a key factor of disruption in brain development and many neurodevelopmental disorders of motor and cognitive dysfunction have their origins in the antenatal period (2, 3). Specifically, intra-uterine growth restriction (IUGR), defined as the inability of a fetus to reach its genetically determined size is closely linked to neurodevelopmental deficits. Indeed, infants exposed to IUGR conditions are at high risk not only for neonatal death and cerebral palsy (4), but also for other neurodevelopmental morbidities including mental retardation, a wide spectrum of learning disabilities and developmental behavioral disorders associated with the onset of neuropsychiatric disorders later in life (5–7). Several of these neurodevelopmental impairments are associated not only with deleterious effect of brain undergrowth but also with IUGR-related injury of the developing brain. Magnetic resonance imaging (MRI) has clearly revealed alterations of brain development in growth-restricted infants, involving both white and gray matter (8, 9) and including altered neural circuitry identified by diffusion MRI connectomics (10, 11) that correlate with functional cognitive, motor, and psychiatric deficits later in life (12, 13).

Hormonal balance has a crucial role in fetal growth and maturation, parturition, neonatal adaptation, and brain development (14). Hormones act as maturational and nutritional signals controlling tissue development and differentiation and closely interact with the *in utero* environment. Imbalance between hormones due to placental dysfunction or antenatal chronic stress conditions don't only impair fetal maturation and growth but could also induce obstetrical, perinatal and neonatal complications including cesarean section, perinatal asphyxia, respiratory distress syndrome, abnormal glycemic regulation or inappropriate adrenal function, and hypothalamus pituitary axis (HPA) responsiveness (5).

This review recapitulates state-of-the art data based on a search in the PubMed library in English for the key words "intra-uterine growth restriction," "hormones," and "brain development." The last search was done in October 2018. No restriction of year and authors were applied and review papers were used as references only for the general concepts. We identified 6 dysregulated hormones in case of IUGR, as a cause or as a result, closely related to brain development and future neurobehavioral outcomes, including glucocorticoids and oxytocin, estrogens and progesterone, insulin growth factor, and thyroid hormones.

FETAL GROWTH RESTRICTION AND CHRONIC EXPOSURE TO ENDOGENOUS GLUCOCORTICOSTEROIDS

Fetal Growth Restriction, Chronic Antenatal Stress, and Glucocorticoid Exposure

Glucocorticoids (GCs) are key mediators of stress responses involved during fetal development in the regulation of fetal growth and maturation of fetal tissues and organs (15, 16). Experimental and clinical evidence indicates that increased exposure of the fetus to GCs is associated with adverse outcomes including IUGR (17), postnatal hypertension, and cardiovascular disease (18, 19), postnatal glucose intolerance, increased postnatal activity in the HPA axis (20), and interference with fetal brain development (21, 22). Conversely, placental vascular diseases leading to IUGR were found to be associated with higher plasma cortisol and lower ACTH levels compared to eutrophic fetuses (23).

Besides high concentrations of GCs observed in pregnancies complicated by IUGR, their biological effects are dependent on glucocorticoid receptors (GR), mineralocorticoid receptors, and 11beta-hydroxysteroid dehydrogenase 1/2 (11β –HSD1/2) whose expression varies over time during the antenatal period. Speirs et al. demonstrated critical periods of GC sensitivity related to changes in the expression of these molecules during antenatal development in the mouse (24). Using *in situ* hybridization they showed that GR mRNA levels were very low at embryonic day (E9.5) in the fetus but not in the placenta, and then variably rose during gestation in several tissues, including the central nervous system (CNS). In humans, both GR and the MR are highly expressed in the hippocampus from 24 weeks of gestation (25).

Fetal 11β-HSD1 mRNA expression, which could enhance GC levels locally was detected at low levels in a few brain regions, including the hippocampus only after E16.5 in mice (24). In sheep, a specific increase in the expression of 11β-HSD1 mRNA in growth-restricted fetuses in late gestation has been reported (26). In the rat, placental 11β-HSD2 is considered as a "barrier" to endogenous GCs and genetic mutations of this enzyme were found to be associated with low birthweights (27). In humans, the 11β-HSD2 gene mutation also produces IUGR which is associated with reduced placental activity of this enzyme also highly expressed in the developing brain (28). Altogether, these data, both in animals and in humans, strongly suggest that the effects of high circulating cortisol levels associated with IUGR could be potentiated by specific changes in gene expression involved in their biological response in many tissues including CNS.

Glucocorticoids, Developing Brain, and Microglia Phenotypes

In humans, GCs regulate several developmental processes in the CNS, including hippocampal neurogenesis with variable effects on proliferation of progenitor cells, neurogenesis and astrogliogenesis in response to either low or high concentrations of cortisol (29). Low cortisol was found to increase proliferation and differentiation of progenitors into S100beta-positive astrocytes, and decrease neurogenesis. High cortisol was found to decrease proliferation and differentiation into neuronal cells without regulating astrogliogenesis. Inappropriate exposure to high levels of GCs early in pregnancy could therefore interfere with overall brain maturation. This programming effect of endogenous GCs affecting notably the HPA axis has been related to gene methylation and histone modifications associated with IUGR (30, 31) and can lead to long-lasting effects on the developing brain (32). IUGR also has sex-specific, persistent effects on hippocampal GR expression and its variants, a mechanism involved in HPA axis reprogramming, mostly in males (30).

GCs confer anti-inflammatory and immunosuppressive effects but are also able to potentiate, at high concentrations, inflammatory responses both at central and peripheral levels (33). In a model of restraint prenatal stress associated with higher levels of corticosterone investigated in juvenile and adult rats, a shift of the immune response toward a pro-inflammatory phenotype has been observed in adult rats (34). The change of GC receptor expression or function induced by IUGR could also change the microglia response toward pro-inflammatory insults associated with intensive care of growth-restricted infants, according to a multiple hit concept (35).

Extensive literature has demonstrated that chronic stress and GC exposure can impair the developing brain facing a large variety of insults, including hypoxia-ischemia, hypoglycemia, oxygen radical accumulation, all conditions potentially observed associated to IUGR (36). In preclinical models, IUGR-associated brain damage is usually associated with neuro-inflammation (5, 37–39), a key feature related to exacerbated activation of microglia, the resident macrophages of the CNS, able to sensitize the developing brain to a secondary insult (40, 41). Microglial cells can acquire distinct phenotypes in response to perinatal stimuli that allow them to either disrupt developmental processes, i.e., myelination, synaptic pruning or axonal growth, or support repair, and regeneration. These diverse roles make microglia critical modulators of brain injury and GC exposure which are able to modulate microglial phenotype both in the developing and mature brain (42–45). In the developing brain, Gómez-González et al. showed that exposure to prenatal stress alters microglia maturation leading to an imbalance between immature and ramified microglia 1 day after birth in rat (46), and increased microglial activation in the hippocampus in juvenile animals (47, 48).

Balance Between GCs and Oxytocin

Oxytocin (OXT), an essential hormone during the perinatal period and parturition, is a neuropeptide released by the paraventricular nucleus and by the supraoptic nucleus of the hypothalamus, which is also known to be balanced against GCs. Indeed, studies carried out in rodents and in humans showed a close link between HPA axis activity and OXT release. OXT is also implicated in autism (49–51) and in the down-regulation of the central inflammatory response to injury in the mature brain (52, 53). In the developing brain, an association between IUGR, low expression of OXT and neuroinflammation, leading to defective myelination and abnormal brain function has been recently reported (54). Pharmacological treatment using carbetocin, a brain permeable long-lasting OXT receptor (OXTR) agonist, was found to be associated with a significant reduction of microglial activation and provided long-term neuroprotection. OTX also alleviated the HPA axis activation reducing GC release (55, 56), supporting the hypothesis of indirect anti-inflammatory action of OXT. These findings make OXT a promising candidate for neuroprotection, in particular in the context of IUGR.

SEX STEROID HORMONES

Sex Steroids in Human Pregnancy and Placenta

Estradiol (E2) and progesterone (P4) are highly expressed during pregnancy (57). Sex steroids are excreted by syncitiotrophoblasts into the intervillous chambers, entering the maternal circulation, and also the fetal vessels after crossing layers of cytotrophoblasts and stromal cells. While fetal circulating E2 and P4 are mainly of placental origin, hormonal concentrations differ between maternal and fetal circulation (58), implying that some of these hormones are converted in the villi (59, 60). 17β-hydroxysteroid dehydrogenase-2 (HSD17β2) converts E2, testosterone and Δ4-androstenedione (Δ4-dione) into estrone (E1), P4, and 20α-dihydroprogesterone, respectively (61, 62). These conversions could be involved in a protective effect from excessive fetal feminization or virilization, but could also play other roles (63). In primary culture of rat hippocampal neurons, it has been shown that E2 confers protection against excitotoxic-induced cell death (64), and some E2 metabolites have various effects on fetal brain development through their receptors by promoting neurite outgrowth, myelination, and synaptogenesis (3, 65, 66) as well as neuroprotective roles (67). P4 is already used as a treatment in human adult traumatic brain injury (68).

Interestingly, recent human studies have suggested that maternal serum concentrations of E2, P4 and some of their metabolites are modified during human pregnancy complicated by preeclampsia and/or IUGR with lower placental aromatization and E2 levels and higher P4 inactivation (20α hydroxylation) (69–75).

While growing evidence demonstrates that steroidogenic enzymes are highly expressed in the CNS, below, we describe data suggesting that changes in P4 and E2 induced by IUGR could have an impact on fetal brain development and adaptation to hypoxic stress.

Progesterone and Allopregnanolone and the Fetal Brain

Both in rodents and in humans, a large variety of brain structures (including olfactory bulb, hypothalamus, striatum, hippocampus, cerebral cortex, and cerebellum) and cell types (including glial, Purkinje, and Schwann cells) synthetize P4 (76, 77). Its 3α,5α-tetrahydroprogesterone (allopregnanolone) metabolite is mainly expressed in the cerebellum of neonatal rats (78). Progesterone receptors are expressed in rats by Purkinje cells and in the cerebellum.

Both P4 and allopregnanolone have a recognized role in neuroprotection (79). P4 has been found to induce inhibition of voltage-gated calcium channels (80) in the rat brain. Allopregnanolone found at high concentrations in maternal (81) and fetal sheep circulation (82) has been shown to have neurotrophic effects on neurons and glial cells (83, 84) in the ovine fetal brain (85).

In humans, available studies comparing controls and preeclamptic women reported conflicting results with unchanged, or higher maternal P4 concentrations (69, 74, 75). Using a reliable gas chromatography/mass spectrometry technique, no difference in maternal blood P4 and allopregnanolone concentrations was reported in women with vascular IUGR with or without preeclampsia compared to normal pregnancy (69). In contrast, in pregnant women with preexisting chronic hypertension, the development of preeclampsia was associated with higher allopregenalone concentrations (75).

In a model of IUGR developed in guinea pigs subjected to partial devascularization of the uterine horns during pregnancy, decreased allopregnanolone concentrations have been observed in fetal plasma and brain (79, 86). Moreover, in this model, despite increased expression of progesterone receptors in the brain, myelination was found to be decreased in the hippocampal region (87). Nevertheless, further studies are needed to better assess changes in P4 and its metabolite concentrations and signaling pathways involved in the adaptive response of the fetal brain to stress.

Estradiol

In rats, estradiol (E2) is synthetized by the hippocampus (88) and cerebellum (89) and potentially by other parts of the brain with some gender differences (90). E2 effects on the brain are not yet well understood as both protecting (64, 91) and damaging effects (90, 92) have been described in primary cultures of rat hippocampal neurons. This hormone has been shown to promote axonal growth notably in cell cultures of fetal rat neurons derived from the ventromedial nucleus of the hypothalamus (93). In the oligodendroglial lineage, E2 also promotes the proliferation of immature oligodendrocytes, their differentiation into myelinating oligodendrocytes, and strongly reduces apoptotic cell death and neuro-inflammation in response to insult (94). On the other hand, as a potent regulator of the depolarizing actions of GABA, E2 can insult fetal brains subjected to hypoxic conditions by increasing the response to excessive GABA release via excess of free intracellular calcium (90).

Aromatase is a key enzyme for estrogen synthesis and several studies suggested a placental aromatase reduced activity in pregnancy with preeclampsia (70–75, 95) or with IUGR (69). As placenta is the major source of fetal estrogens, significantly lower maternal concentrations of E2, E1, or E1/Δ4-dione were reported in these pregnancies which may affect fetal estrogen levels. It can be hypothesized that during an IUGR pregnancy, a lack of fetal estrogens could disturb brain development. However, to our knowledge, no fetal or neonatal blood estrogen profile has been reported yet. Whether this abnormal placental steroidogenesis might induce changes in the steroid profile in the fetal compartment with potential brain insult remains to be determined. In addition, it is important to keep in mind that the developing brain itself has the capability to synthesize and convert sex steroids adding complexity to the interpretation of blood level data.

Despite these limitations, current evidence increasingly supports that E2, P4, and allopregnanolone play a key role in brain development and might be important modulators of brain vulnerability in the fetus with IUGR.

ROLE OF THE GLUCOSE-INSULIN-INSULIN-LIKE GROWTH FACTOR I (IGF-I) AXIS IN PLACENTAL AND FETAL GROWTH

Regulation of IGF Signaling in Growth Restricted Fetuses

The regulation of fetal growth depends not only on the nutrients available to the fetus but also on the regulation of Insulin-IGF/IGF binding protein 3 (IGFBP-3) axis (96, 97). The IGF factors I and II work together to control fetal growth through changes in size and function of the placenta. IGF-II is important for placental growth and development, and therefore allows more nutrients to reach the fetus. IGF-I acts as a "nutrient sensor" and finely regulates nutrient transfer across the placenta according to both the maternal environment and fetal demand. The production of IGF-I, particularly sensitive to maternal undernutrition and parental imprinting, regulates its signaling through its receptor (98). Disruption of this imprinting causes growth disorders including Beckwith–Wiedemann syndrome, associated with fetal overgrowth, and Silver-Russell syndrome, associated with IUGR (99). Several studies have shown that infants born growth restricted have lower levels of IGF-I, IGFBP-3, and insulin compared to appropriate for gestational age infants (100–102). The IGF system, IGF-I and IGF-II in particular, plays a critical role in fetal and placental growth. Disruption of the IGF-I, IGF-II, or IGF-IR gene induces IUGR, whereas disruption of IGF-IIR or overexpression of IGF-II enhances fetal growth (103).

Placenta and IGF Signaling

Many metabolic adaptations of pregnancy are regulated by placental hormones which undergo dramatic changes during gestation including placental estrogen and progesterone (104). Placental hormone expression is supposed to interact with fetal growth through polymorphic or epigenetic regulation of placental growth hormone (PGH) and human chorionic somatomammotropin (CSH) expression could alter the expression of other critical hormones including insulin or IGF-I (105). However, definitive evidence supporting that specific placental hormones are required for normal pregnancy and fetal growth is currently lacking. It is possible that other hormones of maternal origin, such as pituitary GH and/or prolactin, might partially compensate for reduced expression of placental hormones.

Defective IGF Signaling and Neurodevelopment

Abnormal fetal growth could also be associated with medically-induced preterm delivery (106). Low IGF-1 levels in very preterm infants and IUGR neonates were reported to be associated with high risk factor for adverse outcomes including chronic lung disease and retinopathy of prematurity. IGF-1 also plays crucial roles in the development and maturation (107) of the CNS with potent effects on cellular neuroplasticity, learning and memory, and confers neuroprotection following brain injury. IGF-1 acts at several sites to induce cellular plasticity through its receptor IGF-1R in neuronal and non-neuronal cells. IGF-1R is known to induce cellular plasticity by acting on glutamate receptors including AMPA/kaïnate-R, NMDA-R, calcium channels, and neurotransmitter release (108). Abnormal excitatory synaptic transmission observed in genetic diseases associated with behavioral disorders can be corrected by restoring SHANK3 expression or by treating neurons with IGF-1 (109). Regarding microglial activation, a major factor of brain injury, aging-related decrease in IGF-1 may contribute to the defective switch of microglia toward immunomodulatory and repair phenotype (110). During development, the IGF-1 level in cerebral spinal fluid is high, consistently with its important role in brain development, neuronal growth promotion, cellular proliferation, and differentiation (111). Finally, IGF-1 induces anti-inflammatory properties both in the developing and mature brain related to down-regulation of brain cytokine expression (112–114). Studies investigating the effects of intra-nasal IGF-1 demonstrated neuroprotection in models of LPS-induced white matter injury in the developing rat brain (115), cerebral hypoxic-ischemic injury (116, 117), and other neurodegenerative damages (118), probably through the phophatidylinositol-3 kinase/Akt pathway (119). However, the causality between low IGF-1 levels and neuroinflammation associated with IUGR remains to be confirmed.

THYROID HORMONES

Thyroid hormones are essential for fetal brain development and maturation. Severe but also mild or subclinical neonatal hypothyroidism has been associated with neurodevelopmental impairment (120–124). However, all neonates with subclinical or mild hypothyroidism are not identified by newborn screening programs (Guthrie test). Factors associated with neonatal hypothyroidism include prematurity and IUGR (125, 126). IUGR and/or preeclampsia can be the consequences of placental insufficiency associated with overexpression of sFlt-1 (soluble fms-like tyrosine kinase-1) a soluble form of the vascular endothelial growth factor- type 1 (VEGFR-1) (127), several weeks before the beginning of maternal clinical signs (128). sFlt-1 has anti-mitogenic properties on endothelial cells (129) by trapping VEGF and placental growth factor (PlGF) leading to hypertension and proteinuria (127, 130). When IUGR occurs in human, higher sFlt-1 or sFlt-1/PlGF ratio concentrations in maternal blood have also been observed compared to the control group (131, 132). A nested case control study showed that preeclampsia predisposes to reduced maternal thyroid function (transient or permanent) (133) as others report (134). This thyroid insufficiency seems to be mediated by sFlt-1 which impairs fenestrated capillary endothelium present in endocrine glands (135). By disrupting VEGF/VEGF-R signaling in adult mice, Kamba et al. showed capillary regression in different organs, the amount of regression was dose- and organ-dependent with the highest effect in thyroid (135). Recovery of thyroid capillary density has been observed within 2 weeks after cessation of treatment. Since sFlt-1 crosses the placenta, an impact of fetal thyroid function could also be suspected with risk of subsequent neurodevelopmental impairment. Cord blood sFlt1 concentrations have been found to be inversely correlated to birthweight (136) and free T4 and positively correlated with thyroid stimulating hormone (TSH) (137). However, conflicting findings have been reported regarding the effect of IUGR on fetal serum concentration of thyroid hormones. In a series of 49 growth-restricted fetuses who had cordocentesis during pregnancy, higher concentrations of TSH and lower concentrations of free T4 have been found compared to fetuses with appropriate growth for gestational age, and changes in TSH concentrations were correlated to fetal hypoxia and academia (138). In contrast, others reported unchanged or low TSH levels in IUGR cord blood compared to controls (139–142). Variability in fetal exposure to sFlt1 could be involved in TSH regulation and may partly explain these conflicting findings.

In summary, IUGR leads to neuropathological consequences for the developing brain with heterogeneous features and long-term neurocognitive and behavioral consequences (5, 143). Many factors contribute to the vulnerability of the developing brain, including age of delivery, severity of *in utero* compromise, co-morbidities occurring during the perinatal period, complications associated with medically-induced preterm delivery. Changes in several hormones strongly involved in the regulation of brain development and maturation are likely to play a key role. More research is needed to better understand these crosstalks.

AUTHOR CONTRIBUTIONS

OB and NB did the literature review and collectively analyzed articles selected in this review paper. OB wrote paragraphs related to introduction, glucocorticoids, oxytocin, and IGF1. NB wrote paragraphs related to sex steroids and thyroid hormones.

ACKNOWLEDGMENTS

The authors thank Audrey Toulotte-Aebi for editing the manuscript.

REFERENCES

1. Burton GJ, Jauniaux E. Pathophysiology of placental-derived fetal growth restriction. *Am J Obstet Gynecol.* (2018) 218:S745–61. doi: 10.1016/j.ajog.2017.11.577
2. Levine TA, Grunau RE, McAuliffe FM, Pinnamaneni R, Foran A, Alderdice FA. Early childhood neurodevelopment after intrauterine growth restriction: a systematic review. *Pediatrics.* (2015) 135:126–41. doi: 10.1542/peds.2014-1143
3. Miranda A, Sousa N. Maternal hormonal milieu influence on fetal brain development. *Brain Behav.* (2018) 8:e00920. doi: 10.1002/brb3.920
4. Jarvis S, Glinianaia SV, Torrioli MG, Platt MJ, Miceli M, Jouk PS, et al. Cerebral palsy and intrauterine growth in single births: European collaborative study. *Lancet.* (2003) 362:1106–11. doi: 10.1016/S0140-6736(03)14466-2
5. Colella M, Frerot A, Novais ARB, Baud O. Neonatal and long-term consequences of fetal growth restriction. *Curr Pediatr Rev.* (2018) 14:212–8. doi: 10.2174/1573396314666180712114531
6. Guellec I, Marret S, Baud O, Cambonie G, Lapillonne A, Roze JC, et al. Intrauterine growth restriction, head size at birth, and outcome in very preterm infants. *J Pediatr.* (2015) 167:975–81 e2. doi: 10.1016/j.jpeds.2015.08.025
7. Wiles NJ, Peters TJ, Heron J, Gunnell D, Emond A, Lewis G. Fetal growth and childhood behavioral problems: results from the ALSPAC cohort. *Am J Epidemiol.* (2006) 163:829–37. doi: 10.1093/aje/kwj108
8. Padilla N, Junque C, Figueras F, Sanz-Cortes M, Bargallo N, Arranz A, et al. Differential vulnerability of gray matter and white matter to intrauterine growth restriction in preterm infants at 12 months corrected age. *Brain Res.* (2014) 1545:1–11. doi: 10.1016/j.brainres.2013.12.007
9. Dubois J, Benders M, Borradori-Tolsa C, Cachia A, Lazeyras F, Ha-Vinh Leuchter R, et al. Primary cortical folding in the human newborn: an early marker of later functional development. *Brain.* (2008) 131:2028–41. doi: 10.1093/brain/awn137
10. Batalle D, Eixarch E, Figueras F, Munoz-Moreno E, Bargallo N, Illa M, et al. Altered small-world topology of structural brain networks in infants with intrauterine growth restriction and its association

with later neurodevelopmental outcome. *Neuroimage.* (2012) 60:1352–66. doi: 10.1016/j.neuroimage.2012.01.059

11. Fischi-Gomez E, Vasung L, Meskaldji DE, Lazeyras F, Borradori-Tolsa C, Hagmann P, et al. Structural brain connectivity in school-age preterm infants provides evidence for impaired networks relevant for higher order cognitive skills and social cognition. *Cereb Cortex.* (2015) 25:2793–805. doi: 10.1093/cercor/bhu073
12. Tolsa CB, Zimine S, Warfield SK, Freschi M, Sancho Rossignol A, Lazeyras F, et al. Early alteration of structural and functional brain development in premature infants born with intrauterine growth restriction. *Pediatr Res.* (2004) 56:132–8. doi: 10.1203/01.PDR.0000128983.54614.7E
13. Egana-Ugrinovic G, Sanz-Cortes M, Figueras F, Couve-Perez C, Gratacos E. Fetal MRI insular cortical morphometry and its association with neurobehavior in late-onset small-for-gestational-age fetuses. *Ultrasound Obstet Gynecol.* (2014) 44:322–9. doi: 10.1002/uog.13360
14. Murphy VE, Smith R, Giles WB, Clifton VL. Endocrine regulation of human fetal growth: the role of the mother, placenta, and fetus. *Endocr Rev.* (2006) 27:141–69. doi: 10.1210/er.2005-0011
15. Lesage J, Blondeau B, Grino M, Breant B, Dupouy JP. Maternal undernutrition during late gestation induces fetal overexposure to glucocorticoids and intrauterine growth retardation, and disturbs the hypothalamo-pituitary adrenal axis in the newborn rat. *Endocrinology.* (2001) 142:1692–702. doi: 10.1210/endo.142.5.8139
16. Sutherland AE, Crossley KJ, Allison BJ, Jenkin G, Wallace EM, Miller SL. The effects of intrauterine growth restriction and antenatal glucocorticoids on ovine fetal lung development. *Pediatr Res.* (2012) 71:689–96. doi: 10.1038/pr.2012.19
17. Bloom SL, Sheffield JS, McIntire DD, Leveno KJ. Antenatal dexamethasone and decreased birth weight. *Obstet Gynecol.* (2001) 97:485–90. doi: 10.1097/00006250-200104000-00001
18. Benediktsson R, Lindsay RS, Noble J, Seckl JR, Edwards CR. Glucocorticoid exposure *in utero*: new model for adult hypertension. *Lancet.* (1993) 341:339–41. doi: 10.1016/0140-6736(93)90138-7
19. Barker DJ. Fetal nutrition and cardiovascular disease in later life. *Br Med Bull.* (1997) 53:96–108. doi: 10.1093/oxfordjournals.bmb.a011609
20. de Vries A, Holmes MC, Heijnis A, Seier JV, Heerden J, Louw J, et al. Prenatal dexamethasone exposure induces changes in nonhuman primate offspring cardiometabolic and hypothalamic-pituitary-adrenal axis function. *J Clin Invest.* (2007) 117:1058–67. doi: 10.1172/JCI30982
21. Matthews SG. Antenatal glucocorticoids and programming of the developing CNS. *Pediatr Res.* (2000) 47:291–300. doi: 10.1203/00006450-200003000-00003
22. Uno H, Eisele S, Sakai A, Shelton S, Baker E, DeJesus O, et al. Neurotoxicity of glucocorticoids in the primate brain. *Horm Behav.* (1994) 28:336–48. doi: 10.1006/hbeh.1994.1030
23. Economides DL, Nicolaides KH, Linton EA, Perry LA, Chard T. Plasma cortisol and adrenocorticotropin in appropriate and small for gestational age fetuses. *Fetal Ther.* (1988) 3:158–64. doi: 10.1159/000263348
24. Speirs HJ, Seckl JR, Brown RW. Ontogeny of glucocorticoid receptor and 11beta-hydroxysteroid dehydrogenase type-1 gene expression identifies potential critical periods of glucocorticoid susceptibility during development. *J Endocrinol.* (2004) 181:105–16. doi: 10.1677/joe.0.1810105
25. Noorlander CW, De Graan PN, Middeldorp J, Van Beers JJ, Visser GH. Ontogeny of hippocampal corticosteroid receptors: effects of antenatal glucocorticoids in human and mouse. *J Comp Neurol.* (2006) 499:924–32. doi: 10.1002/cne.21162
26. McMillen IC, Warnes KE, Adams MB, Robinson JS, Owens JA, Coulter CL. Impact of restriction of placental and fetal growth on expression of 11beta-hydroxysteroid dehydrogenase type 1 and type 2 messenger ribonucleic acid in the liver, kidney, and adrenal of the sheep fetus. *Endocrinology.* (2000) 141:539–43. doi: 10.1210/endo.141.2.7338
27. Seckl JR, Cleasby M, Nyirenda MJ. Glucocorticoids, 11beta-hydroxysteroid dehydrogenase, and fetal programming. *Kidney Int.* (2000) 57:1412–7. doi: 10.1046/j.1523-1755.2000.00984.x
28. Wyrwoll CS, Holmes MC, Seckl JR. 11beta-hydroxysteroid dehydrogenases and the brain: from zero to hero, a decade of progress. *Front Neuroendocrinol.* (2011) 32:265–86. doi: 10.1016/j.yfrne.2010.12.001
29. Anacker C, Cattaneo A, Luoni A, Musaelyan K, Zunszain PA, Milanesi E, et al. Glucocorticoid-related molecular signaling pathways regulating hippocampal neurogenesis. *Neuropsychopharmacology.* (2013) 38:872–83. doi: 10.1038/npp.2012.253
30. Ke X, Schober ME, McKnight RA, O'Grady S, Caprau D, Yu X, et al. Intrauterine growth retardation affects expression and epigenetic characteristics of the rat hippocampal glucocorticoid receptor gene. *Physiol Genomics.* (2010) 42:177–89. doi: 10.1152/physiolgenomics.00201.2009
31. Filiberto AC, Maccani MA, Koestler D, Wilhelm-Benartzi C, Avissar-Whiting M, Banister CE, et al. Birthweight is associated with DNA promoter methylation of the glucocorticoid receptor in human placenta. *Epigenetics.* (2011) 6:566–72. doi: 10.4161/epi.6.5.15236
32. Wood CE. Development and programming of the hypothalamus-pituitary-adrenal axis. *Clin Obstet Gynecol.* (2013) 56:610–21. doi: 10.1097/GRF.0b013e31829e5b15
33. Yeager MP, Rassias AJ, Pioli PA, Beach ML, Wardwell K, Collins JE, et al. Pretreatment with stress cortisol enhances the human systemic inflammatory response to bacterial endotoxin. *Crit Care Med.* (2009) 37:2727–32. doi: 10.1097/CCM.0b013e3181a592b3
34. Vanbesien-Mailliot CC, Wolowczuk I, Mairesse J, Viltart O, Delacre M, Khalife J, et al. Prenatal stress has pro-inflammatory consequences on the immune system in adult rats. *Psychoneuroendocrinology.* (2007) 32:114–24. doi: 10.1016/j.psyneuen.2006.11.005
35. Leviton A, Fichorova RN, O'Shea TM, Kuban K, Paneth N, Dammann O, et al. Two-hit model of brain damage in the very preterm newborn: small for gestational age and postnatal systemic inflammation. *Pediatr Res.* (2013) 73:362–70. doi: 10.1038/pr.2012.188
36. Sorrells SF, Sapolsky RM. An inflammatory review of glucocorticoid actions in the CNS. *Brain Behav Immun.* (2007) 21:259–72. doi: 10.1016/j.bbi.2006.11.006
37. Baud O, Daire JL, Dalmaz Y, Fontaine RH, Krueger RC, Sebag G, et al. Gestational hypoxia induces white matter damage in neonatal rats: a new model of periventricular leukomalacia. *Brain Pathol.* (2004) 14:1–10. doi: 10.1111/j.1750-3639.2004.tb00492.x
38. Olivier P, Baud O, Evrard P, Gressens P, Verney C. Prenatal ischemia and white matter damage in rats. *J Neuropathol Exp Neurol.* (2005) 64:998–1006. doi: 10.1097/01.jnen.0000187052.81889.57
39. Olivier P, Baud O, Bouslama M, Evrard P, Gressens P, Verney C. Moderate growth restriction: deleterious and protective effects on white matter damage. *Neurobiol Dis.* (2007) 26:253–63. doi: 10.1016/j.nbd.2007.01.001
40. Rideau Batista Novais A, Pham H, Van de Looij Y, Bernal M, Mairesse J, Zana-Taieb E, et al. Transcriptomic regulations in oligodendroglial and microglial cells related to brain damage following fetal growth restriction. *Glia.* (2016) 64:2306–20. doi: 10.1002/glia.23079
41. Fleiss B, Gressens P. Tertiary mechanisms of brain damage: a new hope for treatment of cerebral palsy? *Lancet Neurol.* (2012) 11:556–66. doi: 10.1016/S1474-4422(12)70058-3
42. Frank MG, Hershman SA, Weber MD, Watkins LR, Maier SF. Chronic exposure to exogenous glucocorticoids primes microglia to pro-inflammatory stimuli and induces NLRP3 mRNA in the hippocampus. *Psychoneuroendocrinology.* (2014) 40:191–200. doi: 10.1016/j.psyneuen.2013.11.006
43. Nair A, Bonneau RH. Stress-induced elevation of glucocorticoids increases microglia proliferation through NMDA receptor activation. *J Neuroimmunol.* (2006) 171:72–85. doi: 10.1016/j.jneuroim.2005.09.012
44. Wu CH, Chien HF, Chang CY, Chen SH, Huang YS. Response of amoeboid and differentiating ramified microglia to glucocorticoids in postnatal rats: a lectin histochemical and ultrastructural study. *Neurosci Res.* (2001) 40:235–44. doi: 10.1016/S0168-0102(01)00231-0
45. Tentillier N, Etzerodt A, Olesen MN, Rizalar FS, Jacobsen J, Bender D, et al. Anti-inflammatory modulation of microglia via CD163-targeted glucocorticoids protects dopaminergic neurons in the 6-OHDA Parkinson's disease model. *J Neurosci.* (2016) 36:9375–90. doi: 10.1523/JNEUROSCI.1636-16.2016
46. Gomez-Gonzalez B, Escobar A. Prenatal stress alters microglial development and distribution in postnatal rat brain. *Acta Neuropathol.* (2010) 119:303–15. doi: 10.1007/s00401-009-0590-4

47. Roque A, Ochoa-Zarzosa A, Torner L. Maternal separation activates microglial cells and induces an inflammatory response in the hippocampus of male rat pups, independently of hypothalamic and peripheral cytokine levels. *Brain Behav Immun.* (2016) 55:39–48. doi: 10.1016/j.bbi.2015.09.017
48. Slusarczyk J, Trojan E, Glombik K, Budziszewska B, Kubera M, Lason W, et al. Prenatal stress is a vulnerability factor for altered morphology and biological activity of microglia cells. *Front Cell Neurosci.* (2015) 9:82. doi: 10.3389/fncel.2015.00082
49. Tyzio R, Nardou R, Ferrari DC, Tsintsadze T, Shahrokhi A, Eftekhari S, et al. Oxytocin-mediated GABA inhibition during delivery attenuates autism pathogenesis in rodent offspring. *Science.* (2014) 343:675–9. doi: 10.1126/science.1247190
50. Tyzio R, Cossart R, Khalilov I, Minlebaev M, Hubner CA, Represa A, et al. Maternal oxytocin triggers a transient inhibitory switch in GABA signaling in the fetal brain during delivery. *Science.* (2006) 314:1788–92. doi: 10.1126/science.1133212
51. Penagarikano O, Lazaro MT, Lu XH, Gordon A, Dong H, Lam HA, et al. Exogenous and evoked oxytocin restores social behavior in the Cntnap2 mouse model of autism. *Sci Transl Med.* (2015) 7:271ra8. doi: 10.1126/scitranslmed.3010257
52. Yuan L, Liu S, Bai X, Gao Y, Liu G, Wang X, et al. Oxytocin inhibits lipopolysaccharide-induced inflammation in microglial cells and attenuates microglial activation in lipopolysaccharide-treated mice. *J Neuroinflamm.* (2016) 13:77. doi: 10.1186/s12974-016-0541-7
53. Zinni M, Colella M, Batista Novais AR, Baud O, Mairesse J. Modulating the oxytocin system during the perinatal period: a new strategy for neuroprotection of the immature brain? *Front Neurol.* (2018) 9:229. doi: 10.3389/fneur.2018.00229
54. Mairesse J, Zinni M, Pansiot J, Hassan-Abdi R, Demene C, Colella M, et al. Oxytocin receptor agonist reduces perinatal brain damage by targeting microglia. *Glia.* (2018) 67:345–59. doi: 10.1002/glia.23546
55. Jurek B, Slattery DA, Hiraoka Y, Liu Y, Nishimori K, Aguilera G, et al. Oxytocin regulates stress-induced Crf gene transcription through CREB-regulated transcription coactivator 3. *J Neurosci.* (2015) 35:12248–60. doi: 10.1523/JNEUROSCI.1345-14.2015
56. Windle RJ, Kershaw YM, Shanks N, Wood SA, Lightman SL, Ingram CD. Oxytocin attenuates stress-induced c-fos mRNA expression in specific forebrain regions associated with modulation of hypothalamo-pituitary-adrenal activity. *J Neurosci.* (2004) 24:2974–82. doi: 10.1523/JNEUROSCI.3432-03.2004
57. Abbassi-Ghanavati M, Greer LG, Cunningham FG. Pregnancy and laboratory studies: a reference table for clinicians. *Obstet Gynecol.* (2009) 114:1326–31. doi: 10.1097/AOG.0b013e3181c2bde8
58. Hill M, Parizek A, Cibula D, Kancheva R, Jirasek JE, Jirkovska M, et al. Steroid metabolome in fetal and maternal body fluids in human late pregnancy. *J Steroid Biochem Mol Biol.* (2010) 122:114–32. doi: 10.1016/j.jsbmb.2010.05.007
59. Gurpide E, Marks C, de Ziegler D, Berk PD, Brandes JM. Asymmetric release of estrone and estradiol derived from labeled precursors in perfused human placentas. *Am J Obstet Gynecol.* (1982) 144:551–5. doi: 10.1016/0002-9378(82)90226-5
60. Drolet R, Simard M, Plante J, Laberge P, Tremblay Y. Human type 2 17 beta-hydroxysteroid dehydrogenase mRNA and protein distribution in placental villi at mid and term pregnancy. *Reprod Biol Endocrinol.* (2007) 5:30. doi: 10.1186/1477-7827-5-30
61. Blomquist CH. Kinetic analysis of enzymic activities: prediction of multiple forms of 17 beta-hydroxysteroid dehydrogenase. *J Steroid Biochem Mol Biol.* (1995) 55:515–24. doi: 10.1016/0960-0760(95)00200-6
62. Wu L, Einstein M, Geissler WM, Chan HK, Elliston KO, Andersson S. Expression cloning and characterization of human 17 beta-hydroxysteroid dehydrogenase type 2, a microsomal enzyme possessing 20 alpha-hydroxysteroid dehydrogenase activity. *J Biol Chem.* (1993) 268:12964–9.
63. Moghrabi N, Head JR, Andersson S. Cell type-specific expression of 17 beta-hydroxysteroid dehydrogenase type 2 in human placenta and fetal liver. *J Clin Endocrinol Metab.* (1997) 82:3872–8.
64. Hilton GD, Nunez JL, Bambrick L, Thompson SM, McCarthy MM. Glutamate-mediated excitotoxicity in neonatal hippocampal neurons is mediated by mGluR-induced release of Ca++ from intracellular stores and is prevented by estradiol. *Eur J Neurosci.* (2006) 24:3008–16. doi: 10.1111/j.1460-9568.2006.05189.x
65. Garcia-Segura LM, Melcangi RC. Steroids and glial cell function. *Glia.* (2006) 54:485–98. doi: 10.1002/glia.20404
66. Haraguchi S, Sasahara K, Shikimi H, Honda S, Harada N, Tsutsui K. Estradiol promotes purkinje dendritic growth, spinogenesis, and synaptogenesis during neonatal life by inducing the expression of BDNF. *Cerebellum.* (2012) 11:416–7. doi: 10.1007/s12311-011-0342-6
67. Xiao Q, Luo Y, Lv F, He Q, Wu H, Chao F, et al. Protective effects of 17beta-estradiol on hippocampal myelinated fibers in ovariectomized middle-aged rats. *Neuroscience.* (2018) 385:143–53. doi: 10.1016/j.neuroscience.2018.06.006
68. Xiao G, Wei J, Yan W, Wang W, Lu Z. Improved outcomes from the administration of progesterone for patients with acute severe traumatic brain injury: a randomized controlled trial. *Crit Care.* (2008) 12:R61. doi: 10.1186/cc6887
69. Berkane N, Liere P, Lefevre G, Alfaidy N, Nahed RA, Vincent J, et al. Abnormal steroidogenesis and aromatase activity in preeclampsia. *Placenta.* (2018) 69:40–9. doi: 10.1016/j.placenta.2018.07.004
70. Hertig A, Liere P, Chabbert-Buffet N, Fort J, Pianos A, Eychenne B, et al. Steroid profiling in preeclamptic women: evidence for aromatase deficiency. *Am J Obstet Gynecol.* (2010) 203:477 e1-9. doi: 10.1016/j.ajog.2010.06.011
71. Jobe SO, Tyler CT, Magness RR. Aberrant synthesis, metabolism, and plasma accumulation of circulating estrogens and estrogen metabolites in preeclampsia implications for vascular dysfunction. *Hypertension.* (2013) 61:480–7. doi: 10.1161/HYPERTENSIONAHA.111.201624
72. Bussen S, Bussen D. Influence of the vascular endothelial growth factor on the development of severe pre-eclampsia or HELLP syndrome. *Arch Gynecol Obstet.* (2011) 284:551–7. doi: 10.1007/s00404-010-1704-x
73. Yin G, Zhu X, Guo C, Yang Y, Han T, Chen L, et al. Differential expression of estradiol and estrogen receptor alpha in severe preeclamptic pregnancies compared with normal pregnancies. *Mol Med Rep.* (2013) 7:981–5. doi: 10.3892/mmr.2013.1262
74. Walsh SW. Progesterone and estradiol production by normal and preeclamptic placentas. *Obstet Gynecol.* (1988) 71:222–6.
75. Luisi S, Petraglia F, Benedetto C, Nappi RE, Bernardi F, Fadalti M, et al. Serum allopregnanolone levels in pregnant women: changes during pregnancy, at delivery, and in hypertensive patients. *J Clin Endocrinol Metab.* (2000) 85:2429–33. doi: 10.1210/jcem.85.7.6675
76. Schumacher M, Hussain R, Gago N, Oudinet JP, Mattern C, Ghoumari AM. Progesterone synthesis in the nervous system: implications for myelination and myelin repair. *Front Neurosci.* (2012) 6:10. doi: 10.3389/fnins.2012.00010
77. Tsutsui K. Neurosteroids in the Purkinje cell: biosynthesis, mode of action and functional significance. *Mol Neurobiol.* (2008) 37:116–25. doi: 10.1007/s12035-008-8024-1
78. Tsutsui K, Ukena K. Neurosteroids in the cerebellar Purkinje neuron and their actions (review). *Int J Mol Med.* (1999) 4:49–56. doi: 10.3892/ijmm.4.1.49
79. Brunton PJ, Russell JA, Hirst JJ. Allopregnanolone in the brain: protecting pregnancy and birth outcomes. *Prog Neurobiol.* (2014) 113:106–36. doi: 10.1016/j.pneurobio.2013.08.005
80. Luoma JI, Kelley BG, Mermelstein PG. Progesterone inhibition of voltage-gated calcium channels is a potential neuroprotective mechanism against excitotoxicity. *Steroids.* (2011) 76:845–55. doi: 10.1016/j.steroids.2011.02.013
81. Pennell KD, Woodin MA, Pennell PB. Quantification of neurosteroids during pregnancy using selective ion monitoring mass spectrometry. *Steroids.* (2015) 95:24–31. doi: 10.1016/j.steroids.2014.12.007
82. Nguyen PN, Billiards SS, Walker DW, Hirst JJ. Changes in 5alpha-pregnane steroids and neurosteroidogenic enzyme expression in fetal sheep with umbilicoplacental embolization. *Pediatr Res.* (2003) 54:840–7. doi: 10.1203/01.PDR.0000088066.47755.36
83. Wang JM. Allopregnanolone and neurogenesis in the nigrostriatal tract. *Front Cell Neurosci.* (2014) 8:224. doi: 10.3389/fncel.2014.00224
84. Pluchino N, Russo M, Genazzani AR. The fetal brain: role of progesterone and allopregnanolone. *Horm Mol Biol Clin Investig.* (2016) 27:29–34X. doi: 10.1515/hmbci-2016-0020

85. Nguyen PN, Billiards SS, Walker DW, Hirst JJ. Changes in 5alpha-pregnane steroids and neurosteroidogenic enzyme expression in the perinatal sheep. *Pediatr Res.* (2003) 53:956–64. doi: 10.1203/01.PDR.0000064905.64688.10
86. Kelleher MA, Palliser HK, Walker DW, Hirst JJ. Sex-dependent effect of a low neurosteroid environment and intrauterine growth restriction on foetal guinea pig brain development. *J Endocrinol.* (2011) 208:301–9. doi: 10.1677/JOE-10-0248
87. Palliser HK, Kelleher MA, Tolcos M, Walker DW, Hirst JJ. Effect of postnatal progesterone therapy following preterm birth on neurosteroid concentrations and cerebellar myelination in guinea pigs. *J Dev Orig Health Dis.* (2015) 6:350–61. doi: 10.1017/S2040174415001075
88. Fester L, Prange-Kiel J, Jarry H, Rune GM. Estrogen synthesis in the hippocampus. *Cell Tissue Res.* (2011) 345:285–94. doi: 10.1007/s00441-011-1221-7
89. Dean SL, McCarthy MM. Steroids, sex and the cerebellar cortex: implications for human disease. *Cerebellum.* (2008) 7:38–47. doi: 10.1007/s12311-008-0003-6
90. McCarthy MM. The two faces of estradiol: effects on the developing brain. *Neuroscientist.* (2009) 15:599–610. doi: 10.1177/1073858409340924
91. Pansiot J, Pham H, Dalous J, Chevenne D, Colella M, Schwendimann L, et al. Glial response to 17beta-estradiol in neonatal rats with excitotoxic brain injury. *Exp Neurol.* (2016) 282:56–65. doi: 10.1016/j.expneurol.2016.05.024
92. Nunez JL, McCarthy MM. Resting intracellular calcium concentration, depolarizing Gamma-Aminobutyric Acid and possible role of local estradiol synthesis in the developing male and female hippocampus. *Neuroscience.* (2009) 158:623–34. doi: 10.1016/j.neuroscience.2008.09.061
93. Cambiasso MJ, Colombo JA, Carrer HF. Differential effect of oestradiol and astroglia-conditioned media on the growth of hypothalamic neurons from male and female rat brains. *Eur J Neurosci.* (2000) 12:2291–8. doi: 10.1046/j.1460-9568.2000.00120.x
94. Pansiot J, Mairesse J, Baud O. Protecting the developing brain by 17betaestradiol. *Oncotarget.* (2017) 8:12544–5. doi: 10.18632/oncotarget.14819
95. Berkane N, Liere P, Oudinet JP, Hertig A, Lefevre G, Pluchino N, et al. From pregnancy to preeclampsia: a key role for estrogens. *Endocr Rev.* (2017) 38:123–44. doi: 10.1210/er.2016-1065
96. Beltrand J, Verkauskiene R, Nicolescu R, Sibony O, Gaucherand P, Chevenne D, et al. Adaptive changes in neonatal hormonal and metabolic profiles induced by fetal growth restriction. *J Clin Endocrinol Metab.* (2008) 93:4027–32. doi: 10.1210/jc.2008-0562
97. Gluckman PD. Clinical review 68: the endocrine regulation of fetal growth in late gestation: the role of insulin-like growth factors. *J Clin Endocrinol Metab.* (1995) 80:1047–50.
98. Boucher J, Charalambous M, Zarse K, Mori MA, Kleinridders A, Ristow M, et al. Insulin and insulin-like growth factor 1 receptors are required for normal expression of imprinted genes. *Proc Natl Acad Sci USA.* (2014) 111:14512–7. doi: 10.1073/pnas.1415475111
99. Netchine I, Rossignol S, Azzi S, Brioude F, Le Bouc Y. Imprinted anomalies in fetal and childhood growth disorders: the model of Russell-Silver and Beckwith-Wiedemann syndromes. *Endocr Dev.* (2012) 23:60–70. doi: 10.1159/000341750
100. Leger J, Oury JF, Noel M, Baron S, Benali K, Blot P, et al. Growth factors and intrauterine growth retardation. I. Serum growth hormone, insulin-like growth factor (IGF)-I, IGF-II, and IGF binding protein 3 levels in normally grown and growth-retarded human fetuses during the second half of gestation. *Pediatr Res.* (1996) 40:94–100. doi: 10.1203/00006450-199607000-00017
101. Leger J, Noel M, Limal JM, Czernichow P. Growth factors and intrauterine growth retardation. II. Serum growth hormone, insulin-like growth factor (IGF) I, and IGF-binding protein 3 levels in children with intrauterine growth retardation compared with normal control subjects: prospective study from birth to two years of age. Study Group of IUGR. *Pediatr Res.* (1996) 40:101–7. doi: 10.1203/00006450-199607000-00018
102. Godfrey KM, Hales CN, Osmond C, Barker DJ, Taylor KP. Relation of cord plasma concentrations of proinsulin, 32-33 split proinsulin, insulin and C-peptide to placental weight and the baby's size and proportions at birth. *Early Hum Dev.* (1996) 46:129–40. doi: 10.1016/0378-3782(96)01752-5
103. Gicquel C, Le Bouc Y. Hormonal regulation of fetal growth. *Horm Res.* (2006) 65(Suppl 3):28–33. doi: 10.1159/000091503
104. Freemark M. Regulation of maternal metabolism by pituitary and placental hormones: roles in fetal development and metabolic programming. *Horm Res.* (2006) 65(Suppl 3):41–9. doi: 10.1159/000091505
105. McIntyre HD, Zeck W, Russell A. Placental growth hormone, fetal growth and the IGF axis in normal and diabetic pregnancy. *Curr Diabetes Rev.* (2009) 5:185–9. doi: 10.2174/157339909788920947
106. Zeitlin J, Ancel PY, Saurel-Cubizolles MJ, Papiernik E. The relationship between intrauterine growth restriction and preterm delivery: an empirical approach using data from a European case-control study. *BJOG.* (2000) 107:750–8. doi: 10.1111/j.1471-0528.2000.tb13336.x
107. Dyer AH, Vahdatpour C, Sanfeliu A, Tropea D. The role of Insulin-Like Growth Factor 1 (IGF-1) in brain development, maturation and neuroplasticity. *Neuroscience.* (2016) 325:89–99. doi: 10.1016/j.neuroscience.2016.03.056
108. Mattson MP. Glutamate and neurotrophic factors in neuronal plasticity and disease. *Ann N Y Acad Sci.* (2008) 1144:97–112. doi: 10.1196/annals.1418.005
109. Shcheglovitov A, Shcheglovitova O, Yazawa M, Portmann T, Shu R, Sebastiano V, et al. SHANK3 and IGF1 restore synaptic deficits in neurons from 22q13 deletion syndrome patients. *Nature.* (2013) 503:267–71. doi: 10.1038/nature12618
110. Labandeira-Garcia JL, Costa-Besada MA, Labandeira CM, Villar-Cheda B, Rodriguez-Perez AI. Insulin-like growth factor-1 and neuroinflammation. *Front Aging Neurosci.* (2017) 9:365. doi: 10.3389/fnagi.2017.00365
111. Fernandez AM, Torres-Aleman I. The many faces of insulin-like peptide signalling in the brain. *Nat Rev Neurosci.* (2012) 13:225–39. doi: 10.1038/nrn3209
112. Park SE, Lawson M, Dantzer R, Kelley KW, McCusker RH. Insulin-like growth factor-I peptides act centrally to decrease depression-like behavior of mice treated intraperitoneally with lipopolysaccharide. *J Neuroinflamm.* (2011) 8:179. doi: 10.1186/1742-2094-8-179
113. Tien LT, Lee YJ, Pang Y, Lu S, Lee JW, Tseng CH, et al. Neuroprotective effects of intranasal IGF-1 against neonatal lipopolysaccharide-induced neurobehavioral deficits and neuronal inflammation in the substantia nigra and locus coeruleus of juvenile rats. *Dev Neurosci.* (2017) 39:443–59. doi: 10.1159/000477898
114. Pang Y, Zheng B, Campbell LR, Fan LW, Cai Z, Rhodes PG. IGF-1 can either protect against or increase LPS-induced damage in the developing rat brain. *Pediatr Res.* (2010) 67:579–84. doi: 10.1203/PDR.0b013e3181dc240f
115. Cai Z, Fan LW, Lin S, Pang Y, Rhodes PG. Intranasal administration of insulin-like growth factor-1 protects against lipopolysaccharide-induced injury in the developing rat brain. *Neuroscience.* (2011) 194:195–207. doi: 10.1016/j.neuroscience.2011.08.003
116. Lin S, Fan LW, Rhodes PG, Cai Z. Intranasal administration of IGF-1 attenuates hypoxic-ischemic brain injury in neonatal rats. *Exp Neurol.* (2009) 217:361–70. doi: 10.1016/j.expneurol.2009.03.021
117. Wood TL, Loladze V, Altieri S, Gangoli N, Levison SW, Brywe KG, et al. Delayed IGF-1 administration rescues oligodendrocyte progenitors from glutamate-induced cell death and hypoxic-ischemic brain damage. *Dev Neurosci.* (2007) 29:302–10. doi: 10.1159/000105471
118. Lopes C, Ribeiro M, Duarte AI, Humbert S, Saudou F, Pereira de Almeida L, et al. IGF-1 intranasal administration rescues Huntington's disease phenotypes in YAC128 mice. *Mol Neurobiol.* (2014) 49:1126–42. doi: 10.1007/s12035-013-8585-5
119. Ribeiro M, Rosenstock TR, Oliveira AM, Oliveira CR, Rego AC. Insulin and IGF-1 improve mitochondrial function in a PI-3K/Akt-dependent manner and reduce mitochondrial generation of reactive oxygen species in Huntington's disease knock-in striatal cells. *Free Radic Biol Med.* (2014) 74:129–44. doi: 10.1016/j.freeradbiomed.2014.06.023
120. Meijer WJ, Verloove-Vanhorick SP, Brand R, van den Brande JL. Transient hypothyroxinaemia associated with developmental delay in very preterm infants. *Arch Dis Child.* (1992) 67:944–7. doi: 10.1136/adc.67.7.944
121. Den Ouden AL, Kok JH, Verkerk PH, Brand R, Verloove-Vanhorick SP. The relation between neonatal thyroxine levels and neurodevelopmental outcome at age 5 and 9 years in a national cohort of very preterm

and/or very low birth weight infants. *Pediatr Res.* (1996) 39:142–5. doi: 10.1203/00006450-199601000-00021

122. Leviton A, Paneth N, Reuss ML, Susser M, Allred EN, Dammann O, et al. Hypothyroxinemia of prematurity and the risk of cerebral white matter damage. *J Pediatr.* (1999) 134:706–11. doi: 10.1016/S0022-3476(99) 70285-4
123. Delahunty C, Falconer S, Hume R, Jackson L, Midgley P, Mirfield M, et al. Levels of neonatal thyroid hormone in preterm infants and neurodevelopmental outcome at 5 1/2 years: millennium cohort study. *J Clin Endocrinol Metab.* (2010) 95:4898–908. doi: 10.1210/jc.2010-0743
124. Ghassabian A, Bongers-Schokking JJ, Henrichs J, Jaddoe VW, Visser TJ, Visser W, et al. Maternal thyroid function during pregnancy and behavioral problems in the offspring: the generation R study. *Pediatr Res.* (2011) 69:454–9. doi: 10.1203/PDR.0b013e3182125b0c
125. Fisher DA. Thyroid system immaturities in very low birth weight premature infants. *Semin Perinatol.* (2008) 32:387–97. doi: 10.1053/j.semperi.2008.09.003
126. Kanike N, Davis A, Shekhawat PS. Transient hypothyroidism in the newborn: to treat or not to treat. *Transl Pediatr.* (2017) 6:349–58. doi: 10.21037/tp.2017.09.07
127. Maynard SE, Min JY, Merchan J, Lim KH, Li J, Mondal S, et al. Excess placental soluble fms-like tyrosine kinase 1 (sFlt1) may contribute to endothelial dysfunction, hypertension, and proteinuria in preeclampsia. *J Clin Invest.* (2003) 111:649–58. doi: 10.1172/JCI 17189
128. Levine RJ, Maynard SE, Qian C, Lim KH, England LJ, Yu KF, et al. Circulating angiogenic factors and the risk of preeclampsia. *N Engl J Med.* (2004) 350:672–83. doi: 10.1056/NEJMoa0 31884
129. Kendall RL, Thomas KA. Inhibition of vascular endothelial cell growth factor activity by an endogenously encoded soluble receptor. *Proc Natl Acad Sci USA.* (1993) 90:10705–9. doi: 10.1073/pnas.90.22.10705
130. Koga K, Osuga Y, Tajima T, Hirota Y, Igarashi T, Fujii T, et al. Elevated serum soluble fms-like tyrosine kinase 1 (sFlt1) level in women with hydatidiform mole. *Fertil Steril.* (2010) 94:305–8. doi: 10.1016/j.fertnstert.2009.02.015
131. Savvidou MD, Yu CK, Harland LC, Hingorani AD, Nicolaides KH. Maternal serum concentration of soluble fms-like tyrosine kinase 1 and vascular endothelial growth factor in women with abnormal uterine artery Doppler and in those with fetal growth restriction. *Am J Obstet Gynecol.* (2006) 195:1668–73. doi: 10.1016/j.ajog.2006.03.065
132. Di Martino D, Cetin I, Frusca T, Ferrazzi E, Fuse F, Gervasi MT, et al. Italian Advisory Board: sFlt-1/PlGF ratio and preeclampsia, state of the art and developments in diagnostic, therapeutic and clinical management. *Eur J Obstet Gynecol Reprod Biol.* (2016) 206:70–3. doi: 10.1016/j.ejogrb.2016.08.036
133. Levine RJ, Vatten LJ, Horowitz GL, Qian C, Romundstad PR, Yu KF, et al. Pre-eclampsia, soluble fms-like tyrosine kinase 1, and the risk of reduced thyroid function: nested case-control and population based study. *BMJ.* (2009) 339:b4336. doi: 10.1136/bmj.b4336
134. Mannisto T, Karumanchi SA, Pouta A, Vaarasmaki M, Mendola P, Miettola S, et al. Preeclampsia, gestational hypertension and subsequent hypothyroidism. *Pregnancy Hypertens.* (2013) 3:21–7. doi: 10.1016/j.preghy.2012.09.001
135. Kamba T, Tam BY, Hashizume H, Haskell A, Sennino B, Mancuso MR, et al. VEGF-dependent plasticity of fenestrated capillaries in the normal adult microvasculature. *Am J Physiol Heart Circ Physiol.* (2006) 290:H560–76. doi: 10.1152/ajpheart.00133.2005
136. Voller SB, Chock S, Ernst LM, Su E, Liu X, Farrow KN, et al. Cord blood biomarkers of vascular endothelial growth (VEGF and sFlt-1) and postnatal growth: a preterm birth cohort study. *Early Hum Dev.* (2014) 90:195–200. doi: 10.1016/j.earlhumdev.2014.01.003
137. Korevaar TI, Steegers EA, Schalekamp-Timmermans S, Ligthart S, de Rijke YB, Visser WE, et al. Soluble Flt1 and placental growth factor are novel determinants of newborn thyroid (dys)function: the generation R study. *J Clin Endocrinol Metab.* (2014) 99:E1627–34. doi: 10.1210/jc.2014-1884
138. Thorpe-Beeston JG, Nicolaides KH, McGregor AM. Fetal thyroid function. *Thyroid.* (1992) 2:207–17. doi: 10.1089/thy.1992.2.207
139. Mahajan SD, Aalinkeel R, Singh S, Shah P, Gupta N, Kochupillai N. Endocrine regulation in asymmetric intrauterine fetal growth retardation. *J Matern Fetal Neonatal Med.* (2006) 19:615–23. doi: 10.1080/14767050600799901
140. Nieto-Diaz A, Villar J, Matorras-Weinig R, Valenzuela-Ruiz P. Intrauterine growth retardation at term: association between anthropometric and endocrine parameters. *Acta Obstet Gynecol Scand.* (1996) 75:127–31. doi: 10.3109/00016349609033303
141. Fetter WP, Waals-Van de Wal CM, Van Eyck J, Samson G, Bongers-Schokking JJ. Thyroid hormone concentrations in preterm infants born to pre-eclamptic women with placental insufficiency. *Acta Paediatr.* (1998) 87:186–90. doi: 10.1111/j.1651-2227.1998.tb00973.x
142. Ryckman KK, Spracklen CN, Dagle JM, Murray JC. Maternal factors and complications of preterm birth associated with neonatal thyroid stimulating hormone. *J Pediatr Endocrinol Metab.* (2014) 27:929–38. doi: 10.1515/jpem-2013-0366
143. Miller SL, Huppi PS, Mallard C. The consequences of fetal growth restriction on brain structure and neurodevelopmental outcome. *J Physiol.* (2016) 594:807–23. doi: 10.1113/JP271402

3

Fetal Growth Restriction Alters Cerebellar Development in Fetal and Neonatal Sheep

Tamara Yawno[1,2], Amy E. Sutherland[1], Yen Pham[1], Margie Castillo-Melendez[1], Graham Jenkin[1,2] and Suzanne L. Miller[1,2]*

[1]*The Ritchie Centre, Hudson Institute of Medical Research, Monash University, Clayton, VIC, Australia,*
[2]*Department of Obstetrics and Gynaecology, Monash University, Clayton, VIC, Australia*

Correspondence:
Tamara Yawno
tamara.yawno@monash.edu

Fetal growth restriction (FGR) complicates 5–10% of pregnancies and is associated with increased risks of perinatal morbidity and mortality. The development of cerebellar neuropathology *in utero*, in response to chronic fetal hypoxia, and over the period of high risk for preterm birth, has not been previously studied. Therefore, the objective of this study was to examine the effects of FGR induced by placental insufficiency on cerebellar development at three timepoints in ovine fetal and neonatal development: (1) 115 days gestational age (d GA), (2) 124 d GA, and (3) 1-day-old postnatal age. We induced FGR *via* single umbilical artery ligation (SUAL) at ~105 d GA in fetal sheep, term is ~147 d GA. Animals were sacrificed at 115 d GA, 124 d GA, and 1-day-old postnatal age; fetuses and lambs were weighed and the cerebellum collected for histopathology. FGR lambs demonstrated neuropathology within the cerebellum after birth, with a significant, ~18% decrease in the number of granule cell bodies (NeuN+ immunoreactivity) within the internal granular layer (IGL) and an ~80% reduction in neuronal extension and branching (MAP+ immunoreactivity) within the molecular layer (ML). Oxidative stress (8-OHdG+ immunoreactivity) was significantly higher in FGR lambs within the ML and the white matter (WM) compared to control lambs. The structural integrity of neurons was already aberrant in the FGR cerebellum at 115 d GA, and by 124 d GA, inflammatory cells (Iba-1+ immunoreactivity) were significantly upregulated and the blood-brain barrier (BBB) was compromised (Pearls, albumin, and GFAP+ immunoreactivity). We confirm that cerebellar injuries develop antenatally in FGR, and therefore, interventions to prevent long-term motor and coordination deficits should be implemented either antenatally or perinatally, thereby targeting neuroinflammatory and oxidative stress pathways.

Keywords: cerebellum, preterm, term, fetal sheep, fetal growth restriction, brain injury, blood-brain barrier

INTRODUCTION

Fetal growth restriction (FGR) complicates 5–10% of pregnancies and is associated with increased risks of perinatal morbidity and mortality (Bernstein et al., 2000). FGR is linked to adverse perinatal outcomes, including stillbirth, prematurity, and need for neonatal intensive care; as well as long-term adverse outcomes including metabolic syndromes, hypertension, and neurological deficits (Baschat, 2011; Mayer and Joseph, 2013; Albu et al., 2014; Drost et al., 2018). FGR is principally caused by placental insufficiency, which results in reduced utero-placental transfer of oxygen and nutrients to the developing fetus (Figueras and Gardosi, 2011). FGR can be induced experimentally to examine the neuropathology associated with FGR (Swanson and David, 2015). In sheep, restricted placental growth and function can be induced by surgical removal of the major endometrial caruncles from sheep before mating, causing a 31% reduction in body weight (Robinson et al., 1979; Harding et al., 1985). In rodents, uterine artery ligation models have been widely described in pregnant rats, guinea pigs, and mice (Basilious et al., 2015). Regardless of the experimental model, the fetus responds to chronic hypoxic challenge with a redistribution of cardiac output to favor the brain - termed brain sparing - but this does not ensure normal brain development (Miller et al., 2016). Chronic hypoxia results in widespread cerebral cellular and axonal lipid peroxidation, and white matter (WM) hypomyelination and axonal damage (Miller et al., 2014). FGR in lambs also induces cerebrovascular changes in the WM and causes disruption to the blood-brain barrier (BBB) (Castillo-Melendez et al., 2017). Developmental delays in motor and behavioral function are also present soon after birth in FGR lambs (Miller et al., 2014). These may be attributed to mal-development of the motor and coordination center within the brain, the cerebellum (Volpe, 2009). However, the *in utero* effects of placental insufficiency, chronic hypoxia, and FGR on cerebellar structure and development are not well understood.

The cerebellum is one of the first brain structures to differentiate, but one of the last to mature (Triulzi et al., 2005). In the last trimester of human gestation, and often coinciding with preterm birth in FGR offspring, cerebellar development undergoes a phase of rapid growth and interconnection with other cerebral structures (Volpe, 2009), which then continues into the first postnatal year (Abraham et al., 2001). Therefore, chronic hypoxia and/or preterm birth in the last pregnancy trimester may adversely impact cerebellar maturation and may also alter connectivity and subsequent development of other brain regions (Limperopoulos et al., 2010). The development of the cerebellum and cerebellar morphology has been described in fetal sheep (Rees et al., 1988, 1997). Purkinje cells are present by 100 days gestational age (d GA; term is 145–148 d GA) and branching of their dendritic tree is attained by 140 d GA. However, the presence of immature and mature dendritic neuronal markers indicates that considerable remodeling of Purkinje cell branching is still occurring in late gestation. Rat and guinea pig models of FGR show altered postnatal development of the cerebellum, including deficits in neuronal and glial formation (Mallard et al., 2000; So et al., 2013; McDougall et al., 2017). The ontogeny of cerebellar neuropathology *in utero*, in response to placental insufficiency and chronic fetal hypoxia, and over the period of high risk for preterm birth, has not been previously studied.

Therefore, the objective of this study was to examine the effects of FGR induced by placental insufficiency on cerebellar development. We induced late-onset FGR in fetal sheep *via* single umbilical artery ligation, which causes chronic fetal hypoxia and hypoglycemia but does not routinely cause preterm birth, as per late-onset FGR in the human (Baschat, 2014). We examined the cerebellum at three timepoints in ovine fetal and neonatal development; aim: (1) 115 d GA, (2) 124 d GA, and (3) 1-day-old postnatal age. Although the ontogeny of sheep cerebellar development is not well characterized with respect to human cerebellar development, we selected these timepoints to broadly correspond to human brain cerebrum and cerebellar development from 28 weeks through to infancy in the human (Rees et al., 1997; Back et al., 2012).

MATERIALS AND METHODS

Animal Surgery

The surgical and experimental procedures undertaken in this project were approved by Monash Medical Centre Animal Ethics Committee A (MMCA2010/03). Surgery was performed on 26 Border-Leicester-cross pregnant ewes carrying twins (Aims 1 and 2) or a single fetus (Aim 3; **Table 1**) to induce late-onset FGR *via* SUAL, as previously described (Miller et al., 2012; Alves de Alencar Rocha et al., 2017). Briefly, anesthetized ewes underwent surgery to instrument each fetus with a femoral artery catheter and an amniotic catheter for determination of blood gases and to administer antibiotics, respectively. The SUAL procedure was performed by ligating one of the umbilical arteries with two tight silk ligatures (FGR) and, in the sham procedure, the umbilical cord was exposed but not ligated. SUAL induces necrosis of approximately half of the placental cotyledons, thereby resulting in chronic placental insufficiency with reduced transfer of oxygen and glucose to the developing fetus (Miller et al., 2014). A maternal jugular vein catheter was inserted for antibiotic administration prior to recovery of the ewe.

Experimental Timeline

All animals were monitored daily from surgery until the day of postmortem. The ewe and fetuses were euthanased at three different ages to allow for comparisons of brain development and injury. At 115 and 124 d GA, animals were killed with maternal injection of pentobarbitone (Lethabarb; Virbac, Peakhurst, Australia) and the fetuses were removed, weighed, and brains were collected for analysis. In the third cohort, lambs were born naturally at term (~145 d GA) and at 24 h of age, lambs were euthanased with an intravenous injection of pentobarbitone; the lamb was weighed and brains were collected for analysis. The cerebellum of each animal was divided into right and left halves. The right half of the cerebellum was fixed by immersion in 4% buffered paraformaldehyde (PFA; ProSciTech, Thuringowa, QLD, Australia) for 3 days and transferred to 70% ethanol overnight, prior to embedding in paraffin. Subsequently, 10-µm coronal sections were cut for analyses.

Immunohistochemistry and Histological Stains

Sections were dewaxed and rehydrated through graded ethanol transfer before commencing the procedures described below. All washes were carried out in phosphate-buffered saline

TABLE 1 | Fetal and neonatal outcomes.

	115 d GA		124 d GA		1-day-old lamb	
	Control	FGR	Control	FGR	Control	FGR
Number of ewes	6		5		8	7
Number of fetuses	6	6	5	5	8	7
GA at surgery	107 ± 1.0	107 ± 1.0	104 ± 0.6	104 ± 0.8	105 ± 1.2	105 ± 0.9
Male:female	4:2	4:2	2:3	2:3	4:4	3:4
Body weight (kg)	1.9 ± 0.2	1.6 ± 0.1	3.5 ± 0.1	2.5 ± 0.2*	4.8 ± 0.5	3.5 ± 0.5*
Brain weight (g)	34.3 ± 1.6	34.4 ± 1.9	48.3 ± 2.0	43.9 ± 1.6	55.6 ± 2.7	51.3 ± 2.7
Brain:body weight (g/kg)	18.1 ± 1.3	21.8 ± 2.2	13.8 ± 0.5	17.0 ± 1.1*	11.8 ± 0.4	16.1 ± 1.8*
Blood gas parameters (average across gestation)						
Arterial oxygen saturation (%)	59 ± 1.3	52 ± 1.3*	70 ± 0.8	58 ± 0.8*	62 ± 1.5	43 ± 2.0*
Cerebellum						
Cross-sectional area (mm^2)	$1.3 \times 10^5 \pm 1.2 \times 10^4$	$1.3 \times 10^5 \pm 1.1 \times 10^4$	$1.6 \times 10^5 \pm 1.6 \times 10^4$	$1.8 \times 10^5 \pm 1.6 \times 10^4$	$2.1 \times 10^5 \pm 1.9 \times 10^4$	$2.2 \times 10^5 \pm 1.3 \times 10^4$
Cross-sectional area:body weight (mm^2/kg)	$7.4 \times 10^4 \pm 1.0 \times 10^4$	$8.1 \times 10^4 \pm 6.0 \times 10^3$	$4.7 \times 10^4 \pm 4.7 \times 10^3$	$7.1 \times 10^4 \pm 1.0 \times 10^4$	$4.7 \times 10^4 \pm 4.7 \times 10^3$	$6.2 \times 10^4 \pm 4.3 \times 10^3$*
EGL width (Mm)	22.0 ± 1.6	29.6 ± 2.6*	21.7 ± 2.3	21.5 ± 3.3	14.1 ± 0.7	14.0 ± 0.9
ML width (mm)	142 ± 6	112 ± 5*	160 ± 12	150 ± 11	173 ± 8	195 ± 5*
WM:cross-sectional area (mm^2)	0.1 ± 0.01	0.1 ± 0.02	0.1 ± 0.01	0.1 ± 0.02	0.2 ± 0.02	0.2 ± 0.01
The number of Purkinje cells (mm)	0.016 ± 0.002	0.016 ± 0.001	0.015 ± 0.001	0.013 ± 0.001	0.015 ± 0.001	0.016 ± 0.001

Mean ± SEM are presented for each group.$p \leq 0.05$ vs. control.*
d GA, days gestational age; FGR, fetal growth restriction; EGL, external granular layer; ML, molecular layer; WM, white matter.

(PBS, 0.1 M, pH 7.4). For each immunohistochemical protocol, duplicate sections of the cerebellum from all treatment groups were included in a single run to eliminate variations between runs.

Glial fibrillary acidic protein (GFAP) was used to visualize astrocytes and astrocytic end-feet. Ionized calcium binding adaptor molecule 1 (Iba-1) was used to identify microglia. The DNA adduct 8-hydroxy-2-deoxyguanosine (8-OHdG) was used as a marker of oxidative DNA damage. NEUronal nuclei, clone A60 (NeuN), was used to identify neuronal nuclei; microtubule-associated protein 2 (MAP-2) was used to examine neuronal filaments, and albumin was used to detect blood protein extravasation. GFAP, Iba-1, 8-OHdG, NeuN, MAP-2, and albumin were identified using the following: monoclonal mouse anti-GFAP (1:400; Sigma-Aldrich), rabbit anti-Iba1 (1:1,000; Wako Pure Chemical Industries Ltd., Osaka, Japan), mouse anti-NeuN (1:200; Millipore Corporation, USA), mouse anti-MAP-2 (1:200; Thermo Fisher Scientific, Waltham, Massachusetts, USA), and rabbit anti-sheep albumin (1:1,000; Accurate Chemical and Scientific Corp., Westbury, NY, USA), respectively. Antibodies were diluted in PBS. All sections were treated with a secondary antibody (1:200; biotinylated anti-rabbit or anti-mouse IgG antibody; Vector Laboratories, Burlingame, CA, USA) and immunolabeling was visualized using 3,3-diaminobenzidine (DAB; Pierce Biotechnology, Rockford, IL, USA). Positive and negative control sections were included in each run. Sections were viewed at 400× magnification using a light microscope (Olympus BX-41, Japan).

Perls' Prussian Blue

Perls' staining was used to observe the presence of microbleeds (which presented as free iron) within the cerebellum. Following dewaxing, the slides were rehydrated in distilled water for 5 min. While this took place, a solution of equal parts 4% aqueous potassium ferrocyanide and 4% hydrochloric acid was mixed, and then heated to 60°C in a microwave that was placed within a fumehood to prevent exposure to hydrogen cyanide fumes. Slides were then placed into the heated solution for 40 min and then allowed to cool. The sections were rinsed in running distilled water for 2 min and then placed into a dish and counter-stained with Nuclear Fast Red for 4 min. Following this, the slides were rinsed for another 2 min under running distilled water, and then dehydrated in ascending alcohol concentrations, cleared in xylene, and cover-slipped. Sections were examined for the presence of microbleeds using a light microscope (Olympus BX-41, Japan). All areas of the cerebellum were examined, and bleeds were counted manually.

Image Analysis

Densitometric calculations for GFAP, 8-OHdG (internal granular layer; IGL), and MAP-2-positive immunoreactivity was performed using a computerized image analysis system (ImageJ version 10.2, NIH, Bethesda, Maryland, USA) that reads optical density as gray levels, at 400× magnification. An investigator (TY), blinded to the experimental groups, selected the threshold levels of detection, where nonspecific background was identified and the threshold level was then kept constant for all images within a given immunohistochemistry run. For cell counts and scoring, two sections of the cerebellum per animal were examined, and the number of immunopositive cells for 8-OHdG [molecular layer (ML) and WM] and NeuN, or percentage area occupied by Iba-1-positive cells, was calculated using an average of three fields of view per area, and the results were averaged across the animals in each group. Analysis for cresyl violet and acid fuchsin staining, Purkinje cells, IGL and ML width, GFAP, 8-OHdG, Iba-1, MAP-2, and NeuN immunohistochemistry was performed in the anterior and posterior lobules (II, VI, and VIII), in three randomly selected fields of view. Analysis for microbleeds and albumin extravasation was performed on the entire section of the cerebellum, including all folia. The number of incidences for microbleeds and albumin extravasation was counted and averaged per section in duplicate across all animals in each group. Neuronal cell morphology was assessed using cresyl violet and acid fuchsin staining; cells that displayed swelling of organelles, loss of cell wall, and/or nuclear membrane integrity were considered abnormal. The cross-sectional area of the entire cerebellum and the WM were performed on the cresyl violet and acid fuchsin-stained sections using Image J to trace around each area, and data for cerebellar WM are presented per total area. The IGL and ML width were measured using the same program and data presented as μm (**Figure 1**).

Data Analysis

Data are presented as the mean ± standard error of the mean (SEM). Statistical analysis was performed with GraphPad Prism 7 (GraphPad Software, San Diego, United States). An unpaired nonparametric *t*-test was performed to compare between the control and FGR group at each gestational age. Significance was accepted when $p \leq 0.05$.

RESULTS

We induced late-onset placental insufficiency in fetal sheep (refer to **Table 1** for *n* numbers), which resulted in chronic fetal hypoxia that worsened compared to control fetuses over the course of gestation; 115 d GA 52 vs. 59% FaO_2, 124 d 58 vs. 70%, and 142 d GA 43 vs. 62% FaO_2 (**Table 1**). The success rate for fetal survival after FGR surgery was 83%, with all fetal deaths occurring within the first 24 h post-surgery. Body weights were reduced in FGR fetuses compared to age-matched controls, and this was statistically significant at 124 d GA and in 1-day-old lambs (**Table 1**). Brain weight was spared in FGR fetuses and lambs, such that the brain to body weight ratio was significantly increased at 124 d GA and in 1-day-old FGR lambs. The total area of the cerebellum to body weight ratio was also significantly increased in the FGR 1-day-old lambs compared to controls. FGR had no effect on the area of cerebellar WM (**Table 1**).

Morphological Changes in the Cerebellum

We first assessed basic cerebellar morphology in the control animals. Cresyl violet and acid fuchsin staining showed that, at 115 d GA, a prominent external granular cell layer (EGL) was apparent in control brains (**Table 1**), which actively proliferates over the preterm period studied, wherein the cells migrate inward to form the IGL (Volpe, 2009). After 124 d GA, the EGL was less prominent, and was further decreased in width in 1-day-old control lambs (EGL at 115 d: GA 22.0 ± 1.6 μm, at 124 d: GA 21.7 ± 2.3 μm, and in 1-day-old lambs: 14.1 ± 0.7 μm). By contrast, the width of the ML in control animals increased as gestation progressed (**Table 1**). At 115 d GA, the width of the EGL in FGR fetuses was significantly thicker than control fetuses (**Figures 1A,B**), but this difference was no longer seen at 124 d GA and in 1-day-old lambs. In FGR animals compared to control animals, the width of the ML was significantly reduced at 115 d GA; no difference was observed at 124 d GA, but then became significantly wider in 1-day-old lambs (**Figures 1C,D**).

At 115 d GA, Purkinje cell bodies were evident in control brains, and the number of Purkinje cells remained relatively consistent from 115 d GA through to 1-day-old postnatal lambs (**Table 1**). The IGL had a dense population of neurons, and the boundaries between IGL and the WM were also apparent at 115 d GA. Qualitative analysis revealed that the population of cells in the IGL appeared to be increased by 124 d GA and even further in 1-day-old lambs, and sharp boundaries were formed between the IGL and WM, such that the two layers were highly distinguishable.

There was no evidence of gross lesions within the FGR brains, but at 115 d GA, FGR fetuses showed evidence of neurons with abnormally shaped, darkly stained nuclei, vacuolization, and patchy coverage in parenchymal WM tissue (**Figure 1F**); this was also evident in FGR fetuses at 124 d GA and in 1-day-old lambs. We noted that the cerebellar Purkinje cells exhibited altered cellular morphology and arrangement in FGR brains, as evidenced by intensely stained Purkinje cell bodies of abnormal shape and Purkinje cell disorganization, most apparent in 1-day-old lambs (**Figure 1H**).

We investigated the presence of microbleeds within the cerebellar tissue (**Figure 2A**), visualized as bright blue patches (Perls' positive staining), counter-stained with nuclear fast red (**Figures 2D,H,L**). Control fetuses did not exhibit any blue staining; (**Figures 2C,G,K**) however, microbleeds were present in 4/8 control lambs. In FGR brains, blue staining was present in 4/6 fetuses at 115 d GA, and 5/5 fetuses at 124 d GA, with microbleeds present within the ML, IGL, and WM. Microbleeds were also identified in 5/7 FGR lambs.

The absence of immunoreactive albumin within the brain is indicative of a functional BBB, and albumin was not observed within control fetal and lamb brains (**Figures 2B,E,I,M**), with the exception of albumin extravasation in one of five control animals at 124 d GA. In FGR brains, the occurrence of albumin extravasation from blood vessels (BVs) was observed in all regions of the cerebellum (**Figure 2B**). Where albumin was present in FGR brains, intense immunoreactivity was predominantly observed in brain parenchyma adjacent to BVs (**Figures 2F,J,N**).

Immunohistochemistry

GFAP-positive astrocytes were present in the cerebellar ML, GL, and the WM of control and FGR brain. At 115 d GA,

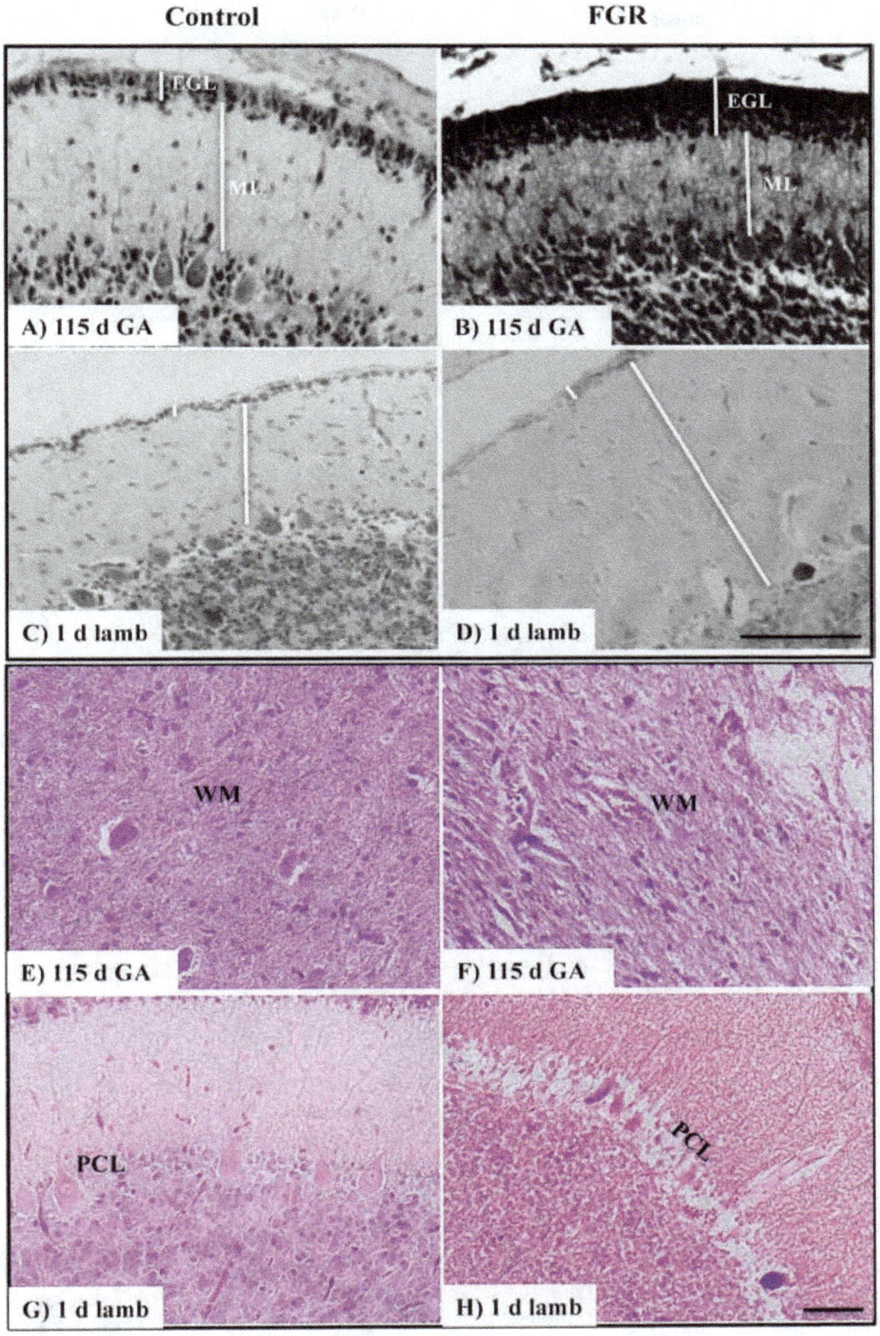

FIGURE 1 | Representative micrographs of cresyl violet and acid fuchsin staining in a 115 d GA fetus and 1-day-old lamb of control **(A,C,E,G)** and FGR **(B,D,F,H)** brain. **(A–D)** show measurements of EGL and ML on each image. Within FGR brains, note the presence of vacuolization in parenchymal WM tissue **(F)** and Purkinje neurons with abnormally shaped, darkly stained nuclei **(H)**. EGL, external granular layer; ML, molecular layer; PCL, Purkinje cell layer; WM, white matter. Scale bar for **(A–D)** in **(D)** = 100 μm and **(E–H)** in **(H)** = 50 μm.

astrocytes were not affected by FGR. However, the density of the astrocytic cell bodies and processes appeared to be reduced in all FGR brains at 124 d GA and 1-day-old lambs compared to control animals but this was only statistically significant in the IGL and WM at 124 d GA (**Figures 3A–C**). Furthermore, we observed very few end-feet of astrocytes associated with BVs in FGR animals (**Figures 3D,E**). The association of astrocytic end-feet to BVs is critical for maintenance of the BBB, and therefore, in this situation, a decrease in astrocyte density and end-feet attachment has likely compromised the BBB in FGR offspring.

We quantified microglial cells, and found that in FGR fetuses at 124 d GA, there was an overall increase in the percentage area coverage of microglia that was significant in the GL and

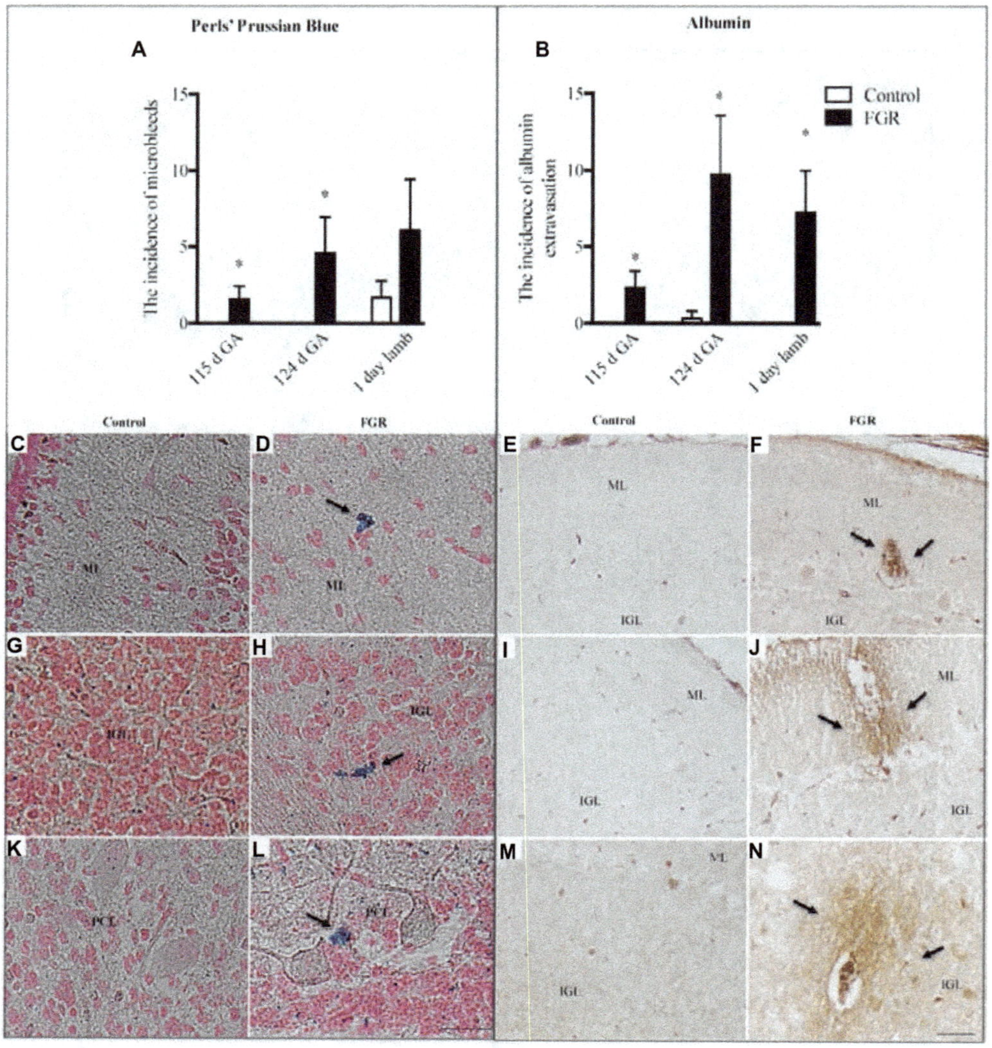

FIGURE 2 | The number of microbleeds **(A)** and albumin extravasation from blood vessels (BVs) **(B)** in the cerebellum of the fetal brain at 115 d GA, 124 d GA, and 1-day-old lamb of control and FGR animals. Each bar represents the mean ± SEM; $^*p \leq 0.05$ versus control. Representative micrographs showing Perls' Prussian Blue staining and albumin immunohistochemistry in a 115 d GA fetus **(C–F)**, 125 d GA **(G–J)**, and 1–day-old lamb **(K–N)** brains. Microbleeds were visualized as bright blue patches that were counter-stained with nuclear fast red. Arrows indicate the sites of microbleeds/albumin extravasation. FGR, fetal growth restriction; PCL, Purkinje cell layer; ML, molecular layer; IGL, internal granular layer. Scale bar for Perls in **(L)** = 25 μm. Scale bar for albumin in **(N)** = 50 μm.

WM (**Figures 4A–C**). There was no difference in microglial cell coverage in FGR (**Figure 4H**) and control (**Figure 4G**) animals at 115 d GA and 1-day-old lambs.

We next examined whether oxidative stress was upregulated in the FGR cerebellum. Cells that were positive for 8-OHdG immunoreactivity were present in control and FGR brains (**Figures 4I,J**). The number of cells that were positive for 8-OHdG was significantly increased in FGR 1-day-old lambs within the ML and WM compared to control brains (**Figures 4D–F**).

We examined neuronal cell number (NeuN) and the morphology of neuronal filaments (MAP-2) within the cerebellum. We utilized NeuN as a neuronal-specific nuclear protein (Mullen et al., 1992) and, as expected, NeuN-positive cells were localized to the cerebellar IGL and not the ML and WM, which is consistent with published data (Zimatkin and Karniushko, 2016), indicative that we had appropriately labeled for mature IGL neurons. The number of mature neurons was significantly reduced in FGR brains of 1-day-old lambs within the IGL compared to control lambs (**Figures 5A,C,D**). When we examined the expression of the MAP-2-positive immunoreactivity within the ML, a region where neuronal filaments extend to other areas in the cerebellum, we observed an overall decrease in the expression of MAP-2 at all gestational ages in the FGR animals, but this decrease was statistically significant at 115 d GA and 1-day-old lambs, compared to control (**Figures 5B,E,F**).

DISCUSSION

Here, we examined the effects of placental insufficiency, chronic fetal hypoxia, and FGR on cerebellar development at three timepoints corresponding to the last trimester of human

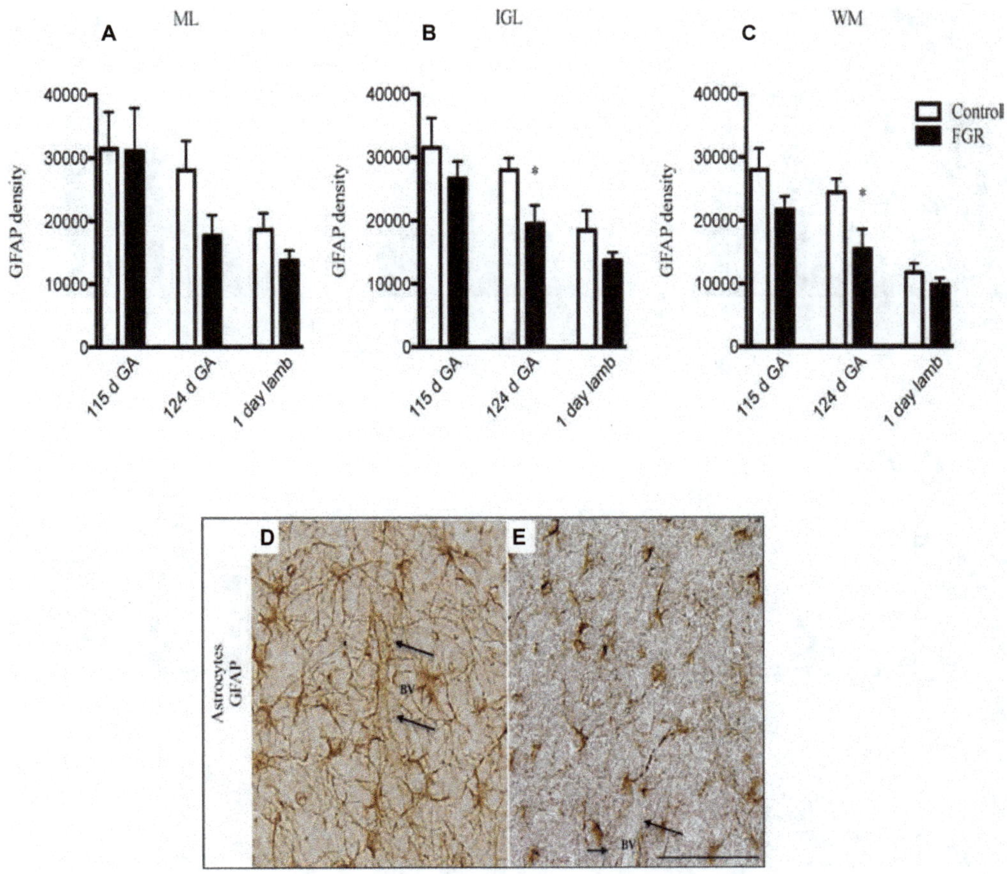

FIGURE 3 | Glial fibrillary acidic protein (GFAP) density in the molecular layer [ML **(A)**], internal granular layer [IGL **(B)**], and white matter [WM **(C)**] in the fetal brain at 115 d GA, 124 d GA, and 1-day-old lamb of control and FGR animals. Comparisons are made within the same brain region at the same gestation and not across regions or across gestation. Each bar represents the mean ± SEM; $^{*}p \leq 0.05$. Representative micrographs showing GFAP-positive immunoreactivity in the fetal IGL at 124 d GA of control **(D)** and FGR **(E)** brain. Arrows pointing to a blood vessel (BV), showing the damaged astrocytic end-feet. FGR, fetal growth restriction. Scale bar = 50 μm.

pregnancy and into the neonatal period. We show that cerebellar growth and development are adversely affected soon after the onset of hypoxia, and that chronic fetal hypoxia leads to a progressively altered developmental profile of the cerebellum. This is the first study to characterize maturation of normal and abnormal morphology within cerebellum from appropriately grown and growth-restricted fetuses and neonates. Most strikingly, newborn FGR lambs demonstrated neuropathology within the cerebellum after birth, with a significant, ~18% decrease, in the number of granule cell bodies within the IGL and an ~80% reduction in neuronal extension and branching within the ML. The foundations of neonatal cerebellar neuropathology were laid down soon after the onset of placental insufficiency and fetal hypoxia. The structural integrity of neurons was already aberrant in the FGR cerebellum at 115 d GA, and by 124 d GA, inflammatory cells were upregulated and the BBB was compromised. These neuropathologies occurred in the absence of gross cerebellar abnormalities; the cross-sectional area of the whole cerebellum and the WM were not different in size compared to control, and no cystic lesions were present in the brain of FGR offspring. Thus, we show that chronic *in utero* compromise leads to progressive maturational deficits in the cerebellum of FGR offspring, likely to have significant functional implications.

We induced late-onset placental insufficiency to mimic the clinical situation of FGR that is most commonly observed (Baschat, 2014). This ovine model of late-onset FGR did not significantly affect body weight 10 days after induction of placental insufficiency (115 d GA); however, body weight was significantly reduced in FGR offspring at 19 days (124 d GA) and 43 days (1-day-old lamb) following the onset of placental dysfunction. This was accompanied by a significant increase in brain to body weight ratio, a finding that supports our previous work (Miller et al., 2009, 2014) and reflects asymmetric growth in response to chronic hypoxia (Baschat, 2014; Miller et al., 2016).

It was interesting to note that, while body weight was not yet affected at 115 d GA, FGR fetuses were already experiencing significant hypoxia, and this was associated with early signs of cerebellar neuropathology. At 115 d GA, many cerebellar granule cells in FGR animals were abnormally shaped, with darkly stained nuclei – not observed in control fetuses – and similar cellular abnormalities remained evident at 124 d GA and in 1-day-old lambs. This supports previous work showing that both acute and chronic hypoxia result in cerebellar

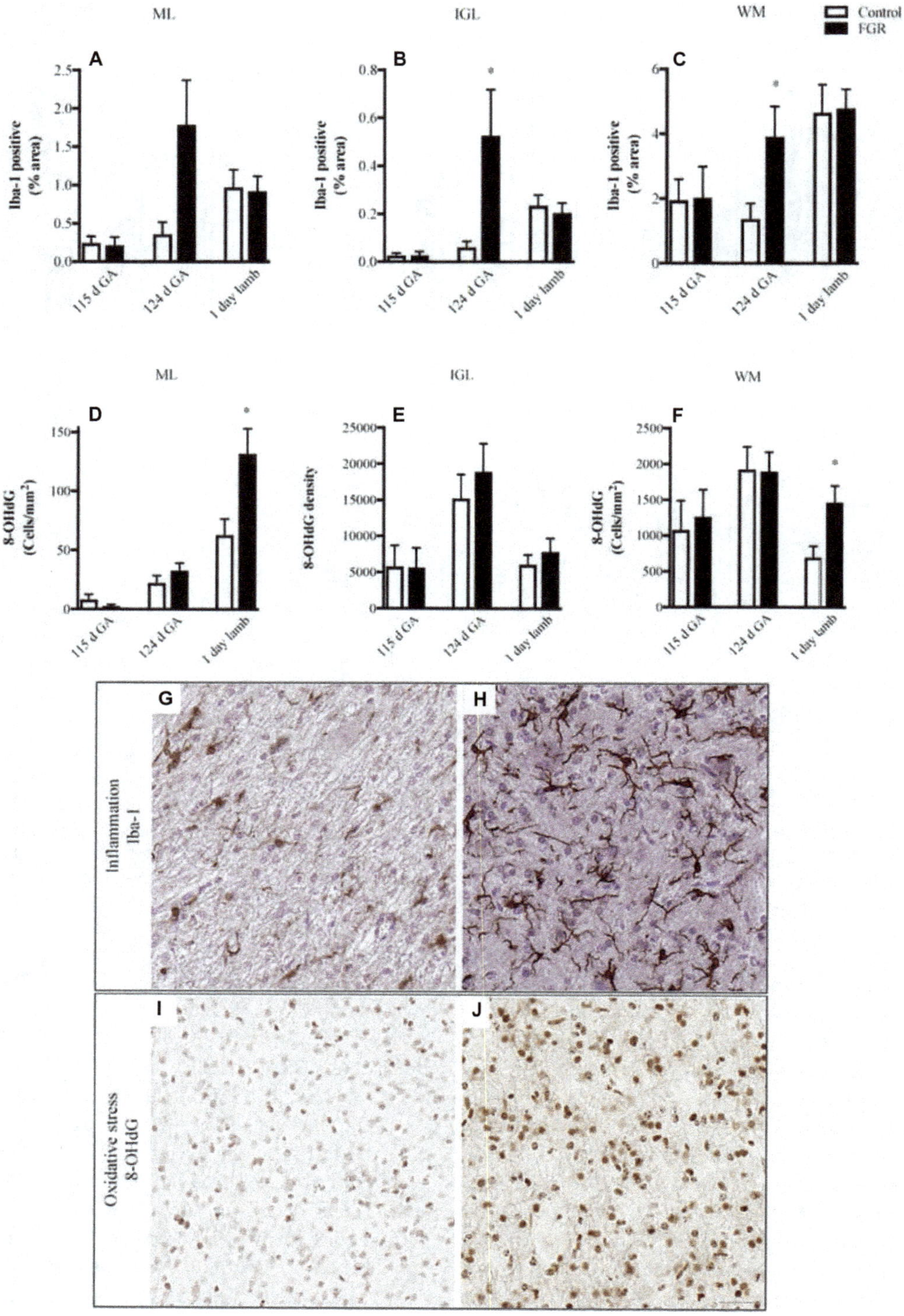

FIGURE 4 | The number of Iba-1-positive cells **(A–C)** and 8-hydroxy-2-deoxyguanosine (8-OHdG)-positive cells **(D–F)** in the molecular layer (ML), internal granular layer (IGL), and white matter (WM) in the fetal brain at 115 d GA, 124 d GA, and 1-day-old lamb of control and FGR animals. Each bar represents the mean ± SEM; *$p \leq 0.05$ versus control. Representative micrographs showing Iba-1- **(G,H)** and 8-OHdG- **(I,J)** positive immunoreactivity in the WM in 124 d GA **(G,H)** and 1-day-old lambs **(I,J)**. Images from control **(G,I)** and FGR **(H,J)** animals are shown. FGR, fetal growth restriction. Scale bar = 25 μm.

neuropathology, as described in fetal sheep (Yawno et al., 2009), rats (McDougall et al., 2017), and guinea pigs (Tolcos et al., 2018); however, these studies did not examine the ontogeny of the cerebellum. Structurally, at 115 d GA, the width of the EGL in FGR animals was significantly increased, and this was associated with a significant decrease in the width of the ML compared to control animals. The changes in the EGL and ML were resolved at 124 d GA. However, in 1-day-old FGR

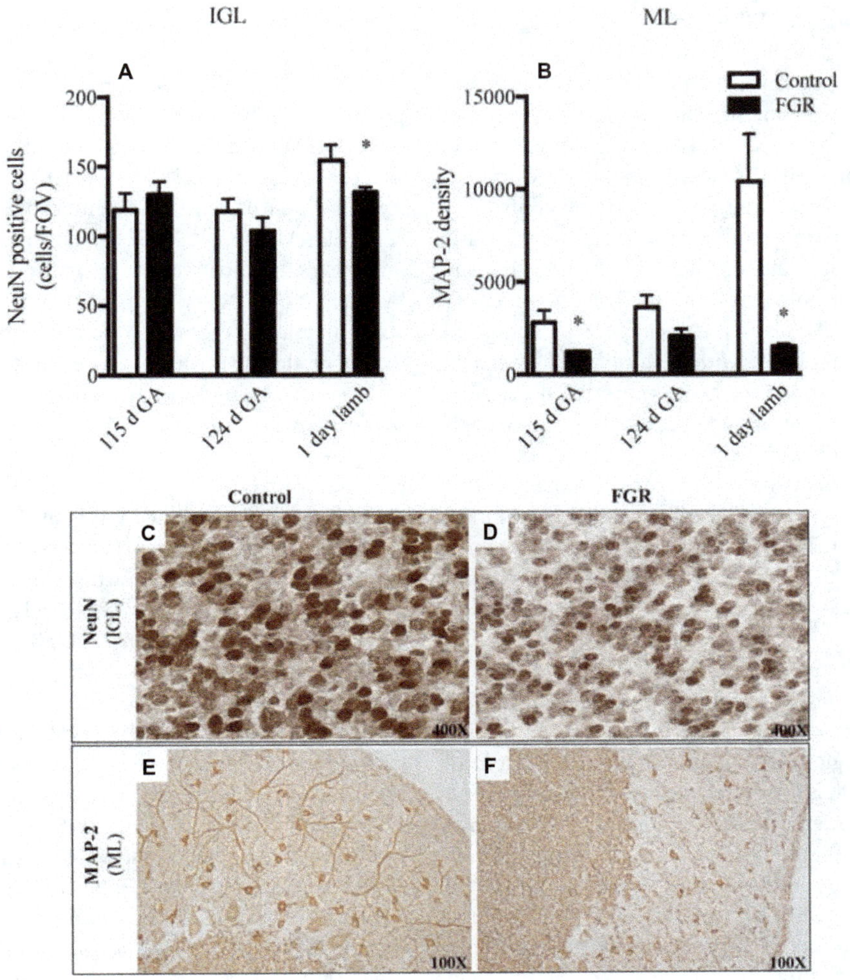

FIGURE 5 | The number of NeuN-positive cells per field of view **(A)** and MAP-2 density **(B)** in the internal granular layer (IGL) and molecular layer (ML) in the fetal brain at 115 d GA, 124 d GA, and 1-day-old lamb of control and FGR animals. Each bar represents the mean ± SEM; $^*p \leq 0.05$ versus control. Representative micrographs showing NeuN-positive immunoreactivity in the IGL **(C,D)** and MAP-2 in the ML **(E,F)** in 1-day-old lambs. Images from control **(C,E)** and FGR **(D,F)** animals are shown. FGR, fetal growth restriction.

lambs, the width of the ML was significantly increased compared to control lambs. These findings support previous results from other models of FGR (McDougall et al., 2017; Tolcos et al., 2018), where it was suggested that the increase in EGL width maybe due to impaired granule cell migration out of the EGL, increased cell proliferation, and reduced granule cell apoptosis. Even if these structural changes were corrected at 124 d GA, alterations were still evident in 1 day-old FGR lambs, which could lead to changes in cellular connectivity and cerebellar circuitry. Hence, further investigations on cell migration, proliferation, and apoptosis are warranted.

We noted that Purkinje cell bodies were morphologically abnormal, and the Purkinje cell layer was highly disorganized in 1-day-old FGR lambs only, thereby suggesting that progression of neuropathology over the course of late gestation had a direct effect on the Purkinje cell layer. Reduction in Purkinje cell number has been reported in the cerebellum of growth restricted guinea pigs and was associated with neurological and behavioral deficits postnatally (Mallard et al., 2000). While we did not see a change in the total number of Purkinje cell in our FGR offspring, it is known that Purkinje cells receive excitatory inputs from injured granule cells within the IGL (Sarna and Hawkes, 2003), thereby potentially making them more susceptible to abnormal development and injury.

A notable observation in the current study was the susceptibility of the cerebellum of FGR animals to hemorrhage. More than 80% of FGR fetuses (both 115 d and 124 d) showed evidence of brain bleeds, compared to no bleeds within control fetuses. In addition, we observed the presence of immunoreactive albumin adjacent to BVs within the brains of all FGR animals (115 d, 124 d, and 1-day-old lambs). This result is likely due to altered cerebrovascular development and suboptimal integrity of the BBB. We have previously examined cerebrovascular development within the subcortical and periventricular WM of the cerebrum, and shown specific cerebrovascular deficits within the FGR brain that include decreased basal lamina area, reduced vascular endothelial growth factor (VEGF), fewer endothelial cells, and reduced BBB integrity (Castillo-Melendez et al., 2015, 2017). The structural and functional features of the BBB are normally maintained by the contribution and cellular interactions of the endothelial cells, pericytes, and astrocytic end-feet contacts (Kim et al., 2013). In particular, close astrocyte association with BVs is important in development as it provides functional and structural support by controlling inflammatory cell infiltration and maintaining homeostasis (Farhy-Tselnicker and Allen, 2018). Thus, our finding that the FGR brain showed reduced expression of astrocytic density from 124 d GA potentially plays a critical role in abnormal brain development. In addition, with reduced glial support, neuronal function may be even further compromised (Laming et al., 2000). It is worth noting that the presence of microbleeds (Perls' stain) in our control lamb brains was unexpected; we are unsure to why this has happened; however, all lambs in this cohort were delivered naturally which could induce temporary instability of the BBB *via* hypoxia at birth, but it is also important to note that the albumin data show that control lambs did not show any albumin extravasation and an indication of a more stable BBB.

Concomitantly with altered BBB function at 124 d GA, we also saw a neuroinflammatory response within the cerebellum of FGR fetuses in this age group, with a large increase in microglial cells in all cerebellar regions examined, compared to control brains. This finding fits with growing knowledge of the contribution of neuroinflammation toward neuropathology in FGR animal studies (Wixey et al., 2018) and in human preterm infants (Buser et al., 2010). Inflammation-induced brain injury is associated with WM damage, acute BBB dysfunction, and neurovascular unit injury, and in turn linked with behavioral alterations (Stolp et al., 2011). It is interesting to note that an elevation in neuroinflammation was only observed within the FGR brain at 124 d GA, and this was linked with an altered astrocyte profile at this age, and high susceptibility to hemorrhage. Previous work has shown that injured glial cells release factors that act on target cells to initiate responses of activated immune cells in the periphery, in turn leading to inflammatory cell infiltration of tissues. These events usually occur when there has been destruction or compromise of the BBB (Streit et al., 1998; Sroga et al., 2003). Taken together, these results are indicative that this developmental timepoint (roughly equivalent to 34 weeks in human cerebellar development) is particularly vulnerable for BBB dysfunction linked with upregulation of neuroinflammation. It is of interest to note that clinically, rates of intraventricular hemorrhage (IVH) are not increased in FGR infants born preterm at 28 weeks compared to appropriately grown infants, but IVH rates are significantly elevated in human infants born late preterm (>34 weeks) (Gilbert and Danielsen, 2003; Ortigosa Rocha et al., 2010), indicative of the vulnerability of the BBB in late gestation (Wixey et al., 2018). It is, however, worth noting that the marker we used to identify inflammatory cells does not discriminate between resting and activated microglia. Therefore, it would be of interest to further phenotype the inflammatory cells to examine whether late-onset FGR induces a pro-inflammatory environment within the cerebellum, which may be amenable to treatment.

We examined the presence of oxidative DNA damage (8-OHdG) to indicate whether oxidative stress was upregulated in the cerebellum of FGR animals and contributed to the neuropathology observed (Yawno et al., 2017). During fetal gestation, both control and FGR animals showed cellular oxidative stress to be present within the cerebellum, with no differences seen between the groups. In 1-day-old lambs, oxidative cell damage was significantly upregulated within the cerebellar ML and WM of FGR offspring, compared to control animals. All lambs were born naturally at term and cared for by their mother after birth, with no need for intervention or supplemental oxygen. Therefore, the observation of increased oxidative damage within the brain of newborn FGR lambs may represent a response to birth. Potentially, this is contributed by relative hyperoxia experienced by FGR lambs after birth compared to control lambs, given their *in utero* conditions of chronic hypoxia. It may also be due to the reduced anti-oxidant defense capabilities in the FGR lamb. We have previously shown that in FGR offspring, circulating malondialdehyde concentration (a marker of oxidative stress) was elevated compared to appropriately grown offspring (Polglase et al., 2017) and that the same FGR offspring had significantly increased levels of oxidative stress within the brain, in both neuronal cell bodies of the cortex and fiber tracts within the periventricular WM (Miller et al., 2014). This is the first study to show that oxidative stress is upregulated in the FGR cerebellum, appearing to affect granule cell axons and migrating neurons within the ML. Oxidative DNA damage might be a precursor to cell death, which would require substantiation in long-term studies.

Mature IGL neurons (NeuN-positive cells) were significantly reduced in the neonatal FGR brains compared to control lambs but no difference was apparent at earlier timepoints, thereby suggesting that cerebellar neuropathology resulting from late-onset FGR takes time to manifest. This finding is in agreement with other literature showing a reduction in the density of cells undergoing mitosis in the cerebellar granular layer of hypoxemic fetal sheep compared to controls (Rees et al., 1997) and suggests that chronic hypoxia is causing an arrested maturational profile in IGL neurons or that mature neurons have not completed migration into the IGL. In addition to reduced total number of neurons in the granular layer, we also observed a decrease in the expression of MAP-2 across gestation in the ML of all FGR animals, indicative of disrupted dendritic branching. MAP-2 is critical for neurite extension and branching, and for cessation of cell division (Johnson and Jope, 1992). In rodents, it has been shown that loss of MAP-2 expression is associated with neuronal degeneration, which has short- (Kinugasa-Taniguchi et al., 2010) and long-term (Matesic and Lin, 1994) effects on cognition and anxiety-related behavior (Matesic and Lin, 1994). Fundamentally, loss of neurons and altered neuronal morphology of existing neurons may well underlie deficits in spatial motor function and coordination, which are present in children who were growth restricted at birth (Tolsa et al., 2004).

A noted limitation of the current study is that we did not have sufficient numbers of animals to examine potential sex differences. A recent review has described important female versus male differences in fetal growth and sex-specific response to preterm birth and compromised placental function (Alur, 2019). In further studies, it would be of interest to examine cerebral and cerebellar development in males and females following compromised intrauterine environment, with the potential for tailored therapeutics.

Cerebellar injuries are often overlooked in experimental and clinical studies of brain neuropathology associated with acute or chronic hypoxia. Here, we demonstrate the progressive nature of developmental deficits in the cerebellum, associated with increasing placental insufficiency, chronic hypoxia, and FGR. These results suggest that the period of suboptimal *in utero* environment contributes to cerebellar pathology in late gestation fetal sheep. These results also indicate that late preterm age in sheep is a time of high risk for glial disturbances. Glial cells play an important function in the survival and maintenance of the neurovascular unit, and conversely, altered glial number or function can cause disruption to the BBB and brain developmental more broadly. We confirm that cerebellar injuries develop antenatally in FGR, and therefore, interventions to prevent long-term motor and coordination deficits should be implemented antenatally and/or perinatally, potentially targeting neuroinflammatory and oxidative stress pathways.

AUTHOR CONTRIBUTIONS

TY performed the experiments and data analysis, and wrote the original draft of the manuscript. GJ, MC-M, and SM provided funding, designed the experimental protocol, and helped draft the manuscript. AS assisted with animal experiments and data analysis, and helped draft the manuscript. YP assisted with data analysis.

REFERENCES

1. Abraham, H., Tornoczky, T., Kosztolanyi, G., and Seress, L. (2001). Cell formation in the cortical layers of the developing human cerebellum. *Int. J. Dev. Neurosci.* 19, 53–62. doi: 10.1016/S0736-5748(00)00065-4
2. Albu, A. R., Anca, A. F., Horhoianu, V. V., and Horhoianu, I. A. (2014). Predictive factors for intrauterine growth restriction. *J. Med. Life* 7, 165–171.
3. Alur, P. (2019). Sex differences in nutrition, growth, and metabolism in preterm infants. *Front. Pediatr.* 7:22. doi: 10.3389/fped.2019.00022
4. Alves de Alencar Rocha, A. K., Allison, B. J., Yawno, T., Polglase, G. R., Sutherland, A. E., Malhotra, A., et al. (2017). Early- versus late-onset fetal growth restriction differentially affects the development of the fetal sheep brain. *Dev. Neurosci.* 39, 141–155. doi: 10.1159/000456542
5. Back, S. A., Riddle, A., Dean, J., and Hohimer, A. R. (2012). The instrumented fetal sheep as a model of cerebral white matter injury in the premature infant. *Neurotherapeutics* 9, 359–370. doi: 10.1007/s13311-012-0108-y
6. Baschat, A. A. (2011). Neurodevelopment following fetal growth restriction and its relationship with antepartum parameters of placental dysfunction. *Ultrasound Obstet. Gynecol.* 37, 501–514. doi: 10.1002/uog.9008
7. Baschat, A. A. (2014). Neurodevelopment after fetal growth restriction. *Fetal Diagn. Ther.* 36, 136–142. doi: 10.1159/000353631
8. Basilious, A., Yager, J., and Fehlings, M. G. (2015). Neurological outcomes of animal models of uterine artery ligation and relevance to human intrauterine growth restriction: a systematic review. *Dev. Med. Child Neurol.* 57, 420–430. doi: 10.1111/dmcn.12599
9. Bernstein, I. M., Horbar, J. D., Badger, G. J., Ohlsson, A., and Golan, A. (2000). Morbidity and mortality among very-low-birth-weight neonates with intrauterine growth restriction. The Vermont Oxford Network. *Am. J. Obstet. Gynecol.* 182, 198–206.
10. Buser, J. R., Segovia, K. N., Dean, J. M., Nelson, K., Beardsley, D., Gong, X., et al. (2010). Timing of appearance of late oligodendrocyte progenitors coincides with enhanced susceptibility of preterm rabbit cerebral white matter to hypoxia-ischemia. *J. Cereb. Blood Flow Metab.* 30, 1053–1065. doi: 10.1038/ jcbfm.2009.286
11. Castillo-Melendez, M., Yawno, T., Allison, B. J., Jenkin, G., Wallace, E. M., and Miller, S. L. (2015). Cerebrovascular adaptations to chronic hypoxia in the growth restricted lamb. *Int. J. Dev. Neurosci.* 45, 55–65. doi: 10.1016/j.ijdevneu.2015.01.004
12. Castillo-Melendez, M., Yawno, T., Sutherland, A., Jenkin, G., Wallace, E. M., and Miller, S. L. (2017). Effects of antenatal melatonin treatment on the cerebral vasculature in an ovine model of fetal growth restriction. *Dev. Neurosci.* 39, 323–333. doi: 10.1159/000471797
13. Drost, F. J., Keunen, K., Moeskops, P., Claessens, N. H. P., Van Kalken, F., Isgum, I., et al. (2018). Severe retinopathy of prematurity is associated with reduced cerebellar and brainstem volumes at term and neurodevelopmental deficits at 2 years. *Pediatr. Res.* 83, 818–824. doi: 10.1038/pr.2018.2
14. Farhy-Tselnicker, I., and Allen, N. J. (2018). Astrocytes, neurons, synapses: a tripartite view on cortical circuit development. *Neural Dev.* 13, 7–19. doi: 10.1186/s13064-018-0104-y
15. Figueras, F., and Gardosi, J. (2011). Intrauterine growth restriction: new concepts in antenatal surveillance, diagnosis, and management. *Am. J. Obstet. Gynecol.* 204, 288–300. doi: 10.1016/j.ajog.2010.08.055
16. Gilbert, W. M., and Danielsen, B. (2003). Pregnancy outcomes associated with intrauterine growth restriction. *Am. J. Obstet. Gynecol.* 188, 1596–1599. discussion 1599–1601. doi: 10.1067/mob.2003.384
17. Harding, J. E., Jones, C. T., and Robinson, J. S. (1985). Studies on experimental growth retardation in sheep. The effects of a small placenta in restricting transport to and growth of the fetus. *J. Dev. Physiol.* 7, 427–442.
18. Johnson, G. V., and Jope, R. S. (1992). The role of microtubule-associated protein 2 (MAP-2) in neuronal growth, plasticity, and degeneration. *J. Neurosci. Res.* 33, 505–512. doi: 10.1002/jnr.490330402
19. Kim, J. H., Byun, H. M., Chung, E. C., Chung, H. Y., and Bae, O. N. (2013). Loss of integrity: impairment of the blood-brain barrier in heavy metal-associated ischemic stroke. *Toxicol. Res.* 29, 157–164. doi: 10.5487/ TR.2013.29.3.157
20. Kinugasa-Taniguchi, Y., Tomimatsu, T., Mimura, K., Kanagawa, T., Shimoya, K., Murata, Y., et al. (2010). Human C-reactive protein enhances vulnerability of immature rats to hypoxic-ischemic brain damage: a preliminary study. *Reprod. Sci.* 17, 419–425. doi: 10.1177/1933719110361379
21. Laming, P. R., Kimelberg, H., Robinson, S., Salm, A., Hawrylak, N., Muller, C., et al. (2000). Neuronal-glial interactions and behaviour. *Neurosci. Biobehav. Rev.* 24, 295–340. doi: 10.1016/S0149-7634(99)00080-9
22. Limperopoulos, C., Chilingaryan, G., Guizard, N., Robertson, R. L., and Du Plessis, A. J. (2010). Cerebellar injury in the premature infant is associated with impaired growth of specific cerebral regions. *Pediatr. Res.* 68, 145–150. doi: 10.1203/PDR.0b013e3181e1d032
23. Mallard, C., Loeliger, M., Copolov, D., and Rees, S. (2000). Reduced number of neurons in the hippocampus and the cerebellum in the postnatal guinea-pig following intrauterine growth-restriction. *Neuroscience* 100, 327–333. doi: 10.1016/S0306-4522(00)00271-2
24. Matesic, D. F., and Lin, R. C. (1994). Microtubule-associated protein 2 as an early indicator of ischemia-induced neurodegeneration in the gerbil forebrain. *J. Neurochem.* 63, 1012–1020. doi: 10.1046/j.1471-4159.1994.63031012.x
25. Mayer, C., and Joseph, K. S. (2013). Fetal growth: a review of terms, concepts and issues relevant to obstetrics. *Ultrasound Obstet. Gynecol.* 41, 136–145. doi: 10.1002/uog.11204
26. McDougall, A. R. A., Wiradjaja, V., Azhan, A., Li, A., Hale, N., Wlodek, M. E., et al. (2017). Intrauterine growth restriction alters the postnatal development of the rat cerebellum. *Dev. Neurosci.* 39, 215–227. doi: 10.1159/000470902

27. Miller, S. L., Huppi, P. S., and Mallard, C. (2016). The consequences of fetal growth restriction on brain structure and neurodevelopmental outcome. *J. Physiol.* 594, 807–823. doi: 10.1113/JP271402
28. Miller, S. L., Supramaniam, V. G., Yawno, T., Castillo-Melendez, M., Walker, D. W., Jenkin, G., et al. (2009). Neuropathology in intrauterine growth restricted (IUGR) lambs is associated with delayed attainment of behavioural milestones in the newborn period. *Reprod. Sci.* 16:109A.
29. Miller, S. L., Sutherland, A. E., Supramaniam, V. G., Walker, D. W., Jenkin, G., and Wallace, E. M. (2012). Antenatal glucocorticoids reduce growth in appropriately grown and growth-restricted ovine fetuses in a sex-specific manner. *Reprod. Fertil. Dev.* 24, 753–758. doi: 10.1071/RD11143
30. Miller, S. L., Yawno, T., Alers, N. O., Castillo-Melendez, M., Supramaniam, V. G., Vanzyl, N., et al. (2014). Antenatal antioxidant treatment with melatonin to decrease newborn neurodevelopmental deficits and brain injury caused by fetal growth restriction. *J. Pineal Res.* 56, 283–294. doi: 10.1111/jpi.12121
31. Mullen, R. J., Buck, C. R., and Smith, A. M. (1992). NeuN, a neuronal specific nuclear protein in vertebrates. *Development* 116, 201–211.
32. Ortigosa Rocha, C., Bittar, R. E., and Zugaib, M. (2010). Neonatal outcomes of late-preterm birth associated or not with intrauterine growth restriction. *Obstet. Gynecol. Int.* 2010, 1-5. doi: 10.1155/2010/231842
33. Polglase, G. R., Barbuto, J., Allison, B. J., Yawno, T., Sutherland, A. E., Malhotra, A., et al. (2017). Effects of antenatal melatonin therapy on lung structure in growth-restricted newborn lambs. 123, 1195–1203. *J. Appl. Physiol.* doi: 10.1152/japplphysiol.00783.2016
34. Rees, S., Bocking, A. D., and Harding, R. (1988). Structure of the fetal sheep brain in experimental growth retardation. *J. Dev. Physiol.* 10, 211–225.
35. Rees, S., Stringer, M., Just, Y., Hooper, S. B., and Harding, R. (1997). The vulnerability of the fetal sheep brain to hypoxemia at mid-gestation. *Brain Res. Dev. Brain Res.* 103, 103–118. doi: 10.1016/S0165-3806(97)81787-7
36. Robinson, J. S., Kingston, E. J., Jones, C. T., and Thorburn, G. D. (1979). Studies on experimental growth retardation in sheep. The effect of removal of a endometrial caruncles on fetal size and metabolism. *J. Dev. Physiol.* 1, 379–398.
37. Sarna, J. R., and Hawkes, R. (2003). Patterned Purkinje cell death in the cerebellum. *Prog. Neurobiol.* 70, 473–507. doi: 10.1016/S0301-0082(03)00114-X So, K., Chung, Y., Lee, H., Kim, E., and Jeon, Y. (2013). The effect of chronic prenatal hypoxia on the development of mature neurons in the cerebellum. *J. Neurodev. Disord.* 5:17. doi: 10.1186/1866-1955-5-17
38. Sroga, J. M., Jones, T. B., Kigerl, K. A., Mcgaughy, V. M., and Popovich, P. G. (2003). Rats and mice exhibit distinct inflammatory reactions after spinal cord injury. *J. Comp. Neurol.* 462, 223–240. doi: 10.1002/cne.10736
39. Stolp, H. B., Johansson, P. A., Habgood, M. D., Dziegielewska, K. M., Saunders, N. R., and Ek, C. J. (2011). Effects of neonatal systemic inflammation on blood-brain barrier permeability and behaviour in juvenile and adult rats. *Cardiovasc. Psychiatry Neurol.* 2011, 1–10. doi: 10.1155/2011/469046
40. Streit, W. J., Semple-Rowland, S. L., Hurley, S. D., Miller, R. C., Popovich, P. G., and Stokes, B. T. (1998). Cytokine mRNA profiles in contused spinal cord and axotomized facial nucleus suggest a benefi al role for inflammation and gliosis. *Exp. Neurol.* 152, 74–87. doi: 10.1006/exnr.1998.6835
41. Swanson, A. M., and David, A. L. (2015). Animal models of fetal growth restriction: considerations for translational medicine. *Placenta* 36, 623–630. doi: 10.1016/j.placenta.2015.03.003
42. Tolcos, M., Mcdougall, A., Shields, A., Chung, Y., O'dowd, R., Turnley, A., et al. (2018). Intrauterine growth restriction affects cerebellar granule cells in the developing guinea pig brain. *Dev. Neurosci.* 40, 162–174. doi: 10.1159/000487797 Tolsa, C. B., Zimine, S., Warfield, S. K., Freschi, M., Sancho Rossignol, A., Lazeyras, F., et al. (2004). Early alteration of structural and functional brain development in premature infants born with intrauterine growth restriction. *Pediatr. Res.* 56, 132–138. doi: 10.1203/01.PDR.0000128983.54614.7E
43. Triulzi, F., Parazzini, C., and Righini, A. (2005). MRI of fetal and neonatal cerebellar development. *Semin. Fetal Neonatal Med.* 10, 411–420. doi: 10.1016/j. siny.2005.05.004
44. Volpe, J. J. (2009). Cerebellum of the premature infant: rapidly developing, vulnerable, clinically important. *J. Child Neurol.* 24, 1085–1104. doi: 10.1177/0883073809338067
45. Wixey, J. A., Chand, K. K., Pham, L., Colditz, P. B., and Bjorkman, S. T. (2018). Therapeutic potential to reduce brain injury in growth restricted newborns. *J. Physiol.* 596, 5675–5686. doi: 10.1113/JP275428
46. Yawno, T., Hirst, J. J., Castillo-Melendez, M., and Walker, D. W. (2009). Role of neurosteroids in regulating cell death and proliferation in the late gestation fetal brain. *Neuroscience* 163, 838–847. doi: 10.1016/j. neuroscience.2009.07.009 Yawno, T., Mahen, M., Li, J., Fahey, M. C., Jenkin, G., and Miller, S. L. (2017).
47. The beneficial effects of melatonin administration following hypoxia-ischemia in preterm fetal sheep. *Front. Cell. Neurosci.* 11:296. doi: 10.3389/fncel.2017.00296 Zimatkin, S. M., and Karniushko, O. A. (2016). Expression of doublecortin and NeuN in the developing cerebellar neurons in rat. *Morfologiia* 149, 38–42. doi: 10.1007/s11055-016-0374-y

4

Impaired Progesterone-Responsiveness of CD11c^{+} Dendritic Cells Affects the Generation of CD4^{+} Regulatory T Cells and is Associated with Intrauterine Growth Restriction in Mice

Kristin Thiele[1], Alexandra Maximiliane Hierweger[1], Julia Isabel Amambay Riquelme[1], María Emilia Solano[1], John P. Lydon[2] and Petra Clara Arck[1]**

[1] *Division of Experimental Feto-Maternal Medicine, Department of Obstetrics and Fetal Medicine, University Medical Center Hamburg-Eppendorf, Hamburg, Germany,*
[2] *Department of Molecular and Cellular Biology, Baylor College of Medicine, Houston, TX, United States*

***Correspondence:**
Kristin Thiele
k.thiele@uke.de
Petra Clara Arck
p.arck@uke.de

Up to 10% of pregnancies in Western societies are affected by intrauterine growth restriction (IUGR). IUGR reduces short-term neonatal survival and impairs long-term health of the children. To date, the molecular mechanisms involved in the pathogenesis of IUGR are largely unknown, but the failure to mount an adequate endocrine and immune response during pregnancy has been proposed to facilitate the occurrence of IUGR. A cross talk between the pregnancy hormone progesterone and innate immune cell subsets such as dendritic cells (DCs) is vital to ensure adequate placentation and fetal growth. However, experimental strategies to pinpoint distinct immune cell subsets interacting with progesterone *in vivo* have long been limited. In the present study, we have overcome this limitation by generating a mouse line with a specific deletion of the progesterone receptor (PR) on CD11c^{+} DCs. We took advantage of the cre/loxP system and assessed reproductive outcome in Balb/c-mated C57Bl/6 PR$^{flox/flox}$CD11c$^{cre/wt}$ females. Balb/c-mated C57Bl/6 PR$^{wt/wt}$CD11c$^{cre/wt}$ females served as controls. In all dams, fetal growth and development, placental function and maternal immune and endocrine adaptation were evaluated at different gestational time points. We observed a significantly reduced fetal weight on gestational day 13.5 and 18.5 in PR$^{flox/flox}$CD11c$^{cre/wt}$ females. While frequencies of uterine CD11c^{+} cells were similar in both groups, an increased frequency of co-stimulatory molecules was observed on DCs in PR$^{flox/flox}$CD11c$^{cre/wt}$ mice, along with reduced frequencies of CD4^{+} FoxP3^{+} and CD8^{+} CD122^{+} regulatory T (Treg) cells. Placental histomorphology revealed a skew toward increased junctional zone at the expense of the labyrinth in implantations of PR$^{flox/flox}$CD11c$^{cre/wt}$ females, accompanied by increased plasma progesterone concentrations. Our results support that DCs are highly responsive to progesterone, subsequently adapting to a tolerogenic phenotype. If such cross talk between progesterone and DCs is impaired, the generation of pregnancy-protective immune cells subsets such as $CD4^+$ and $CD8^+$ Treg cells is reduced, which is associated with poor placentation and IUGR in mice.

Keywords: dendritic cells, IUGR, placenta, progesterone, Tregs

INTRODUCTION

In Western societies, up to 10% of pregnancies are affected by intrauterine growth restriction (IUGR) (1), which is defined as a pathological delay in fetal growth. IUGR reduces short-term survival due to immediate neonatal complications such as asphyxia, hypothermia, hypoglycemia and immunodeficiency (2). Moreover, child development and long-term health is impaired. Thus, IUGR children have an increased risk for metabolic, immunologic and neurodevelopmental impairments (3–5). In addition, clinical studies also reveal an association between IUGR and a significantly higher incidence of metabolic, renal and cardiovascular diseases later in life of the children (6). The molecular mechanisms involved in the pathogenesis of IUGR are largely unknown. However, various pathways have been proposed to contribute to the development of IUGR including maternal, fetal, genetic, and placental factors (2).

In order to ensure adequate placentation and subsequently fetal growth, the maternal immune, and endocrine system needs to actively adapt to the semiallogenic fetus. One key features of this tailored immune response are tolerogenic dendritic cells (tDC) present at the feto-maternal interphase during early pregnancy. The tDCs are characterized by a reduced expression of co-stimulatory molecules and enhanced IL-10 production. Functionally, tDCs promote the generation of regulatory T (Treg) cells (7–9). A number of markers with immunomodulatory potential including Galectin-1 or steroid hormones have been suggested to initiate the generation of tDCs from the less stable subset of immature DCs and sustains their ability to produce IL-10 (8, 10, 11). However, due to technical limitations, it is still unknown which immunomodulatory marker directly triggers the generation of tDCs.

It was the aim of this study to overcome these limitations and address this gap in knowledge. We hereby focussed on the role of progesterone in modulating DC functions by utilizing a cell-specific knockout of the intracellular progesterone receptor (PR) on DCs, as such approach allows to investigate the direct effect of progesterone on dendritic cells and its role in pregnancy outcome.

MATERIALS AND METHODS

Generation of $PR^{flox/flox}CD11c^{cre/wt}$ Mice

$PR^{flox/flox}$ and $CD11c^{cre/wt}$ mice were kindly provided by John P. Lydon from Baylor College of Medicine, Houston, Texas, US and Manuel Friese from University Medical Center Hamburg-Eppendorf, Hamburg, Germany, respectively. In order to generate female mice with a selective KO of the PR on CD11c dendritic cells, $PR^{flox/flox}$ females, and $CD11c^{cre/wt}$ males were mated in the Animal Facility of the University Medical Center Hamburg-Eppendorf (**Figure 1A**). Subsequently, male $PR^{flox/wt}$ $CD11c^{cre/wt}$ and female $PR^{flox/wt}$ $CD11c^{wt/wt}$ offspring were mated in order to generate $PR^{flox/flox}$ $CD11c^{cre/wt}$ and $PR^{wt/wt}$ $CD11c^{cre/wt}$ animals. Experimental mice were obtained by mating male mice with a genotype of $PR^{flox/flox}$ $CD11c^{cre/wt}$ and $PR^{wt/wt}$ $CD11c^{cre/wt}$ with $PR^{flox/flox}$ $CD11c^{wt/wt}$ and $PR^{wt/wt}$ $CD11c^{wt/wt}$ females, respectively. Hence, the cre expression was always transmitted from the father to avoid a premature potential impact of an impaired Progesterone-DC-crosstalk.

Isolation of $CD11c^+$ and $CD11^{neg}$ Cells

In order to confirm the selective KO of the PR on CD11c dendritic cells, the spleen was harvested from WT, $PR^{neg}CD11c$, and $PR^{flox/wt}$ $CD11c^{cre/wt}$ mice. Single cell suspensions were obtained as described previously (12). In brief: the tissue was mashed with the plunger of a sterile disposable syringe in circles through a 40 µm cell strainer (Falcon Cell Strainer 40 µm, BD Bioscience, VWR, Germany). The resulting cell suspension was centrifuged for 8 min with 450 × g at 4°C and the supernatant was discarded. Subsequently, a red cell blood (RBC) lysis was performed using RBC lysis buffer (eBioscience, San Diego, CA) according to the manufacturer's instruction. After centrifugation the cell pellet was resuspended in MACS-Buffer (1xPBS, 0.5% BSA. 2 mM EDTA). $CD11c^+$ cells were enriched by magnetic cell separation using the CD11c MicroBeads UltraPure mouse kit (MACS®, Miltenyi Biotec, Bergisch-Gladbach, Germany) according to the manufacturer's instruction. Finally, fluorescence-activated cell sorting of $CD11c^+$ and $CD11^{neg}$ cells was performed to achieve highest purity.

DNA Isolation and Polymerase Chain Reaction (PCR)

DNA was isolated from mouse tail and $CD11c^+$ and $CD11^{neg}$ cells obtained from WT, $PR^{neg}CD11c$ and $PR^{flox/wt}$ $CD11c^{cre/wt}$ mice using the DNeasy Kit (Qiagen) according to the manufacturer's protocol.

PCR analysis was performed as 3-Primer-PCR in 50 µl reactions using the Mastercycler® nexus GX2 (Eppendorf). Primer sequences used were previously published (13) and ordered from TIB Molbiol. The PCR program consisted of initial 94°C for 10 min followed by 30 cycles: 94°C for 1 min, 55°C for 1 min, and 72°C for 2 min. Amplicons were visualized using Agarose gel electrophoresis. Expected band sizes were 226bp for the wildtype allele, 260 bp for the floxed allele and 381 bp for the KO allele.

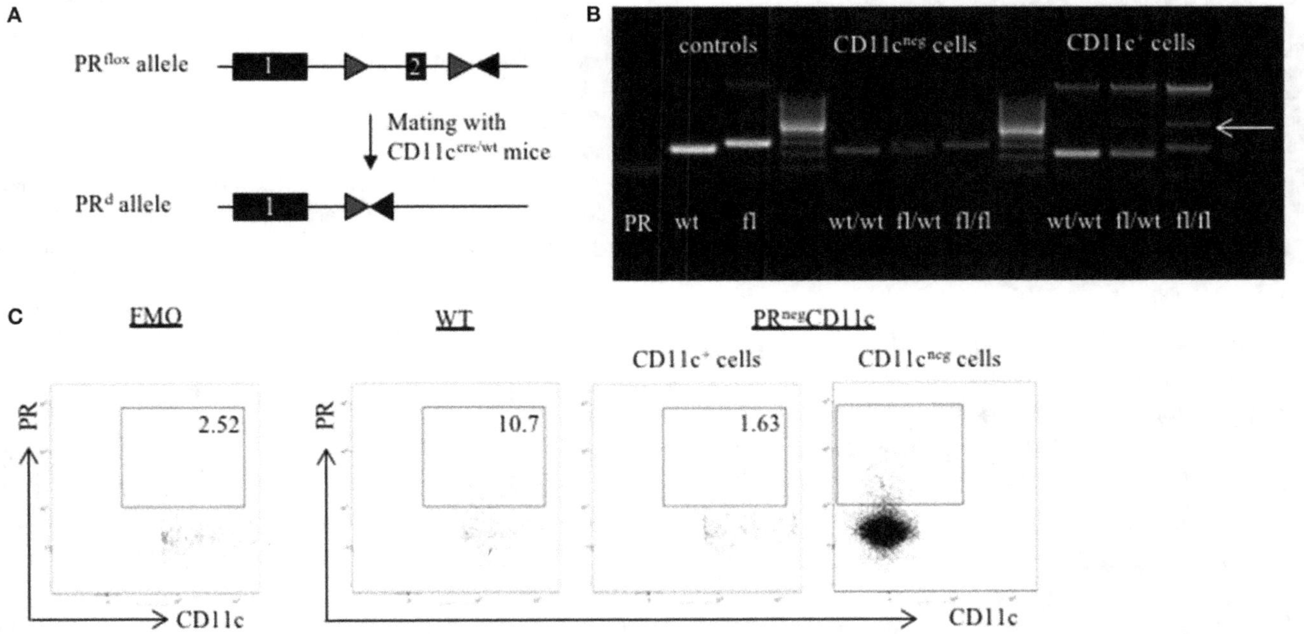

FIGURE 1 | Generation of a selective knockout (KO) of the progesterone receptor (PR) on CD11c dendritic cells (DCs): **(A)** $PR^{flox/flox}$ mice were crossed with $CD11c^{cre/wt}$ transgenic mice resulting in recombination of the PRflox allele to a PR null allele (PRd) on $CD11c^{+}$ cells. **(B)** The selective KO of the PR on $CD11c^{+}$ cells was confirmed on DNA level. PCR amplicons were visualized using agarose gel electrophoresis and band sizes were 226 bp for the wildtype allele, 260 bp for the floxed allele, and 381 bp for the KO allele, respectively. **(C)** The selective KO of the PR on $CD11c^{+}$ DCs harvested from WT and $PR^{neg}CD11c$ mice was confirmed on protein level by means of flow cytometry. The first dot plot on the left side is a fluorescence minus one (FMO) control for the PR antibody.

Timed Pregnancies

Eight to ten weeks old $PR^{flox/flox}CD11c^{cre/wt}$ female mice with a C57Bl/6 background were mated to Balb/c male mice. Aged-matched Balb/c-mated $PR^{wt/wt}CD11c^{cre/wt}$ females served as controls in order to control for unwanted side effects due to the expression of the cre. For simplicity we will refer to $PR^{flox/flox}CD11c^{cre/wt}$ mice as $PR^{neg}CD11c$ and to $PR^{wt/wt}CD11c^{cre/wt}$ control mice as WT.

The presence of a vaginal plug in the morning was considered as gestation day (gd) 0.5. Maternal weight control on gd 8.5 and 10.5 was conducted to confirm pregnancy. Animals were kept under 12 h light/ dark cycles and received food and water *ad libitum*. All experiments were performed in accordance with the animal ethics approval given by the State Authority of Hamburg (ORG_763).

Tissue Harvesting

On gd 13.5 and 18.5, mice were anesthetized by carbon dioxide ventilation, a blood sample was collected by retro bulbar puncture and subsequently mice were sacrificed by cervical dislocation. The abdomen was opened and the uterus-draining lymph node was harvested and kept in PBS on ice. The uterus was removed and stored in HBSS on ice immediately after the fetuses were isolated from the amniotic membranes to determine fetal weight. Placentas were either stored at −20°C in RNAlater (Ambion by Life Technologies GmbH) or embedded in biopsy cassettes and stored in 4% Formaldehyde solution (36.5–38%, Sigma-Aldrich, St, Louis, US) for 24 h before transfer into 1% Formaldehyde solution for long-term storage. Maternal ovaries were also preserved in RNAlater.

Pregnancy Outcome

Number of implantations and abortions was assessed per pregnant female. The abortion rate refers to the number of fetuses resorbed per litter using the following equation: (number of abortions/number of implantations) * 100.

Tissue Processing

Single cell suspensions of maternal lymph nodes and uteri were obtained as described before (14). In brief, maternal lymph nodes were passed through a cell strainer and after centrifugation at 450 g for 8 min at 4°C, the cell pellet was resuspended in PBS. The uterus was enzymatically digested using 200 U/mL hyaluronidase (Sigma-Aldrich), 1 mg/mL collagenase VIII type (Sigma-Aldrich), and 1 mg/mL bovine serum albumin fraction V (Sigma-Aldrich) dissolved in 5 mL HBSS. Subsequently, the uterus was incubated twice for 20 min in a 37°C water bath with agitation. Intermediately, the solution was recovered and filtered through a mesh. The solution was centrifuged at 450 × g for 10 min at 4°C and resuspended PBS.

Number of viable leukocytes in both tissues was obtained by counting the cells using a Neubauer chamber upon adding Trypan Blue stain (0.4 %, Life Technologies GmbH, Darmstadt, Germany).

TABLE 1 | Summary of antibodies used in the present study.

Target antigen	Fluorochrome	Clone	Dilution	Source
anti-CD45	Allophycocyanin (APC)-Cyanine (Cy)7	30-F11	1:400	BD
anti-CD3	R-phycoerythrin (PE) Cy7	145-2C11	1:200	Biolegend
anti-CD8	Brilliant Violet (BV) 650	53-6.7	1:100	Biolegend
anti-CD4	Pacific Blue	RM4-5	1:400	Biolegend
anti-FoxP3	PE	FJK-16s	1:200	eBioscience
anti-CD122	PerCP eFluor 710	TM-b1	1:100	eBioscience
F4/80	BV421	BM8	1:100	Biolegend
anti-CD11c	BV785	N418	1:100	Biolegend
MHCII	APC	M5/144.15.2	1:200	BD
anti-CD80	BV605	16-10A1	1:100	Biolegend
anti-CD86	BV605	GL-1	1:100	Biolegend

Flow Cytometry

For flow cytometric analyses, 1.0×10^6 maternal lymph node and uterus cells were used. Non-specific binding was blocked by rat anti-mouse CD16/CD32 Mouse Fragment crystallizable (Fc) Block (1:200, BD Bioscience) and Normal Rat Serum (1:100, eBioscience) for 15 min at 4°C. Subsequently, the cells were incubated with the respective antibodies for 30 min for surface and intracellular stainings. Antibodies used in this study are displayed in **Table 1**. In case of solely surface staining, 7-amino-actinomycin D (7AAD, 1:400, Biolegend) was used to identify dead cells. For intracellular staining, cells were fixed and permeabilized using Foxp3 Fixation/Permeabilization Concentrate and Diluent (eBioscience). Dead/live staining was performed with eFluor 506 viability dye (eBioscience).

In order to quantify the expression of the PR by flow cytometry, cells were stained with the respective surface markers and subsequently permeabilized with Cytofix/Cytoperm (eBioscience) according to the manufacturer's instructions. Afterwards, cells were blocked with mouse serum preventing non-specific binding of antibodies to intracellular proteins and then incubated with Progesterone Receptor Monoclonal Antibody (R.809.9, Invitrogen) for 30 min. A FITC-conjugated secondary antibody (1:200) was added for additional 20 min.

Flow cytometric data were acquired using a BD LSRFortessa II (BD Biosciences) and analyzed using FlowJo (Tree Star, Ashland, OR, USA).

Placenta Histology

Placentas harvested on gd 13.5 and 18.5 were embedded in paraffin. Subsequently, 4 μm thick histological sections were prepared at the mid-sagittal plane using a microtome (SM2010R, Leica, Bensheim, Germany). Slides were dewaxed and rehydrated using xylene and ethanol. Masson-Goldner trichrome staining was performed following standard protocol (15). Subsequently slides were also scanned with a Mirax Midi Slide Scanner. Histomorphological analyses of placental areas were performed by two independent observers using Pannoramic Viewer (3DHistech Kft. Budapest, Hungary).

Progesterone Analysis

Maternal blood samples were centrifuged at 10,000 g for 20 min at 4°C and the supernatant plasma was immediately frozen at −20°C. For progesterone analysis, plasma samples were diluted 1:200 using ELISA Buffer and measured with a competitive immunoassay (Progesterone ELISA Kit, Cayman Chemical, Michigan, USA) on a NanoQuant (Tecan Group AG, Männedorf, Switzerland) according to manufacturer's instructions.

Theiler Scoring of Fetuses on gd13.5

Fetal development of mouse embryos was evaluated by observation of Bouin-fixed fetuses under a Zeiss Stemi 2000-C stereomicroscope according to Theiler's description (16). Main criteria to differentiate the developmental stages at gd 13.5 have been the formation of the pinna, fingers and feet, and the presence or absence of 5 rows of whiskers.

RNA Isolation and cDNA Synthesis

Following tissue harvesting, half of the placentas were preserved in RNAlater at −20°C. Tissue homogenization was carried out using micro packaging vials with ceramic beads (1.4 mm) in a Precellys® 24 Tissue Homogenizer (Peqlab). RNA isolation and DNA digestion were conducted by use of RNeasy Plus Universal Mini Kit (QIAGEN) and DNA-free Kit (Applied Biosystems by Thermo Fisher), respectively. cDNA synthesis was performed with random primers (Invitrogen by Thermo Fisher). Concentration and purity of RNA and cDNA were assessed employing NanoQuant (Tecan).

Quantitative Real-Time Polymerase Chain Reaction (qRT-PCR)

Gene expression analyses of ovarian tissue was performed using gene expression assays (Applied Biosystems by Thermo Fisher) for steroidogenic acute regulatory protein (Star, Mm00441558_m1), 3β-hydroxysteroid dehydrogenase (Hsd3b1, Mm01261921_mH), and 20αHSD (Akr1c18, Mm00506289_m1). Beta-actin (Actb) and ubiquitin C (Ubc) served as endogenous control to normalize cDNA content. Gene expression analyses of placental tissue were carried out using gene expression assays (Applied Biosystems by Thermo Fisher) for the following targets: insulin like growth factor 1 (Igf1, Mm00439560_m1), hydroxysteroid 11-beta dehydrogenase (Hsd11b) 1 and 2 (Mm00476182_m1 and Mm01251104_m1), placental growth factor (Plgf, Mm00435613_m1), epidermal growth factor (Egf, Mm00438696_m1), vascular endothelial growth factor A (Vegf, Mm00437306_m1), B cell leukemia/lymphoma 2 (Bcl2, Mm00477631_m1) and soluble FMS-like tyrosine kinase 1 (sFlt1, Mm00438980_m1), heme oxygenase 1 (Hmox1, Mm00516005_m1), galectin-1 (Gal-1, Mm00839408_g1), and placental lactogen II (Prl3b1, Mm00435852_m1). RNA polymerase II subunit A (Polr2a, Mm00839502_m1) and ubiquitin C (Ubc, Mm02525934_g1) served as endogenous controls (17). All reactions were performed in 50 cycles using a standard two-step RT-PCR: initial 50°C for 2 min and 95°C for 10 min, 15 s denaturation at 95°C and 60 s annealing and extension at 60°C with the NanoQuant5 Real-Time PCR System (Applied Biosystems) and the corresponding software. The fold change of PR^{neg}CD11c over WT control expression was calculated employing the $\Delta\Delta$Ct method (18).

Statistical Analysis

Statistical analysis was performed using GraphPad Prism version 7.0 (GraphPad Software, La Jolla, CA, USA). All results are expressed as means ± standard error of the mean (SEM). Means between groups were compared using unpaired *t*-test. Welch's *t*-test was used in case of unequal standard deviation and unequal sample sizes between groups (19).

RESULTS

Confirmation of the Selective Knockout of the PR on CD11c$^+$ DCs

In order to confirm the selective knockout of the PR on CD11c$^+$ DCs on a DNA level, we performed genotyping of tail biopsies and CD11c$^+$ and CD11^{neg} cells of WT, $PR^{flox/wt}CD11c^{cre/wt}$ and PR^{neg}CD11c mice, respectively. The agarose gel shows the amplicons of tail biopsies from WT mice at the expected band size of 226 bp and from PR^{neg}CD11c at 260 bp. PCR of sorted CD11c^{neg} spleen cells from the respective genotypes resulted also in a 226 bp amplicon for WT and in a 260 bp amplicon for PR^{neg}CD11c while cells from heterozygote mice showed both bands. Equally, PCR of sorted CD11c$^+$ spleen cells from WT mice resulted in a 226 pb amplicon. CD11c$^+$ spleen cells from $PR^{flox/wt}CD11c^{cre/wt}$ and PR^{neg}CD11c animals exhibit a band of 381 bp for the KO allele (**Figure 1B**). In order to confirm this selective KO also on the protein level, we used a monoclonal antibody against the PR for detection by flow cytometry. CD11c$^+$ cells harvested from PR^{neg}CD11c mice showed a lower frequency of the PR on DC compared to cells isolated from WT mice (**Figure 1C**). A positive PR expression could be confirmed on CD11c^{neg} cells from PR^{neg}CD11c mice. However, as we also detected CD11c^{pos} PR^{pos} cells at low frequencies among cells isolated from PR^{neg}CD11c mice, unspecific binding of the secondary antibody must be assumed. Alternatively, the cre recombinase may not exhibit 100% efficiency.

Impaired Progesterone-Responsiveness of CD11c$^+$ DCs Affects Fetal Growth

Pregnancy rate did not significantly differ between WT and PRnegCD11c female mice (**Figure 2A**). Pregnancy outcome was assessed on gd 13.5 as well as 18.5. We could not identify any modification with regards to number of implantations (**Figures 2B,E**) and abortion rate (**Figures 2C,F**) in litters from WT and PR^{neg}CD11c females. However, we observed a significantly reduced fetal weight on gestational day 13.5 and 18.5 in litters of PR^{neg}CD11c females (**Figures 2D,G**) along with a minor tendency toward a decreased placental weight on gd 18.5 (**Figure 2H**). We did not observe sex-specific effects, as a similar fetal weight could be observed in male and female offspring (**Figure 2J**). Further, the chosen mating combination yields to two fetal genotypes: $PR^{flox/wt}CD11c^{cre/wt}$ and $PR^{flox/wt}CD11c^{wt/wt}$. In order to exclude an impact of the fetal expression of the cre recombinase on the fetal weight, we assessed the fetal genotype from 2 litters and could exclude that the fetal genotype caused alterations of the fetal weight (**Figure 2K**). Using Theiler staging as a criterion to assess fetal development, we observed only a minor delay in fetuses from PR^{neg}CD11c mother (**Figure 2L**). A representative photographic image of fetuses from WT and PR^{neg}CD11c mice in shown in **Figure 2M**.

Impaired Progesterone-Responsiveness of CD11c$^+$ DCs Affects Maternal Immune Adaptation

Flow cytometry analysis from the uterus of gd 13.5 revealed similar frequencies of uterine CD11c$^+$ cells in both groups (**Figure 3A**). While the co-expression of MHCII was not different between groups (data not shown), we observed increased frequencies of DCs expression co-stimulatory molecules CD80 or CD86 in PR^{neg}CD11c mice (**Figure 3B**). Further, we identified reduced frequencies of CD4$^+$ FoxP3$^+$ and CD8$^+$ CD122$^+$ regulatory T (Treg) cells in uteri of PR^{neg}CD11c dams (**Figures 3C,D**). Representative dot plots are shown in **Figures 3E–G**. We made similar observations of unaltered CD11c frequencies and increased co-expression of CD80 and CD86 in cells isolated from uterus-draining lymph nodes (**Figures 3H,J**), whereas no significant differences were detectable for CD4$^+$ FoxP3$^+$ Treg cell frequencies (**Figure 3K**) and CD8$^+$ CD122$^+$ Treg cells (**Figure 3L**) between WT and PR^{neg}CD11c dams.

Placental Histomorphology and Plasma Progesterone Levels Was Modulated on gd 13.5

Placenta morphology was assessed on gd 13.5 and 18.5 by Masson-Goldner trichrome staining on mid-sagittal sections. The overall placental surface area did not differ between groups (**Figures 4A,E**). However, a skew toward an increased junctional zone at the expense of the labyrinth could be detected in PR^{neg}CD11c females compared to WT females on gd 13.5 (**Figures 4B,C**), which resulted in a significantly decreased placental ratio (labyrinth/junctional zone, **Figure 4D**), a proxy for placental function (20). The same observation could be made when analyzing the placentas from gd 18.5, but it did not reach statistical significance (**Figures 4F–H**). Representative photomicrographs from gd 13.5 and 18.5 placentas are shown in **Figure 4J**.

We also determined plasma progesterone concentrations and observed a significant increase in PR^{neg}CD11c mice compared to WT controls on gd 13.5 (**Figure 5A**). Subsequent qPCR analysis of maternal ovaries on gd 13.5 revealed no differences in gene expression of the ovarian steroidogenic acute regulatory protein (Star) (**Figure 5B**) and 3β-hydroxysteroid dehydrogenase (Hsd3b1), which converts pregnenolone to progesterone (**Figure 5C**). Progesterone metabolism was also not modulated in the KO line, suggested by the low, unaltered

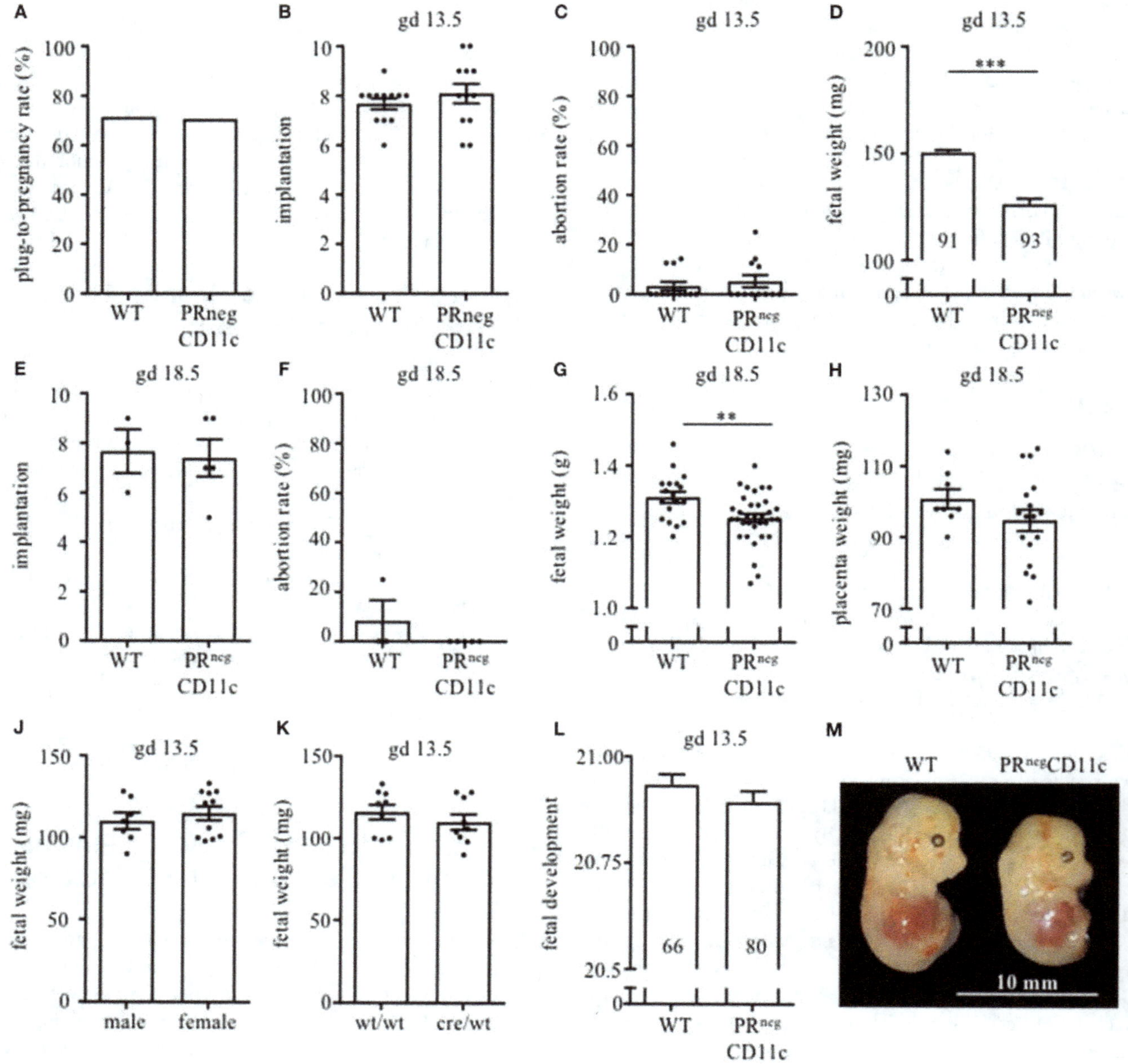

FIGURE 2 | Impaired progesterone-responsiveness of CD11c$^+$ dendritic cells affects fetal growth: WT and PR^{neg}CD11c female mice were allogenically mated to Balb/c males and pregnancy outcome was assessed, maternal phenotype is always indicated below: **(A)** Plug-to-pregnancy rate. On gestational day (gd) 13.5, we assessed number implantation **(B)**, abortion rate **(C)** and fetal weight **(D)**. For gd 18.5, number implantation **(E)**, abortion rate **(F)**, fetal weight **(G),** and placental weight **(H)** were determined. Fetal weight of fetuses from PR^{neg}CD11c dams is further shown dependent on fetal sex **(J)** and fetal genotype **(K)**. **(L)** Fetal development was scored on gd13.5 according to Theiler criteria and a representative picture from gd 13.5 fetuses of WT (left) and PR^{neg}CD11c (right) mice is shown in **(M)**, white line in the picture denote 10 mm. Data are represented as mean ± SEM. $^{***}p \le 0.001$, $^{**}p \le 0.01$.

ovarian expression of 20α-hydroxysteroid dehydrogenase (Akr1c18) (**Figure 5D**).

We also analyzed the differential expression of placental genes that has been linked to the pathogenesis of IUGR (**Figure 5E**) and could demonstrate that placental growth factor (Plgf) was significantly increased in placentas from PR^{neg}CD11c mothers. In contrast, significantly decreased placental expression was observed for epidermal growth factor (Egf), vascular endothelial growth factor A (Vegfa) and insulin like growth factor 1 (Igf1). In addition, hydroxysteroid 11-beta dehydrogenase 2 (Hsd11b2) and placental lactogen II (Prl3b1) showed a trend toward reduced expression in PR^{neg}CD11c placentas, but did not reach levels of significance. B cell leukemia/lymphoma 2 (Bcl-2), soluble FMS-like tyrosine kinase 1 (sFlt1), heme oxygenase 1 (Hmox), and galectin-1 (Gal-1) were not affected by the selective KO of the PR.

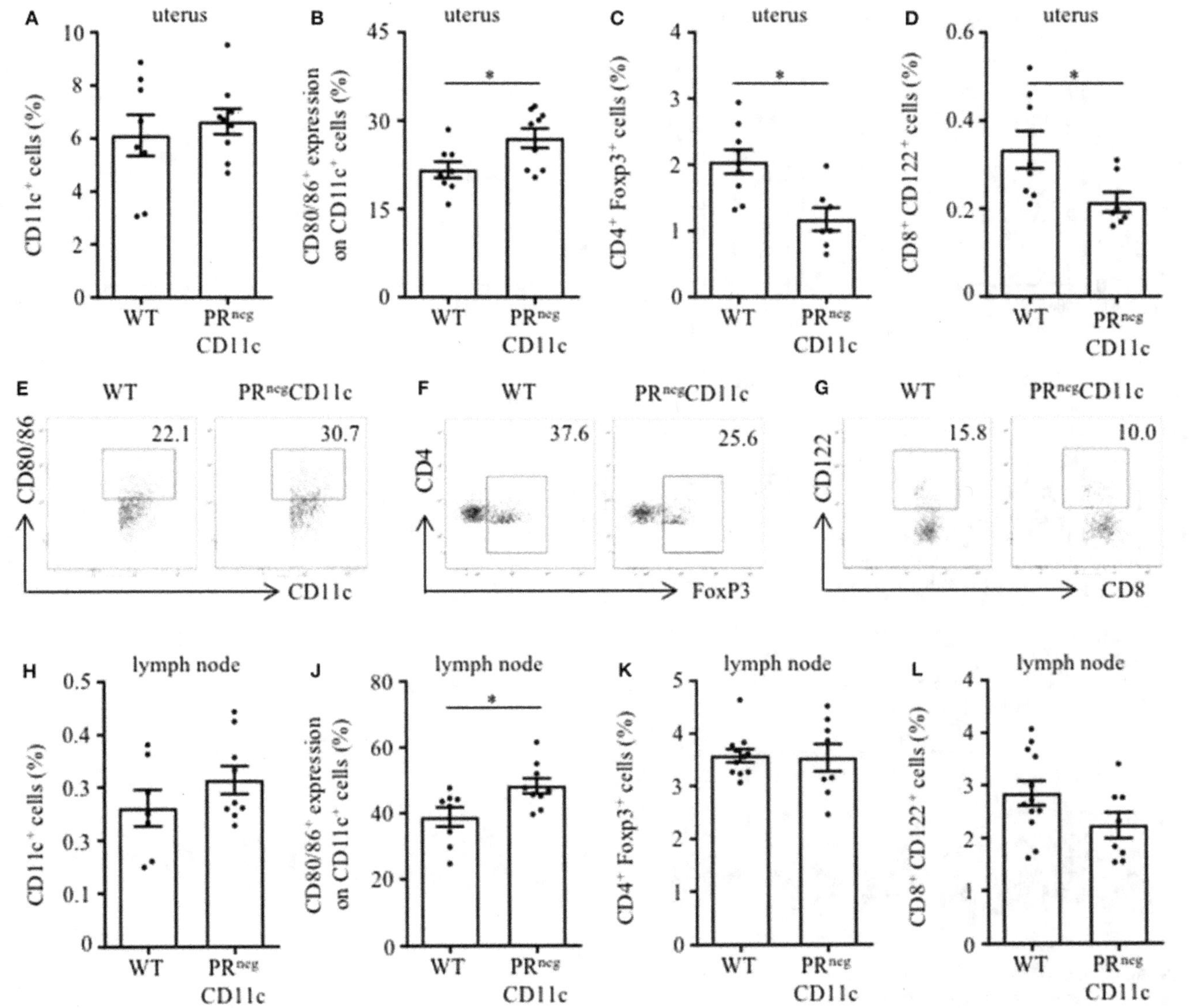

FIGURE 3 | Impaired progesterone-responsiveness of CD11c$^+$ dendritic cells (DCs) affects maternal immune adaptation: WT and PR^{neg}CD11c female mice were allogenically mated and flow cytometric analysis was performed on gestation day 13.5. Graphs present the frequencies of **(A)** CD11c$^+$ DCs, **(B)** the co-expression of CD80 and CD86, **(C)** CD4$^+$FoxP3$^+$ Treg cells, and **(D)** CD8$^+$CD122$^+$ T cells in uteri harvested from WT and PR^{neg}CD11c dams. Representative dot plots display CD80/86 expression on CD11c$^+$ cells **(E)**, FoxP3$^+$ expression on CD4$^+$ cells **(F)**, and CD122$^+$ expression in CD8$^+$ T cells **(G)** of WT and PR^{neg}CD11c mice. Respective cell frequencies in the right corner are expressed as percentage of CD11c$^+$, CD4$^+$ and CD8$^+$ cells, respectively. **(H–L)** Flow cytometric analysis of CD11c$^+$ DCs **(H)**, the co-expression of CD80 and CD86 **(J)**, CD4$^+$FoxP3$^+$ Treg cells **(K)**, and CD8$^+$CD122$^+$ T cells **(L)** in uterus-draining lymph node harvested from WT and PR^{neg}CD11c dams. Bars represent mean ± SEM. *$p \leq 0.05$, unless otherwise stated, cell frequencies are expressed as percentage of living CD45$^+$ cells.

DISCUSSION

The steroid hormone progesterone is known to be indispensable for successful reproduction, as demonstrated in mice carrying a null mutation of the PR gene (PR-KO mice) (21). Here, male mice do not show any abnormalities, but female mice display significant functional defects in all reproductive tissues, including the inability to ovulate, uterine hyperplasia and inflammation and severely limited mammary gland development (21).

Due to the complexity of endocrine-immune cross talk particularly in the context of steroid actions, the generation of a mouse model enabling conditional excision of PR function (PRflox mice) in a cell- or tissue-specific manner provides a useful tool to study progesterone-dependent pathways and processes (13). Using such approach in the present study, we observed that mice devoid of PR on DCs do not exhibit major reproductive abnormalities, such as an altered plug-to-pregnancy rate or increased fetal loss rate. However, the offspring of such PR^{neg}CD11c dams were severely affected by IUGR, as fetal weight was ~15% lower compared to WT dams on gd 13.5. This result was not compromised by possible alterations of the viable litter size, by fetal sex or fetal genotype as such effects were not

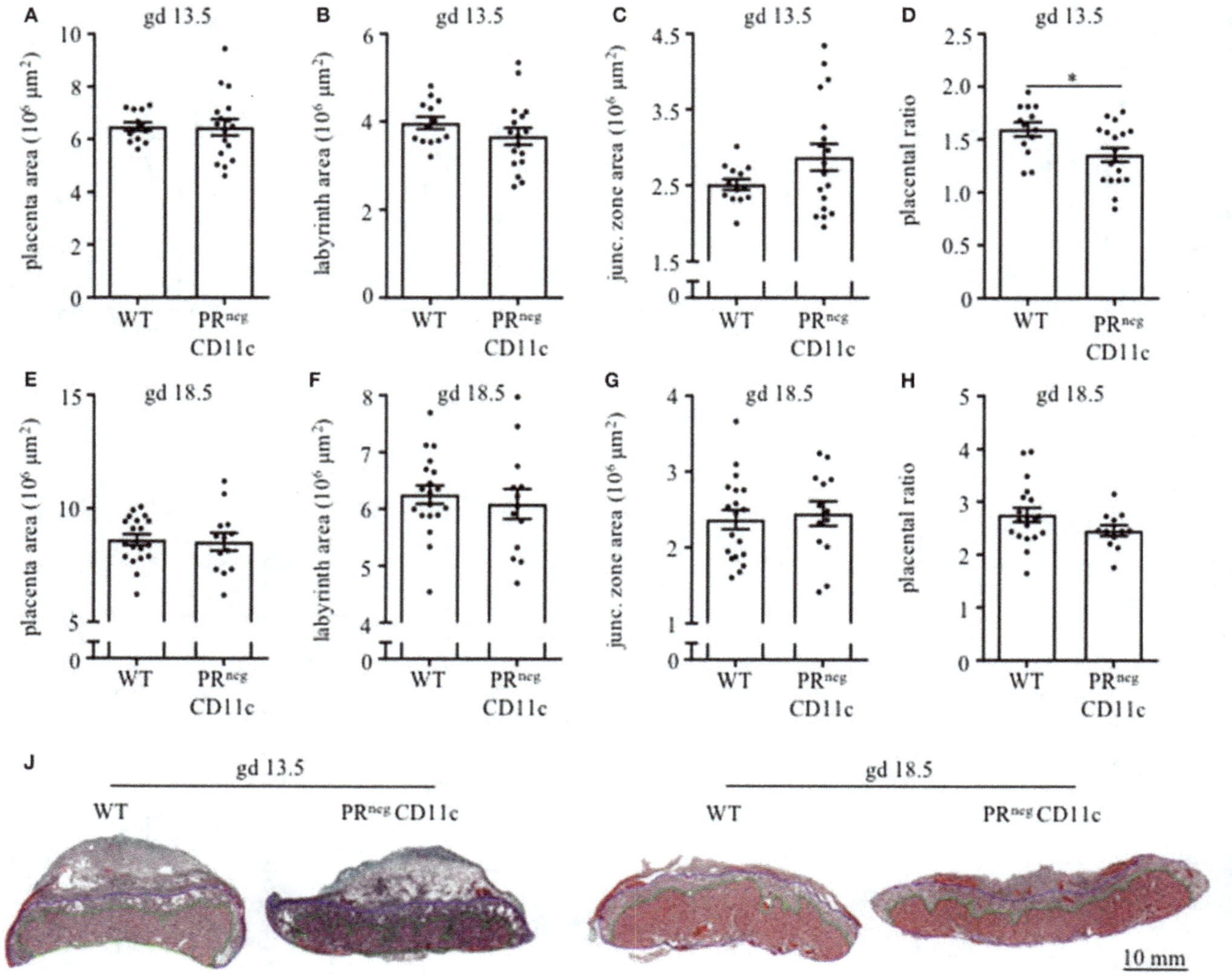

FIGURE 4 | Impaired progesterone-responsiveness of CD11c$^+$ dendritic cells affects placental morphology: WT and PR^{neg}CD11c female mice were allogenically mated and placentas harvested on gestation day (gd) 13.5 und 18.5 were evaluated by Masson-Goldner trichrome staining allowing the differentiation of the labyrinth and junctional zone. **(A,E)** show total placenta area on gd 13.5 and 18.5, respectively. Area of the labyrinth **(B,F)** and the junctional zone **(C,G)** have been assessed and the placental ratio **(D,H)** was calculated. **(J)** Representative photomicrographs illustrating mid-sagittal sections of gd 13.5 and 18.5 placental tissue from WT (left) and PR^{neg}CD11c (right) mothers, black line in the picture denotes 10 mm, green lines encircle the labyrinth, blue lines surround the junctional zone. Data are represented as mean ± SEM. *$p \leq 0.05$.

detectable between the groups and could therefore be excluded as potential confounder. A graphical summary of the main finding is presented in **Figure 6**.

Our data further provide strong evidence that progesterone is directly involved in arresting DCs in a tolerogenic phenotype, mirrored by the increased expression of the co-stimulatory molecules CD80/CD86 in mice where the PR is lacking on DCs. This sheds new light on the recent recognition that progesterone promotes tolerance of the adaptive immune system during gestation via glucocorticoid receptor-dependent pathways (22) and suggests that progesterone modulates innate immune response during gestation through the PR by inducing a tolerogenic phenotype in DCs. However, the extrapolation of cellular functions solely based on the expression of cell surface markers is limited. Thus, the presumed tolerogenic function of DCs during pregnancy—or lack thereof in the absence of the PR—requires confirmation upon functional in-depth characterization in future experiments.

Such tDC may then account for the generation of CD4$^+$ Treg cells, which has been suggested by published data (7–9, 23, 24). Our data support that progesterone considerably induces the generation of CD4$^+$ Treg cells via DC-dependent pathways rather than direct effects on CD4$^+$ T cells. However, in order to prove this causality, it will be necessary to perform adoptive transfer experiments demonstrating that replenishing Tregs in mice devoid of the PR on CD11c cells will prevent the development of the observed IUGR. Similarly, we provide evidence that the generation of a newly identified CD8$^+$

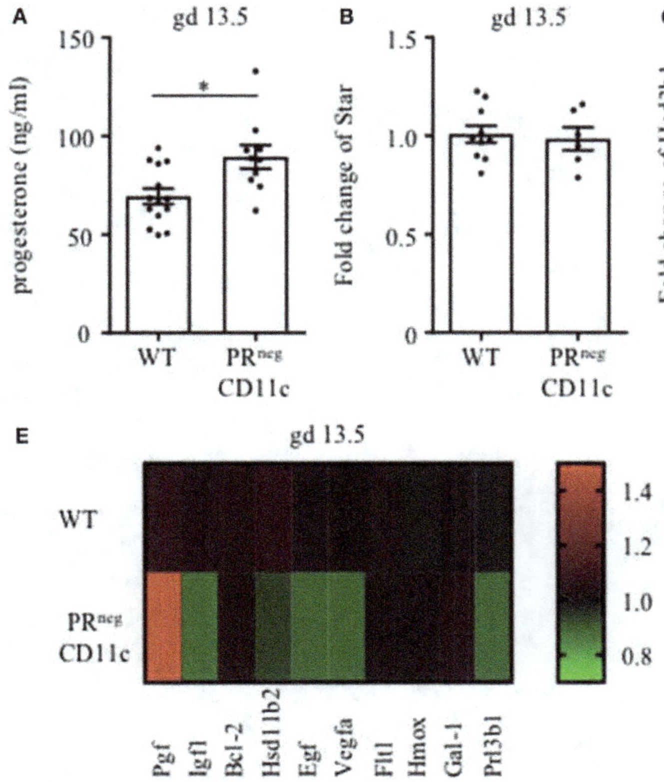

FIGURE 5 | Selective knockout of the progesterone receptor (PR) on CD11c^{+} dendritic cells affects gene expression analysis of ovarian and placental tissue: **(A)** Plasma progesterone levels of WT and PR^{neg}CD11c female mice on gd 13.5 as analyzed by ELISA. **(B–D)** Ovarian expression of steroidogenic acute regulatory protein (Star), 3β-hydroxysteroid dehydrogenase (Hsd3b1), and 20αHSD (Akr1c18) was assessed by qPCR from tissue harvested on gd 13.5. The fold change over WT control expression was calculated using beta-actin (Actb) and ubiquitin C (Ubc) as endogenous control and employing the ΔΔCt method. **(E)** Heatmap summarizing the placental expression of placental growth factor (Plgf), insulin like growth factor 1 (Igf1), B cell leukemia/lymphoma 2 (Bcl2), hydroxysteroid 11-beta dehydrogenase (Hsd11b2), epidermal growth factor (Egf), vascular endothelial growth factor A (Vegfa), soluble FMS-like tyrosine kinase 1 (sFlt1), heme oxygenase 1 (Hmox1), Galectin-1 (Gal-1), and placental lactogen II (Prl3b1) calculated by qPCR from gd 13.5 placentas. The fold change over WT control expression was calculated using RNA polymerase II subunit A (Polr2a) and Ubc as endogenous control and employing the ΔΔCt method. Bars represent mean ± SEM. $^{*}p \leq 0.05$.

CD122^{+} Treg cell subset involved in promoting fetal growth (15) is also critically dependent on the possibility of DCs to respond to progesterone. It has been suggested that progesterone upregulates placental Hmoxl expression, hereby promoting the generation of CD8^{+} CD122^{+} T cells. However, since placental expression of Hmoxl was not altered in mice lacking the PR on DCs, we propose that placental Hmoxl as well as tDCs may independently promote the generation of CD8^{+} CD122^{+} T cells.

As CD11c cells are involved in a variety of functions, e.g., thymic T cell development, one might suspect that the missing PR on CD11c cells may have an impact on the adaptive immune response even outside the context of pregnancy, but progesterone levels are rather low in pre-adolescent female mice and also during the menstrual cycle. Further, reduced CD4^{+} Treg frequencies were exclusively observed locally in the uterus of PRnegCD11c mice, whereas CD4^{+} Treg frequencies in secondary lymphoid organs or peripherally were unaffected. Hence, an effect of the missing PR on CD11c cells on the adaptive immune system in a non-pregnant state can largely be excluded.

We could pinpoint the cause for IUGR to the lack of the PR on DCs in the mother rather than the fetal genotype, as modulation was not dependent on the fetal genotype and only affected by the maternal PR expression on DCs. Modulation of fetal weight loss can result from placental insufficiency, a known contributor to IUGR (25). We could confirm such effect, as poor placental development was present in litters of PR^{neg}CD11c dams. Whilst placental size and weight was unaffected by the maternal genotype, the junctional zone was increased at the expense of the labyrinth at implantation sites of PR^{neg}CD11c dams. Such skew of placental functional areas might impair fetal supply with nutrients and oxygen (26).

Normally, impaired fetal growth and poor placentation is accompanied by reduced progesterone levels, as seen in response to prenatal challenges (14, 15). Hence, we were rather intrigued by the high progesterone levels in PR^{neg}CD11c dams. This overproduction of progesterone, which appears to be an attempt to compensate for its failure to interact with DC, may lead to other placental modifications contributing to the development of IUGR, such as placental vasculogenesis and angiogenesis. Both are modulated by endothelium-specific molecules such as PlGF and VEGF (27, 28) which compete for the same cell surface tyrosine kinase receptors, VEGFR-1/Flt-1, but

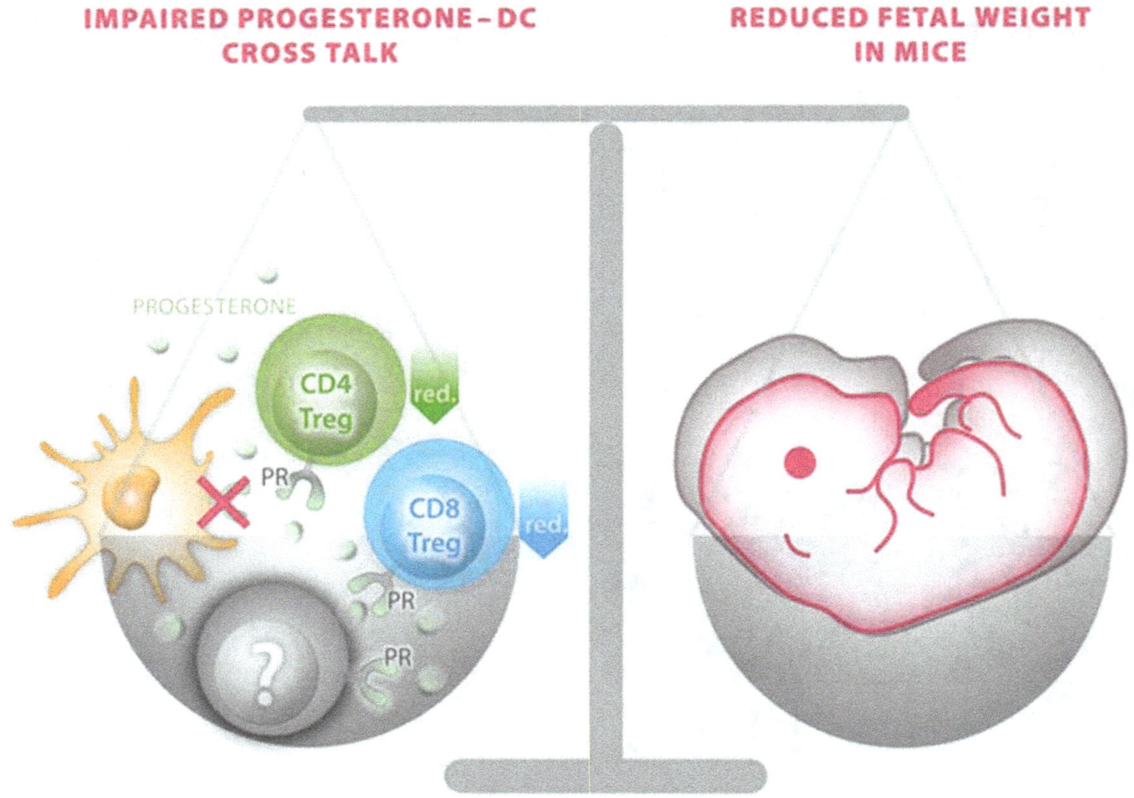

FIGURE 6 | Graphical scenario depicting the impact of the selective knockout of the progesterone receptor on CD11c$^+$ dendritic cells (DCs) and its consequences for fetal growth. An impaired progesterone-DC cross talk disturbs the fine-tuned balance of a functional immune response of DCs to progesterone by affecting CD4 and CD8 Treg populations (and potentially also on yet to be identified immune cells marked in gray) on one site and fetal outcome on the other side.

differentially induce angiogenesis; VEGF controls branching of blood vessels, while PlGF promotes a low resistance vascular network during mid- to late pregnancy (28). However, both factors are sensitive for changes in the microenvironment. As progesterone release is reduced in hypoxic condition (29), it could be speculated that high progesterone favors a hyperoxic environment. In this case, placental PlGF is increased while VEGF is decreased (30), similar to the gene expression we observed in our study. Consequently, superfluous progesterone could result in the decreased vascular branching, along with an increase in fetoplacental flow impedance via differential modulation of PlGF and VEGF (31). Moreover, the decrease of VEGF we observed in dams lacking the PR on DCs is even more striking as the competition for the same receptor should normally increase the quantity of VEGF then acting via the VEGFR-2 which is a major mediator of angiogenic responses (32). On the other hand, there are many studies postulating a decrease of PlGF in IUGR placenta (33–35). Hence, one might speculate that Plgf expression is not dependent on a functional PR-DC crosstalk and the observed over-expression is initiated to support placentation and angiogenesis. An altered placental gene expression in IUGR was reported for EGF (36), which we could also observe in placentas from PR^{neg}CD11c females. Hence, EGF may be a target that requires a communication between progesterone and DCs and a lack of this communication impairs placental vascularization and consequently fetal nourishment. Additionally, IGF1 is known to facilitate the transport of glucose and amino acids across the placenta to the fetus and placental expression is reduced in IUGR and SGA fetuses associated with DNA methylation alterations (37). Our results support that the reduced placental Igf-1 expression observed in PR^{neg}CD11c dams contribute to development of IUGR (38, 39). Taken together, these qPCR results pinpoint the need to characterize the mechanisms underlying placental vascularization in PR^{neg}CD11c mice in future studies.

One limitation of the mouse model we here describe is that we chose CD11c-cre mice to target gene expression in DC (40). Although CD11c is widely accepted as a pan marker for conventional DCs (cDCs), CD11c is also expressed on macrophages and monocytes (41), plasmacytoid DCs and marginally on some lymphocyte subsets (42). Therefore, the CD11c cell specific deletion of the PR we here describe is not fully DC specific. A better option may be the recently generated cDC-restricted cre mouse (zDCcre) using a zinc finger transcription factor, zDC (Zbtb46, Btbd4), which is not expressed by monocytes, pDCs, or other immune cell populations (43, 44). These zDCcre mice could be used in future investigation to knock out the PR in cDCs in order to verify and compare to the present results. Nevertheless, as the large majority of $CD11c^+$ cells are cDCs, our results provide strong evidence of a critical crosstalk between progesterone and DCs to ensure reproductive success.

Further, the cre-lox system itself shows certain limitations, such as the efficiency of target gene deletion, cre-mediated toxicity and undesired deletions (45). In order to avoid the two latter confounding factors, we used $PR^{wt/wt}CD11c^{cre/wt}$ mice as controls. Even if the CD11c-cre exhibits unwanted side effects, we can exclude an impact on our result, as both groups share the same potential cre-mediated toxicity burden. Upon detection of the PR gene on DNA and protein level, we observe an incomplete gene deletion on DCs. This may result from cell contamination during MACS and sorting, unspecific binding of the secondary antibody, but also be due to a minor deficiency of PR gene target deletion on $CD11c^+$ cells. Although PR deletion might be incomplete, this mouse model has proven to be a suitable tool to investigate progesterone-dependent pathways in DCs.

In summary, we utilized the Cre-Lox recombination to successfully generate a DC-specific knockout of the PR in mice. We could demonstrate that a progesterone-responsiveness of dendritic cells is critical for fetal growth and facilitates the generation of pregnancy-protective $CD4^+$ and $CD8^+$ Tregs and adequate placentation. An association between diseases of insufficient placentation and the maturity of DCs have also been demonstrated in human placenta (46). In addition, human pregnancies complicated by IUGR were shown to exhibit peripheral blood DCs with an altered state of activation (47). These findings highlight the importance that an in-depth understanding of modulators that yield to such DC alterations must be gained, as addressed in the present manuscript.

AUTHOR CONTRIBUTIONS

KT and PA: conceptualization; KT, AH, JL, and MS: methodology; KT, AH, and JR: Investigation; KT, JL, and PA: resources; KT and PA: writing—original draft; All authors: comments on manuscript.

ACKNOWLEDGMENTS

We would like to thank JL, Francesco J. DeMayo and Manuel A. Friese for providing the $PR^{flox/flox}$ and $CD11c^{cre/wt}$ mice, respectively. We also thank Agnes Wieczorek, Christopher Urbschat, and Thomas Andreas (Department of Obstetrics and Fetal Medicine, University Medical Center Hamburg) for their technical assistance. The flow cytometers used in this study were provided by the FACS Core Unit of the University Medical Center Hamburg-Eppendorf.

REFERENCES

1. Romo A, Carceller R, Tobajas J. Intrauterine growth retardation (IUGR): epidemiology and etiology. *Pediatr Endocrinol Rev.* (2009) 6(Suppl. 3):332–6.
2. Sharma D, Shastri S, Sharma P. Intrauterine growth restriction: antenatal and postnatal aspects. *Clin Med Insights Pediatr.* (2016) 10:67–83. doi: 10.4137/CMPed.S40070
3. Guellec I, Lapillonne A, Renolleau S, Charlaluk M-L, Roze J-C, Marret S, et al. Neurologic outcomes at school age in very preterm infants born with severe or mild growth restriction. *Pediatrics* (2011) 127:e883 LP–91. doi: 10.1542/peds.2010-2442
4. Nepomnyaschy L, Reichman NE. Low birthweight and asthma among young urban children. *Am J Public Health* (2006) 96:1604–10. doi: 10.2105/AJPH.2005.079400
5. Longo S, Bollani L, Decembrino L, Di Comite A, Angelini M, Stronati M. Short-term and long-term sequelae in intrauterine growth retardation (IUGR). *J Matern Neonatal Med.* (2013) 26:222–5. doi: 10.3109/14767058.2012.715006
6. Menendez-Castro C, Rascher W, Hartner A. Intrauterine growth restriction - impact on cardiovascular diseases later in life. *Mol Cell Pediatr.* (2018) 5:4. doi: 10.1186/s40348-018-0082-5
7. Kämmerer U, Eggert AO, Kapp M, McLellan AD, Geijtenbeek TBH, Dietl J, et al. Unique appearance of proliferating antigen-presenting cells expressing DC-SIGN (CD209) in the decidua of early human pregnancy. *Am J Pathol.* (2003) 162:887–96. doi: 10.1016/S0002-9440(10)63884-9
8. Blois SM, Ilarregui JM, Tometten M, Garcia M, Orsal AS, Cordo-Russo R, et al. A pivotal role for galectin-1 in fetomaternal tolerance. *Nat Med.* (2007) 13:1450–7. doi: 10.1038/nm1680
9. Segerer SE. MIC-1 (a multifunctional modulator of dendritic cell phenotype and function) is produced by decidual stromal cells and trophoblasts. *Hum Reprod.* (2012) 27:200–9. doi: 10.1093/humrep/der358
10. Blois SM, Kammerer U, Soto CA, Tometten MC, Shaikly V, Barrientos G, et al. Dendritic cells: key to fetal tolerance? *Biol Reprod.* (2007) 77:590–8. doi: 10.1095/biolreprod.107.060632
11. Blois SM. Lineage, maturity, and phenotype of uterine murine dendritic cells throughout gestation indicate a protective role in maintaining pregnancy. *Biol Reprod.* (2004) 70:1018–23. doi: 10.1095/biolreprod.103.022640
12. Thiele K, Holzmann C, Solano ME, Zahner G, Arck PC. Comparative sensitivity analyses of quantitative polymerase chain reaction and flow cytometry in detecting cellular microchimerism in murine tissues. *J Immunol Methods* (2014) 406:74–82. doi: 10.1016/j.jim.2014.03.009
13. Fernandez-Valdivia R, Jeong J, Mukherjee A, Soyal SM, Li J, Ying Y, et al. A mouse model to dissect progesterone signaling in the female reproductive tract and mammary gland. *Genesis* (2010) 48:106–13. doi: 10.1002/dvg.20586
14. Thiele K, Solano ME, Huber S, Flavell RA, Kessler T, Barikbin R, et al. Prenatal acetaminophen application affects maternal immune and endocrine adaptation to pregnancy, induces placental damage and impairs fetal development in mice. *Am J Pathol.* (2015) 185:2805–18. doi: 10.1016/j.ajpath.2015.06.019
15. Solano ME, Kowal MK, O'Rourke GE, Horst AK, Modest K, Plösch T, et al. Progesterone and HMOX-1 promote fetal growth by CD8+ T cell modulation. *J Clin Invest.* (2015) 125:1726–38. doi: 10.1172/JCI68140
16. Theiler K. *The House Mouse Atlas of Embryonic Development.* 2. New York, NY; Berlin; Heidelberg: Springer-Verlag (1989).
17. Solano ME, Thiele K, Kowal MK, Arck PC. Identification of suitable reference genes in the mouse placenta. *Placenta* (2016) 39:7–15. doi: 10.1016/j.placenta.2015.12.017
18. Livak KJ, Schmittgen TD. Analysis of relative gene expression data using real-time quantitative PCR and the 2-ΔΔCT method. *Methods* (2001) 25:402–8. doi: 10.1006/meth.2001.1262
19. Ruxton GD. The unequal variance t-test is an underused alternative to Student's t-test and the Mann–Whitney U test. *Behav Ecol.* (2006) 17:688–90. doi: 10.1093/beheco/ark016

20. Sferruzzi-Perri AN, Macpherson AM, Roberts CT, Robertson SA. Csf2 null mutation alters placental gene expression and trophoblast glycogen cell and giant cell abundance in mice1. *Biol Reprod.* (2009) 81:207–21. doi: 10.1095/biolreprod.108.073312
21. Lydon JP, DeMayo FJ, Funk CR, Mani SK, Hughes AR, Montgomery CA, et al. Mice lacking progesterone receptor exhibit pleiotropic reproductive abnormalities. *Genes Dev.* (1995) 9:2266–78. doi: 10.1101/gad.9.18.2266
22. Engler JB, Kursawe N, Solano ME, Patas K, Wehrmann S, Heckmann N, et al. Glucocorticoid receptor in T cells mediates protection from autoimmunity in pregnancy. *Proc Natl Acad Sci USA.* (2017) 114:E181–90. . doi: 10.1073/pnas.1617115114
23. Darrasse-Jèze G, Deroubaix S, Mouquet H, Victora GD, Eisenreich T, Yao K, et al. Feedback control of regulatory T cell homeostasis by dendritic cells *in vivo. J Exp Med.* (2009) 206:1853–62. doi: 10.1084/jem.20090746
24. Yogev N, Frommer F, Lukas D, Kautz-Neu K, Karram K, Ielo D, et al. Dendritic cells ameliorate autoimmunity in the CNS by controlling the homeostasis of PD-1 receptor^{+} regulatory T cells. *Immunity* (2012) 37:264–75. doi: 10.1016/j.immuni.2012.05.025
25. Murthi P, Kalionis B, Rajaraman G, Keogh RJ, Da Silva Costa F. The role of homeobox genes in the development of placental insufficiency. *Fetal Diagn Ther.* (2012) 32:225–30. doi: 10.1159/000339657
26. Watson ED, Cross JC. Development of structures and transport functions in the mouse placenta. *Physiology* (2005) 20:180–93. doi: 10.1152/physiol.00001.2005
27. Gale NW, Yancopoulos GD. Growth factors acting via endothelial cell-specific receptor tyrosine kinases: VEGFs, Angiopoietins, and ephrins in vascular development. *Genes Dev.* (1999) 13:1055–66.
28. Vrachnis N, Kalampokas E, Sifakis S, Vitoratos N, Kalampokas T, Botsis D, et al. Placental growth factor (PlGF): a key to optimizing fetal growth. *J Matern Neonatal Med.* (2013) 26:995–1002. doi: 10.3109/14767058.2013.766694
29. Esterman A, Finlay TH, Dancis J. The effect of hypoxia on term trophoblast: hormone synthesis and release. *Placenta* (1996) 17:217–22. doi: 10.1016/S0143-4004(96)90041-7
30. Khaliq A, Dunk C, Jiang J, Shams M, Li X, Acevedo C, et al. Hypoxia down-regulates placenta growth factor, whereas fetal growth restriction up-regulates placenta growth factor expression: molecular evidence for "placental hyperoxia" in intrauterine growth restriction. *Lab Invest.* (1999) 79:151–70.
31. Ahmed A, Dunk C, Ahmad S, Khaliq A. Regulation of Placental Vascular Endothelial Growth Factor (VEGF) and Placenta Growth Factor (PlGF) and Soluble Flt-1 by Oxygen— A Review. *Placenta* (2000) 21:S16–24. doi: 10.1053/plac.1999.0524
32. Carmeliet P, Moons L, Luttun A, Vincenti V, Compernolle V, De Mol M, et al. Synergism between vascular endothelial growth factor and placental growth factor contributes to angiogenesis and plasma extravasation in pathological conditions. *Nat Med.* (2001) 7:575. doi: 10.1038/87904
33. Alahakoon TI, Zhang W, Arbuckle S, Zhang K, Lee V. Reduced angiogenic factor expression in intrauterine fetal growth restriction using semiquantitative immunohistochemistry and digital image analysis. *J Obstet Gynaecol Res.* (2018) 44:861–72. doi: 10.1111/jog.13592
34. Hoeller A, Ehrlich L, Golic M, Herse F, Perschel FH, Siwetz M, et al. Placental expression of sFlt-1 and PlGF in early preeclampsia vs. early IUGR vs. age-matched healthy pregnancies. *Hypertens Pregnancy* (2017) 36:151–60. doi: 10.1080/10641955.2016.1273363
35. Joó JG, Rigó J, Börzsönyi B, Demendi C, Kornya L. Placental gene expression of the placental growth factor (PlGF) in intrauterine growth restriction. *J Matern Neonatal Med.* (2017) 30:1471–5. doi: 10.1080/14767058.2016.1219993
36. Rab A, Szentpéteri I, Kornya L, Börzsönyi B, Demendi C, Joó JG. Placental gene expression patterns of epidermal growth factor in intrauterine growth restriction. *Eur J Obstet Gynecol Reprod Biol.* (2013) 170:96–9. doi: 10.1016/j.ejogrb.2013.05.020
37. Nawathe AR, Christian M, Kim SH, Johnson M, Savvidou MD, Terzidou V. Insulin-like growth factor axis in pregnancies affected by fetal growth disorders. *Clin Epigenetics* (2016) 8:11. doi: 10.1186/s13148-016-0178-5
38. Sferruzzi-Perri AN, Owens JA, Pringle KG, Robinson JS, Roberts CT. Maternal insulin-like growth factors-I and -II act via different pathways to promote fetal growth. *Endocrinology* (2006) 147:3344–55. doi: 10.1210/en.2005-1328
39. Agrogiannis GD, Sifakis S, Patsouris ES, Konstantinidou AE. Insulin-like growth factors in embryonic and fetal growth and skeletal development (Review). *Mol Med Rep.* (2014) 10:579–84. doi: 10.3892/mmr.2014.2258
40. Caton ML, Smith-Raska MR, Reizis B. Notch–RBP-J signaling controls the homeostasis of CD8^{-} dendritic cells in the spleen. *J Exp Med.* (2007) 204:1653–64. doi: 10.1084/jem.20062648
41. Schittenhelm L, Hilkens CM, Morrison VL. β(2) Integrins as regulators of dendritic cell, monocyte, and macrophage function. *Front Immunol.* (2017) 8:1866. doi: 10.3389/fimmu.2017.01866
42. Winslow GM, Papillion AM, Kenderes KJ, Levack RC. CD11c+ T-bet+ memory B cells: Immune maintenance during chronic infection and inflammation? *Cell Immunol.* (2017) 321:8–17. doi: 10.1016/j.cellimm.2017.07.006
43. Meredith MM, Liu K, Darrasse-Jeze G, Kamphorst AO, Schreiber HA, Guermonprez P, et al. Expression of the zinc finger transcription factor zDC (Zbtb46, Btbd4) defines the classical dendritic cell lineage. *J Exp Med.* (2012) 209:1153–65. doi: 10.1084/jem.20112675
44. Loschko J, Schreiber HA, Rieke GJ, Esterházy D, Meredith MM, Pedicord VA, et al. Absence of MHC class II on cDCs results in microbial-dependent intestinal inflammation. *J Exp Med.* (2016) 213:517–34. doi: 10.1084/jem.20160062
45. Schmidt-Supprian M, Rajewsky K. Vagaries of conditional gene targeting. *Nat Immunol.* (2007) 8:665. doi: 10.1038/ni0707-665
46. Scholz C, Toth B, Santoso L, Kuhn C, Franz M, Mayr D, et al. Original article: distribution and maturity of dendritic cells in diseases of insufficient placentation. *Am J Reprod Immunol.* (2008) 60:238–45. doi: 10.1111/j.1600-0897.2008.00619.x
47. Cappelletti M, Giannelli S, Martinelli A, Cetin I, Colombo E, Calcaterra F, et al. Lack of activation of peripheral blood dendritic cells in human pregnancies complicated by intrauterine growth restriction. *Placenta* (2013) 34:35–41. doi: 10.1016/j.placenta.2012.10.016

5

Molecular Principles of Intrauterine Growth Restriction in *Plasmodium falciparum* Infection

Johanna Seitz[1†], Diana Maria Morales-Prieto[1†], Rodolfo R. Favaro[1†], Henning Schneider[2,3] and Udo Rudolf Markert[1]*

[1] Placenta Lab, Department of Obstetrics, Jena University Hospital, Jena, Germany, [2] Institute of Biochemistry and Molecular Medicine, University of Bern, Bern, Switzerland, [3] Department of Obstetrics and Gynecology, Inselspital, Bern University Hospital, University of Bern, Bern, Switzerland

***Correspondence:**
Udo Rudolf Markert
markert@med.uni-jena.de

† These authors have contributed equally to this work

Malaria in pregnancy still constitutes a particular medical challenge in tropical and subtropical regions. Of the five *Plasmodium* species that are pathogenic to humans, infection with *Plasmodium falciparum* leads to fulminant progression of the disease with massive impact on pregnancy. Severe anemia of the mother, miscarriage, stillbirth, preterm delivery and intrauterine growth restriction (IUGR) with reduced birth weight are frequent complications that lead to more than 10,000 maternal and 200,000 perinatal deaths annually in sub-Saharan Africa alone. *P. falciparum* can adhere to the placenta via the expression of the surface antigen VAR2CSA, which leads to sequestration of infected erythrocytes in the intervillous space. This process induces a placental inflammation with involvement of immune cells and humoral factors. Especially, monocytes get activated and change the release of soluble mediators, including a variety of cytokines. This proinflammatory environment contributes to disorders of angiogenesis, blood flow, autophagy, and nutrient transport in the placenta and erythropoiesis. Collectively, they impair placental functions and, consequently, fetal growth. The discovery that women in endemic regions develop a certain immunity against VAR2CSA-expressing parasites with increasing number of pregnancies has redefined the understanding of malaria in pregnancy and offers strategies for the development of vaccines. The following review gives an overview of molecular processes in *P. falciparum* infection in pregnancy which may be involved in the development of IUGR.

Keywords: malaria, plasmodium, pregnancy, placenta, intrauterine growth restriction, small for gestational age, anemia

INTRODUCTION

Pregnant women are more susceptible to infection with *Plasmodium falciparum* and present a more severe form of the disease than non-pregnant women (1). The probability of suffering from severe malaria infections is three times higher—with a mortality rate of up to 50% (2, 3). Other complications involve severe anemia, cerebral malaria, and massive pregnancy disorders (4). The increased susceptibility is attributed to two main factors: firstly, physiological processes during pregnancy, such as the altered hormone constellation with suppression of certain immune reactions, and increased body temperature, which makes pregnant women more attractive to Anopheles mosquitoes (5, 6); secondly, the sequestration of *P. falciparum*-infected erythrocytes in the placenta (7).

In placental malaria, *P. falciparum* expresses a special Plasmodium falciparum erythrocyte membrane protein 1 (PfEMP-1), the VAR2CSA antigen, which can bind to chondroitin sulfate A (CSA) produced by trophoblast cells. This interaction promotes the retention of parasites in the intervillous space triggering an inflammatory reaction known as intervillitis. Women in endemic regions often have developed humoral immunity reflected by the production of antibodies against different PfEMP-1 expressing *P. falciparum* strains. However, as the VAR2CSA appears only in pregnancy, primiparous women have no antibodies against this antigen yet, and again, are at high risk for a new *P. falciparum* infection. Infections in further pregnancies are usually less severe due to previous contact with VAR2CSA-expressing *P. falciparum* strains and increasing immunity to VAR2CSA (8). By accumulation in the placenta, *P. falciparum* also evades elimination processes in the spleen. In endemic regions, the peripheral infection can be controlled mostly with acquired partial immunity against *P. falciparum*, while the plasmodia may persist unrecognized in the placenta and can cause maternal anemia as well as fetal developmental disorders (9). In addition to *P. falciparum*, *P. vivax* can also lead to pregnancy complications. However, the consequences are generally less severe and are not presented in this review (4, 10).

Various measures and antimalarials can be taken to prevent and treat malaria during pregnancy but there is a lack of information regarding their safety, efficacy and pharmacokinetics. In all regions affected by malaria, early diagnosis and treatment as well as the use of ITNs (insecticide-treated nets) are crucial. In regions with endemic malaria, intermittent preventive treatment (IPTp) starting at the second trimester with the antimalarial drug sulfadoxine-pyrimethamine is additionally recommended for pregnant women by the World Health Organization (11). A metadata analysis confirmed that this therapy reduces the risk of low birth weight (LBW) when 3 or more doses are administrated, compared to the standard 2-doses regimen (12), but among the estimated 35 million pregnant women eligible for IPTp therapy, in 2017, <50% received two, and only ~22% received three or more doses of IPTp (11). Further efforts are needed to improve the coverage and access to IPTp for this vulnerable population.

Currently, the most effective first-line treatment recommended by the WHO for the general population is an artemisin-based combination therapy (11). This therapy resulted embryotoxic in animal studies. Therefore, less efficient and less well-tolerated medicines such us quinine and clindamycin have been recommended for women in first trimester pregnancy (13). However, the embryo exposure and toxic effects to artemisins may be different or lower in humans due to their specific placenta morphology (14). This may be supported by growing evidence that artemisins in first trimester pregnancy do not increase the risk of miscarriage, stillbirth or malformations when compared to quinine-based treatment (13, 14). For these reasons a clear conclusion of the risk/benefit ratio of antimalarials medicines cannot be drawn until further studies on pharmacokinetics and safety in humans will be conducted.

Finally, an additional approach to prevent malaria is based on current studies focused on the identification of the most immunogenic epitopes of the VAR2CSA antigen for vaccine development against placental malaria in pregnancy (see below) (15).

P. FALCIPARUM INFECTION IN PREGNANCY

It has been estimated that, in 2007, out of 85.3 million pregnant women in areas at risk for *P. falciparum* malaria, about 2/3 lived in regions with stable (endemic) malaria (16). In these areas, one out of four women at delivery had evidence of placental infection (4). In sub-Saharan Africa alone, malaria was responsible for more than 10,000 maternal and 200,000 perinatal deaths annually until 2009 (2). In 2015, it has been estimated that 900,000 newborns suffer from reduced birth weight due to placental malaria (17). The exact incidence of *P. falciparum* malaria in pregnancy and the resulting IUGR cases remain unknown.

During pregnancy, the clinical appearance of a *P. falciparum* infection depends largely on the maternal immune status, which in turn is associated with the geographical region. If the woman has already acquired immunity, which is usually the case in areas with stable malaria, the infection is often asymptomatic. High fever and complications such as cerebral malaria, hypoglycemia, or pulmonary edema are rare. However, especially in their first pregnancy, women are not protected against placental infection. As the infection may persist undetected, it can lead to pronounced maternal anemia and serious consequences for the unborn child.

Low birth weight (defined as birth weight <2,500 g) is the largest risk factor for infant and child mortality in Africa (18). Independently of malaria infection, growth restricted babies have nine times higher risk of dying within the first month of life than normal weight newborns (19). Annually, around 100,000 children die in Africa as result of malaria-associated LBW (19). The major causes are premature birth and IUGR (20).

It is still unclear which period of infection during pregnancy is the most detrimental for fetal growth. In a recent study including 1190 pregnant women in Burkina Faso, maternal infection after the sixth month of pregnancy was significantly related to higher risk of LBW, while only a trend was found between early infection (≤4 months of pregnancy) and LBW (21). Conversely, a second study reported higher risk of LBW after infection in the second compared to third trimester or at delivery (22). And in a Benin cohort, only infection in early pregnancy was associated with LBW and maternal anemia at delivery (23). Remarkably, a high number of infections during pregnancy leads to an increased risk of LBW independently of the timing (22, 24). As the maternal immunological reactions change during pregnancy, more studies are needed to fully understand the interaction between infection and host response depending on the stage of pregnancy, and how this impare fetal growth.

Since severe maternal anemia and placental malaria are the major mechanisms responsible for malaria-related IUGR, they will be comprehensively addressed in the following sections.

Maternal Anemia in Malaria

Severe anemia (defined as hemoglobin concentration Hb < 7 g/dl) is the main complication of maternal *P. falciparum* infections in regions with stable malaria. In the sub-Saharan region, between 200,000 and 500,000 pregnant women are estimated to develop malaria-associated severe anemia (25–27). Severe anemia can lead to death even if only slight blood loss occurs during delivery. Circulation problems with an increased risk of heart failure and pulmonary edema may also occur (2, 9). In addition to malaria, other causes such as iron, vitamins (e.g., folate, vitamin A, and vitamin B-12) and trace element deficiency or worm infections may further contribute to the occurrence of anemia (28–30).

The pathogenesis of anemia in malaria is generally multifactorial, even in non-pregnant women, and includes (I) hemolysis or phagocytosis of infected and non-infected erythrocytes, (II) disturbed development of erythrocytes from their precursor cells (dyserythropoiesis) due to hemozoin deposits in the bone marrow and (III) suppression of erythropoiesis as a result of a chronic inflammatory reaction (**Figure 1**) (31). (I) The elimination of non-infected erythrocytes is estimated to be almost 10 times higher than that of infected erythrocytes and thus plays also an important role in the development of anemia (32). Several potential reasons for this phenomenon are under discussion: hypersplenism and the increased activation of macrophages contribute to generally increased phagocytosis and cell lysis (33–36); non-infected erythrocytes also exhibit reduced deformability and are thus degraded in the spleen (37, 38); and the deposition of immune complexes and complement factors on non-infected erythrocytes that may cause receptor-mediated phagocytosis by macrophages (39–41).

(II) The malaria pigment hemozoin directly stimulates the apoptosis of erythrorid progenitor cells (42–44). *In vivo*, elevated plasma hemozoin concentration is associated with anemia and suppression of reticulocytes. The number of pigmented precursor cells in bone marrow correlates with the degree of abnormal erythrocyte development (43). Hemozoin also indirectly impairs erythropoiesis through inflammatory mediators such as TNF and nitric oxide (NO) from activated mononuclear cells (42). In *in vitro* experiments, NO synthesis in monocytes is stimulated by hemozoin. Increased nitric oxide production is associated with decreased hemoglobin levels in children with malaria anemia (45). In contrast, macrophages seem to protect the bone marrow from toxic effects of hemozoin (44).

(III) A further aspect in the development of malaria anemia is the suppression of erythropoiesis due to an inflammatory reaction. Malaria anemia is mainly caused by dysregulation of pro- and anti-inflammatory cytokines, chemokines, growth factors and effector molecules (31). Increased levels of TNF, IL-6 and IL-8 as well as decreased IL-10:TNF or TGF-β1:TNF ratios are associated with anemia (46–51). Proinflammatory cytokines also lead to hypoferremia with reduced hemopoiesis, a major mechanism of inflammatory anemia (52, 53). IL-6 stimulates the synthesis of the iron regulatory peptide hepcidin in the liver, which inhibits intestinal iron resorption and the release of iron from hepatocytes and reticuloendothelial cells (54, 55). In an experimental study on *P. falciparum* infection in five voluntarily participating adults, only slightly elevated levels of IL-6 and hepcidin were measured in serum, but a clear hypoferremia with strongly reduced hemoglobin concentration in the reticulocytes has been reported. The results suggest that the inflammatory disorder of iron hemostasis promotes the development of malaria anemia (56).

Several studies have described a link between maternal anemia and fetal development disorders (27, 29, 57). The reduced number of red blood cells (RBCs) together with altered properties of parasitized RBCs (PRBCs) result in deficient transport of oxygen and CO_2 in the bloodstream. As consequences, chronic hypoxia and elevated oxidative stress arise in the maternal-fetal interface contributing to the occurrence of IUGR (58, 59) (**Figure 1**).

Placental Malaria

Placental malaria is characterized by sequestration of peripheral erythrocytes in the intervillous space and the activation of immune responses leading to inflammation. The manifestation and extent of IUGR have been associated with the severity of placental damage promoted by *P. falciparum* infection. Numerous mechanisms are associated with placental dysfunction and IUGR, including inadequate trophoblast functions, disturbed transport of nutrients, morphological changes, and abnormal angiogenesis. In the following sections, the association between *P. falciparum* infection and these processes will be further discussed in the context of placental malaria. **Figure 1** illustrates the pathogenic mechanisms of maternal anemia and placental malaria that contribute to IUGR.

STRUCTURAL, CELLULAR, AND MOLECULAR MECHANISMS LINKING PLACENTAL MALARIA AND IUGR

Histopathological Changes in the Placenta

Decreased placental weight was detected in women with malaria infection and associated with the presence of placental inflammation and damage (60). In histological samples from patients with active *P. falciparum* infection, erythrocytes in the intervillous space are packed with parasites. In case of past infections, but especially in active chronic infection, the malaria pigment hemozoin can be detected in migrated monocytes or in fibrin deposits (61). Hemozoin deposits without parasitemia indicate an inactive infection (7, 62). Acute infection is more likely to be associated with preterm birth, whilst chronic infection is associated with maternal anemia and reduced birth weight due to IUGR (63). Further histological changes, especially in chronic inflammation, are fibrin deposition, clumping of syncytiotrophoblast cells, reduction of their microvilli, focal necrosis, and thickening of the trophoblast basal membrane (61, 62, 64, 65). These deposits can disturb blood flow in the placenta causing hypoxia and contributing to IUGR (**Figure 1**).

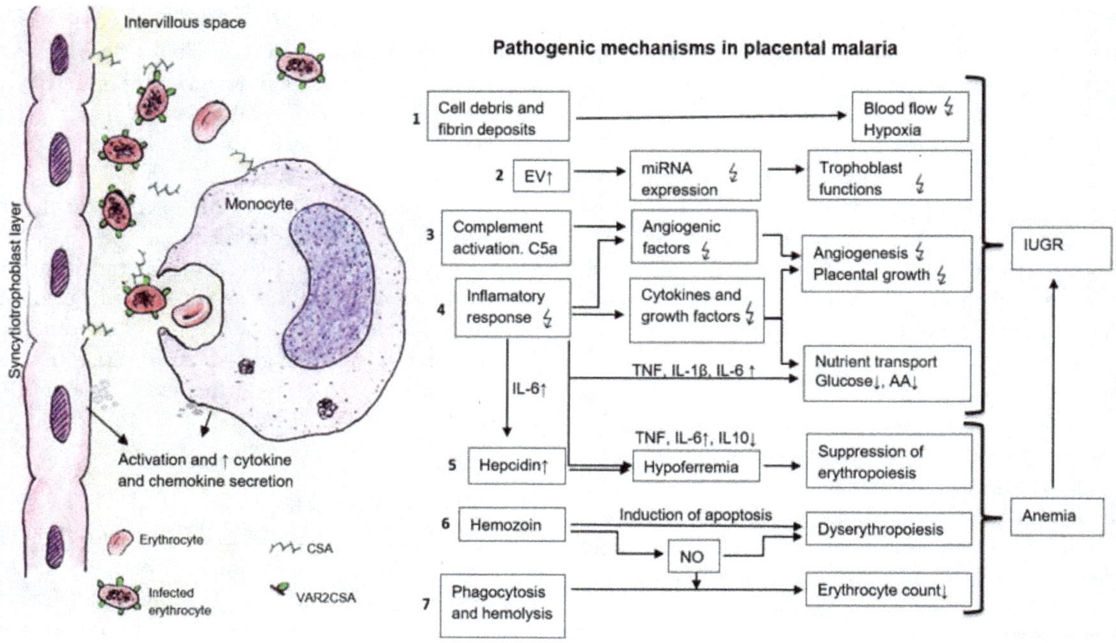

FIGURE 1 | Pathogenetic processes potentially contributing to the development of IUGR in placental malaria. The sequestration of infected erythrocytes expressing VAR2CSA in the intervillous space occurs through the binding to placental chondroitin sulfate (CSA). This process leads to the activation of syncytiotrophoblast cells and local monocytes. These cells secrete chemokines and cytokines, which attract further immune cells which contribute to the pathogenesis of fetal growth restriction. 1. Cell debris and fibrin deposits can disrupt placental blood flow and lead to hypoxia. 2. Elevated EV may carry modified patterns of miRNAs disturbing trophoblast functions. 3–4. Activated complement factors (C5a) and inflammatory responses alter the concentration of cytokines, angiogenic and growth factors, affecting vascularization and placental growth. Cytokines and decreased growth factors impact placental nutrient transporters, resulting in decreased amino acid and glucose transport. 5. The suppressed erythropoiesis is caused either directly via cytokines or indirectly via increased hepatic hepcidin and lowered iron levels. 6. Dyserythropoiesis is a consequence of hemozoin deposits in the bone marrow, which disturb blood formation directly via apoptosis induction or indirectly via inflammatory mediators such as nitric oxide (NO). 7. Phagocytosis and hemolysis reduce erythrocyte numbers contributing to anemia. Together with placental alterations, maternal anemia leads to fetal growth restriction. ϟ, disturbed; ↑, increased; ↓, decreased; AA, amino acids; C5a, activated complement factor 5; CSA, chondroitin sulfate A, EV, extracellular vesicles; IL, interleukin; NO, nitric oxide; TNF, tumor necrosis factor.

Altered Inflammatory Response in the Placenta

Infection with *P. falciparum* leads to an inflammatory reaction in the placenta that shifts the balance between Th1 and Th2 immune responses toward the Th1 pathway leading to release of proinflammatory cytokines and migration of immune cells (5, 66). In dual *ex vivo* perfusion experiments on isolated human placental cotyledons *P. falciparum* induces upregulation of transcription factor c-fos gene expression and release of the macrophage migration inhibitory factor (MIF), whereas expression of other chemokines and proinflammatory cytokines has been discussed as unspecific responses to oxidative and hypoxic stress. The observed release of placental chemokines and cytokines has been directed toward the maternal compartment while only trace amounts have been detected in the fetal circuit (67). By sequestration of infected erythrocytes in the intervillous space, syncytiotrophoblast and local maternal immune cells express elevated levels of chemokines [e.g., macrophage-inflammatory protein 1 (MIP1), monocyte chemoattractant protein 1 (MCP1) and interferon-gamma induced protein 10 (IP10)], which cause an increased migration of monocytes (68–71). By means of phagocytosis, cytokine secretion and antigen presentation to T cells, they contribute strongly to the elimination of the pathogens (72). On the other hand, excessive monocyte infiltration contributes to malaria pathogenesis and correlates in numerous studies with negative consequences such as reduced birth weight, premature birth and maternal anemia (73–78). The role of natural killer cells (NK cells) in the placental immune response is controversially discussed. A complete absence of NK cells in the intervillous space of malaria infected placentas has been described, which may be partly responsible for reduced parasite elimination (78). Pregnant women with *P. falciparum* infection have significantly lower levels of INFγ-producing NK cells in the placenta than aparasitemic pregnant women (79). Moreover, the cytotoxicity of NK cells against infected erythrocytes is lower in primiparous women, who are particularly susceptible to malaria, than in multiparous mothers (80). These results suggest that a higher number of INFγ-producing NK cells protects against infection (79, 80). In another study, however, NK cells in infected placentas are elevated and associated with low HLA-G production in trophoblast cells, which may contribute to a negative pregnancy outcome (81).

Monocytes secrete cytokines for the differentiation and activation of further immune cells. The following proinflammatory cytokines can be found elevated in peripheral and/or placental blood of infected pregnant women: TNF

(50, 51, 66, 71, 82–87), IFNγ (50, 51, 66, 71, 82, 83, 85, 88, 89), IL-1/β (66, 84, 86, 89), IL-2 (50, 82) and IL-6 (51, 66). In addition, elevated concentrations of antiinflammatory cytokines such as IL-4 and IL-10 have been detected (51, 66, 71, 82, 84, 85, 90). In some studies IL-2, IL-4, IL-6, IL-10, and TGFβ have been reported as decreased (50, 66, 86). Increased concentrations of TNF are associated with high placental parasite density and pregnancy complications such as LBW, IUGR, preterm birth and maternal anemia (50, 86, 87, 91). In one study, elevated IFNγ has been associated with reduced birth weight (50), while another study did not find this correlation (87) and a further study has shown that reduced IFNγ is associated with reduced birth weight (90). Other authors have found elevated IFNγ in non-infected multiparous women which is associated with the absence of infection and conclude an important role of IFNγ in protecting against infection (85, 89).

Increased IL-10 levels are associated with parasitemia, reduced birth weight and premature birth. The authors assume that IL-10 impedes adequate control of the pathogen (91, 92). In contrast, other authors claim that high IL-10 levels are important to counteract an excessive cellular inflammatory response and to protect against negative pregnancy outcome (50, 66). Since in placental infections IL-10 is also highly elevated in peripheral blood, it has been discussed as a potential biomarker for the diagnosis of infection with *P. falciparum* in pregnancy (84, 90). Furthermore, elevated levels of IL-6 and IL-8 may be associated with high parasite density and anemia, IL-8 with intrauterine growth restriction and IL-7 with absence of infection (51, 86, 89). Lower expression of IL-5 is associated with reduced birth weight (90). **Table 1** summarizes the most important associations of elevated cytokines caused by *P. falciparum* infection with clinical parameters.

Alterations in the levels of placental Th1 and Th2 cytokines and growth factors as a response to *P. falciparum* infection may result in a disbalance which potentially impacts placental functions contributing to IUGR (**Figure 1**).

TABLE 1 | Associations of cytokines with clinical parameters in *P. falciparum* infections in pregnancy.

Elevated cytokine	Association with	References
TNF	High parasite density and monocyte infiltration	(50, 87)
	Low birth weight	(87)
	Premature birth	(91)
	Intrauterine growth restriction	(86)
	Maternal anemia	(50)
	Fetal death in mice	(93)
IFNγ	Low birth weight	(50)
	Fetal death in mice	(93)
	Absence of infection	(85, 89)
	No association with low birth weight	(87)
Low IFNγ	Correlation with low birth weight	(90)
IL-10	Parasitemia and low birth weight	(92)
	Premature birth	(71)
	Control of inflammation	(50, 66)
IL-8	High parasite density and low Hb	(51)
	Intrauterine growth retardation	(86)
IL-7	Absence of infection	(89)
IL-6	High parasite density and low Hb	(51)
Low IL-5	Correlation with low birth weight	(90)

Disruption of Hormonal Balance

Several of the critical hormones in pregnancy are altered in malaria infections, such as the steroid hormones estrogen and progesterone. In addition to their effects on placental development and function, they contribute to the adaptation of the maternal immune system to pregnancy which is crucial for establishing maternal-fetal immunotolerance and prevention of fetal rejection (5, 94). Cortisol, which is secreted by the adrenal glands and associated with stress responses, also performs physiological functions on the placenta and suppresses immune responses (95, 96). The polypeptide hormone prolactin exerts a plethora of effects on maternal metabolism and immune system. It is expressed by the pituitary gland, decidua, myometrium, and immune cells (97).

In infection with *P. falciparum, the* steroid hormones estrogen and progesterone, prolactin and cortisol are altered (89, 98–100). In malaria, estrogen (estradiol, E2) has been found decreased in third trimester peripheral blood (100), and in another study increased in the placenta (89). In the latter study, low levels of estrogen are found especially in multiparous women and are associated with the absence of infection. Pregnancy-maintaining progesterone correlates positively with maternal Hb and child birth weight and is reduced in malaria infection (89). Prolactin has been described as either unchanged or decreased in infected pregnant women (98, 99). Being regulated by progesterone, the dropping of prolactin levels may be related to progesterone shortfall. The concentration of glucocorticoids such as cortisol is significantly increased and associated with high parasite loads (98, 99). Cortisol also correlates with a low number of NK cells and inhibits their cytotoxicity (80, 101).

Changes in the levels of endocrine hormones ocurring in women with malaria may contribute to impaired placental functions and, hence, IUGR. Likewise, hormones have also the potential to interfere with maternal immune responses against the parasite, which potentially influences placental and fetal complications (**Figure 1**). The consequences of the observed hormonal imbalances, however, are poorly understood, and require further investigations.

Disturbed Angiogenesis and Placenta Development

Doppler sonography studies of *P. falciparum* infected pregnant women (32–35 weeks of pregnancy) show abnormal uteroplacental blood flow associated with preterm birth, LBW and perinatal death (102). The underlying pathogenetic processes are complex and not fully understood. Growth and vascularization of the placenta are regulated by various growth factors such as IGF and angiogenesis factors such as angiopoetin (ANG-1/-2), VEGF and its soluble receptor (sVEGFR1) (103).

Altered expression of these factors can severely impair the development of the placenta and the fetus (**Figure 1**). In malaria infected mice, decreased levels of ANG-1, an increased ANG-2/ANG-1 ratio and growth disorders of the fetus have been described (104). Dysregulation of angiopoetin can also be detected in exposed primiparous women and is associated with reduced birth weight (104). Reduced levels of ANG-1 are also associated with various histopathological changes of the placenta in infected pregnant women in areas with low malaria transmission (105). The activation of the complement system, particularly the factor C5, seems to be significantly involved in the pathogenesis of disturbed angiogenesis. In mice, activated C5 (C5a) leads to an increased release of sVEGFR-1 from monocytes, which binds VEGF and makes it ineffective. Important growth stimuli for placental vessels are missing, as a result rejection and fetal growth restriction can occur (106, 107). In case-control studies of pregnant women from Kenya and Malawi, C5a is significantly elevated in placental malaria infection (108, 109). Increased levels of C5a are associated with altered angiogenesis parameters and with babies small for gestational age (109). Levels of IGF-1, an essential growth factor, are significantly reduced in infected pregnant women compared to non-infected ones. Decreased IGF-1 levels also correlate with decreased birth weight (110).

Malaria infection and pre-eclampsia or pregnancy-associated hypertension have some similarities (111). For instance, there is reduced placental perfusion in both pregnancy complications (102, 112). Biomarkers for pre-eclampsia, such as sVEGFR1 and soluble endoglin, are often elevated also in placental *P. falciparum* infection (113–115). An increased risk of hypertension in young primiparous women with chronic malaria infection has been described (114). A similar link between placental infection and pregnancy hypertension has been reported also in a hypoendemic region in Senegal (116). Malaria in pregnancy seems to contribute to the development of pre-eclampsia by placental inflammatory processes with increased cytokine secretion (114–116). Subsequently, preeclampsia constitutes a risk factor for fetal growth restriction (117).

Disorders of Nutrient Transport

Several studies support the hypothesis that in malaria infection, dysregulation of placental nutrient transporters contributes to fetal growth restriction (**Figure 1**). System A transporter, one of the most important amino acid transporters in the placenta, is downregulated in malaria infection (118, 119). In several studies, a reduced function of this transporter has been associated with fetal growth disorders (120–122). Its activity is particularly reduced in placental inflammation with monocyte infiltrate (118). In placental malaria infection, inflammatory mediators inhibit essential signal transduction pathways (119). *In vitro* studies show that proinflammatory cytokines such as 1β, IL-6, and TNF lead to System A transporter dysregulation (123, 124). As described above, they are elevated in malaria infections and associated with reduced birth weight. In addition, growth factors such as IGF-1, which stimulate placental amino acid uptake, are reduced in *P. falciparum infections* (110, 125). In infected placentas, the expression of GLUT-1, a transporter important for basal glucose supply, is also downregulated (126, 127). The GLUT-1 expression at the basal membrane shows a positive correlation with birth weight and a strongly negative correlation with the density of the monocyte infiltrate. These results suggest that the inflammatory response in the intervillous space leads to fetal growth restriction due to impaired transplacental glucose transport (126). In general, increased TNF levels, decreased IGF-1 levels and placental hypoxia are associated with dysregulation of glucose transport (128–130).

Extracellular Vesicles (EV) Containing microRNAs in Malaria

In recent years, extracellular vesicles (EV) have reached the spotlight of intercellular communication, particularly in the maternofetal relationship. Current studies demonstrate that placenta-derived EV are able, for instance, to modulate maternal immune cells (131), platelets (132), and vascular cells (133, 134).

EV are packed with non-coding RNAs, including microRNAs (miRNAs), mRNAs, proteins and lipids, which after internalization, influence the behavior of recipient cells. Several pathological conditions, including preeclampsia (131), IUGR (135), and malaria (136) have been associated with alterations of EV content and functions.

The human placenta possesses a unique profile of miRNA which is dynamically expressed to supply the specific needs of the respective gestational age (137). The study of miRNA expression patterns in placenta tissue has revealed dominant expression of oncogenic, angiogenic, and antiapoptotic miRNAs during the first trimester of pregnancy, whereas the third-trimester is characterized by prevailing expression of miRNAs related to cell differentiation and tumor suppression (138).

Despite the accumulating reports of miRNA expression in IUGR or small for gestational age (SGA) cases associated with preeclampsia (139–141), only few studies have investigated alteration in absence of preeclampsia. Interestingly, these publications suggest an important role of placenta-specific and placenta-associated miRNAs in the development of IUGR. For instance, a report on the placenta-associated miR-141, which is highly enriched in maternal plasma, has shown its overexpression in placentas complicated with IUGR and confirmed the miR-141 target pleiomorphic adenoma gene 1 (PLAG1), which may contribute to the development of this pathology (142). Likewise, seven members of the Chromosome 19 miRNA Cluster (C19MC) are downregulated in placentas from IUGR pregnancies (143).

C19MC is a placenta-specific cluster, low expressed at the beginning of pregnancy, but highly expressed at term (137). Members of C19MC have emerged as important players in the regulation of trophoblast invasion, proliferation and differentiation (144, 145), and more recently, in the immune response to viral infections in pregnancy (146, 147). It has been proposed that C19MC members confer antiviral immunity to trophoblast cells (148) but their role in defense to bacterial or parasite infections remains unknown.

Only a handful of studies have been carried out to investigate the changes in levels of circulating placental EV and miRNAs as response to malaria infection. Most of these studies have used animal models or had very low number of patients, and thus, have not been included in this review. To our knowledge a single report has been published analyzing expression of these and other placental-miRNAs in plasma EV of pregnant women with malaria (136). The concentration of total and placental-derived microparticles in plasma, characterized by the presence of Pregnancy-Specific Glycoprotein1 (PSG1) on their surface, remains unaltered in women with malaria and increased in those carrying HIV. Independently of malaria or HIV infection, women who delivered growth restricted neonates have higher quantities of both total and placental-derived EV. Furthermore, the level of miRNA-517c, a miRNA belonging to C19MC, is elevated in vesicles isolated from patients with malaria compared to uninfected controls (136). miRNA-517c is also associated with the development of preeclampsia and *in vitro* studies have demonstrated its involvement in decreasing trophoblast invasion and angiogenesis, as well as in increased production sFLT1 contributing to placenta dysfunction (149).

In human subjects, peripheral erythrocytes from malaria infected patients produce higher amounts of EV than from uninfected individuals. The severity of malaria infection and efficacy of anti-malaria therapies can be assessed based on plasma EV content (150, 151). A set of miRNAs is dysregulated during the blood stage of *P. falciparum* infection in adults compared to uninfected subjects. Four miRNAs: miR-1246, miR-6780b-5p, miR-3135b, and miR-6126 were reported as of great importance to malaria pathogenesis due to their involvement in multiple processes, such as cell defense response, immune response, TNF signaling pathway, and T cell receptor signaling pathway (152). A broader analysis of the consensus disease phenocode revealed a group of miRNAs commonly altered in a diverse spectrum of human diseases including autoimmune and infectious diseases. Eighty-eight percent of the miRNAs of the consensus set have the potential to target the principal components of the nuclear import and the inflammasome pathways including KPNA1, NLRP1 (NALP1), and NLRP3 (NALP3) genes. After being upregulated in malaria, these genes return to normal levels in PBMC from patients treated with chloroquine (153), a drug considered in the antimalaria drug policy of the WHO (154) and used for malaria prophylaxis during pregnancy due to its relatively high safety (155).

New miRNA functions have been explored regarding the infection and propagation of malaria. Several studies have demonstrated that *P. falciparum* lack miRNA sequences in its genome, presumably by absence of argonaute and dicer genes (156, 157). However, the presence of approximately 100 human miRNAs was detected within the parasites suggesting a unidirectional transfer (158). During the blood stage of *P. falciparum* malaria infection, uninfected erythrocytes enhance the release of EV which mainly target infected erythrocytes and the parasites therein. An *in vitro* study demonstrated that these EV contain hAgo2-miRNA complexes including those of miR-451 and miR-140, which after internalization by the parasites result in effective downregulation of the essential malaria antigen, PfEMP1 expression (159). This finding supports a report on erythrocytes of sickle cell anemia patients, showing enriched human miR-451 and let-7i in erythrocytes, which are transferred to parasites and target cAMP-dependent protein kinase PKA-R mRNA. This results in inhibition of *P. falciparum* blood stage development and contributes to malaria resistance (158). Monocytes, macrophages, and neutrophils also become activated after being exposed to peripheral erythrocyte EV, indicating their contribution to inflammatory processes taking place during malaria infection (160). These findings highlight the role of miRNAs in the innate resistance of erythrocytes to malaria infection as a host mechanism to minimize disease severity. The study of miRNA in placental infection is also worth to be pursued since the expression of miR-451 and other six placenta-associated miRNAs is altered in primary trophoblast cells exposed to hypoxia and in plasma of pregnant women with IUGR (161).

It is tempting to speculate that EVs produced by *P. falciparum*-infected cells or other cells affected during the infection (e.g., immune cells) as well as their secreted miRNAs may play a role in the pathogenesis of placental malaria and IUGR (**Figure 1**). However, the potential effects and biological mechanisms by which these EV may influence trophoblast cell functions constitute a yet unexplored field. Despite being still at its beginning, the study of EVs and miRNA expression during malaria may contribute to identify novel biomarkers, to understand host immunoregulation and to develop new vaccination and treatments strategies.

INTERACTION BETWEEN VAR2CSA AND CSA IN *P. FALCIPARUM* INFECTION IN THE PLACENTA

The pathogenesis of pregnancy malaria is mainly due to the fact that erythrocytes infected with *P. falciparum* bind to receptors in the placenta and accumulate in the intervillous space (sequestration). According to current research, the interaction between the VAR2CSA protein, a special variant of PfEMP-1 on the surface of infected erythrocytes, and CSA in the intervillous space of the placenta is regarded as the most important binding (162).

Sequestration of infected erythrocytes in the placenta mediated specifically by VAR2CSA has been confirmed using dual side *ex vivo* placenta perfusion (67, 163). Only *P. falciparum* infected erythrocytes expressing VAR2CSA but not those binding to endothelial protein C receptor (EPCR) or lacking PfEMP1 disappear from the maternal circulation and accumulate in the perfused tissue, mostly in the intervillous space and to a less extend on the syncytiotrophoblast (163). Therefore, understanding the molecular and structural processes of VAR2CSA-CSA binding and the mechanisms to inhibit this interaction may offer new intervention options, in particular for vaccine development.

Chondroitin Sulfate a (CSA): Function, Occurrence, and Structure

CSA is a glycosaminoglycan, a sugar chain made up of disaccharide units which, bound to a protein, forms a proteoglycan (164). In 1996, CSA was described as a target structure for the adhesion of *P. falciparum* infected erythrocytes in the placenta (165). It has been detected by immunohistochemistry in the intervillous space and to a lesser extent at the syncytiotrophoblastic layer. It has been discussed that CSA is produced by the fetus and secreted into the intervillous space (166). In placenta infected with *P. falciparum* significantly higher concentrations of CSA have been found (166, 167). Since it is assumed that proteoglycans are involved in the mobilization of cytokines, hormones and growth factors in tissues, an increased expression of CSA may negatively influence placental functions and promote the development of complications through increased adhesion of parasites (167–169).

The understanding of the exact molecular and structural composition of CSA is fundamental to analyze its interaction with VAR2CSA (164). In addition, it is important for the development of novel therapeutic approaches, such as chondroitin sulfate oligomers that bind to VAR2CSA with a higher affinity than CSA and thus impede the sequestration of infected erythrocytes in the placenta (170).

The *var2csa* Gene in *P. falciparum* Infection

In the presence of a placenta, a *P. falciparum* subpopulation switches to the expression of the *var2csa* gene, one of 60 var genes of PfEMP-1 (171). In contrast to the other var genes, which differ greatly between the strains, *var2csa* is widely conserved (172–175). The *var2csa* gene is detected in the analysis of the genome of *P. falciparum* isolates from different regions in almost all strains (173, 175, 176). Of the 60 var genes, only three, including *var2csa*, seem to be expressed in all three examined *P. falciparum* strains (3D7, IT4, and HB3 strains).

In earlier studies, *var2csa* and other var genes, such as *var1csa* and *varcs2*, have been associated with the adhesion of infected erythrocytes in addition to *var2csa*, but this could not be confirmed in more recent studies (171, 177–180). However, studies investigating the genome and protein synthesis of placental parasites have revealed other highly regulated genes and proteins that might be indirectly involved in the pathogenesis of placental malaria (181–185). While the disruption of the *var2csa* gene leads to the loss of CSA binding capacity (179, 186), no other highly regulated var genes are directly related to placental adhesion (187).

VAR2CSA Protein in *P. falciparum* Infection

VAR2CSA is selectively expressed on the surface of *P. falciparum* infected erythrocytes in the placenta. It was discovered in 2003 by Salanti et al. and confirmed in numerous further studies as the most important ligand of CSA (175, 179, 180, 186–189). VAR2CSA is a large (350 kDa) transmembrane polypeptide. The extracellular part consists of six Duffy binding-like domains (three DBL domains each of class x and ε, omitted in the further text for reasons of clarity), a cysteine-rich interdomain (ID2a/b) and further short interdomain segments (ID1, ID4; **Figure 2** and **Table 2**) (198). VAR2CSA is structurally and functionally very different from other PfEMP-1 proteins. For example, specific domains necessary for the recognition of vascular receptors such as CD36 and ICAM-1 are missing (162, 175). Rosetting—an otherwise important pathogenesis factor that describes accumulation of infected erythrocytes—is also atypical in placental malaria infections (199–201).

The VAR2CSA Duffy Binding-Like Domains

Due to the size and complexity of VAR2CSA, only the quaternary structure of individual domains, but not that of the entire protein, has been described so far (202, 203). The best-known structure is that of the DBL3x domain (DBL3), which binds CSA *in vitro* and has been described in detail in two crystallographic studies (204, 205). DBL3 consists of an α helix with numerous inserted loops and can be divided into three subdomains. A loop between the second and third subdomain, which is disordered in the unbound state, assumes an organized structure in the presence of sulfate or disaccharides and forms a sulfate binding pocket (204). The conformational change creates a positively charged region that attracts the negatively charged CSA. It has been shown that mutations in these areas strongly affect the binding of CSA to DBL3 (205, 206). The flexible loop and other surrounding structures are located on the domain surface, are polymorphic and may protect the CSA binding site from recognition by the immune system (204).

VAR2CSA has numerous polymorphic areas compared to non-var proteins, leading to a high antigenic diversity and different placental *P. falciparum* strains (176, 207). Polymorphisms are important mechanisms for immune evasion and arise under selection pressure through exposure to the host immune system (176, 190, 192). They are mostly located on the protein surface, protect conserved areas from immune defense and hinder the formation of cross-strain antibodies (208–210). By analyzing the amino acid sequence of VAR2CSA and by comparing VAR2CSA sequences of different *P. falciparum* strains, conserved and polymorphic areas can be identified and the DBL domains of VAR2CSA can be further characterized. For instance, the DBL3 domain consists of four highly conserved sequences (C1-4) and three variable sequences (V1-3). Some of the conserved areas are also located on the protein surface and are target structures of naturally acquired antibodies (196, 197) (**Table 2**).

The sequence of the DBL2 region of VAR2CSA shows a so-called "dimorphic" structural motif of 26 amino acid length, which divides the strains into two phylogenetic groups (the FCR3 and the 3D7 strains) (207). Another dimorphic region of 167 amino acid length has been detected in the interdomain 1 (ID1), with 76% of placental isolates from Benin containing the first variant (cluster 1) and 24% the second variant (cluster 2). *P. falciparum* isolates with cluster 2 are associated with both multiple pregnancy and high parasitemia (192). The dimorphic areas seem to assume an essential function in pathogenesis, as they contain important elements for CSA binding and have remained stable for a long time in evolutionary history (192, 207).

The analysis of nearly full-length *var2csa* sequences from parasite isolates form around the world and also those reported at the GenBank and the *P. falciparum* genome sequencing projects (in total 106 *var2csa* sequences) revealed that the six DBL domains differ in amino acid conservation between 61 and 88%

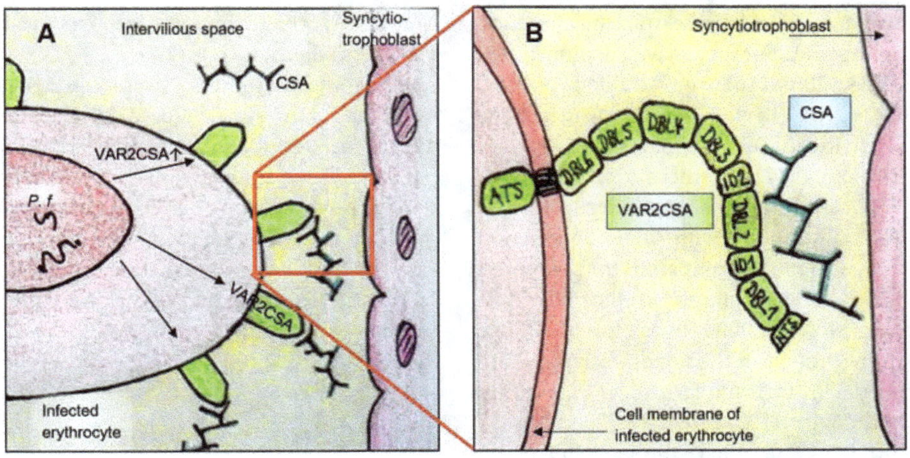

FIGURE 2 | Simplified illustration of the interaction between VAR2CSA and CSA in the placenta. **(A)** *P. falciparum* expresses VAR2CSA on the surface of infected erythrocytes, which in turn binds to CSA in the intervillous space. Pf, *P. falciparum* within a parasitophorous vacuole; CSA, chondroitin sulfate A. **(B)** Enlarged view of **(A)**. VAR2CSA binds to CSA with its N-terminal domains. ATS, Acidic terminal segment; DBL, Duffy-binding-like domain; ID, Interdomain; NTS, N-terminal segment.

TABLE 2 | Structure and sequence polymorphism of VAR2CSA domains relevant for CSA interaction and sequestration of *P. falciparum* in the placenta.

Domain	Structure and sequence polymorphism	Strains in which domain binds to CSA	Strains in which multidomains bind to CSA
DBL1	7 VBs, 4 SCBs (190)	Does not bind to CSA	
Interdomain 1 (ID1)	Dimorphic region of 167 amino acid length; 78% variant (cluster 1) and 24% the second variant (cluster 2) (192)	Does not bind to CSA	3D7 (191)
DBL2	8 VBs, 4 SCBs (190) Dimorphic structural motif of 26 amino acid length, which classifies two phylogenetic groups (the FCR3 and the 3D7 strain) (194)	3D7, FCR3	FCR3 (193) FCR3 (195)
Interdomain 2 (ID2)	Not described	Not described	
DBL3	5 VBs, 4 SCBs (190) 3 variable sequences (V1-3) and four highly conserved sequences (C1-4) (196, 197)	3D7, FCR3	
DBL4	5 VBs, 4 SCBs (190)	Does not bind to CSA	
DBL5	7 VBs, 4 SCBs (190)	3D7	
DBL6	6 VBs, 4 SCBs (190)	3D7	

VB, variable block; SCB, semi-conserved blocks.

and are also structured into variable blocks (VB) and semi-conserved blocks (SCB, block B, D, F, and H) (190). DBL6 is the least conserved VAR2CSA domain with seven variable blocks consisting of a limited number of consensus sequences, i.e., similar or identical sequence patterns (211). Within DBL-6, the variable blocks 1 and 5 (VB1, VB5) from different parasite strains are recognized cross-reactively by antibodies from the plasma of exposed pregnant women (202, 212) (**Table 2**).

The gene diversity of *var2csa* is based on a high rate of self-recombination with a limited repertoire of sequences. In many variable regions the polymorphism is limited by already known or similar structural motifs (176, 190, 213, 214). As they may cause cross-reactive antibody production, these globally shared structural motifs as well as the conserved surface-exposed areas of VAR2CSA are of particular interest for the vaccine development (190, 196, 213). A summary of the structure and gene polymorphisms of individual DBL motifs are presented in **Table 2**.

Interaction of VAR2CSA and CSA

To test if individual domains of VAR2CSA can independently bind to CSA, the DBL domains of two *P. falciparum* laboratory strains, the 3D7 and FCR3 strains, have been produced recombinantly and their binding to immobilized CSA has been measured *in vitro*. Four domains (DBL2, DBL3, DBL5, and DBL6) which bind to CSA have been found (**Table 2**). However, the results vary depending on the study and strain: from the 3D7 strain DBL2 (188, 215–218), DBL3 (196, 206, 216, 218), DBL5 (215, 218), and DBL6 (188, 206, 215, 217) and from the FCR3 strain, only DBL2 (188, 217) and DBL3 (188, 196, 205, 217) bind to CSA (**Table 2**).

Binding specificity and affinity of individual DBL domains also differ greatly from that of the entire extracellular section of VAR2CSA. Although some authors have demonstrated CSA-specific binding (188, 205, 216), the addition of CSC (chondroitin sulfate C) or HA (hyaluron sulfate) affects the binding to CSA of individual DBL domains but not of the entire VAR2CSA protein (217). Furthermore, DBL3 and DBL6 domains of the 3D7 strain bind nonspecifically various glycosaminoglycans, especially those with high sulfonation and many negative charges (206). Compared to the entire extracellular part of VAR2CSA, the affinity of the individual domains to CSA is up to 100,000 times lower. While concentrations of the entire protein in the nanomolar range are sufficient to bind >50% of CSA, micromolar concentrations are necessary for individual domains (191, 219, 220). These results suggest that individual domains do not have the same functional capacity as the entire VAR2CSA protein and that a specific and highly affine CSA binding requires multiple domains. This has been supported by studies demonstrating that combined domains in the N-terminal region of VAR2CSA can bind CSA with similar affinity as the whole protein (191, 196). According to Clausen et al., the minimal CSA binding region is located in the small ID1-DBL2b range, with DBL2b reaching up to 93 amino acids into the ID2a segment. Since ID1-DBL2 does not bind to CSA and ID1-DBL2b binds with high affinity, these 93 amino acids of ID2a appear to play an important role in the interaction with CSA. Although the ID1 region does not seem to be essential for direct binding, it is essential for the formation of a functional CSA binding protein (193). In two other studies, the core region of binding was found in the multidomains DBL1-DBL2/DBL3 (191) and DBL2-ID2b (195). Except for DBL2-ID2b and DBL1-ID2b all VAR2CSA fragments show specificity for CSA (193, 195). In summary, by combining several N-terminal domains around DBL2, a high CSA specificity and affinity can be achieved (**Figure 2** and **Table 2**).

The spatial structure of VAR2CSA is very complex. In order to establish highly specific and affine binding to low sulfonated CSA, several domains of VAR2CSA appear to come into contact with each other and form a quaternary structure (210, 219, 220). This creates specific pockets, loops and structures that interact with the various functional groups of CSA (164). It can be assumed that VAR2CSA is an allosteric protein with positive cooperativity. This means that the binding of a functional CSA group to a domain of VAR2CSA changes the conformation of the protein in a way that the binding affinity for further CSA groups increases progressively (198).

Further Relevant Binding Structures

It is under discussion whether other receptors besides CSA, including hyaluron sulfate (HA) and the Fc part of non-specific antibodies, contribute to the pathogenesis of pregnancy malaria (221, 222). Placental isolates can also bind to HA *in vitro* and at least some *P. falciparum* strains recognize both CSA and HA (221, 223). Placental isolates from Uganda show binding to CSA, HA and non-specific IgG and IgM (224). Further studies confirm the binding of the Fc part of IgM to VAR2CSA, which supports the hypothesis of immune evasion via unspecific blocking (200, 225–227). Other studies did not find significant binding of placenta isolates to HA or IgG antibodies (187, 219, 220, 228). Furthermore, HA does not appear in intervillous space, indicating that an essential role in pathogenesis is unlikely (167). As CSA is currently considered the main receptor for placental parasites, vaccine development focusses on inhibiting CSA-VAR2CSA interaction (193, 228). However, additional interactions, such as the immune evasion of parasites by shielding with IgM, can strongly influence the success of a vaccine or may lead to development of novel targets (163, 225).

VAR2CSA for Vaccine Development

VAR2CSA is the leading candidate for a vaccine against malaria in pregnancy. Besides other preventive strategies the vaccine may be given to girls before puberty. This contact with the VAR2CSA protein leads to immunity against VAR2CSA-expressing *P. falciparum* which, in pregnancy, prevents the sequestration in the placenta (229).

Polymorphism and size (350 kDA) of VAR2CSA protein remain two major challenges that, thus far, have prevented the production of the entire protein for vaccination purposes (230). Therefore, the focus of current research is the identification of the minimal binding area within VAR2CSA, which has a high CSA binding affinity and specificity similar to that of the entire protein, and which simultaneously, induces broad binding-inhibitory antibody production (213).

As described before, this minimal binding region is located in the N-terminal region of VAR2CSA (191, 193, 195). Further studies have examined naturally acquired antibodies in multigravida in endemic regions (231–234) or the expression of antibodies against the VAR2CSA-CSA complex in laboratory animals and *in vitro* (195, 235–239). Two multidomains (ID1-ID2a, DBL1-DBL2) of VAR2CSA have been found as promising vaccine candidates (191, 193, 236, 238–240). They are part of two placental malaria vaccine projects, the PlacMalVac and PRIMALVAC project, which started phase I clinical trials in 2013 and 2016, respectively (241, 242). According to current information, PlacMalVac is safe, well-tolerated and a phase II clinical trial is under preparation (242, 243).

CONCLUSIONS

P. falciparum infection in pregnancy leads to a specific involvement of the placenta where infected erythrocytes express the unique antigen VAR2CSA which binds to CSA in the intervillous space leading to their sequestration. This process induces an inflammatory reaction of the placenta that activates monocytes to switch the release pattern of soluble factors. The consequences are manifold and include disorders of erythropoiesis, angiogenesis, blood flow, and nutrient transport which together impact placental growth, and finally, fetal growth.

The knowledge on the specific VAR2CSA expression and its detailed structure and binding to placental CSA has led to the development of novel vaccine strategies which have a high potential to reduce *P. falciparum* induced pregnancy disorders and IUGR in the near future.

AUTHOR CONTRIBUTIONS

UM has coordinated the writing and has done revisions and corrections on the manuscript. JS has written most parts of the manuscript. RF and DM-P have added the chapter on EV and miRNA and have done several modifications of the text. HS has critically read and corrected the manuscript.

REFERENCES

1. Brabin BJ. An analysis of malaria in pregnancy in Africa. *Bull World Health Organ.* (1983) 61:1005–16.
2. Schantz-Dunn J, Nour NM. Malaria and pregnancy: a global health perspective. *Rev Obstet Gynecol.* (2009) 2:186–92.
3. WHO. *Guidelines for the Treatment of Malaria.* Geneva: World Health Organization (2006).
4. Desai M, ter Kuile FO, Nosten F, McGready R, Asamoa K, Brabin B, et al. Epidemiology and burden of malaria in pregnancy. *Lancet Infect Dis.* (2007) 7:93–104. doi: 10.1016/S1473-3099(07)70021-X
5. Robinson DP, Klein SL. Pregnancy and pregnancy-associated hormones alter immune responses and disease pathogenesis. *Horm Behav.* (2012) 62:263–71. doi: 10.1016/j.yhbeh.2012.02.023
6. Lindsay S, Ansell J, Selman C, Cox V, Hamilton K, Walraven G. Effect of pregnancy on exposure to malaria mosquitoes. *Lancet.* (2000) 355:1972. doi: 10.1016/S0140-6736(00)02334-5
7. Rogerson SJ, Hviid L, Duffy PE, Leke RF, Taylor DW. Malaria in pregnancy: pathogenesis and immunity. *Lancet Infect Dis.* (2007) 7:105–17. doi: 10.1016/S1473-3099(07)70022-1
8. Rogerson SJ, Mwapasa V, Meshnick SR. Malaria in pregnancy: linking immunity and pathogenesis to prevention. *Am J Trop Med Hyg.* (2007) 77:14–22.
9. Warrell DA, Gilles HM. *Essential Malariology.* London: Arnold (2002).
10. McLean AR, Ataide R, Simpson JA, Beeson JG, Fowkes FJ. Malaria and immunity during pregnancy and postpartum: a tale of two species. *Parasitology.* (2015) 142:999–1015. doi: 10.1017/S0031182015000074
11. World Health Organization. *World Malaria Report 2018.* Geneva (2018).
12. Kayentao K, Garner P, van Eijk AM, Naidoo I, Roper C, Mulokozi A, et al. Intermittent preventive therapy for malaria during pregnancy using 2 vs 3 or more doses of sulfadoxine-pyrimethamine and risk of low birth weight in Africa: systematic review and meta-analysis. *JAMA.* (2013) 309:594–604. doi: 10.1001/jama.2012.216231
13. Saito M, Gilder ME, McGready R, Nosten F. Antimalarial drugs for treating and preventing malaria in pregnant and lactating women. *Expert Opin Drug Saf.* (2018) 17:1129–44. doi: 10.1080/14740338.2018.1535593
14. Moore KA, Simpson JA, Paw MK, Pimanpanarak M, Wiladphaingern J, Rijken MJ, et al. Safety of artemisinins in first trimester of prospectively followed pregnancies: an observational study. *Lancet Infect Dis.* (2016) 16:576–83. doi: 10.1016/S1473-3099(15)00547-2
15. Saveria T, Duffy PE, Fried M. Evaluation of pregnancy malaria vaccine candidates: the binding inhibition assay. *Methods Mol Biol.* (2015) 1325:231–9. doi: 10.1007/978-1-4939-2815-6_19
16. Dellicour S, Tatem AJ, Guerra CA, Snow RW, ter Kuile FO. Quantifying the number of pregnancies at risk of malaria in 2007: a demographic study. *PLoS Med.* (2010) 7:e1000221. doi: 10.1371/journal.pmed.1000221
17. Meeting of the Strategic Advisory Group of Experts on immunization, October 2015 - conclusions and recommendations. *Wkly Epidemiol Rec.* (2015) 90:681–99.
18. WHO. *WHA Global Nutrition Targets 2025: Low Birth Weight Policy Brief.* World Health Organisation, World Health Assembly, Geneva (2012).
19. Guyatt HL, Snow RW. Impact of malaria during pregnancy on low birth weight in sub-Saharan Africa. *Clin Microbiol Rev.* (2004) 17:760–9, table of contents. doi: 10.1128/CMR.17.4.760-769.2004
20. Oraneli BU, Okeke OC, Ubachukwu PO. Effect of placental malaria on birth weight of babies in Nnewi, Anambra state, Nigeria. *J Vector Borne Dis.* (2013) 50:13–7.
21. Cottrell G, Mary JY, Barro D, Cot M. The importance of the period of malarial infection during pregnancy on birth weight in tropical Africa. *Am J Trop Med Hyg.* (2007) 76:849–54. doi: 10.4269/ajtmh.2007.76.849
22. Kalilani L, Mofolo I, Chaponda M, Rogerson SJ, Meshnick SR. The effect of timing and frequency of *Plasmodium falciparum* infection during pregnancy on the risk of low birth weight and maternal anemia. *Trans R Soc Trop Med Hyg.* (2010) 104:416–22. doi: 10.1016/j.trstmh.2010.01.013
23. Huynh BT, Fievet N, Gbaguidi G, Dechavanne S, Borgella S, Guezo-Mevo B, et al. Influence of the timing of malaria infection during pregnancy on birth weight and on maternal anemia in Benin. *Am J Trop Med Hyg.* (2011) 85:214–20. doi: 10.4269/ajtmh.2011.11-0103
24. Landis SH, Lokomba V, Ananth CV, Atibu J, Ryder RW, Hartmann KE, et al. Impact of maternal malaria and under-nutrition on intrauterine growth restriction: a prospective ultrasound study in Democratic Republic of Congo. *Epidemiol Infect.* (2009) 137:294–304. doi: 10.1017/S0950268808000915
25. Steketee RW, Nahlen BL, Parise ME, Menendez C. The burden of malaria in pregnancy in malaria-endemic areas. *Am J Trop Med Hyg.* (2001) 64:28–35. doi: 10.4269/ajtmh.2001.64.28
26. Guyatt HL, Snow RW. The epidemiology and burden of *Plasmodium falciparum*-related anemia among pregnant women in sub-Saharan Africa. *Am J Trop Med Hyg.* (2001) 64:36–44. doi: 10.4269/ajtmh.2001.64.36
27. Uneke CJ. Impact of placental *Plasmodium falciparum* malaria on pregnancy and perinatal outcome in sub-Saharan Africa: part III: placental malaria, maternal health, public health. *Yale J Biol Med.* (2008) 81:1–7.
28. Achidi EA, Kuoh AJ, Minang JT, Ngum B, Achimbom BM, Motaze SC, et al. Malaria infection in pregnancy and its effects on haemoglobin levels in women from a malaria endemic area of Fako Division, South West Province, Cameroon. *J Obstet Gynaecol.* (2005) 25:235–40. doi: 10.1080/01443610500060628
29. Adam I, Elhassan EM, Haggaz AE, Ali AA, Adam GK. A perspective of the epidemiology of malaria and anaemia and their impact on maternal and perinatal outcomes in Sudan. *J Infect Dev Ctries.* (2011) 5:83–7. doi: 10.3855/jidc.1282
30. van den Broek NR, Letsky EA. Etiology of anemia in pregnancy in south Malawi. *Am J Clin Nutr.* (2000) 72:247S–56S.
31. Perkins DJ, Were T, Davenport GC, Kempaiah P, Hittner JB, Ong'echa JM. Severe malarial anemia: innate immunity and pathogenesis. *Int J Biol Sci.* (2011) 7:1427–42. doi: 10.7150/ijbs.7.1427
32. Jakeman GN, Saul A, Hogarth WL, Collins WE. Anaemia of acute malaria infections in non-immune patients primarily results from destruction of uninfected erythrocytes. *Parasitology.* (1999) 119(Pt 2):127–33. doi: 10.1017/S0031182099004564
33. Mohan K, Dubey ML, Ganguly NK, Mahajan RC. *Plasmodium falciparum*: role of activated blood monocytes in erythrocyte membrane damage and red cell loss during malaria. *Exp Parasitol.* (1995) 80:54–63. doi: 10.1006/expr.1995.1007
34. Ekvall H. Malaria and anemia. *Curr Opin Hematol.* (2003) 10:108–14. doi: 10.1097/00062752-200303000-00002

35. Biemba G, Gordeuk VR, Thuma PE, Mabeza GF, Weiss G. Prolonged macrophage activation and persistent anaemia in children with complicated malaria. *Trop Med Int Health.* (1998) 3:60–65. doi: 10.1046/j.1365-3156.1998.00168.x
36. Schofield L, Grau GE. Immunological processes in malaria pathogenesis. *Nat Rev Immunol.* (2005) 5:722–35. doi: 10.1038/nri1686
37. Dondorp AM, Angus BJ, Chotivanich K, Silamut K, Ruangveerayuth R, Hardeman MR, et al. Red blood cell deformability as a predictor of anemia in severe falciparum malaria. *Am J Trop Med Hyg.* (1999) 60:733–7. doi: 10.4269/ajtmh.1999.60.733
38. Dondorp AM, Angus BJ, Hardeman MR, Chotivanich KT, Silamut K, Ruangveerayuth R, et al. Prognostic significance of reduced red blood cell deformability in severe falciparum malaria. *Am J Trop Med Hyg.* (1997) 57:507–11. doi: 10.4269/ajtmh.1997.57.507
39. Waitumbi JN, Opollo MO, Muga RO, Misore AO, Stoute JA. Red cell surface changes and erythrophagocytosis in children with severe plasmodium falciparum anemia. *Blood.* (2000) 95:1481–6.
40. Odhiambo CO, Otieno W, Adhiambo C, Odera MM, Stoute JA. Increased deposition of C3b on red cells with low CR1 and CD55 in a malaria-endemic region of western Kenya: implications for the development of severe anemia. *BMC Med.* (2008) 6:23. doi: 10.1186/1741-7015-6-23
41. Kai OK, Roberts DJ. The pathophysiology of malarial anaemia: where have all the red cells gone? *BMC Med.* (2008) 6:24. doi: 10.1186/1741-7015-6-24
42. Awandare GA, Kempaiah P, Ochiel DO, Piazza P, Keller CC, Perkins DJ. Mechanisms of erythropoiesis inhibition by malarial pigment and malaria-induced proinflammatory mediators in an *in vitro* model. *Am J Hematol.* (2011) 86:155–62. doi: 10.1002/ajh.21933
43. Casals-Pascual C, Kai O, Cheung JO, Williams S, Lowe B, Nyanoti M, et al. Suppression of erythropoiesis in malarial anemia is associated with hemozoin *in vitro* and *in vivo*. *Blood.* (2006) 108:2569–77. doi: 10.1182/blood-2006-05-018697
44. Lamikanra AA, Theron M, Kooij TW, Roberts DJ. Hemozoin (malarial pigment) directly promotes apoptosis of erythroid precursors. *PLoS ONE.* (2009) 4:e8446. doi: 10.1371/journal.pone.0008446
45. Keller CC, Kremsner PG, Hittner JB, Misukonis MA, Weinberg JB, Perkins DJ. Elevated nitric oxide production in children with malarial anemia: hemozoin-induced nitric oxide synthase type 2 transcripts and nitric oxide in blood mononuclear cells. *Infect Immun.* (2004) 72:4868–73. doi: 10.1128/IAI.72.8.4868-4873.2004
46. Kurtzhals JA, Adabayeri V, Goka BQ, Akanmori BD, Oliver-Commey JO, Nkrumah FK, et al. Low plasma concentrations of interleukin 10 in severe malarial anaemia compared with cerebral and uncomplicated malaria. *Lancet.* (1998) 351:1768–72. doi: 10.1016/S0140-6736(97)09439-7
47. Lyke KE, Burges R, Cissoko Y, Sangare L, Dao M, Diarra I, et al. Serum levels of the proinflammatory cytokines interleukin-1 beta (IL-1beta), IL-6, IL-8, IL-10, tumor necrosis factor alpha, and IL-12(p70) in Malian children with severe *Plasmodium falciparum* malaria and matched uncomplicated malaria or healthy controls. *Infect Immun.* (2004) 72:5630–7. doi: 10.1128/IAI.72.10.5630-5637.2004
48. Perkins DJ, Weinberg JB, Kremsner PG. Reduced interleukin-12 and transforming growth factor-beta1 in severe childhood malaria: relationship of cytokine balance with disease severity. *J Infect Dis.* (2000) 182:988–92. doi: 10.1086/315762
49. Othoro C, Lal AA, Nahlen B, Koech D, Orago AS, Udhayakumar V. A low interleukin-10 tumor necrosis factor-alpha ratio is associated with malaria anemia in children residing in a holoendemic malaria region in western Kenya. *J Infect Dis.* (1999) 179:279–82. doi: 10.1086/314548
50. Fried M, Muga RO, Misore AO, Duffy PE. Malaria elicits type 1 cytokines in the human placenta: IFN-gamma and TNF-alpha associated with pregnancy outcomes. *J Immunol.* (1998) 160:2523–30.
51. Chandrasiri UP, Randall LM, Saad AA, Bashir AM, Rogerson SJ, Adam I. Low antibody levels to pregnancy-specific malaria antigens and heightened cytokine responses associated with severe malaria in pregnancy. *J Infect Dis.* (2014) 209:1408–17. doi: 10.1093/infdis/jit646
52. Ludwiczek S, Aigner E, Theurl I, Weiss G. Cytokine-mediated regulation of iron transport in human monocytic cells. *Blood.* (2003) 101:4148–54. doi: 10.1182/blood-2002-08-2459
53. Nweneka CV, Doherty CP, Cox S, Prentice A. Iron delocalisation in the pathogenesis of malarial anaemia. *Trans R Soc Trop Med Hyg.* (2010) 104:175–84. doi: 10.1016/j.trstmh.2009.08.007
54. Ganz T, Nemeth E. Hepcidin and iron homeostasis. Biochim Biophys Acta (2012) 1823:1434–43. doi: 10.1016/j.bbamcr.2012.01.014
55. Nemeth E, Rivera S, Gabayan V, Keller C, Taudorf S, Pedersen BK, et al. IL-6 mediates hypoferremia of inflammation by inducing the synthesis of the iron regulatory hormone hepcidin. *J Clin Invest.* (2004) 113:1271–6. doi: 10.1172/JCI200420945
56. de Mast Q, van Dongen-Lases EC, Swinkels DW, Nieman AE, Roestenberg M, Druilhe P, et al. Mild increases in serum hepcidin and interleukin-6 concentrations impair iron incorporation in haemoglobin during an experimental human malaria infection. *Br J Haematol.* (2009) 145:657–64. doi: 10.1111/j.1365-2141.2009.07664.x
57. Kidanto HL, Mogren I, Lindmark G, Massawe S, Nystrom L. Risks for preterm delivery and low birth weight are independently increased by severity of maternal anaemia. *S Afr Med J.* (2009) 99:98–102.
58. Boeuf P, Tan A, Romagosa C, Radford J, Mwapasa V, Molyneux ME, et al. Placental hypoxia during placental malaria. *J Infect Dis.* (2008) 197:757–65. doi: 10.1086/526521
59. Kozuki N, Lee AC, Katz J. Child Health Epidemiology Reference Group. Moderate to severe, but not mild, maternal anemia is associated with increased risk of small-for-gestational-age outcomes. *J Nutr.* (2012) 142:358–62. doi: 10.3945/jn.111.149237
60. Uneke CJ. Impact of placental *Plasmodium falciparum* malaria on pregnancy and perinatal outcome in sub-Saharan Africa: II: effects of placental malaria on perinatal outcome; malaria and HIV. *Yale J Biol Med.* (2007) 80:95–103.
61. Ismail MR, Ordi J, Menendez C, Ventura PJ, Aponte JJ, Kahigwa E, et al. Placental pathology in malaria: a histological, immunohistochemical, and quantitative study. *Hum Pathol.* (2000) 31:85–93. doi: 10.1016/S0046-8177(00)80203-8
62. Walter PR, Garin Y, Blot P. Placental pathologic changes in malaria. A histologic and ultrastructural study. *Am J Pathol.* (1982) 109:330–42.
63. Brabin BJ, Romagosa C, Abdelgalil S, Menendez C, Verhoeff FH, McGready R, et al. The sick placenta-the role of malaria. *Placenta.* (2004) 25:359–78. doi: 10.1016/j.placenta.2003.10.019
64. Bulmer JN, Rasheed FN, Francis N, Morrison L, Greenwood BM. Placental malaria. I. Pathological classification. *Histopathology.* (1993) 22:211–8. doi: 10.1111/j.1365-2559.1993.tb00110.x
65. Yamada M, Steketee R, Abramowsky C, Kida M, Wirima J, Heymann D, et al. *Plasmodium falciparum* associated placental pathology: a light and electron microscopic and immunohistologic study. *Am J Trop Med Hyg.* (1989) 41:161–8. doi: 10.4269/ajtmh.1989.41.161
66. Fievet N, Moussa M, Tami G, Maubert B, Cot M, Deloron P, et al. *Plasmodium falciparum* induces a Th1/Th2 disequilibrium, favoring the Th1-type pathway, in the human placenta. *J Infect Dis.* (2001) 183:1530–4. doi: 10.1086/320201
67. King C. L., May K., Mostertz J., Paprotka K., Fraunholz M., Grube M, et al. Adherence of plasmodium falciparum infected red cells to the trophoblast and placental inflammatory response studied by dual *ex vivo* perfusion of an isolated cotyledon. *Placenta.* (2010) 117.
68. Abrams ET, Brown H, Chensue SW, Turner GD, Tadesse E, Lema VM, et al. Host response to malaria during pregnancy: placental monocyte recruitment is associated with elevated beta chemokine expression. *J Immunol.* (2003) 170:2759–64. doi: 10.4049/jimmunol.170.5.2759
69. Chaisavaneeyakorn S, Moore JM, Mirel L, Othoro C, Otieno J, Chaiyaroj SC, et al. Levels of macrophage inflammatory protein 1 alpha (MIP-1 alpha) and MIP-1 beta in intervillous blood plasma samples from women with placental malaria and human immunodeficiency virus infection. *Clin Diagn Lab Immunol.* (2003) 10:631–6.
70. Lucchi NW, Peterson DS, Moore JM. Immunologic activation of human syncytiotrophoblast by *Plasmodium falciparum*. *Malar J.* (2008) 7:42. doi: 10.1186/1475-2875-7-42
71. Suguitan AL Jr, Leke RG, Fouda G, Zhou A, Thuita L, Metenou S, et al. Changes in the levels of chemokines and cytokines in the placentas of women with *Plasmodium falciparum* malaria. *J Infect Dis.* (2003) 188:1074–82. doi: 10.1086/378500

72. Chua CL, Brown G, Hamilton JA, Rogerson S, Boeuf P. Monocytes and macrophages in malaria: protection or pathology? *Trends Parasitol.* (2013) 29:26–34. doi: 10.1016/j.pt.2012.10.002
73. Muehlenbachs A, Fried M, McGready R, Harrington WE, Mutabingwa TK, Nosten F, et al. A novel histological grading scheme for placental malaria applied in areas of high and low malaria transmission. *J Infect Dis.* (2010) 202:1608–16. doi: 10.1086/656723
74. Rogerson SJ, Pollina E, Getachew A, Tadesse E, Lema VM, Molyneux ME. Placental monocyte infiltrates in response to *Plasmodium falciparum* malaria infection and their association with adverse pregnancy outcomes. *Am J Trop Med Hyg.* (2003) 68:115–9. doi: 10.4269/ajtmh.2003.68.1.0680115
75. Rogerson SJ, Mkundika P, Kanjala MK. Diagnosis of *Plasmodium falciparum* malaria at delivery: comparison of blood film preparation methods and of blood films with histology. *J Clin Microbiol.* (2003) 41:1370–4. doi: 10.1128/JCM.41.4.1370-1374.2003
76. Shulman CE, Marshall T, Dorman EK, Bulmer JN, Cutts F, Peshu N, et al. Malaria in pregnancy: adverse effects on haemoglobin levels and birthweight in primigravidae and multigravidae. *Trop Med Int Health.* (2001) 6:770–8. doi: 10.1046/j.1365-3156.2001.00786.x
77. Menendez C, Ordi J, Ismail MR, Ventura PJ, Aponte JJ, Kahigwa E, et al. The impact of placental malaria on gestational age and birth weight. *J Infect Dis.* (2000) 181:1740–5. doi: 10.1086/315449
78. Ordi J, Menendez C, Ismail MR, Ventura PJ, Palacin A, Kahigwa E, et al. Placental malaria is associated with cell-mediated inflammatory responses with selective absence of natural killer cells. *J Infect Dis.* (2001) 183:1100–7. doi: 10.1086/319295
79. Othoro C, Moore JM, Wannemuehler KA, Moses S, Lal A, Otieno J, et al. Elevated gamma interferon-producing NK cells, CD45RO memory-like T cells, and CD4 T cells are associated with protection against malaria infection in pregnancy. *Infect Immun.* (2008) 76:1678–85. doi: 10.1128/IAI.01420-07
80. Bouyou-Akotet MK, Issifou S, Meye JF, Kombila M, Ngou-Milama E, Luty AJ, et al. Depressed natural killer cell cytotoxicity against *Plasmodium falciparum*-infected erythrocytes during first pregnancies. *Clin Infect Dis.* (2004) 38:342–7. doi: 10.1086/380646
81. Sartelet H, Schleiermacher D, Le-Hesran JY, Graesslin O, Gaillard D, Fe M, et al. Less HLA-G expression in *Plasmodium falciparum*-infected third trimester placentas is associated with more natural killer cells. *Placenta.* (2005) 26:505–11. doi: 10.1016/j.placenta.2004.08.006
82. Agudelo OM, Aristizabal BH, Yanow SK, Arango E, Carmona-Fonseca J, Maestre A. Submicroscopic infection of placenta by Plasmodium produces Th1/Th2 cytokine imbalance, inflammation and hypoxia in women from north-west Colombia. *Malar J.* (2014) 13:122. doi: 10.1186/1475-2875-13-122
83. Diouf I, Fievet N, Doucoure S, Ngom M, Andrieu M, Mathieu JF, et al. IL-12 producing monocytes and IFN-gamma and TNF-alpha producing T-lymphocytes are increased in placentas infected by *Plasmodium falciparum. J Reprod Immunol.* (2007) 74:152–62. doi: 10.1016/j.jri.2006.10.001
84. Kabyemela ER, Muehlenbachs A, Fried M, Kurtis JD, Mutabingwa TK, Duffy PE. Maternal peripheral blood level of IL-10 as a marker for inflammatory placental malaria. *Malar J.* (2008) 7:26. doi: 10.1186/1475-2875-7-26
85. Moore JM, Nahlen BL, Misore A, Lal AA, Udhayakumar V. Immunity to placental malaria. I. Elevated production of interferon-gamma by placental blood mononuclear cells is associated with protection in an area with high transmission of malaria. *J Infect Dis.* (1999) 179:1218–25. doi: 10.1086/314737
86. Moormann AM, Sullivan AD, Rochford RA, Chensue SW, Bock PJ, Nyirenda T, et al. Malaria and pregnancy: placental cytokine expression and its relationship to intrauterine growth retardation. *J Infect Dis.* (1999) 180:1987–93. doi: 10.1086/315135
87. Rogerson SJ, Brown HC, Pollina E, Abrams ET, Tadesse E, Lema VM, et al. Placental tumor necrosis factor alpha but not gamma interferon is associated with placental malaria and low birth weight in Malawian women. *Infect Immun.* (2003) 71:267–70. doi: 10.1128/IAI.71.1.267-270.2003
88. Bouyou-Akotet MK, Mavoungou E. Natural killer cell IFN-gamma-activity is associated with *Plasmodium falciparum* infection during pregnancy. *Exp Parasitol.* (2009) 123:265–8. doi: 10.1016/j.exppara.2009.07.011
89. Megnekou R, Tenou S, Bigoga JD, Djontu JC, Medou FM, Lissom A. Placental malaria and modulation of immune and hormonal responses in Cameroonian women. *Acta Trop.* (2015) 147:23–30. doi: 10.1016/j.actatropica.2015.04.001
90. Chene A, Briand V, Ibitokou S, Dechavanne S, Massougbodji A, Deloron P, et al. Placental cytokine and chemokine profiles reflect pregnancy outcomes in women exposed to *Plasmodium falciparum* infection. *Infect Immun.* (2014) 82:3783–9. doi: 10.1128/IAI.01922-14
91. Suguitan AL, Jr., Cadigan TJ, Nguyen TA, Zhou A, Leke RJ, Metenou S, et al. Malaria-associated cytokine changes in the placenta of women with pre-term deliveries in Yaounde, Cameroon. *Am J Trop Med Hyg.* (2003) 69:574–81. doi: 10.4269/ajtmh.2003.69.574
92. Megnekou R, Djontu JC, Bigoga JD, Lissom A, Magagoum SH. Role of some biomarkers in placental malaria in women living in Yaounde, Cameroon. *Acta Trop.* (2015) 141:97–102. doi: 10.1016/j.actatropica.2014.10.007
93. Poovassery JS, Sarr D, Smith G, Nagy T, Moore JM. Malaria-induced murine pregnancy failure: distinct roles for IFN-gamma and TNF. *J Immunol.* (2009) 183:5342–9. doi: 10.4049/jimmunol.0901669
94. Napso T, H.Yong EJ, Lopez-Tello J, Sferruzzi-Perri AN. The role of placental hormones in mediating maternal adaptations to support pregnancy and lactation. *Front Physiol.* (2018) 9:1091. doi: 10.3389/fphys.2018.01091
95. Clifton VL, Cuffe J, Moritz KM, Cole TJ, Fuller PJ, Lu NZ, et al. Review: The role of multiple placental glucocorticoid receptor isoforms in adapting to the maternal environment and regulating fetal growth. *Placenta.* (2017) 54:24–29. doi: 10.1016/j.placenta.2016.12.017
96. Calcagni E, Elenkov I. Stress system activity, innate and T helper cytokines, and susceptibility to immune-related diseases. *Ann N Y Acad Sci.* (2006) 1069:62–76. doi: 10.1196/annals.1351.006
97. Díaz L, Díaz-Muñoz M, González L, Lira-Albarrán S, Larrea F, Méndez I. *Prolactin in the Immune System* (2013). p. 53–82.
98. Bayoumi NK, Elhassan EM, Elbashir MI, Adam I. Cortisol, prolactin, cytokines and the susceptibility of pregnant Sudanese women to *Plasmodium falciparum* malaria. *Ann Trop Med Parasitol.* (2009) 103:111–7. doi: 10.1179/136485909X385045
99. Bouyou-Akotet MK, Adegnika AA, Agnandji ST, Ngou-Milama E, Kombila M, Kremsner PG, et al. Cortisol and susceptibility to malaria during pregnancy. *Microbes Infect.* (2005) 7:1217–23. doi: 10.1016/j.micinf.2005.04.008
100. Watkinson M, Rushton DI, Lunn PG. Placental malaria and foetoplacental function: low plasma oestradiols associated with malarial pigmentation of the placenta. *Trans R Soc Trop Med Hyg.* (1985) 79:448–50. doi: 10.1016/0035-9203(85)90059-8
101. Mavoungou E, Bouyou-Akotet MK, Kremsner PG. Effects of prolactin and cortisol on natural killer (NK) cell surface expression and function of human natural cytotoxicity receptors (NKp46, NKp44 and NKp30). *Clin Exp Immunol.* (2005) 139:287–96. doi: 10.1111/j.1365-2249.2004.02686.x
102. Dorman EK, Shulman CE, Kingdom J, Bulmer JN, Mwendwa J, Peshu N, et al. Impaired uteroplacental blood flow in pregnancies complicated by falciparum malaria. *Ultrasound Obstet Gynecol.* (2002) 19:165–70. doi: 10.1046/j.0960-7692.2001.00545.x
103. Umbers AJ, Aitken EH, Rogerson SJ. Malaria in pregnancy: small babies, big problem. *Trends Parasitol.* (2011) 27:168–75. doi: 10.1016/j.pt.2011.01.007
104. Silver KL, Zhong K, Leke RG, Taylor DW. Kain KC. Dysregulation of angiopoietins is associated with placental malaria and low birth weight. *PLoS ONE.* (2010) 5:e9481. doi: 10.1371/journal.pone.0009481
105. Ataide R, Murillo O, Dombrowski JG, Souza RM, Lima FA, Lima GF, et al. Malaria in pregnancy interacts with and alters the angiogenic profiles of the placenta. *PLoS Negl Trop Dis.* (2015) 9:e0003824. doi: 10.1371/journal.pntd.0003824
106. Girardi G. Complement inhibition keeps mothers calm and avoids fetal rejection. *Immunol Invest.* (2008) 37:645–59. doi: 10.1080/08820130802191615
107. Girardi G, Yarilin D, Thurman JM, Holers VM, Salmon JE. Complement activation induces dysregulation of angiogenic factors and causes fetal rejection and growth restriction. *J Exp Med.* (2006) 203:2165–75. doi: 10.1084/jem.20061022
108. Conroy A, Serghides L, Finney C, Owino SO, Kumar S, Gowda DC, et al. C5a enhances dysregulated inflammatory and angiogenic responses to malaria *in*

vitro: potential implications for placental malaria. *PLoS ONE*. (2009) 4:e4953. doi: 10.1371/journal.pone.0004953
109. Conroy AL, Silver KL, Zhong K, Rennie M, Ward P, Sarma JV, et al. Complement activation and the resulting placental vascular insufficiency drives fetal growth restriction associated with placental malaria. *Cell Host Microbe*. (2013) 13:215–26. doi: 10.1016/j.chom.2013.01.010
110. Umbers AJ, Boeuf P, Clapham C, Stanisic DI, Baiwog F, Mueller I, et al. Placental malaria-associated inflammation disturbs the insulin-like growth factor axis of fetal growth regulation. *J Infect Dis*. (2011) 203:561–9. doi: 10.1093/infdis/jiq080
111. Brabin BJ, Johnson PM. Placental malaria and pre-eclampsia through the looking glass backwards? *J Reprod Immunol*. (2005) 65:1–15. doi: 10.1016/j.jri.2004.09.006
112. Roberts JM, Lain KY. Recent Insights into the pathogenesis of pre-eclampsia. *Placenta*. (2002) 23:359–72. doi: 10.1053/plac.2002.0819
113. Gueneuc A, Deloron P, Bertin GI. Usefulness of a biomarker to identify placental dysfunction in the context of malaria. *Malar J*. (2017) 16:11. doi: 10.1186/s12936-016-1664-0
114. Muehlenbachs A, Mutabingwa TK, Edmonds S, Fried M, Duffy PE. Hypertension and maternal-fetal conflict during placental malaria. *PLoS Med*. (2006) 3:e446. doi: 10.1371/journal.pmed.0030446
115. Silver KL, Conroy AL, Leke RG, Leke RJ, Gwanmesia P, Molyneux ME, et al. Circulating soluble endoglin levels in pregnant women in Cameroon and Malawi–associations with placental malaria and fetal growth restriction. *PLoS ONE*. (2011) 6:e24985. doi: 10.1371/journal.pone.0024985
116. Ndao CT, Dumont A, Fievet N, Doucoure S, Gaye A, Lehesran JY. Placental malarial infection as a risk factor for hypertensive disorders during pregnancy in Africa: a case-control study in an urban area of Senegal, West Africa. *Am J Epidemiol*. (2009) 170:847–53. doi: 10.1093/aje/kwp207
117. Xiao R, Sorensen TK, Williams MA, Luthy DA. Influence of pre-eclampsia on fetal growth. *J Matern Fetal Neonatal Med*. (2003) 13:157–62. doi: 10.1080/jmf.13.3.157.162
118. Boeuf P, Aitken EH, Chandrasiri U, Chua CL, McInerney B, McQuade L, et al. *Plasmodium falciparum* malaria elicits inflammatory responses that dysregulate placental amino acid transport. *PLoS Pathog*. (2013) 9:e1003153. doi: 10.1371/journal.ppat.1003153
119. Dimasuay KG, Aitken EH, Rosario F, Njie M, Glazier J, Rogerson SJ, et al. Inhibition of placental mTOR signaling provides a link between placental malaria and reduced birthweight. *BMC Med*. (2017) 15:1. doi: 10.1186/s12916-016-0759-3
120. Jansson N, Pettersson J, Haafiz A, Ericsson A, Palmberg I, Tranberg M, et al. Down-regulation of placental transport of amino acids precedes the development of intrauterine growth restriction in rats fed a low protein diet. *J Physiol*. (2006) 576:935–46. doi: 10.1113/jphysiol.2006.116509
121. Glazier JD, Cetin I, Perugino G, Ronzoni S, Grey AM, Mahendran D, et al. Association between the activity of the system A amino acid transporter in the microvillous plasma membrane of the human placenta and severity of fetal compromise in intrauterine growth restriction. *Pediatr Res*. (1997) 42:514–9. doi: 10.1203/00006450-199710000-00016
122. Jansson T, Ylven K, Wennergren M, Powell TL. Glucose transport and system A activity in syncytiotrophoblast microvillous and basal plasma membranes in intrauterine growth restriction. *Placenta*. (2002) 23:392–9. doi: 10.1053/plac.2002.0826
123. Jones HN, Jansson T, Powell TL. IL-6 stimulates system A amino acid transporter activity in trophoblast cells through STAT3 and increased expression of SNAT2. *Am J Physiol Cell Physiol*. (2009) 297:C1228-35. doi: 10.1152/ajpcell.00195.2009
124. Thongsong B, Subramanian RK, Ganapathy V, Prasad PD. Inhibition of amino acid transport system a by interleukin-1beta in trophoblasts. *J Soc Gynecol Investig*. (2005) 12:495–503. doi: 10.1016/j.jsgi.2005.06.008
125. Karl PI. Insulin-like growth factor-1 stimulates amino acid uptake by the cultured human placental trophoblast. *J Cell Physiol*. (1995) 165:83–8. doi: 10.1002/jcp.1041650111
126. Chandrasiri UP, Chua CL, Umbers AJ, Chaluluka E, Glazier JD, Rogerson SJ, et al. Insight into the pathogenesis of fetal growth restriction in placental malaria: decreased placental glucose transporter isoform 1 expression. *J Infect Dis*. (2014) 209:1663–7. doi: 10.1093/infdis/jit803
127. Alberts B, Johnson A, Lewis J, Morgan D, Raff M, Roberts K, et al. *Molekularbiologie der Zelle*. New York, NY: John Wiley & Sons (2011).
128. Gordon MC, Zimmerman PD, Landon MB, Gabbe SG, Kniss DA. Insulin and glucose modulate glucose transporter messenger ribonucleic acid expression and glucose uptake in trophoblasts isolated from first-trimester chorionic villi. *Am J Obstet Gynecol*. (1995) 173:1089–97. doi: 10.1016/0002-9378(95)91332-7
129. Hotamisligil GS, Murray DL, Choy LN, Spiegelman BM. Tumor necrosis factor alpha inhibits signaling from the insulin receptor. *Proc Natl Acad Sci USA*. (1994) 91:4854–8. doi: 10.1073/pnas.91.11.4854
130. Zamudio S, Baumann MU, Illsley NP. Effects of chronic hypoxia *in vivo* on the expression of human placental glucose transporters. *Placenta*. (2006) 27:49–55. doi: 10.1016/j.placenta.2004.12.010
131. Ospina-Prieto S, Chaiwangyen W, Herrmann J, Groten T, Schleussner E, Markert UR, et al. MicroRNA-141 is upregulated in preeclamptic placentae and regulates trophoblast invasion and intercellular communication. *Transl Res*. (2016) 172:61–72. doi: 10.1016/j.trsl.2016.02.012
132. Tannetta DS, Hunt K, Jones CI, Davidson N, Coxon CH, Ferguson D, et al. Syncytiotrophoblast extracellular vesicles from pre-eclampsia placentas differentially affect platelet function. *PLoS ONE*. (2015) 10:e0142538. doi: 10.1371/journal.pone0142538
133. Cronqvist T, Tannetta D, Morgelin M, Belting M, Sargent I, Familari M, et al. Syncytiotrophoblast derived extracellular vesicles transfer functional placental miRNAs to primary human endothelial cells. *Sci Rep*. (2017) 7:4558. doi: 10.1038/s41598-017-04468-0
134. Tong M, Stanley JL, Chen Q, James JL, Stone PR, Chamley LW. Placental nano-vesicles target to specific organs and modulate vascular tone *in vivo*. *Hum Reprod*. (2017) 32:2188–98. doi: 10.1093/humrep/dex310
135. Miranda J, Paules C, Nair S, Lai A, Palma C, Scholz-Romero K, et al. Placental exosomes profile in maternal and fetal circulation in intrauterine growth restriction - Liquid biopsies to monitoring fetal growth. *Placenta*. (2018) 64:34–43. doi: 10.1016/j.placenta.2018.02.006
136. Moro L, Bardají A, Macete E, Barrios D, Morales-Prieto DM, España C, et al. Placental microparticles and microRNAs in pregnant women with *Plasmodium falciparum* or HIV infection. *PLoS ONE*. (2016) 11:e0146361. doi: 10.1371/journal.pone.0146361
137. Morales-Prieto DM, Chaiwangyen W, Ospina-Prieto S, Schneider U, Herrmann J, Gruhn B, et al. MicroRNA expression profiles of trophoblastic cells. *Placenta*. (2012) 33:725–34. doi: 10.1016/j.placenta.2012.05.009
138. Gu Y, Sun J, Groome LJ, Wang Y. Differential miRNA expression profiles between the first and third trimester human placentas. *Am J Physiol Endocrinol Metab*. (2013) 304:E836–43. doi: 10.1152/ajpendo.00660.2012
139. Morales-Prieto DM, Ospina-Prieto S, Schmidt A, Chaiwangyen W, Markert UR. Elsevier Trophoblast Research Award Lecture: origin, evolution and future of placenta miRNAs. *Placenta*. (2014) 35(Suppl.):S39–45. doi: 10.1016/j.placenta.2013.11.017
140. Maccani MA, Padbury JF, Marsit CJ. miR-16 and miR-21 expression in the placenta is associated with fetal growth. *PLoS ONE*. (2011) 6:e21210. doi: 10.1371/journal.pone.0021210
141. Chiofalo B, Laganà AS, Vaiarelli A, La Rosa VL, Rossetti D, Palmara V, et al. Do miRNAs play a role in fetal growth restriction? A fresh look to a busy corner. *Biomed Res Int*. (2017) 2017:6073167. doi: 10.1155/2017/6073167
142. Tang Q, Wu W, Xu X, Huang L, Gao Q, Chen H, et al. miR-141 contributes to fetal growth restriction by regulating PLAG1 expression. *PLoS ONE*. (2013) 8:e58737. doi: 10.1371/journal.pone.0058737
143. Higashijima A, Miura K, Mishima H, Kinoshita A, Jo O, Abe S, et al. Characterization of placenta-specific microRNAs in fetal growth restriction pregnancy. *Prenat Diagn*. (2013) 33:214–22. doi: 10.1002/pd.4045
144. Xie L, Sadovsky Y. The function of miR-519d in cell migration, invasion, and proliferation suggests a role in early placentation. *Placenta*. (2016) 48:34–37. doi: 10.1016/j.placenta.2016.10.004
145. Zhang M, Muralimanoharan S, Wortman AC, Mendelson CR. Primate-specific miR-515 family members inhibit key genes in human trophoblast differentiation and are upregulated in preeclampsia. *Proc Natl Acad Sci USA*. (2016) 113:E7069–76. doi: 10.1073/pnas.1607849113
146. Ouyang Y, Bayer A, Chu T, Tyurin VA, Kagan VE, Morelli AE, et al. Isolation of human trophoblastic extracellular vesicles and

characterization of their cargo and antiviral activity. *Placenta.* (2016) 47:86–95. doi: 10.1016/j.placenta.2016.09.008

147. Bayer A, Lennemann NJ, Ouyang Y, Sadovsky E, Sheridan MA, Roberts RM, et al. Chromosome 19 microRNAs exert antiviral activity independent from type III interferon signaling. *Placenta.* (2018) 61:33–38. doi: 10.1016/j.placenta.2017.11.004
148. Mouillet JF, Ouyang Y, Bayer A, Coyne CB, Sadovsky Y. The role of trophoblastic microRNAs in placental viral infection. *Int J Dev Biol.* (2014) 58:281–9. doi: 10.1387/ijdb.130349ys
149. Anton L, Olarerin-George AO, Hogenesch JB, Elovitz MA. Placental expression of miR-517a/b and miR-517c contributes to trophoblast dysfunction and preeclampsia. *PLoS ONE.* (2015) 10:e0122707. doi: 10.1371/journal.pone.0122707
150. Nantakomol D, Dondorp AM, Krudsood S, Udomsangpetch R, Pattanapanyasat K, Combes V, et al. Circulating red cell-derived microparticles in human malaria. *J Infect Dis.* (2011) 203:700–6. doi: 10.1093/infdis/jiq104
151. Sahu U, Sahoo PK, Kar SK, Mohapatra BN, Ranjit M. Association of TNF level with production of circulating cellular microparticles during clinical manifestation of human cerebral malaria. *Hum Immunol.* (2013) 74:713–21. doi: 10.1016/j.humimm.2013.02.006
152. Li JJ, Huang MJ, Li Z, Li W, Wang F, Wang L, et al. Identification of potential whole blood MicroRNA biomarkers for the blood stage of adult imported falciparum malaria through integrated mRNA and miRNA expression profiling. *Biochem Biophys Res Commun.* (2018) 506:471–7. doi: 10.1016/j.bbrc.2018.10.072
153. Glinsky GV. SNP-guided microRNA maps (MirMaps) of 16 common human disorders identify a clinically accessible therapy reversing transcriptional aberrations of nuclear import and inflammasome pathways. *Cell Cycle.* (2008) 7:3564–76. doi: 10.4161/cc.7.22.7073
154. World Health Organization. *The World Malaria Report 2017.* Geneva (2017).
155. Levy M, Buskila D, Gladman DD, Urowitz MB, Koren G. Pregnancy outcome following first trimester exposure to chloroquine. *Am J Perinatol.* (1991) 8:174–8. doi: 10.1055/s-2007-999371
156. Rathjen T, Nicol C, McConkey G, Dalmay T. Analysis of short RNAs in the malaria parasite and its red blood cell host. *FEBS Lett.* (2006) 580:5185–8. doi: 10.1016/j.febslet.2006.08.063
157. Xue X, Zhang Q, Huang Y, Feng L, Pan W. No miRNA were found in Plasmodium and the ones identified in erythrocytes could not be correlated with infection. *Malar J* .(2008) 7:47. doi: 10.1186/1475-2875-7-47
158. LaMonte G, Philip N, Reardon J, Lacsina JR, Majoros W, Chapman L, et al. Translocation of sickle cell erythrocyte microRNAs into *Plasmodium falciparum* inhibits parasite translation and contributes to malaria resistance. *Cell Host Microbe.* (2012) 12:187–99. doi: 10.1016/j.chom.2012.06.007
159. Wang Z, Xi J, Hao X, Deng W, Liu J, Wei C, et al. Red blood cells release microparticles containing human argonaute 2 and miRNAs to target genes of *Plasmodium falciparum. Emerg Microbes Infect.* (2017) 6:e75. doi: 10.1038/emi.2017.63
160. Mantel PY, Hoang AN, Goldowitz I, Potashnikova D, Hamza B, Vorobjev I, et al. Malaria-infected erythrocyte-derived microvesicles mediate cellular communication within the parasite population and with the host immune system. *Cell Host Microbe.* (2013) 13:521–534. doi: 10.1016/j.chom.2013.04.009
161. Mouillet JF, Chu T, Hubel CA, Nelson DM, Parks WT, Sadovsky Y. The levels of hypoxia-regulated microRNAs in plasma of pregnant women with fetal growth restriction. *Placenta.* (2010) 31:781–4. doi: 10.1016/j.placenta.2010.07.001
162. Doritchamou J, Sossou-tchatcha S, Cottrell G, Moussiliou A, Hounton Houngbeme C, Massougbodji A, et al. Dynamics in the cytoadherence phenotypes of *Plasmodium falciparum* infected erythrocytes isolated during pregnancy. *PLoS ONE.* (2014) 9:e98577. doi: 10.1371/journal.pone.0098577
163. Pehrson C, Mathiesen L, Heno KK, Salanti A, Resende M, Dzikowski R, et al. Adhesion of *Plasmodium falciparum* infected erythrocytes in *ex vivo* perfused placental tissue: a novel model of placental malaria. *Malar J.* (2016) 15:292. doi: 10.1186/s12936-016-1342-2
164. Goel S, Gowda DC. How specific is *Plasmodium falciparum* adherence to chondroitin 4-sulfate? *Trends Parasitol.* (2011) 27:375–81. doi: 10.1016/j.pt.2011.03.005
165. Fried M, Duffy PE. Adherence of *Plasmodium falciparum* to chondroitin sulfate A in the human placenta. *Science.* (1996) 272:1502–4. doi: 10.1126/science.272.5267.1502
166. Muthusamy A, Achur RN, Bhavanandan VP, Fouda GG, Taylor DW, Gowda DC. *Plasmodium falciparum*-infected erythrocytes adhere both in the intervillous space and on the villous surface of human placenta by binding to the low-sulfated chondroitin sulfate proteoglycan receptor. *Am J Pathol.* (2004) 164:2013–25. doi: 10.1016/S0002-9440(10)63761-3
167. Muthusamy A, Achur RN, Valiyaveettil M, Botti JJ, Taylor DW, Leke RF, et al. Chondroitin sulfate proteoglycan but not hyaluronic acid is the receptor for the adherence of *Plasmodium falciparum*-infected erythrocytes in human placenta, infected red blood cell adherence up-regulates the receptor expression. *Am J Pathol.* (2007) 170:1989–2000. doi: 10.2353/ajpath.2007.061238
168. Achur RN, Valiyaveettil M, Gowda DC. The low sulfated chondroitin sulfate proteoglycans of human placenta have sulfate group-clustered domains that can efficiently bind *Plasmodium falciparum*-infected erythrocytes. *J Biol Chem.* (2003) 278:11705–13. doi: 10.1074/jbc.M211015200
169. Nietfeld JJ, Huber-Bruning O, Bylsma JW. Cytokines and proteoglycans. *EXS.* (1994) 70:215–42. doi: 10.1007/978-3-0348-7545-5_13
170. Beaudet JM, Mansur L, Joo EJ, Kamhi E, Yang B, Clausen TM, et al. Characterization of human placental glycosaminoglycans and regional binding to VAR2CSA in malaria infected erythrocytes. *Glycoconj J.* (2014) 31:109–16. doi: 10.1007/s10719-013-9506-6
171. Scherf A, Hernandez-Rivas R, Buffet P, Bottius E, Benatar C, Pouvelle B, et al. Antigenic variation in malaria: in situ switching, relaxed and mutually exclusive transcription of var genes during intra-erythrocytic development in *Plasmodium falciparum. EMBO J.* (1998) 17:5418–26. doi: 10.1093/emboj/17.18.5418
172. Fried M, Duffy PE. Two DBLgamma subtypes are commonly expressed by placental isolates of *Plasmodium falciparum. Mol Biochem Parasitol.* (2002) 122:201–10. doi: 10.1016/S0166-6851(02)00103-2
173. Rowe JA, Kyes SA, Rogerson SJ, Babiker HA, Raza A. Identification of a conserved *Plasmodium falciparum* var gene implicated in malaria in pregnancy. *J Infect Dis.* (2002) 185:1207–11. doi: 10.1086/339684
174. Salanti A, Jensen AT, Zornig HD, Staalsoe T, Joergensen L, Nielsen MA, et al. A sub-family of common and highly conserved *Plasmodium falciparum* var genes. *Mol Biochem Parasitol.* (2002) 122:111–5. doi: 10.1016/S0166-6851(02)00080-4
175. Salanti A, Staalsoe T, Lavstsen T, Jensen AT, Sowa MP, Arnot DE, et al. Selective upregulation of a single distinctly structured var gene in chondroitin sulphate A-adhering *Plasmodium falciparum* involved in pregnancy-associated malaria. *Mol Microbiol.* (2003) 49:179–91. doi: 10.1046/j.1365-2958.2003.03570.x
176. Trimnell AR, Kraemer SM, Mukherjee S, Phippard DJ, Janes JH, Flamoe E, et al. Global genetic diversity and evolution of var genes associated with placental and severe childhood malaria. *Mol Biochem Parasitol.* (2006) 148:169–80. doi: 10.1016/j.molbiopara.2006.03.012
177. Buffet PA, Gamain B, Scheidig C, Baruch D, Smith JD, Hernandez-Rivas R, et al. *Plasmodium falciparum* domain mediating adhesion to chondroitin sulfate A: a receptor for human placental infection. *Proc Natl Acad Sci USA.* (1999) 96:12743–8. doi: 10.1073/pnas.96.22.12743
178. Jensen AT, Zornig HD, Buhmann C, Salanti A, Koram KA, Riley EM, et al. Lack of gender-specific antibody recognition of products from domains of a var gene implicated in pregnancy-associated *Plasmodium falciparum* malaria. *Infect Immun.* (2003) 71:4193–6. doi: 10.1128/IAI.71.7.4193-4196.2003
179. Viebig NK, Gamain B, Scheidig C, Lepolard C, Przyborski J, Lanzer M, et al. A single member of the *Plasmodium falciparum* var multigene family determines cytoadhesion to the placental receptor chondroitin sulphate A. *EMBO Rep.* (2005) 6:775–81. doi: 10.1038/sj.embor.7400466
180. Tuikue Ndam NG, Salanti A, Bertin G, Dahlback M, Fievet N, Turner L, et al. High level of var2csa transcription by *Plasmodium falciparum* isolated from the placenta. *J Infect Dis.* (2005) 192:331–5. doi: 10.1086/430933

181. Francis SE, Malkov VA, Oleinikov AV, Rossnagle E, Wendler JP, Mutabingwa TK, et al. Six genes are preferentially transcribed by the circulating and sequestered forms of *Plasmodium falciparum* parasites that infect pregnant women. *Infect Immun.* (2007) 75:4838–50. doi: 10.1128/IAI.00635-07
182. Tuikue Ndam N, Bischoff E, Proux C, Lavstsen T, Salanti A, Guitard J, et al. *Plasmodium falciparum* transcriptome analysis reveals pregnancy malaria associated gene expression. *PLoS ONE.* (2008) 3:e1855. doi: 10.1371/journal.pone.0001855
183. Bertin GI, Sabbagh A, Guillonneau F, Jafari-Guemouri S, Ezinmegnon S, Federici C, et al. Differential protein expression profiles between *Plasmodium falciparum* parasites isolated from subjects presenting with pregnancy-associated malaria and uncomplicated malaria in Benin. *J Infect Dis.* (2013) 208:1987–97. doi: 10.1093/infdis/jit377
184. Fried M, Hixson KK, Anderson L, Ogata Y, Mutabingwa TK, Duffy PE. The distinct proteome of placental malaria parasites. *Mol Biochem Parasitol.* (2007) 155:57–65. doi: 10.1016/j.molbiopara.2007.05.010
185. Goel S, Valiyaveettil M, Achur RN, Goyal A, Mattei D, Salanti A, et al. Dual stage synthesis and crucial role of cytoadherence-linked asexual gene 9 in the surface expression of malaria parasite var proteins. *Proc Natl Acad Sci USA.* (2010) 107:16643–8. doi: 10.1073/pnas.1002568107
186. Duffy MF, Maier AG, Byrne TJ, Marty AJ, Elliott SR, O'Neill MT, et al. VAR2CSA is the principal ligand for chondroitin sulfate A in two allogeneic isolates of *Plasmodium falciparum*. *Mol Biochem Parasitol.* (2006) 148:117–24. doi: 10.1016/j.molbiopara.2006.03.006
187. Viebig NK, Levin E, Dechavanne S, Rogerson SJ, Gysin J, Smith JD, et al. Disruption of var2csa gene impairs placental malaria associated adhesion phenotype. *PLoS ONE.* (2007) 2:e910. doi: 10.1371/journal.pone.0000910
188. Gamain B, Trimnell AR, Scheidig C, Scherf A, Miller LH, Smith JD. Identification of multiple chondroitin sulfate A (CSA)-binding domains in the var2CSA gene transcribed in CSA-binding parasites. *J Infect Dis.* (2005) 191:1010–3. doi: 10.1086/428137
189. Salanti A, Dahlback M, Turner L, Nielsen MA, Barfod L, Magistrado P, et al. Evidence for the involvement of VAR2CSA in pregnancy-associated malaria. *J Exp Med.* (2004) 200:1197–203. doi: 10.1084/jem.20041579
190. Bockhorst J, Lu F, Janes JH, Keebler J, Gamain B, Awadalla P, et al. Structural polymorphism and diversifying selection on the pregnancy malaria vaccine candidate VAR2CSA. *Mol Biochem Parasitol.* (2007) 155:103–12. doi: 10.1016/j.molbiopara.2007.06.007
191. Srivastava A, Gangnard S, Dechavanne S, Amirat F, Lewit Bentley A, Bentley GA, et al. Var2CSA minimal CSA binding region is located within the N-terminal region. *PLoS ONE.* (2011) 6:e20270. doi: 10.1371/journal.pone.0020270
192. Doritchamou J, Sabbagh A, Jespersen JS, Renard E, Salanti A, Nielsen MA, et al. Identification of a major dimorphic region in the functionally critical N-terminal ID1 domain of VAR2CSA. *PLoS ONE.* (2015) 10:e0137695. doi: 10.1371/journal.pone.0137695
193. Clausen TM, Christoffersen S, Dahlback M, Langkilde AE, Jensen KE, Resende M, et al. Structural and functional insight into how the *Plasmodium falciparum* VAR2CSA protein mediates binding to chondroitin sulfate A in placental malaria. *J Biol Chem.* (2012) 287:23332–45. doi: 10.1074/jbc.M112.348839
194. Rovira-Vallbona E, Monteiro I, Bardaji A, Serra-Casas E, Neafsey DE, Quelhas D, et al. VAR2CSA signatures of high *Plasmodium falciparum* parasitemia in the placenta. *PLoS ONE.* (2013) 8:e69753. doi: 10.1371/journal.pone.0069753
195. Dahlback M, Jorgensen LM, Nielsen MA, Clausen TM, Ditlev SB, Resende M, et al. The chondroitin sulfate A-binding site of the VAR2CSA protein involves multiple N-terminal domains. *J Biol Chem.* (2011) 286:15908–17. doi: 10.1074/jbc.M110.191510
196. Dahlback M, Rask TS, Andersen PH, Nielsen MA, Ndam NT, Resende M, et al. Epitope mapping and topographic analysis of VAR2CSA DBL3X involved in P. falciparum placental sequestration. *PLoS Pathog.* (2006) 2:e124. doi: 10.1371/journal.ppat.0020124
197. Talundzic E, Shah S, Fawole O, Owino S, Moore JM, Peterson DS. Sequence polymorphism, segmental recombination and toggling amino acid residues within the DBL3X domain of the VAR2CSA placental malaria antigen. *PLoS ONE.* (2012) 7:e31565. doi: 10.1371/journal.pone.0031565
198. Rieger H, Yoshikawa HY, Quadt K, Nielsen MA, Sanchez CP, Salanti A, et al. Cytoadhesion of *Plasmodium falciparum*-infected erythrocytes to chondroitin-4-sulfate is cooperative and shear enhanced. *Blood.* (2015) 125:383–91. doi: 10.1182/blood-2014-03-561019
199. Rogerson SJ, Beeson JG, Mhango CG, Dzinjalamala FK, Molyneux ME. *Plasmodium falciparum* rosette formation is uncommon in isolates from pregnant women. *Infect Immun.* (2000) 68:391–3. doi: 10.1128/IAI.68.1.391-393.2000
200. Stevenson L, Huda P, Jeppesen A, Laursen E, Rowe JA, Craig A, et al. Investigating the function of Fc-specific binding of IgM to *Plasmodium falciparum* erythrocyte membrane protein 1 mediating erythrocyte rosetting. *Cell Microbiol.* (2015) 17:819–31. doi: 10.1111/cmi.12403
201. Maubert B, Fievet N, Tami G, Boudin C, Deloron P. *Plasmodium falciparum*-isolates from Cameroonian pregnant women do not rosette. *Parasite.* (1998) 5:281–3. doi: 10.1051/parasite/1998053281
202. Gangnard S, Badaut C, Ramboarina S, Baron B, Ramdani T, Gamain B, et al. Structural and immunological correlations between the variable blocks of the VAR2CSA domain DBL6epsilon from two *Plasmodium falciparum* parasite lines. *J Mol Biol.* (2013) 425:1697–711. doi: 10.1016/j.jmb.2013.02.014
203. Gangnard S, Lewit-Bentley A, Dechavanne S, Srivastava A, Amirat F, Bentley GA, et al. Structure of the DBL3X-DBL4epsilon region of the VAR2CSA placental malaria vaccine candidate: insight into DBL domain interactions. *Sci Rep.* (2015) 5:14868. doi: 10.1038/srep14868
204. Higgins MK. The structure of a chondroitin sulfate-binding domain important in placental malaria. *J Biol Chem.* (2008) 283:21842–6. doi: 10.1074/jbc.C800086200
205. Singh K, Gittis AG, Nguyen P, Gowda DC, Miller LH, Garboczi DN. Structure of the DBL3x domain of pregnancy-associated malaria protein VAR2CSA complexed with chondroitin sulfate A. *Nat Struct Mol Biol.* (2008) 15:932–8. doi: 10.1038/nsmb.1479
206. Khunrae P, Philip JM, Bull DR, Higgins MK. Structural comparison of two CSPG-binding DBL domains from the VAR2CSA protein important in malaria during pregnancy. *J Mol Biol.* (2009) 393:202–13. doi: 10.1016/j.jmb.2009.08.027
207. Sander AF, Salanti A, Lavstsen T, Nielsen MA, Magistrado P, Lusingu J, et al. Multiple var2csa-type PfEMP1 genes located at different chromosomal loci occur in many *Plasmodium falciparum* isolates. *PLoS ONE.* (2009) 4:e6667. doi: 10.1371/journal.pone.0006667
208. Andersen P, Nielsen MA, Resende M, Rask TS, Dahlback M, Theander T, et al. Structural insight into epitopes in the pregnancy-associated malaria protein VAR2CSA. *PLoS Pathog.* (2008) 4:e42. doi: 10.1371/journal.ppat.0040042
209. Dahlback M, Nielsen MA, Salanti A. Can any lessons be learned from the ambiguous glycan binding of PfEMP1 domains? *Trends Parasitol.* (2010) 26:230–5. doi: 10.1016/j.pt.2010.02.002
210. Khunrae P, Higgins MK. Structural insights into chondroitin sulfate binding in pregnancy-associated malaria. *Biochem Soc Trans.* (2010) 38:1337–41. doi: 10.1042/BST0381337
211. Badaut C, Bertin G, Rustico T, Fievet N, Massougbodji A, Gaye A, et al. Towards the rational design of a candidate vaccine against pregnancy associated malaria: conserved sequences of the DBL6epsilon domain of VAR2CSA. *PLoS ONE.* (2010) 5:e11276. doi: 10.1371/journal.pone.0011276
212. Deloron P, Milet J, Badaut C. *Plasmodium falciparum* variability and immune evasion proceed from antigenicity of consensus sequences from DBL6epsilon; generalization to all DBL from VAR2CSA. *PLoS ONE.* (2013) 8:e54882. doi: 10.1371/journal.pone.0054882
213. Bordbar B, Tuikue Ndam N, Renard E, Jafari-Guemouri S, Tavul L, Jennison C, et al. Genetic diversity of VAR2CSA ID1-DBL2Xb in worldwide *Plasmodium falciparum* populations: impact on vaccine design for placental malaria. *Infect Genet Evol.* (2014) 25:81–92. doi: 10.1016/j.meegid.2014.04.010
214. Hommel M, Elliott SR, Soma V, Kelly G, Fowkes FJ, Chesson JM, et al. Evaluation of the antigenic diversity of placenta-binding *Plasmodium falciparum* variants and the antibody repertoire among pregnant women. *Infect Immun.* (2010) 78:1963–78. doi: 10.1128/IAI.01365-09
215. Avril M, Gamain B, Lepolard C, Viaud N, Scherf A, Gysin J. Characterization of anti-var2CSA-PfEMP1 cytoadhesion inhibitory

mouse monoclonal antibodies. *Microbes Infect.* (2006) 8:2863–71. doi: 10.1016/j.micinf.2006.09.005

216. Bir N, Yazdani SS, Avril M, Layez C, Gysin J, Chitnis CE. Immunogenicity of Duffy binding-like domains that bind chondroitin sulfate A and protection against pregnancy-associated malaria. *Infect Immun.* (2006) 74:5955–63. doi: 10.1128/IAI.00481-06
217. Resende M, Ditlev SB, Nielsen MA, Bodevin S, Bruun S, Pinto VV, et al. Chondroitin sulphate A (CSA)-binding of single recombinant Duffy-binding-like domains is not restricted to *Plasmodium falciparum* Erythrocyte Membrane Protein 1 expressed by CSA-binding parasites. *Int J Parasitol.* (2009) 39:1195–204. doi: 10.1016/j.ijpara.2009.02.022
218. Resende M, Nielsen MA, Dahlback M, Ditlev SB, Andersen P, Sander AF, et al. Identification of glycosaminoglycan binding regions in the *Plasmodium falciparum* encoded placental sequestration ligand, VAR2CSA. *Malar J.* (2008) 7:104. doi: 10.1186/1475-2875-7-104
219. Khunrae P, Dahlback M, Nielsen MA, Andersen G, Ditlev SB, Resende M, et al. Full-length recombinant *Plasmodium falciparum* VAR2CSA binds specifically to CSPG and induces potent parasite adhesion-blocking antibodies. *J Mol Biol.* (2010) 397:826–34. doi: 10.1016/j.jmb.2010.01.040
220. Srivastava A, Gangnard S, Round A, Dechavanne S, Juillerat A, Raynal B, et al. Full-length extracellular region of the var2CSA variant of PfEMP1 is required for specific, high-affinity binding to CSA. *Proc Natl Acad Sci USA.* (2010) 107:4884–9. doi: 10.1073/pnas.1000951107
221. Beeson JG, Rogerson SJ, Cooke BM, Reeder JC, Chai W, Lawson AM, et al. Adhesion of *Plasmodium falciparum*-infected erythrocytes to hyaluronic acid in placental malaria. *Nat Med.* (2000) 6:86–90. doi: 10.1038/71582
222. Flick K, Scholander C, Chen Q, Fernandez V, Pouvelle B, Gysin J, et al. Role of nonimmune IgG bound to PfEMP1 in placental malaria. *Science.* (2001) 293:2098–100. doi: 10.1126/science.1062891
223. Beeson JG, Brown GV. *Plasmodium falciparum*-infected erythrocytes demonstrate dual specificity for adhesion to hyaluronic acid and chondroitin sulfate A and have distinct adhesive properties. *J Infect Dis.* (2004) 189:169–79. doi: 10.1086/380975
224. Rasti N, Namusoke F, Chene A, Chen Q, Staalsoe T, Klinkert MQ, et al. Nonimmune immunoglobulin binding and multiple adhesion characterize *Plasmodium falciparum*-infected erythrocytes of placental origin. *Proc Natl Acad Sci USA.* (2006) 103:13795–800. doi: 10.1073/pnas.0601519103
225. Barfod L, Dalgaard MB, Pleman ST, Ofori MF, Pleass RJ, Hviid L. Evasion of immunity to *Plasmodium falciparum* malaria by IgM masking of protective IgG epitopes in infected erythrocyte surface-exposed PfEMP1. *Proc Natl Acad Sci USA.* (2011) 108:12485–90. doi: 10.1073/pnas.1103708108
226. Creasey AM, Staalsoe T, Raza A, Arnot DE, Rowe JA. Nonspecific immunoglobulin M binding and chondroitin sulfate A binding are linked phenotypes of *Plasmodium falciparum* isolates implicated in malaria during pregnancy. *Infect Immun.* (2003) 71:4767–71. doi: 10.1128/IAI.71.8.4767-4771.2003
227. Semblat JP, Raza A, Kyes SA, Rowe JA. Identification of *Plasmodium falciparum* var1CSA and var2CSA domains that bind IgM natural antibodies. *Mol Biochem Parasitol.* (2006) 146:192–7. doi: 10.1016/j.molbiopara.2005.12.007
228. Fried M, Domingo GJ, Gowda CD, Mutabingwa TK, Duffy PE. *Plasmodium falciparum*: chondroitin sulfate A is the major receptor for adhesion of parasitized erythrocytes in the placenta. *Exp Parasitol.* (2006) 113:36–42. doi: 10.1016/j.exppara.2005.12.003
229. Pehrson C, Salanti A, Theander TG, Nielsen MA. Pre-clinical and clinical development of the first placental malaria vaccine. *Expert Rev Vaccines.* (2017) 16:613–624. doi: 10.1080/14760584.2017.1322512
230. Fried M, Duffy PE. Designing a VAR2CSA-based vaccine to prevent placental malaria. *Vaccine.* (2015) 33:7483–8. doi: 10.1016/j.vaccine.2015.10.011
231. Duffy PE, Fried M. Antibodies that inhibit *Plasmodium falciparum* adhesion to chondroitin sulfate A are associated with increased birth weight and the gestational age of newborns. *Infect Immun.* (2003) 71:6620–3. doi: 10.1128/IAI.71.11.6620-6623.2003
232. Staalsoe T, Shulman CE, Bulmer JN, Kawuondo K, Marsh K, Hviid L. Variant surface antigen-specific IgG and protection against clinical consequences of pregnancy-associated *Plasmodium falciparum* malaria. *Lancet.* (2004) 363:283–9. doi: 10.1016/S0140-6736(03)15386-X
233. Dechavanne S, Srivastava A, Gangnard S, Nunes-Silva S, Dechavanne C, Fievet N, et al. Parity-dependent recognition of DBL1X-3X suggests an important role of the VAR2CSA high-affinity CSA-binding region in the development of the humoral response against placental malaria. *Infect Immun.* (2015) 83:2466–74. doi: 10.1128/IAI.03116-14
234. Tuikue-Ndam N, Deloron P. Developing vaccines to prevent malaria in pregnant women. *Expert Opin Biol Ther.* (2015) 15:1173–82. doi: 10.1517/14712598.2015.1049595
235. Nielsen MA, Pinto VV, Resende M, Dahlback M, Ditlev SB, Theander TG, et al. Induction of adhesion-inhibitory antibodies against placental *Plasmodium falciparum* parasites by using single domains of VAR2CSA. *Infect Immun.* (2009) 77:2482–7. doi: 10.1128/IAI.00159-09
236. Bigey P, Gnidehou S, Doritchamou J, Quiviger M, Viwami F, Couturier A, et al. The NTS-DBL2X region of VAR2CSA induces cross-reactive antibodies that inhibit adhesion of several *Plasmodium falciparum* isolates to chondroitin sulfate A. *J Infect Dis.* (2011) 204:1125–33. doi: 10.1093/infdis/jir499
237. Bordbar B, Tuikue-Ndam N, Bigey P, Doritchamou J, Scherman D, Deloron P. Identification of Id1-DBL2X of VAR2CSA as a key domain inducing highly inhibitory and cross-reactive antibodies. *Vaccine.* (2012) 30:1343–8. doi: 10.1016/j.vaccine.2011.12.065
238. Doritchamou J, Bigey P, Nielsen MA, Gnidehou S, Ezinmegnon S, Burgain A, et al. Differential adhesion-inhibitory patterns of antibodies raised against two major variants of the NTS-DBL2X region of VAR2CSA. *Vaccine.* (2013) 31:4516–22. doi: 10.1016/j.vaccine.2013.07.072
239. Nielsen MA, Resende M, de Jongh WA, Ditlev SB, Mordmuller B, Houard S, et al. The influence of sub-unit composition and expression system on the functional antibody response in the development of a VAR2CSA based *Plasmodium falciparum* placental malaria vaccine. *PLoS ONE.* (2015) 10:e0135406. doi: 10.1371/journal.pone.0135406
240. Doritchamou JY, Herrera R, Aebig JA, Morrison R, Nguyen V, Reiter K, et al. VAR2CSA domain-specific analysis of naturally acquired functional antibodies to *Plasmodium falciparum* placental malaria. *J Infect Dis.* (2016) 214:577–86. doi: 10.1093/infdis/jiw197
241. ClinicalTrials.gov. *Trial to Evaluate the Safety and Immunogenicity of a Placental Malaria Vaccine Candidate (PRIMVAC) in Healthy Adults (PRIMALVAC)* (2016).
242. Nielsen MA. *Final Report Summary - PLACMALVAC (Clinical Development of a VAR2CSA-Based Placental Malaria Vaccine).* Copenhagan (2017).
243. Nielsen MA. *Placental Malaria Vaccine (PlacMalVac), Main Results and Significance.* Copenhagen (2017).

6

School Age Neurological and Cognitive Outcomes of Fetal Growth Retardation or Small for Gestational Age Birth Weight

Brigitte Vollmer [1,2*] *and Caroline J. Edmonds* [3]

[1] *Clinical and Experimental Sciences, Faculty of Medicine, University of Southampton, Southampton, United Kingdom,* [2] *Paediatric and Neonatal Neurology, Southampton Children's Hospital, University Hospital Southampton NHS Foundation Trust, Southampton, United Kingdom,* [3] *School of Psychology, University of East London, London, United Kingdom*

Correspondence:
Brigitte Vollmer
b.vollmer@soton.ac.uk

Children who were growth restricted *in utero* (FGR) and are born small for gestational age (SGA) may experience poorer long term neurological and cognitive outcomes. Those also born preterm may have particular difficulties. The objective of this paper was to review the literature on school age neurocognitive outcome for term and preterm children that was published in the last 15 years. Considering term born children first, there is evidence that these children are at higher risk for Cerebral Palsy (CP) than those born appropriate for gestational age (AGA); information on neuromotor function in the absence of CP is somewhat contradictory. With regards to cognitive outcome, the most common finding was that being born SGA and/or FGR at term does not impact negatively on general intellectual functioning, commonly assessed by IQ scores. There was some indication that they may experience particular problems with attention. With regards to children born preterm, the risk of CP appears not to be increased compared to those preterms born AGA. For preterm children who do not develop CP, motor outcome is more affected by post-natal and post-neonatal brain growth than intrauterine growth. In contrast to term born children, preterm SGA and/or FGR children are at increased risk of cognitive and behavioral difficulties, and in common with term born children, are at higher risk than their AGA counterparts of difficulties with attentional control. In conclusion, preterm born SGA and/or FGR children are at higher risk of neurodevelopmental problems in the school years. It is important to continue to follow up children into the school age years because these difficulties may take time to emerge, and may be more visible in the more demanding school environment.

Keywords: small for gestational age, fetal growth restriction, cognitive outcome, neuromotor outcome, school age

Low birth weight and poor fetal growth affects a significant proportion of newborns and pregnancies worldwide, and have been associated with a risk for impaired neurodevelopment across multiple domains (1, 2) for both individuals born preterm and born term, with a notion that outcomes for those born preterm are likely to be more complex than in those born term.

In the existing literature on neurodevelopmental outcomes, often, small for gestational age (SGA) and fetal growth restriction (FGR) are used interchangeably, but FGR is not the same as SGA.

This makes interpretation and comparison of outcome studies often complicated. Study-specific definitions of FGR, SGA and IUGR are included in the tables.

The definition of small-for gestational age (SGA) by the Royal College of Obstetrics and Gynecology (RCOG; https://www.rcog.org.uk/globalassets/documents/guidelines/gtg_31.pdf) in the UK, and also the American College of Obstetricians and Gynecologists, refers to a newborn with a weight or abdominal circumference at birth at less than the 10th centile, either according to population based growth charts or centiles that take into account factors such as gestational age, sex, ethnicity, and maternal characteristics. Further, this can be divided into normal (i.e., constitutionally small), non-placenta mediated growth restriction (for example, chromosomal abnormalities, syndromes, infections), and placental mediated growth restriction. Fetal growth restriction implies that the fetus cannot achieve its growth potential, and this is often indicated by abnormal Doppler studies. Over half of those who are SGA have appropriate fetal growth ("constitutional" SGA), although the likelihood of also having FGR is higher in SGA. Fetal growth restriction can be classified into symmetrical (both body weight and head circumference are affected) and asymmetrical (body weight and/or length may be affected, head size is normal) and according to the time of onset of FGR (early, i.e., before 28 weeks of gestation, late, i.e., after 28 weeks of gestation) (3). Time of onset of FGR is an important factor since early and late onset FGR are distinct phenotypes in terms of placental dysfunction and effects on the brain. Early and late onset FGR affect the brain at different developmental stages and it is therefore likely that different brain regions are affected in a different way, which may partly explain the different outcomes in these two groups (4). Fetal growth retardation and preterm birth are often associated (5). Preterm birth *per se* poses a risk for long term neurological and developmental impairment and the combination with FGR is likely to add to this risk, however, it may be difficult to disentangle the effects of FGR from the effect of prematurity, and, indeed there have been somewhat inconsistent and contradictory finding in existing studies.

Studies have reported differences for the above described groups in neurodevelopmental outcomes, generally reporting favorable outcomes for those with constitutional SGA, whereas those with placenta-mediated FGR appear to be at risk for cognitive and/or behavioral problems later in life (6). In addition, within the FGR group, differences in outcomes are reported between those with symmetrical and those with asymmetrical FGR (7), although, again, some contradictory study results exist. Overall, existing studies are heterogeneous, for example, with regards to definition of growth restriction and small for gestational age, time of onset of FGR, inclusion and exclusion criteria, outcome measures, all of which makes comparison between studies difficult.

Nevertheless, some common themes emerge and in this narrative literature review we will summarize evidence on neuromotor and cognitive long term outcomes of SGA at birth and after FGR. The focus will be on school age outcomes rather than earlier outcomes as toddler age or adult age outcomes, and this will be described separately for children born at term age and for those born preterm. We considered literature published in the last 15 years. We have excluded studies that included children with underlying chromosomal abnormalities or teratogenic exposure.

MEASURES USED IN STUDIES ON SGA/ FGR OUTCOMES

While the use of standardized assessments makes cross-study comparison possible, some of the assessments used were more individual and depended on the study location and specific sample. For example, some studies used information from military conscription (8), national registers of learning disability (9), and/or and information extracted from medical records (10).

Neuromotor and neurosensory outcomes are described in some, but not all, studies. In the studies that did describe neuromotor outcomes, only seldom a standardized approach was applied for neurological examination. Diagnosis of Cerebral Palsy (CP) was either based on direct neurological examination assessing posture, movements, muscle tone, and reflexes, or on information extracted from medical notes. In a few studies, and when diagnosis was based on examination, the Surveillance of Cerebral Palsy in Europe (SCPE) criteria for CP were used (11). Functional impairment in those with CP was not always defined, but in some studies the Gross Motor Function Classification System (GMFCS, (12) was used for overall motor function classification. In one study, independently of a diagnosis of CP, gross motor function was assessed using the GMFCS, and hand function using the Manual Ability Classification System (13). The most commonly used tool for assessment of motor skills was the Movement ABC for Children (14), a standardized tool, which assesses dexterity, balance skills, and ball skills. Another standardized test, the Peabody Developmental Motor Scales (15), testing reflexes, stationary, locomotion, object manipulation, grasping, and visual-motor integration, has also been used.

Very rarely are visual function and hearing function described specifically, and, if so, this information was mainly extracted from medical records and reported as a binary outcome (impairment/no impairment).

Abbreviations: AGA, appropriate for gestational age; ANT, Amsterdam Neuropsychological Tasks; AGR, asymmetric growth restriction; ARED, absent or reversed end-diastolic blood flow; BW, Birth weight; BL, Birth Length; BRIEF, Behavior Rating Inventory of Executive Function; CLD, Chronic lung disease; CP, Cerebral Palsy; FGR, Fetal growth restriction; FSIQ, Full Scale IQ Score; GA, Gestational age; HC, Head Circumference; HGR, Head growth restriction; ICH, Intracranial hemorrhage; IQ, Intelligence Quotient Score; IUGR, Intrauterine growth restriction; K-ABC, Kaufmann Assessment Battery for Children; M-ABC, Movement ABC for Children; MHPT-Moray House Picture Test; NEPSY, A Developmental Neuropsychological Assessment; PIQ, Performance IQ Score; POBW, Percentage of optimal birth weight; RAVLT, Rey's Auditory Verbal Learning Test; ROYCF-Rey Osterreith Complex Figure test; SES, Socio-economic status; SGA, Small for gestational age; TeaCH, Test of Everyday Attention in Children; VIQ, Verbal IQ score; WASI, Wechsler Abbreviated Scales of Intelligence; w, Week; WGR, Weight growth restriction; WISC, Wechsler Intelligence Scales for Children; WISC-R, Wechsler Intelligence Scale for Children – revised; WPPSI, Wechsler Preschool and Primary Scale of Intelligence; WRAT, Wide Range Achievement Test; y, Year.

For outcome measures used to assess general cognitive abilities and specific cognitive functions, there was a large and heterogeneous range of assessments reported, but most of the outcome measures used were standardized neuropsychological tests and questionnaires. For assessing general intellectual functioning, the most frequently used assessment was the Wechsler Intelligence Scale set, most commonly the Wechsler Intelligence Scales for Children (WISC) (16), but also the Wechsler Abbreviated Scales of Intelligence (WASI) (17), and the Wechsler Preschool and Primary Scale of Intelligence (WPPSI) (18). The Wechsler Scales assess performance across cognitive domains and usually include an overall IQ score, and performance and verbal IQ scores. General intellectual functioning was also assessed using the Kaufman ABC (19). More focused neuropsychological assessments were used to examine specific aspects of performance, including attention (the Test of Everyday Attention in Children—TEA-Ch) (20), memory (Rey's Auditory Verbal Learning Test—RAVALT) (21), and design copying of the Rey Ostereith figure (22). Executive functioning was assessed using the NEPSY (23), and parental ratings of children's behavior were also employed. Children's executive functioning at home and/or at school were assessed using the Behavior Rating Inventory of Executive Function (BRIEF) (24). The Strengths and Difficulties Questionnaire (SDQ) (25), a brief behavior screening questionnaire, has parents and/or teachers rate children on emotional symptoms, conduct problems, hyperactivity/inattention, peer relationship problems, and prosocial behavior.

The development of typical and atypical social behavior was assessed using the Social Responsiveness Scale (SRS) (26), and screeners for autism included the Social Communication Questionnaire (SCQ) (27) and Autism Diagnostic Observation Schedule (ADOS) (28).

SCHOOL AGE OUTCOMES OF SGA AND/OR FGR IN CHILDREN BORN AT TERM

The study of neurocognitive outcome after fetal growth restriction in term infants is not subject to the same confounding factors as that in preterm infants because many of the mechanisms that affect preterm birth do not affect term infants. Nevertheless, with studies using different indicators of growth restriction, such as strict SGA criteria or birth weight as a continuum, it can be difficult to make cross study comparisons. **Table 1** reports study details from studies that examined school age neurocognitive outcome of SGA and/or FGR in the past 15 years. Of these, most studies defined SGA as birth weight <10th centile (9, 10, 32, 37–40, 46, 48, 49). Two studies assessed growth in head circumference from the prenatal period and/or birth to later childhood (34, 36). Three studies defined FGR in relation to birth weight standard deviation scores (8, 44, 48). Thus, there is disparity with the definition of SGA and FGR across studies that could affect the results. Only 2 studies included information on placental insufficiency, which would allow FGR to be identified rather than babies being SGA (38, 40). Furthermore, some of the studies of term born children also include a proportion of preterm babies (8, 40, 44).

Neuromotor Outcomes

Studies assessing only children with CP are reported here and not included in the table (10, 48, 49). An association between Cerebral Palsy (CP) and having been born SGA and/or FGR has been reported for children born at term in outcome studies on SGA and/or FGR, and data from Cerebral Palsy registers support this association (11, 50, 51). Whether FGR leads to CP or whether abnormal brain development that causes CP leads to FGR is debated.

The Surveillance of Cerebral Palsy in Europe (11) group report an increased risk of CP, across the gestational age range, for those born below the 10th centile and above the 97th centile [using the North of England standard (52) and fetal growth standard by Maršál et al. (53)]. Data from the Canadian Cerebral Palsy Registry (10) and from other reports based on CP registry data (49, 50, 54) show that those with CP who were born term and SGA compared to those with CP born AGA had more frequently intrauterine infections, small head circumference at birth, maternal gestational hypertension, placental abnormalities, perinatal asphyxia, and delivery by emergency cesarean section, amongst other risk factors, such as birth defects (congenital microcephaly, teratogenic, genetic, and syndromal) as reported by Blair et al. (48), for the Australian CP register cohort. This illustrates that it has to be kept in mind when interpreting findings on associations between SGA and/or FGR with CP that SGA populations in CP registers tend to include a heterogeneous group of SGA children, i.e., also children who had other risk factors for SGA and/or FGR than placenta-mediated FGR.

Many of the prospective follow-up studies examining neurodevelopmental outcomes of SGA and/or FGR at term excluded children with CP or other co-morbidities, and of those that did not exclude them, few reported on the presence or absence of CP, or neurological signs in the absence of CP. Leitner et al. (40) compared the occurrence of neurological signs in the absence of CP in children who were born with BW <10th centile with a group of children born AGA at age 9 years; all SGA children had onset of FGR in the mid-second to third trimester, verified by fetal ultrasound, and all had asymmetric FGR. They found a significant difference in the quality of neurology between those born after FGR and those born AGA, with poorer scores for to motor coordination, timed coordination performance, grapho-motor skills and lower muscle tone in the FGR group. Similarly, Emond et al. (31), who used the M-ABC at age 8 years found, after controlling for socio-economic variables, significantly lower scores for dynamic balance and eye–hand coordination in those born SGA (<10th BW centile) but similar performance to those born AGA for manual dexterity. Tanis et al. (44), in contrast, did not find a significant difference between a group of children born at term and SGA and a group born AGA at the age of 7 years when assessed with the M-BAC (dexterity, balance, ball skills) and on tests of visuo-motor integration. The findings by Tanis et al are consistent with those by Sommerfelt et al. (42), in 5 years old children born <15th centile (Norwegian Birth Registry standards), who did not find significantly poorer

TABLE 1 | Included studies for term born children.

References	Study type	Definition of fetal growth	Participants	Neurology/Neuromotor function	Cognitive/behavior Outcome measure	Cognitive/behavior findings	Conclusion
Beukers (29)	Prospective follow up study comparing term FGR and term AGA children	BWt ratio <10th centile; BWR calculated as BW/expected weight for GA, using the Gardosi customized fetal growth chart 50th centile values (30)	96 term children with FGR; 32 term and birthweight ≥ 2,500 g BY 200–2003 Age at assessment: 12 y	Not assessed	*Child assessment:* IQ–Wechsler Intelligence Scale for Children (WISC). Executive Functioning–Impulse control (stop task); Verbal working memory (WISC Digit span); Visual working memory (Spatial Temporal Span of the Amsterdam Neuropsychological Tasks–ANT); set shifting (Shifting visual set–ANT); planning (Tower of London). *Parent ratings:*- Behavior Rating Inventory of Executive Functions Dutch version (BRIEF)	No difference in IQ, executive functioning, attention or parent rating of EF between FGR and controls. Parent report FGR children more social and attention problems	Neurocognitive outcomes including IQ, executive function, memory and attention comparable in FGR children AGA controls Parent ratings suggested elevated levels of social and attention problems
Emond (31)	Population based cohort, north east Brazil	Low BW: BW 1,500–2,499 g ($n = 202$) Appropriate BW: BW 3,000–3,499 g ($n = 212$); matched for sex and month of birth	Born ≥37 wGA BY 1993–1994 Age at assessment: 8 y 40% of original cohort assessed ($n = 83$ low birth weight; $n = 81$ appropriate birth weight) Analyses adjusted for socio-economic background variables Additional analyses performed to examine head size at birth, age 6 m and 8 y with IQ at age 8 y	Neurological status (muscle tone, focal neurological signs) M-ABC for neuromotor function *Findings:* No significant difference in frequency of focal neurological signs	WISC-III for Full Scale IQ, Performance IQ, Verbal IQ Memory (auditory and verbal) assessed with WISC-III subtests TeaCH for attention abilities SDQ for behavior	After controlling for socio-economic background no significant difference between BW groups for IQ scores, memory function Significant differences between BW groups for dynamic balance skills and eye-hand coordination, selective attention; peer relationships Head size at birth, age 6 m and 8 y significantly associated with IQ age 8 y	Low birth weight not associated with general cognitive abilities, except selective attention. Neuromotor function poorer in low birth weight children. Post-natal head growth more important than birth weight.
Fattal-Valevski (32)	Prospective follow-up study	BW <10th centile for GA according to Israeli birth weight curves (33); Growth data (weight, height, head circumference) from 1 to 2 y, 2–6 y, and 6–9 y	136 IUGR children BY 1992–2002 Age at assessment: Annual follow-up from birth; current assessment 9–10 y	Neurodevelopmental examination score including soft neurological signs. Score expressed as percentage of optimal items out of the total.	Short term memory, coordination skills; IQ assessed by the Wechsler Intelligence Scale for Children—revised (WISC-R)	BW, BL and GA positively correlated with 9–10 y neurodevelopmental score BW, BL, but not GA, positively correlated with 9–10 y IQ scores Better outcome for those with asymmetric IUGR than symmetric	Correlation of IQ with BW, BL but not GA suggests that there is better outcome for IUGR children delivered early Correlation of GA with neurodevelopmental score, suggests prematurity affects other areas of development

(Continued)

TABLE 1 | Continued

References	Study type	Definition of fetal growth	Participants	Neurology/Neuromotor function	Cognitive/behavior Outcome measure	Cognitive/behavior findings	Conclusion
Gale (34)	Prospective cohort study	HC growth–expressed as Standard Deviation Score (SDS), measured at 18 weeks gestation and birth, and 9 y, using the British 1990 growth reference data (35)	221 children assessed at 18 weeks gestation, births, 9 months and 9 years BY 1992–1994 Age at assessment: 9 y	Not assessed	Wechsler Abbreviated Scales of Intelligence (WASI)—Full Scale IQ (FSIQ), Verbal IQ (VIQ) and Performance IQ (PIQ)	No significant associations between head circumference at 18 weeks gestation or birth and 9 years old IQ scores. Post-natal head group was associated with IQ. After adjusting for sex, FSIQ, VIQ and PIQ increased with each SD increase in head circumference up to 9 months, and to 9 years. The highest FSIQ were observed in children who had large increases in HC between birth and 9 months, and a further increase between 9 months and 9 years. This was not linked to maternal or home characteristics other than maternal education	Post-natal brain growth is more important than prenatal brain growth for IQ Post-natal head growth greater in children of mothers educated to degree level, or of higher SES
Gale (36)	Prospective cohort study – the Avon Longitudinal Study of Parents and Children cohort (ALSPAC). The cohort studied is the Children in Focus cohort – a random 10% selected from ALSPAC.	HC growth - measured at birth, 4, 8, 12, 25, 31, 37, 43, 49, 61, and 96 months. HC in analyses –birth, 1, 4, and 8 years—expressed as z scores obtained from the study group. Growth between time points calculated	633 children BY 1991–1992 Age at assessment: 8 y	Not assessed	IQ assessed by Wechsler Intelligence Scale for Children (WISC) at 8 years	Children with larger HC had higher IQ scores For each 1 SD increase in HC– after adjusting for gender, GA, parental factors—FSIQ, VIQ and PIQ increased age 8 years IQ at 8 years was associated with HG during infancy	Above average head growth during infancy associated with above average IQ scores at 8 years Post-natal brain growth during infancy more important to later IQ than growth at other times Brain growth after infancy may not compensate for slower growth in the first year of life
Geva (37)	Population based prospective follow up study of single center (Tel Aviv, Israel)	BW <10th centile for GA according to Israeli birth weight curves (33), those with genetic disorders and unrelated co-morbidities excluded	110 IUGR children born at term, 63 control AGA children BY 1992–1995 Age at assessment: 9 y	Not assessed	Visual aural digit span test for digit span—aural-oral, visual-oral, aural-written, visual-written; RAVLT (superspan list learning test); Rey Osterreith Complex Figure test (ROYCF)	Learning functions over trials were similar for IUGR and controls on RAVLT. IUGR children performed more poorly than controls on ROYCF. IUGR children worse performance on immediate digit span than controls. Performance on digit span output mode did not differ between IUGR and control. IUGR children have memory problems particularly when the input is aural.	Memory difficulties in children born IUGR in the short term, not observed in later stages of learning (i.e., processing, consolidation and retrieval not affected) Difficulties when recalling both verbal and complex visuo-spatial material

(Continued)

TABLE 1 | Continued

References	Study type	Definition of fetal growth	Participants	Neurology/Neuromotor function	Cognitive/behavior Outcome measure	Cognitive/behavior findings	Conclusion
Geva (38)	Population based prospective follow up study of single center (Tel Aviv, Israel)	BW <10th centile for GA according to Israeli birth weight curves (33), those with genetic disorders and unrelated co-morbidities excluded	138 IUGR children born at term, 64 control AGA children BY 1992–1995 Age at assessment: 9 y	Not assessed	VADS Digit span–aural-oral, visual-oral, aural-written, visual-written; IQ assessed by Wechsler Intelligence Scale for Children–revised (WISC-R)	IQ significantly lower in IUGR group. IUGR children performed worse than controls on verbal STM tasks.	Short term memory difficulties in IUGR children are particularly observed when material presented aurally and oral response required General cognitive performance also poorer in IUGR children relative to controls
Lawlor (39)	Single center, population based prospective birth cohort -Aberdeen Children of the 1950s cohort.	IUG rate measured as BW standardized for gender and GA. SGA calculated as BW < 10th centile, using a customized birthweight-for-gestation standard for the whole cohort	9,792 singleton children and 1,645 sibling pairs BY 1950–1956 Age at assessment: 7, 9 and 11 y	Not assessed	General ability measured by the Moray House picture test (MHPT)	Positive linear association between BW and MHPT, even when adjusted for SES, Maternal height and age, gender and GA. Within sibling comparison of SGA vs. AGA showed no difference in MHPT scores. If AGE compared to SGA outside of sibling pairs, AGA performed more poorly	While BW correlates with general cognitive ability within-sibling analyses suggest that associations between AGA status and cognitive ability in singletons is explained by within family factors, including SES, parental education and intelligence, genetic factors and fixed maternal factors
Leitner (40)	Prospective birth cohort	BW < 10th centile for gestational age, according to the Israeli percentile curves published by Lieberman et al. (33). Late onset IUGR (mid 2nd to 3rd trimester; verified by fetal ultrasound)	123 children with IUGR and 63 AGA controls, 30% of the sample were preterm BY 1992–2002 Age at assessment: 9–10 y Children with CP or severe neurological deficits were excluded	Neurological examination from birth, follow-up and at 9–10 years. 72 item examination. At age 9 years assessment of co-ordination skills, tone, timed performance, graphomotor skills. *Findings:* IUGR group poorer performance in coordination, timed performance, graphomotor skills; lower muscle tone	IQ assessed by Wechsler Intelligence Scale for Children (WISC), School achievement by Kauffman Assessment Battery for Children (K-ABC)	IUGR children performed more poorly than AGA controls on IQ and school achievement, where learning difficulties, particularly language-based difficulties were observed. Attention span, speech and language abilities were poorer in the IUGR group. Subgroup analyses compared IUGR children whose height, weight and head circumference were above ("optimal") or below ("suboptimal") the 10th growth percentile at age 9–10 years–the "suboptimal" catch up group performed worse in neurodevelopmental and cognitive tests than "optimal" group	Children with IUGR perform more poorly than their AGA peers on tests of IQ, school achievement, and neurological examination. Early growth ameliorates these group differences

(Continued)

TABLE 1 | Continued

References	Study type	Definition of fetal growth	Participants	Neurology/Neuromotor function	Cognitive/behavior Outcome measure	Cognitive/behavior findings	Conclusion
Leonard (9)	Population-based record linkage study of children in Western Australia born 1983–1992 with intellectual disability of unknown cause	Percentage of optimal birthweight (POBW) categorized as %-POBW <85% was equivalent to <10th centile of optimal BW based on data from the 1998–2002 Western Australia birth cohort (35)	2,865 children with intellectual disability, including both term and preterm children BY 1983–1992	Not assessed	Registrations with the Disability Services Commission or educational services defined as "mild to moderate" (85.9%), "severe or profound" (7.4%), Autism spectrum disorder (6.7%)	In infants born at term, less than optimal fetal growth (POBW < 85%) was associated with "mild to moderate" intellectual disability, POBW < 75% was associated with "severe" intellectual disability. These were after adjusting for factors including SES and paternal occupation	Less than optimal uterine growth associated with intellectual disability in term born children. This persists after adjusting for sociodemographic factors. Severe growth restriction in term children associated with severe intellectual disability
Lundgren (8)	Population based cohort study of singleton male infants born from 1973 to 1976 and alive aged 18 years	"Light for gestational age" defined as > −2 SDs from mean BW for GA, AGA defined as between −2 and +2 SDS, "heavy for GA" defined as > +2 SDs from mean BW according to Swedish birth standards (41)	168,068 males conscripted for national service BW 1973–1976 Age at assessment: 18–25 y This study includes term and preterm adults	Not assessed	General intellectual performance assessed on four dimensions, logical/inductive, verbal, spatial and theoretical/technical	Being born SGA associated with increased risk of subnormal performance on all outcome measures compared to those born AGA SGA and small HC conferred additional risk of subnormal logical performance, SGA and short adult stature associated with a 40–50% increased risk in all outcome measures	Being born SGA associated with increased risk of impairment on logical/inductive, verbal, spatial and theoretical/technical dimensions of intellectual performance
Sommerfelt (42)	Multicenter study on causes and consequences of *in utero* growth retardation, the NICHD Study of Successive Small-for-Gestational Age Births (NSSSAB) 3 geographical Scandinavian regions; mothers recruited before 20 wGA	SGA = BW were <15th centile for gestation according to reference standards from the Norwegian Birth Registry (43); above 15th centile AGA	321 SGA and 312 AGA (78% of eligible children) Recruitment <20 w GA between January 1986 and March 1988 Age at assessment: 5 y	PDMS for balance, eye-hand coordination, locomotor abilities., Grooved Pegboard test for manual dexterity *Findings:* Motor problems more frequent in SGA group but no significance group difference	WPPSI for IQ scores (Verbal IQ, Performance IQ) Norwegian version of the Illinois Test of Psycholinguistic Abilities for receptive language and short-term memory	No significant difference in IQ scores, memory tests SGA with poorer motor performance lower scores on tests of visuospatial, manual dexterity, and verbal function	SGA group differs little from AGA peers on neuropsychologic profile and neuromotor outcome SGA group weakness in visuo-spatial skills and manual dexterity

(Continued)

TABLE 1 | Continued

References	Study type	Definition of fetal growth	Participants	Neurology/Neuromotor function	Cognitive/behavior Outcome measure	Cognitive/behavior findings	Conclusion
Tanis (44)	Population based regional cohort—subgroup (Longitudinal Preterm Outcome Project study), Netherlands	BW < −1 SD and BW > −1 SD according to GA; Dutch Kloosterman curve (45). Cut-off for SGA (> 1 SD, below the 16th percentile) according to Etude Epidemiologique sur les Petits Ages Gestationnels study	42 SGA children (10 full term) and 336 AGA children (120 full term), Analyses combine MPT and term –GA range is 31–41. Both SGA and AGA groups consisted of mostly preterm children BY 2002–2003 Age at assessment: 7 y	Motor outcomes assessed by Movement Assessment Battery for Children (M-ABC) *Findings:* No significant difference in motor skills between AGA and SGA group	Full Scale IQ scores (FSIQ) from the Wechsler Intelligence Scale for Children (WISC). Selective attention and Attention control assessed by the Test of Everyday Attention in Children (TEA-Ch). Verbal memory assessed using Rey's Auditory Verbal Learning Test (RAVLT). Visuomotor integration assessed by Neuropsychological Assessment. Executive functioning in daily life assessed by the Behavior Rating Inventory of Executive Function (BRIEF)	No differences between AGA and SGA children on FSIQ, attention, verbal memory, visuomotor integration, executive functioning. SGA children 4 times more likely to be in the abnormal range on the Attention Control measure than AGA children	SGA and AGA children similar on IQ, verbal memory, executive functioning and movement tests, but SGA children more likely to be in the abnormal range on attention control
Theodore (46)	Case-control follow up study	SGA defined as BW < 10th centile for GA for New Zealand standards (47)	241 SGA children and 348 aGA controls BY 1995–1996 Age at assessment: 7 y	Not assessed	Full Scale IQ scores (FSIQ) from the Wechsler Intelligence Scale for Children (WISC)	No significant difference in FSIQ between SGA and AGA children. In the whole sample, parental education and birth order were associated with FSIQ	No long term negative effect of being born SGA on FSIQ scores

AGA, appropriate for gestational age; BW, birth weight; BL, Birth Length; BY-birth year; FGR, fetal growth restriction; GA, gestational age; HC, Head Circumference; IUGR, intrauterine growth restriction; POBW, Percentage of optimal birthweight; SES, socio-economic status; SGA, small for gestational age; w, week; y, year. ANT, Amsterdam Neuropsychological Tasks; CP, Cerebral Palsy; BRIEF, Behavior Rating Inventory of Executive Function; K-ABC, Kaufmann Assessment Battery for Children; M-ABC, Movement ABC for Children; MHPT-Moray House Picture Test; NEPSY, A Developmental NEuroPSYchological Assessment; RAVLT, Rey's Auditory Verbal Learning Test; ROYCF-Rey Osterreith Complex Figure test; PDMS, Peabody Developmental Motor Scales; SDQ, Strengths and Difficulties Questionnaire; STM, short term memory; TeaCH, Test of Everyday Attention in Children; VADS, Visual aural digit span test; WASI, Wechsler Abbreviated Scales of Intelligence; WISC, Wechsler Intelligence Scales for Children; WISC-R, Wechsler Intelligence Scale for Children – revised; WPPSI, Wechsler Preschool and Primary Scale of Intelligence; WRAT, Wide Range Achievement Test. IQ, Intelligence Quotient Score; FSIQ, Full Scale IQ Score; PIQ, Performance IQ Score; VIQ, Verbal IQ score. The terms SGA, IUGR, FGR were used as in the study that is described.

performance in the SGA group when compared to the AGA group on testing with the M-ABC.

Cognitive and Behavioral Outcomes

In the reviewed studies, many different measures of neurocognitive outcome were employed, which can lead to difficulties summarizing results across studies. With this in mind, the first outcome to be discussed is that which was most commonly used across the reviewed studies—general intellectual functioning. IQ scores acquired from the Wechsler tests were the most commonly reported general cognitive outcome measures (29, 31, 32, 34, 36, 40, 42, 44, 46). There was some cross-study consensus about the effect of fetal growth restriction at term on Wechsler derived IQ scores, with three studies reporting that term FGR children's IQ scores were no different from those of control children (29, 42, 44, 46). In contrast, one study reported that FGR children's IQ scores were significantly lower than controls (40), but it should be noted that this study included both term and preterm children and thus this finding may not be isolated to term FGR children. One study found significant positive correlations between IQ scores and birth weight (32). A further two studies used head circumference at birth as an indication of fetal growth restriction (34, 36) and found that, for optimal IQ scores in later childhood, post-natal head growth in term born children was more important than prenatal head growth (34). In addition, the amount of post-natal head growth in term born children was greater for children whose mothers had been educated to degree level, or whose families had higher SES, which could be a consequence of cognitive stimulation and could also be linked to better nutrition (34). General intellectual functioning was also assessed by standardized measures other than the Wechsler range of tests, including the Kauffman ABC (40) and the Moray House picture test (39). Term children with FGR showed weaker performance than controls on both these assessments. In addition, higher levels of learning difficulties were reported, particularly language-based difficulties, and these were reflected by parental report of increased incidence of special educational needs interventions, particularly remedial education, neurological follow up, speech therapy and psychological intervention (40). However, this sample included 30% preterm children. While scores on the Moray House picture test were not affected by AGA status, birth weight as a continuous variable was associated with scores (39).

Taken together, the most common finding is that being born SGA at term does not impact significantly negatively on general intellectual functioning. The majority of studies that specifically examine FGR term children report similar performance on IQ-type measures as those found in controls (29, 39, 44, 46). Two studies reported that FGR term children have lower general intellectual functioning than controls (39, 40), but one of these studies also included a minority of preterm children, whose presence could account for these results (40). The other of these two studies (39) reported on children with late onset IUGR (occurring in the second to third trimester), thus it is possible that differences in the timing of growth restriction across studies impacts on the reported outcome; as not all studies reported the time at which growth restriction occurred, this interpretation is speculative. Birth weight correlates with later IQ scores in some studies (32), but not all (31), but other studies have reported that this occurs even in the normal birth weight range and therefore is not specific to FGR children (55).

As well as assessing performance on tasks measuring general intellectual functioning, the reviewed studies considered the effect of being born SGA at term on a range of more specific cognitive processes. However, as there was little consensus in either the aspects of cognition examined or the tests used, it is not possible to draw strong conclusions about specific outcomes, but any trends in the literature are considered here. Three studies examined memory processes (29, 38, 44). There was no difference between FGR term children and AGA term controls on a standard, orally presented digit span test or visual working memory (29), or differences between SGA and AGA children on a verbal list learning task (RAVLT) (44), although it should be noted that this latter study included both preterm and term SGA children. When performance on a digit span test that systematically varied both the presentation and recall of numbers was examined, the performance of FGR children was characterized by particular difficulty when the presentation was aural and children were required to make an oral response (38). While these findings require corroboration, they could have implications for classroom teachers as they suggest it might be more useful for children with FGR ifs teaching materials were non-aural (e.g., written/picture material) and children's responses should not always require them to speak aloud, but perhaps make written responses instead.

Two studies explored whether term born SGA children experience difficulties with executive functions, which describes a range of cognitive functions whose neural correlate lies in the frontal lobes and are involved with cognitive control of behavior (56). Executive functions are assessed both by performance on neurodevelopmental assessments, and also by questionnaire based rating scales, often completed by parents, which given an indication of how poor executive control can affect children's daily lives. The evidence on the effects of FGR on term born children's executive functioning was limited and mixed. For example, no differences in performance between FRG and AGA controls were found on a measure of impulse control (stop task) (29), and no differences between term SGA or term AGA on the parent rating form the BRIEF (44). However, SGA children were four times more likely to be in the abnormal range on TEA-Ch Attention Control compared to AGA children (44), although it should be noted that this sample included children born at term or preterm. Even in term born children without growth restriction, head circumference at birth and head circumference to length ratio at birth were predictive of ADHD symptoms at age 5 to 6 years (57). Term born low birth weight children had particular problems with attention (31). Thus, there is limited evidence in terms of the number of studies and within these studies, there is no reliable pattern of results on executive functions in term born FGR children. There were other measures assessed in individual studies only, with no cross-study comparison possible. For example, the presence of communication problems identified from children's medical charts did not differ between AGA and SGA term children who had CP (10).

Some of these studies of term born SGA children highlight the period of catch up growth that is particularly important for long term neurocognitive outcome. General intellectual functioning in childhood is influenced by early brain growth–indexed by growth in head circumference–that occurs in infancy. For example, IQ score at 8 years was associated with greater than expected head growth during infancy, rather than head circumference at birth (31, 36), catch up growth at 2 years predicted 9–10 years IQ scores (40). Later growth is also important for IQ; children with optimal somatic catch-up growth at age 9–10 years, but not 2 years (defined as >10th centile in height, weight and head circumference) had significantly higher scores on neurodevelopmental and cognitive tests at 9–10 years than children with suboptimal catch-up growth (defined as <10th centile in height, weight or head circumference) (40). However, there seem to be better outcomes for term born children with asymmetric FGR, which favors head growth over the rest of the body, compared to children with symmetric FGR (32); this suggests sparing of the head, a neuroadaptive modification to conserve the developing brain.

SCHOOL AGE OUTCOMES OF SGA AND/OR FGR IN THE CONTEXT OF PRETERM BIRTH

Neurodevelopmental outcome of SGA and/or FGR in preterm (born <37 w GA; very preterm = born <32 w GA; extremely preterm ≤28 wGA at birth) infants is difficult to study since there it is complicated separate the effects of SGA/FGR from the consequences of preterm birth *per se*. The majority of studies investigating school age outcomes of SGA or/and FGR in preterm born children have excluded children with congenital abnormalities, congenital infections, chromosomal abnormalities, or syndromes. However, only in some studies detailed information on antenatal growth is available, and seldom are SGA and FGR clearly distinguished and examined separately; some studies may include constitutionally "small at birth" children. Definitions of SGA and growth references used differ between studies. All this is likely to affect study findings and needs to be kept in mind when interpreting and comparing results from different studies.

Table 2 provides study details from 10 studies on neurocognitive outcomes in preterm school aged children, the majority of which are population based studies that examined outcomes of FGR or SGA published in the past 15 years.

Neuromotor Outcomes

An association between SGA and/or FGR with CP in children born preterm has been reported from CP registers, for example, from the Surveillance of Cerebral Palsy in Europe (SCPE), who found that those born with BW for GA below the 10th percentile (using fetal growth standards) had a higher risk for CP than those with a BW between 25th and 75th centile. This was found for the GA range of 32–41 weeks and was similar for all CP subtypes. The association between SGA at birth and CP, however, was not as clear for those born very or extremely preterm. Interestingly, a higher risk is also reported for those with BW above the 97th centile (11). Similar data are reported from other cohorts. For example, Jacobsson (49), using data from the CP register for West Sweden, after adjustment for maternal height, weight in early pregnancy, parity, ethnic origin and baby's sex, did not find an increased proportion of children who were SGA at birth in the preterm group (born <36+6 wGA), whereas in the term born group children with CP were significantly more likely to have been SGA at birth. It should be kept in mind that these are associations and that this does not necessarily mean that growth restriction causes CP. For very and extremely preterm children, the evidence suggests that other biological risk factors, in particular, focal preterm brain injury, pose a higher risk for severe neuromotor impairment than growth restriction. The findings of the studies reviewed here (**Table 2**) do not suggest that SGA and/or FGR pose a significant independent risk for CP in children born preterm, and this appears to be the case across the preterm gestational age range (7, 49, 58, 61, 66). Post-natal growth appears to be an important factor as, for example, indicated by the study by Franz et al. (58) in school aged children born <30 wGA and BW<1,500 g, who found that neuromotor outcome was associated with post-natal growth but not FGR, and this was still the case once analyses had been adjusted for important other biological risk factors including brain injury.

Neuromotor function in the absence of CP has been reported by several groups. The studies reviewed here report contradictory findings. Tanis (44), examined motor skills with the M-ABC in school aged children born 31–41 weeks of gestation in a population based cohort in the Netherlands, and did not find a difference in motor skills for the moderately preterm group between those who were AGA and those who were SGA at birth. Korzeniewski et al. (64), reported for the extremely preterm born ELGAN cohort no differences in motor function (assessed with the GMFC and MACS) at school age between those born after FGR and those without FGR. In another study in extremely preterm children Kan et al. (63), report M-ABC data from the Victorian Infant Collaborative study, a population based study of children born extremely preterm, and did not find an association between motor skills and FGR. However, they did see a significant association between head circumference at age 2 years and age 8 years with motor skills, suggesting that post-natal and post-neonatal brain growth is a crucial factor for motor outcome at school age, independently of presence of absence of FGR. In contrast to the findings by Kan (63), Tanis, and Korzeniewski (44, 63, 64) from 3 large population based cohorts, Raz et al. (67), report for a single center study of children born <34+6 wGA, using the PDMS-2, poorer gross and fine motor skills as well as performance IQ scores, for those with FGR compared to those born with appropriate for GA birth weight, and, importantly, an association between intrauterine growth and motor skills as well as Performance IQ even in those who had adequate standardized birth weight. Despite these inconsistent findings between studies, it appears to emerge that post-natal and post-neonatal brain growth is more important than intrauterine growth for neuromotor development in those

TABLE 2 | Included studies for preterm born children.

References	Study type	Definition of fetal growth	Participants	Neurology/neuromotor function	Cognitive/behavior Outcome measure	Cognitive/behavior findings	Conclusion
Franz (58)	Single center study (Level 3 Neonatal Unit)	IUGR defined as BW < −2 SD according to British Growth Reference (59) expressed as SDS	Born < 30 wGA and BW < 1,500 g BY 1996–1999 *N* = 297 preterms admitted to neonatal unit Age at assessment: 5.4 y Those with neuromotor and sensory impairment included	Neurological examination: normal, mildly abnormal (minor neurologic signs such as broad gait, dysdiadochokinesis, or dysmetria), severely abnormal (any paresis with or without spasticity, cerebral nerve palsy, or ataxia) GMFCS for level of motor function *Findings:* Neuromotor outcome associated with post-natal growth, not IUGR	K-ABC (Mental Processing Composite, MPC) Analyses adjusted for GA, sex, multiple birth, ICH > Grade 3; PVL, ROP > Grade 3, ventilation > 7 days, language, maternal education	MPC associated with IUGR (BW), early neonatal weight gain, head growth post-discharge	Intrauterine growth (weight) and in-hospital weight gain predictor of cognitive outcome Post-natal weight gain but not IUGR associated with CP HC growth but not weight gain from discharge to follow-up predictor of cognitive outcome Combined contribution of IVH and prolonged mechanical ventilation greater than the combined contribution of growth
Guellec (7)	Population based; EPIPAGE study, 9 regions in France	*N* = 2,846 SGA = <10th centile (9.2%) Mildly SGA (MSGA) = 10th–<20th centile (9.6%) AGA =>20th centile Neonatal internal reference to approach *in utero* growth restriction, similar to Mamelle et al. (60) 2 preterm groups: <28 weeks GA (*n* = 828) 28–32 weeks GA (*n* = 2018) Term born (39/40 wGA) reference group (666 children) included at birth in the same regions	All live borns 24–32 weeks GA, born 1997 in 9 regions in France *n* = 2,846 Age at assessment: 5 y: 77% neurology; 65% cognitive assessment;71% behavior questionnaires 8 y: 61%	Categorized into presence of absence of cerebral palsy (SCPE criteria for CP used) *Findings:* **29-32 weeks GA group:** Cerebral Palsy: AGA 7.7%; MSGA 4.6%; SGA 3.2% **<28 weeks GA group:** Cerebral Palsy: AGA 14%; MSGA 11.1%; SGA 18.2%	**At age 5 years**: K-ABC: Mental processing composite score (IQ equivalent). Moderate cognitive deficiency: score between 70 and 84; severe cognitive deficiency: score <70 Behavioral problems: SDQ: inattention-hyperactivity, conduct, emotional, peer problems; total behavioral difficulties score **At age 8 years**: School questionnaire (school difficulties: special schooling institution or special school, special class in mainstream school, mainstream class) or low grades Analyses adjusted for sex, GA	**29–32 weeks GA group:** Cognitive deficit: AGA 28.7%; MSGA 41.8%; SGA 40.6% Behavioral problems: AGA 19.4%; MSGA 15.7%; SGA 23.5% School difficulties: AGA 18.4%; MSGA 32.18%; SGA 28 % **<28 weeks GA group:** Cognitive deficit: AGA 38.3%; MSGA 32.1%; SGA 37.5% Behavioral problems: AGA 23.7%; MSGA 27.3%; SGA 33.3% School difficulties: AGA 33.2%; MSGA 44.8%; SGA 35.3% Analyses controlled for socio-economic factors and sex	Growth restriction associated with adverse neurodevelopmental outcomes only in the 29- to 32-week GA group; both SGA and MSGA associated with an increase of cognitive deficiency, behavioral problems, and school difficulties. CP not associated with SGA

(Continued)

TABLE 2 | Continued

References	Study type	Definition of fetal growth	Participants	Neurology/neuromotor function	Cognitive/behavior Outcome measure	Cognitive/behavior findings	Conclusion
Guellec (61)	Population based; EPIPAGE study, 9 regions in France	4 categories: Symmetric growth restriction (SGR): HC and BW <20th centile and in the same percentile range; asymmetric growth restriction (AGR): at least 1 of HC and BW <20th centile and the other in a higher decile range. Two forms of AGR: head growth restriction (HGR), weight growth restriction (WGR). AGA: both BW and HC >20th centile	All live borns 26–32 wGA BY 1997 Age at assessment: 5 y (school performance at 8 y)	Categorized into presence of absence of cerebral palsy (SCPE criteria for CP used) *Findings:* No difference between groups for CP	K-ABC: Mental processing composite score (IQ equivalent), Moderate cognitive deficiency: score between 70 and 84; severe cognitive deficiency: score <70 Behavioral problems: SDQ: inattention-hyperactivity, conduct, emotional, peer problems; total behavioral difficulties score	SGR: higher risks of both moderate and severe cognitive deficiency. HGR: only higher risk for severe cognitive deficiency No difference between groups for behavior SGR: higher rate of school difficulties than AGA children Discussion	SGR associated with impaired cognitive and school performance Outcome of AGR differed according to HC: HGR associated with impaired cognitive function; WGR not associated with cognitive outcome No higher risk for CP in SGR
Kallankari (62)	Population based (regional cohort, Finland)	FGR defined as BW < −2 SD from mean of gestation-adjusted birth weight; documented FGR due to placental insufficiency by Doppler ultrasound and histological placental perfusion defect and lack of congenital infections or malformations	Born <32 wGA ($n = 154$); term born controls ($n = 90$) BY 1998–2002 Age at assessment: 9 y $n = 77$ preterms; $n = 18$ (23% FGR), $n = 27$ term controls Only preterms without CP and without cognitive impairment included	N/A	14 subtests from NEPSY II 6 subtests from WISC-III Mean scores for 5 domains calculated: visuospatial–sensorimotor processing, attention–executive functions, language, memory–learning and social perception Analyses controlled for GA, sex, maternal education	FGR only identified risk factor for impairment in language and memory learning skills in the preterm group; no difference between preterm AGA and FGR group for attention, executive functions, visuo-spatial, sensorimotor function	FGR independently predicts poor language, memory and learning skills
Kan (63)	Population based; Victorian Infant Collaborative Study	IUGR defined as BW < −2 SD according to British Growth Reference (59); expresses as Z-score	Born <28 wGA BY 1991–1992 $n = 179$ (2.2% IUGR); Age at assessment: 8 y Those with neurosensory impairment excluded	M-ABC 2 for assessment of motor skills (dexterity, ball skills, balance) *Findings:* HC or BW, or weight catch up in early childhood not associated with outcome, but, HC age 2 y and age 8 y associated with motor outcome	WISC-III for IQ WRAT-II for educational skills (reading, spelling, arithmetic) Analyses adjusted for potential biological and environmental risk factors (IVH grade 3 or 4, cystic PVL, surgery, post-natal steroids; maternal education, social class, other languages than English)	IUGR not associated with outcome at age 8 years HC or weight at birth, or weight catch up in early childhood not associated with outcome, but HC age 2 y and age 8 y associated with cognitive outcome	Intrauterine growth mostly unrelated to cognitive and other outcomes in preterm children without neurosensory impairment, but events between post-birth and age 2 years have an effect on brain growth and function, over and above effects of prematurity

(Continued)

TABLE 2 | Continued

References	Study type	Definition of fetal growth	Participants	Neurology/neuromotor function	Cognitive/behavior Outcome measure	Cognitive/behavior findings	Conclusion
Korzeniewski (64)	Multicenter, prospective, observational study (Extremely Low Gestational Age Newborns, ELGAN)	3 groups according to BW z-score (65) Severe FGR: <-2, Less severe FGR: ≥-2 and <-1 No FGR: ≥-1	Born <28 w GA $N = 889$ (93%) of original cohort BY 2002–2004 $n = 52$ severe FGR $n = 113$ less severe FGR Age at assessment: 10 y	GMFCS for gross motor function MACS for hand function *Findings:* FGR not associated with poorer motor function	DAS-II, NEPSY-II for general and specific cognitive functions (including executive function, memory, attention, verbal reasoning, visuo-motor precision etc.) WIAT-III for academic achievements (reading, spelling, numerical operations) OWLS for language (oral and written), Communication Function Classification Scale, and CCC-2 for communication skills SRS for social abilities, SCQ for screen for autism; ADOS-2 for autism diagnosis Analyses adjusted for sex and racial identity	Both severe and less severe FGR similar in having lower scores than no FGR peers in verbal reasoning, listening, comprehension, visuomotor precision, word reading, working memory, pseudoword decoding, and spelling subtests; more problems with social awareness and social cognition Severe FGR group lower scores than less severe FGR group for measures of auditory attention and response as well as inhibition switching, inhibition naming, as well as having higher scores on autism screen, and a variety of communication problems	Severe FGR poses increased risk of multiple cognitive and behavioral dysfunctions There is a positive relationship between severity of FGR and severity of cognitive impairment and behavior FGR not associated with poorer motor function
Morsing (66)	Single center study, Sweden	BW < -2 SD from mean of Swedish growth standards (53)	46 fetuses with IUGR and ARED umbilical artery blood flow; delivered <30 wGA at level III perinatal center BY 1998–2004 Follow-up: $n = 34$ preterm SGA with IUGR, ARED on umbilical arterial flow antenatally $n = 34$ preterm AGA (matched for sex, GA, BY) $n = 34$ term AGA Age at assessment: 5–8 y Those with CP not excluded	Information on diagnosis of CP and GMFCS level, hearing and visual function collected at time of cognitive assessment *Findings:* No difference in CP frequency	WPPSI-III; WISC-III (IQ) SDQ, Brown ADD Scale (total scores) for socio-emotional functioning and attention difficulties Analyses controlled for parental education, neonatal septicaemia, CLD, ICH>grade 3, PVL, post-natal steroids, ROP grade 3–5	FSIQ and VIQ lower in SGA/IUGR preterms than AGA preterms; PIQ not different; this was driven by poorer performance of male preterm SGA/IUGR children No difference in SDQ and ADD scores	Male preterm SGA children with IUGR and ARED blood flow *in utero* have poorer cognitive outcome than female preterms with IUGR and AERD No higher risk for CP
Raz (67)	Single center study	IUGR defined as BW < 10th centile; Z-score computed as the deviation of BW from the mean BW gestational age group, at delivery	Born 23–34+6 wGA (mean 28.6) BY 1991–2000 $n = 25$ IUGR $n = 118$ AG (appropriate growth) Age at assessment: 3–6 y Those with CP and ICH excluded	PDMS-2 for gross and fine motor skills *Findings:* Difference in gross and fine motor scores with IUGR having poorer motor skills	WPPSI-R for IQ scores PLS-3 for language skills (auditory comprehension and expressive communication) Analyses adjusted for sex, no significant difference in socio-economic class between groups	Full Scale IQ poorer in IUGR group; driven by difference in Performance IQ scores	Association between intrauterine growth and cognitive and motor outcome even within the population of preterm children who had adequate standardized birth weight

(Continued)

TABLE 2 | Continued

References	Study type	Definition of fetal growth	Participants	Neurology/neuromotor function	Cognitive/behavior Outcome measure	Cognitive/behavior findings	Conclusion
Tanis (44)	Population based regional cohort—subgroup (Longitudinal Preterm Outcome Project study), Netherlands	BW < −1 SD and birth weight > −1 SD according to GA; Dutch Kloosterman curve (45). Cut-off for SGA (> 1 SD, below the 16th percentile) according to Etude Epidemiologique sur les Petits Ages Gestationnels study	Born 31–41 wGA. AGA = 336; 216/336 moderately preterm SGA = 42; 216 32/42 moderately preterm BY 2002–2003 Age at assessment: 7 y	M-ABC 2 for assessment of motor skills (dexterity, ball skills, balance) *Findings:* No significant difference between groups	WISC III (Full Scale IQ) TEA-Ch: selective attention and Attention control RAVLT: Verbal memory NEPSY-II: Visuomotor integration BRIEF: Executive functioning in daily life Analyses adjusted for GA and sex	SGA children poorer attentional control, irrespective of GA No significant difference in other outcome measures	SGA children higher risk for difficulties with attentional control, irrespective of GA at birth. General cognitive, executive function, and motor skills not different between AGA and SGA

AGA, appropriate for gestational age; ARED, absent or reversed end-diastolic blood flow; AGR, asymmetric growth restriction; BW, birth weight; CLD, chronic lung disease; FGR, fetal growth restriction; GA, gestational age; HGR, head growth restriction; ICH, intracranial hemorrhage; IUGR, intrauterine growth restriction; PVL, periventricular leukomalacia; ROP, retinopathy of prematurity; SGA, small for gestational age; SGR, symmetric growth restriction; w, week; WGR, weight growth restriction; y, year. ADOS, Autism Diagnostic Observation Schedule; CCL, Children's Communication Scale; CP, Cerebral Palsy; CSI, Child Symptom Inventory; Brown ADD, Brown Attention-Deficit Disorder Scales; BRIEF, Behavior Rating Inventory of Executive Function; CBCL, Child Behavior Checklist;; DAS, Differential Ability Scales; GMFCS, Gross Motor Function Classification Scale; K-ABC, Kaufmann Assessment Battery for Children; MACS, Manual Ability Classification Scale; M-ABC, Movement ABC for Children; MPC, Mental Processing Composite; NEPSY, A Developmental NEuroPSYchological Assessment; OWLS, Oral and Written Language Scales; PDMS, Peabody Developmental Motor Scales; PLS, Preschool Language Scale; RAVLT, Rey's Auditory Verbal Learning Test; SCQ, Social Communication Questionnaire; SDQ, Strengths and Difficulties Questionnaire; TeaCH, Test of Everyday Attention in Children; WIAT, Wechsler Individual Achievement Test; WISC, Wechsler Intelligence Scales for Children; WPPSI, Wechsler Preschool and Primary Scale of Intelligence; WRAT, Wide Range Achievement Test. The terms SGA, IUGR, FGR were used as in the study that is described.

who do not develop CP, which is also supported by Neubauer et al. (68), who examined 448 children born <32 w GA (19.9% SGA), and found that head size at age 3 months was the best predictor for motor (and cognitive) outcome at age 24 months. Visuo-motor skills at age 11 years were examined in the study by Kok et al. (69), for a cohort of preterm children (born <33 wGA) born FGR and who had antenatal Doppler studies performed; comparison was made between the group with and without "brain sparing." No significant differences were see in any of the tests (Beery-Buktencia Developmental test of Visuo-motor Integration, Motor Accuracy Test (MAT), Motor-Free Visual Perception Test (MVPT-R), and the balls skills subtest from the M-ABC).

Cognitive and Behavioral Outcomes

It is well-known that prematurity, in particular, very and extremely preterm birth, poses a risk for impairment of general cognitive abilities as well as difficulties in specific cognitive functions such as memory functions, processing speed, cognitive flexibility, attentional abilities, as well as socio-emotional behavior, all of which will affect for academic progress and peer relationships. Being born preterm and SGA and/or having FGR may be an independent risk factor for impairment of long term cognitive and behavioral outcomes, over and above other relevant biological and social risk factors. Long term outcomes of preterm birth are affected by a number of factors and it is often complicated to establish an independent effect of SGA and/or FGR on long term cognitive outcomes in the context of prematurity. Often, those who are SGA and/or have had FGR, also are those who, compared to those born AGA, have more other neonatal morbidities that have been show to affect outcome (such as chronic lung disease, neonatal sepsis, etc.), which has been illustrated, for example, by the large EPIPAGE study (61). In addition, often, there are no detailed fetal growth measures or information on fetal Doppler studies available, which can make it difficult to establish the exact cause of a preterm infant's SGA birth weight. Direct comparison of study findings is difficult since slightly different criteria for definition of SGA and/or FGR are used in different studies. In addition, although most studies have assessed general cognitive abilities with either the Wechsler Intelligence Scales (44, 62, 63, 66, 67), the Kaufmann ABC (7, 58, 61), or the NEPSY assessment (62, 64), different studies focused on different specific cognitive functions, and there is a large variety of different tests used. Furthermore, in some studies participants with neurosensory impairment were not excluded from analyses on cognitive and behavioral function, which complicates comparison with those studies in which only those without neurosensory impairment were assessed. However, overall, the studies reviewed here suggest that preterm children born SGA and/or having had FGR, compared to their AGA preterm peers, are at increased risk of developing cognitive and behavioral difficulties, although some study findings are inconsistent. With the exception of the study on the Victorian Infant Collaborative Study cohort (63), who did not find an association between FGR and cognitive abilities at school age, but between post-neonatal head growth and cognitive development, the large multicenter or population based studies reviewed here

(7, 44, 61, 64) report an effect of FGR (it has to be kept in mind that in most studies SGA was used as a surrogate marker for FGR) on long term cognitive function, and, in the majority of the studies, this was still the case once other biological and social risk factors are considered. Guellec (7), reported school age outcome data for the EPIPAGE cohort (GA range 24–32 weeks) and divided the SGA participants into 2 groups, mildly SGA and SGA, and also formed 2 GA groups (<28 wGA, 29–32 wGA). They found impaired cognitive function, behavioral problems, and school difficulties at school age were more frequent in both the mildly SGA and the SGA born children in the 29–32 wGA group but not in the more immature GA group.

Korzeniewski et al. (64), examined school age outcomes for the extremely preterm (<28 wGA) born ELGAN cohort, focusing on general and specific cognitive abilities (including executive function, memory, attention, verbal reasoning, visuo-motor precision), communication abilities, and socio-emotional behavior. They did find overall a positive relationship between severity of FGR and severity of cognitive impairment and behavior for most areas assessed, and, in addition, that those with the most severe FGR also had more problems than those with less severe FGR in auditory attention, inhibition switching, inhibition naming, higher scores on autism screen, and a variety of communication problems. Kallankari et al. (62), followed a Finnish cohort of children born at a more mature GA (<32 wGA) for whom FGR due to placental insufficiency was documented by Doppler ultrasound and histological placental perfusion defect. They reported that FGR independently predicted poor language, memory and learning skills, but did not find an effect of FGR on attention, executive function, visuo-spatial, or sensorimotor function. For a cohort with a larger range of GA at birth (31–41 wGA), Tanis et al. (44), established that those born SGA were at higher risk for difficulties with attentional control, irrespective of GA at birth, but that there was no difference to those born AGA for measures of general cognitive abilities, executive function, visuomotor integration, or memory function. These findings on attention difficulties in children born SGA and/or FGR are consistent with those from a large nationwide case-control study in Finland that investigated associations between prematurity and fetal growth in relation to Attention Deficit Hyperactivity Disorder (ADHD) (70). This study found that prematurity was a risk factor for ADHD across the preterm gestational age range, and that with lowest weight for GA (< −2 SD) had the highest risk for ADHD, together with those being more than 2 SD large for GA.

Some studies have investigated childhood outcomes of preterm children born SGA and/or FGR for whom information on umbilical artery blood flow was available. Morsing et al. (66), examined outcome in a cohort of fetuses with FGR and absent or reversed end-diastolic umbilical artery (AERD) blood flow who were delivered before 30 wGA, and compared them to a control group of preterm infants of the same GA born with AGA birth weight. At school age those with AERD had poorer full scale and verbal IQ than those born AGA and this difference was driven by the poor performance of male participants in the FGR/AERD group. These findings are inconsistent with those of Valcamonico et al. (71), who found a higher incidence of severe neurological problems (CP, visual and/or hearing impairment) but no difference in general cognitive abilities in a group of very preterm born (mean GA at birth 33.3 weeks; 35 % SGA with BW <5th centile) school aged children who had AERD when compared to a group of children (mean GA at birth 30.8 weeks; 38% SGA) who did not have AERD. It is possible that the difference in outcomes between these studies are explained by the different proportions of children having been SGA at birth, despite all having had AERD; furthermore there are differences between studies in the methodology of the Doppler studies and definition of SGA and/or fetal growth. van den Broek et al. (72), compared behavior in a large cohort of 11 years old children born preterm (<33 wGA) in whom weekly antenatal Doppler studies were done to assess the ratio between umbilical and cerebral pulsatility index (U/C ration) for assessment of "brain sparing." In this study, rather than using centile curves, fetal growth ratio was defined as the ratio of the observed birth weight to the expected mean birth weight for gestational age, based on Dutch intrauterine growth curves. At age 5 years significant difference in the proportion of those with Full Scale IQ <85 in the group with "brain sparing," but no significant difference for mean FS IQ between the groups. At age 11 years no significant association was seen between parent and teacher rating of behavior on the CBCL and U/C ratio after controlling for neonatal variables and IQ at age 5 years, indicating that "brain sparing" was not an independent risk factor for behavioral difficulties at age 11 y.

Most of the existing studies in term born babies use growth or birth weight <10th centile, often based on different growth standards, as definition of FGR. Using more stringent FGR bands may be useful in future work in order to examine in more detail whether there is an effect of only severe FGR on development. Kan et al. (63) studied long term cognitive outcome in extremely preterm born children, using stricter criteria for FGR (< −2 SD) and did not find an association between FGR and outcome, but strong associations between post-natal head growth and outcome, which emphasizes the importance of head growth, very likely independently of the severity of FGR. The importance of post-neonatal head growth for cognitive development in children born SGA and/or FGR has also been highlighted by the study by Franz et al. (58), who reported for a single center cohort born <30 wGA that FGR, in-hospital weight gain, and post-neonatal head growth (but not weight gain) predicted general cognitive abilities at school age (63).

CONCLUSIONS

Overall, existing studies are heterogeneous, for example, with regards to definitions of growth restriction and small for gestational age, time of onset of FGR, inclusion and exclusion criteria, outcome measures, all of which makes comparison between studies difficult.

However, in summary, the literature reviewed here suggests that cognitive development in term born children is not hugely impacted by them being born SGA or FGR, particularly in the case of general intellectual function, on which the majority of studies have been conducted. There is some limited evidence that term born growth restricted children may experience problems with attention, and such difficulties may have more impact on children's learning and behavior as they progress through school, suggesting that this would be a useful area for further work. The risk for developing CP is higher in children born SGA with FGR; currently there is contradictory information available on neuromotor function in the absence of CP.

In contrast, preterm born SGA and/or FGR children are at great risk of poorer general intellectual functioning than their AGA counterparts. These children are also at risk for difficulties with attentional control, and some studies suggest that memory, executive function, and communication skills are also affected. It does not appear that SGA and/or FGR *per se* pose a higher risk for CP; information on motor outcome in the absence of CP is, similar to the term born children, somewhat contradictory.

Post-neonatal head growth and head growth in infancy and early childhood emerges as an important factor for long term neurodevelopmental outcome.

There is some inconsistency between the conclusions of our review of school aged children and those studies that report follow up data acquired in the toddler years. This could result from certain cognitive difficulties taking time to emerge and/or these being more subtle problems that are nevertheless clinically and functionally important. It is important to continue to follow up children into the school age years because these difficulties may take time to emerge, and may be more visible in the more demanding school environment.

AUTHOR CONTRIBUTIONS

BV and CE have made equal contributions to this work. Both provide approval for publication of the work and agree to be accountable for all aspects of the work.

REFERENCES

1. Murray E, Fernandes M, Fazel M, Kennedy SH, Villar J, Stein A. Differential effect of intrauterine growth restriction on childhood neurodevelopment: a systematic review. *BJOG An Int J Obstet Gynaecol.* (2015) 122:1062–72. doi: 10.1111/1471-0528.13435
2. van Wassenaer A. Neurodevelopmental consequences of being born SGA. *Pediatr Endocrinol Rev.* (2005) 2:372–7.
3. Maulik D. Fetal growth compromise: definitions, standards, and classification. *Clin Obs Gynecol.* (2006) 49:214–8. doi: 10.1097/00003081-200606000-00004
4. Baschat A. Neurodevelopment after fetal growth restriction. *Fetal Diagn Ther.* (2014) 36:136–42. doi: 10.1159/000353631
5. Goldenberg RL, Culhane JF, Iams JD, Romero R. Epidemiology and causes of preterm birth. *Lancet.* (2008) 371:75–84. doi: 10.1016/S0140-6736(08)60074-4
6. Walker D, Marlow N. Neurocognitive outcome following fetal growth restriction. *Arch Dis Child Fetal Neonatal Ed.* (2008) 93:F322–5. doi: 10.1136/adc.2007.120485
7. Guellec I, Lapillonne A, Renolleau S, Charlaluk M, Roze J, Marret S. Neurologic outcomes at school age in very preterm infants born with severe or mild growth restriction. *Pediatrics.* (2011) 127:e883–91. doi: 10.1542/peds.2010-2442
8. Lundgren EM, Cnattingius S, Jonsson B, Tuvemo T. Birth characteristics and different dimensions of intellectual performance in young males: a nationwide population-based study. *Acta Paediatr Int J Paediatr.* (2003) 92:1138–43. doi: 10.1111/j.1651-2227.2003.tb02473.x
9. Leonard H, Nassar N, Bourke J, Blair E, Mulroy S, De Klerk N, et al. Relation between intrauterine growth and subsequent intellectual disability in a ten-year population cohort of children in Western Australia. *Am J Epidemiol.* (2008) 167:103–11. doi: 10.1093/aje/kwm245
10. Freire G, Shevell M, Oskoui M. Cerebral palsy: phenotypes and risk factors in term singletons born small for gestational age. *Eur J Paediatr Neurol.* (2015) 19:218–25. doi: 10.1016/j.ejpn.2014.12.005
11. Jarvis S, Glinianaia S, Torrioli M, Platt M, Miceli M, Jouk P, et al. Surveillance of cerebral palsy in Europe (SCPE) collaboration of European cerebral palsy registers. Cerebral palsy and intrauterine growth in single births: European collaborative study. *Lancet.* (2003) 4:1106–11. doi: 10.1016/S0140-6736(03)14466-2
12. Palisano R, Rosenbaum P, Walter S, Russell D, Wood E, Galuppi B. Development and reliability of a system to classify gross motor function in children with cerebral palsy. *Dev Med Child Neurol.* (1997) 39:214–23. doi: 10.1111/j.1469-8749.1997.tb07414.x
13. Eliasson A, Krumlinde-Sundholm L, Rösblad B, Beckung E, Arner M, Ohrvall A, et al. The manual ability classification system (MACS) for children with cerebral palsy: scale development and evidence of validity and reliability. *Dev Med Child Neurol.* (2006) 48:549–54. doi: 10.1017/S0012162206001162
14. Henderson S, Sugden D, Barnett A. *Movement Assessment Battery for Children—Second Edition (MABC-2).* London: Psychological Corporation (2007).
15. Folio M, Fewell R. *Peabody Developmental Motor Scales-Second Edition.* Austin, TX: Pro-Ed, Inc.
16. Wechsler D. *The Wechsler Intelligence Scale for Children.* 5th edn. Bloomington, MN: Pearson (2014).
17. Wechsler D. *Wechsler Abbreviated Scale of Intelligence.* San Antonio, TX: Psychological Corporation (1999).
18. Wechsler D. *Wechsler Preschool and Primary Scale of Intelligence - Fourth Edition (WPPSITM - IV).* Bloomington, MN: Pearson, Psychological Corporation (2012).
19. Kauffman A, Kauffman N. *Assessment Battery for Children (K-ABC) Hebrew Version.* Jerusalam: Ministry of Education (1996).
20. Manly T, Anderson V, Nimmo-Smith I, Turner A, Watson P, Robertson I. The differential assessment of children's attention: the test of everyday attention for children (TEA-Ch), normative sample and ADHD performance. *J Child Psychol Psychiatry.* (2001) 42:1065–81. doi: 10.1111/1469-7610.00806
21. Vakil E, Blachstein H, Rochberg J, Vardi M. Characterization of memory impairment following closed-head injury in children using the rey auditory verbal learning test (AVLT) child neuropsychology. *Neuropsychol Dev Cogn Sect C.* (2004) 10:57–66. doi: 10.1080/09297040490911078
22. Osterreith P. Le test do copie d'une figure complex. *Arch Psychol.* (1944) 30:206–36.
23. Korkman M, Kirk U, Kemp S. *NEPSY-II: Clinical and Interpretive Manual.* San Antonio, TX: Pearson Education (2007).
24. Gioia G, Isquith PK, Guy SC, Kenworthy L. *Behavior Rating Inventory of Executive Function.* Odessa, FL: Psychological Assessment Resources (2000).
25. Goodman R. The strengths and difficulties questionnaire: a research note. *J Child Psychol Psychiatry.* (1997) 38:581–6. doi: 10.1111/j.1469-7610.1997.tb01545.x
26. Constantino J, Gruber C. *Social Responsiveness Scale (SRS2).* Los Angeles, CA: Western Psychological Services (2012).
27. Rutter M, Bailey A, Lord C. *The Social Communication Questionnaire.* Los Angeles, CA: Western Psychological Services (2003).
28. Lord C, Rutter M, DiLavore P, Risi S, Gotham K, Bishop S. *Autism Diagnostic Observation Schedule.* 2nd ed. Torrance, CA: Western Psychological Services (2012).
29. Beukers F, Aarnoudse-Moens CSH, van Weissenbruch MM, Ganzevoort W, van Goudoever JB, van Wassenaer-Leemhuis AG. Fetal growth restriction

with brain sparing: neurocognitive and behavioral outcomes at 12 years of age. *J Pediatr.* (2017) 188:103–9.e2. doi: 10.1016/j.jpeds.2017.06.003

30. Gardosi J, Mongelli M, Wilcox M, Change A. An adjustable fetal weight standard. *Ultrasound Obstet Gynecol.* (1995) 6:167–74. doi: 10.1046/j.1469-0705.1995.06030168.x
31. Emond A, Lira P, Lima M, Grantham-McGregor, SM Ashworth A. Development and behaviour of low-birthweight term infants at 8 years in northeast Brazil: a longitudinal study. *Acta Paediatr.* (2006) 95:1249–57. doi: 10.1080/08035250600615127
32. Fattal-Valevski A, Toledano-Alhadef H, Leitner Y, Geva R, Eshel R, Harel S. Growth patterns in children with intrauterine growth retardation and their correlation to neurocognitive development. *J Child Neurol.* (2009) 24:846–51. doi: 10.1177/0883073808331082
33. Lieberman J, Fraser D, Weitzman S, Glezerman M. Birthweight curves in southern Israel populations. *Isr J Med Sci.* (1993) 5:198–203.
34. Gale CR, O'Callaghan FJ, Godfrey KM, Law CM, Martyn CN. Critical periods of brain growth and cognitive function in children. *Brain.* (2004) 127:321–9. doi: 10.1093/brain/awh034
35. Blair E, Liu Y, de Klerk N. Optimal fetal growth for the Caucasian singleton and assessment of appropriateness of fetal growth: an analysis of a total population perinatal database. *BMC Pediatr.* (2005) 5:13. doi: 10.1186/1471-2431-5-13
36. Gale CR, O'Callaghan FJ, Bredow M, Martyn CN. The influence of head growth in fetal life, infancy, and childhood on intelligence at the ages of 4 and 8 years. *Pediatrics.* (2006) 118:1486–92. doi: 10.1542/peds.2005-2629
37. Geva R, Eshel R, Leitner Y, Fattal-Valevski A, Harel S. Memory functions of children born with asymmetric intrauterine growth restriction. *Brain Res.* (2006) 1117:186–94. doi: 10.1016/j.brainres.2006.08.004
38. Geva R, Eshel R, Leitner Y, Fattal-Valevski A, Harel S. Verbal short-term memory span in children: long-term modality dependent effects of intrauterine growth restriction. *J Child Psychol Psychiatry.* (2008) 49:1321–30. doi: 10.1111/j.1469-7610.2008.01917.x
39. Lawlor DA. Intrauterine growth and intelligence within sibling pairs: findings from the aberdeen children of the 1950s cohort. *Pediatrics.* (2006) 117:e894–902. doi: 10.1542/peds.2005-2412
40. Leitner Y, Fattal-valevski A, Geva R, Eshel R, Toledano-alhadef H, Rotstein M, et al. Neurodevelopmental outcome of children a longitudinal, 10-year prospective study. *J Child Neurol.* (2009) 22:580–7. doi: 10.1177/0883073807302605
41. Niklasson A, Erison A, Fryer J, Karlberg J, Lawrence C, Karlberg P. An update of the Swedish reference standards for weigh, length and head circumference at birth for given gestational age. *Acta Paediatr Scan.* (1991) 80:756–62. doi: 10.1111/j.1651-2227.1991.tb11945.x
42. Sommerfelt K, Sonnander K, Skranes J, Andersson H, Ahlsten G, Ellertsen B, et al. Neuropsychologic and motor function in small-for-gestation preschoolers. *Pediatr Neurol.* (2002) 26:186–91. doi: 10.1016/S0887-8994(01)00381-2
43. Bakketeig L. Current growth standards, definitions, diag- nosis and classification of fetal growth retardation. *Eur J Clin Nutr.* (1998) 52:1–4.
44. Tanis JC, Van Braeckel KNJA, Kerstjens JM, Bocca-Tjeertes IFA, Reijneveld SA, Bos AF. Functional outcomes at age 7 years of moderate preterm and full term children born small for gestational age. *J Pediatr.* (2015) 166:552–8. doi: 10.1016/j.jpeds.2014.11.043
45. Kloosterman G. On intrauterine growth: the significance of prenatal care. *Int J Gynaecol Obstet.* (1970) 8:895–912. doi: 10.1002/j.1879-3479.1970.tb00313.x
46. Theodore RF, Thompson JMD, Waldie KE, Becroft DMO, Robinson E, Wild CJ, et al. Determinants of cognitive ability at 7 years: a longitudinal case-control study of children born small-for-gestational age at term. *Eur J Pediatr.* (2009) 168:1217–24. doi: 10.1007/s00431-008-0913-9
47. Thompson J, Mitchell E, Borman B. Sex specific birthweight percentiles by gestational age for New Zealand. *N Z Med J.* (1994) 10:1–3.
48. Blair EM, Nelson KB. Fetal growth restriction and risk of cerebral palsy in singletons born after at least 35 weeks' gestation. *Am J Obstet Gynecol.* (2015) 212:520.e1–7. doi: 10.1016/j.ajog.2014.10.1103
49. Jacobsson B, Ahlin K, Francis A, Hagberg G, Hagberg H, Gardosi J. Cerebral palsy and restricted growth status at birth: population-based case-control study. *BJOG An Int J Obstet Gynaecol.* (2008) 115:1250–5. doi: 10.1111/j.1471-0528.2008.01827.x
50. Drummond P, Colver A. Analysis by gestational age of cerebral palsy in singleton births in north-east England 1970-94. *Paediatr Perinat Epidemiol.* (2002) 16:172–80. doi: 10.1046/j.1365-3016.2002.00408.x
51. Himmelmann K, Ahlin K, Jacobsson B, Cans C, Thorsen P. Risk factors for cerebral palsy in children born at term. *Acta Obs Gynecol Scand.* (2011) 90:1070–81. doi: 10.1111/j.1600-0412.2011.01217.x
52. Tin W, Wariyar U, Hey E. Selection biases invalidate current low birthweight for gestation standards. *Br J Obs Gynaecol.* (1997) 104:180–5. doi: 10.1111/j.1471-0528.1997.tb11041.x
53. Maršál K, Persson P, Larsen T, Lilja H, Selbing A, Sultan B. Intrauterine growth curves based on ultrasonically estimated foetal weights. *Acta Paediatr.* (1996) 85:843–8. doi: 10.1111/j.1651-2227.1996.tb14164.x
54. Stoknes M, Andersen G, Elkamil A, Irgens L, Skranes J, Salvesen K, et al. The effects of multiple pre- and perinatal risk factors on the occurrence of cerebral palsy. A Norwegian register based study. *Eur J Paediatr Neurol.* (2012) 16:56–63. doi: 10.1016/j.ejpn.2011.10.004
55. Matte TD, Bresnahan M, Begg MD, Susser E. Influence of variation in birth weight within normal range and within sibships on IQ at age 7 years: cohort study. *BMJ.* (2001) 323:310–4. doi: 10.1136/bmj.323.7308.310
56. Diamond A. Executive functions. *Annu Rev Psychol.* (2013) 64:135–68. doi: 10.1146/annurev-psych-113011-143750
57. Lahti J, Räikkönen K, Kajantie E, Heinonen K, Pesonen A, Järvenpää A, et al. Small body size at birth and behavioural symptoms of ADHD in children aged five to six years. *J Child Psychol Psychiatry.* (2006) 47:1167–74. doi: 10.1111/j.1469-7610.2006.01661.x
58. Franz AR, Pohlandt F, Bode H, Mihatsch WA, Sander S, Kron M, et al. Intrauterine, early neonatal, and postdischarge growth and neurodevelopmental outcome at 5.4 years in extremely preterm infants after intensive neonatal nutritional support. *Pediatrics.* (2009) 123:e101–9. doi: 10.1542/peds.2008-1352
59. Cole T, Freeman J, Preece M. British 1990 growth reference centiles for weight, height, body mass index and head circumference fitted by maximum penalized likelihood. *Stat Med.* (1998) 17:407–29. doi: 10.1002/(SICI)1097-0258(19980228)17:4<407::AID-SIM742>3.0.CO;2-L
60. Mamelle N, Boniol M, Rivière O, Joly M, Mellier G, Maria B, et al. Identification of newborns with Fetal Growth Restriction (FGR) in weight and/or length based on constitutional growth potential. *Eur J Pediatr.* (2006) 165:717–25. doi: 10.1007/s00431-005-0045-4
61. Guellec I, Marret S, Baud O, Cambonie G, Lapillonne A, Roze JC, et al. Intrauterine growth restriction, head size at birth, and outcome in very preterm infants. *J Pediatr.* (2015) 167:975–81e2. doi: 10.1016/j.jpeds.2015.08.025
62. Kallankari H, Kaukola T, Olsén P, Ojaniemi M, Hallman M. Very preterm birth and foetal growth restriction are associated with specific cognitive deficits in children attending mainstream school. *Acta Paediatr Int J Paediatr.* (2015) 104:84–90. doi: 10.1111/apa.12811
63. Kan E, Roberts G, Anderson PJ, Doyle LW. The association of growth impairment with neurodevelopmental outcome at eight years of age in very preterm children. *Early Hum Dev.* (2008) 84:409–16. doi: 10.1016/j.earlhumdev.2007.11.002
64. Korzeniewski SJ, Allred EN, Joseph RM, Heeren T, Kuban KCK, O'Shea TM, et al. Neurodevelopment at age 10 years of children born <28 weeks with fetal growth restriction. *Pediatrics.* (2017) 140:e20170697. doi: 10.1542/peds.2017-0697
65. Yudkin P, Aboualfa M, Eyre J, Redman C, Wilkinson A. New birthweight and head circumference centiles for gestational ages 24 to 42 weeks. *Early Hum Dev.* (1987) 15:45–52. doi: 10.1016/0378-3782(87)90099-5
66. Morsing E, Asard M, Ley D, Stjernqvist K, Marsal K. Cognitive function after intrauterine growth restriction and very preterm birth. *Pediatrics.* (2011) 127:e874–82. doi: 10.1542/peds.2010-1821
67. Raz S, Debastos AK, Newman JB, Batton D. Intrauterine growth and neuropsychological performance in very low birth weight preschoolers. *J Int Neuropsychol Soc.* (2012) 18:200–11. doi: 10.1017/S1355617711001767
68. Neubauer V, Griesmaier E, Pehböck-Walser N, Pupp-Peglow U, Kiechl-Kohlendorfer U. Poor postnatal head growth in very preterm infants is associated with impaired neurodevelopment

outcome. *Acta Paediatr.* (2013) 102:883–8. doi: 10.1111/apa.12319

69. Kok JH, Prick L, Merckel E, Everhard Y, Verkerk GJQ, Scherjon SA. Visual function at 11 years of age in preterm-born children with and without fetal brain sparing. *Pediatrics.* (2007) 119:e1342–50. doi: 10.1542/peds.2005-2857
70. Sucksdorff M, Lehtonen L, Chudal R, Suominen A, Joelsson P, Gissler M, et al. Preterm birth and poor fetal growth as risk factors of attention-deficit/hyperactivity disorder. *Pediatrics.* (2015) 136:e599–608. doi: 10.1542/peds.2015-1043
71. Valcamonico A, Accorsi P, Battaglia S, Soregaroli M, Beretta D, Frusca T. Absent or reverse end-diastolic flow in the umbilical artery: intellectual development at school age. *Eur J Obs Gynecol Reprod Biol.* (2004) 114:23–8. doi: 10.1016/j.ejogrb.2003.09.033
72. van den Broek AJM, Kok JH, Houtzager BA, Scherjon SA. Behavioural problems at the age of eleven years in preterm-born children with or without fetal brain sparing: a prospective cohort study. *Early Hum Dev.* (2010) 86:379–84. doi: 10.1016/j.earlhumdev.2010.04.007

7

Is Umbilical Cord Blood Therapy an Effective Treatment for Early Lung Injury in Growth Restriction?

Beth J. Allison[1,2], Hannah Youn[1,2], Atul Malhotra[1,3], Courtney A. McDonald[1,2], Margie Castillo-Melendez[1,2], Yen Pham[1,2], Amy E. Sutherland[1,2], Graham Jenkin[1,2], Graeme R. Polglase[1,2] and Suzanne L. Miller[1,2]*

[1] The Ritchie Centre, Hudson Institute of Medical Research, Clayton, VIC, Australia, [2] Department of Obstetrics and Gynaecology and Paediatrics, Monash University, Clayton, VIC, Australia, [3] Monash Newborn, Monash Medical Centre, Clayton, VIC, Australia

***Correspondence:**
Beth J. Allison
beth.allison@hudson.org.au

Fetal growth restriction (FGR) and prematurity are often co-morbidities, and both are risk factors for lung disease. Despite advances in early delivery combined with supportive ventilation, rates of ventilation-induced lung injury (VILI) remain high. There are currently no protective treatments or interventions available that target lung morbidities associated with FGR preterm infants. Stem cell therapy, such as umbilical cord blood (UCB) cell administration, demonstrates an ability to attenuate inflammation and injury associated with VILI in preterm appropriately grown animals. However, no studies have looked at the effects of stem cell therapy in growth restricted newborns. We aimed to determine if UCB treatment could attenuate acute inflammation in the first 24 h of ventilation, comparing effects in lambs born preterm following FGR with those born preterm but appropriately grown (AG). Placental insufficiency (FGR) was induced by single umbilical artery ligation in twin-bearing ewes at 88 days gestation, with twins used as control (appropriately grown, AG). Lambs were delivered preterm at ∼126 days gestation (term is 150 days) and randomized to either immediate euthanasia (unventilated controls, AG_{UVC} and FGR_{UVC}) or commenced on 24 h of gentle supportive ventilation (AG_V and FGR_V) with additional cohorts receiving UCB treatment at 1 h (AG_{CELLS}, FGR_{CELLS}). Lungs were collected at post-mortem for histological and biochemical examination. Ventilation caused lung injury in AG lambs, as indicated by decreased septal crests and elastin density, as well as increased inflammation. Lung injury in AG lambs was attenuated with UCB therapy. Ventilated FGR lambs also sustained lung injury, albeit with different indices compared to AG lambs; in FGR, ventilation reduced septal crest density, reduced alpha smooth muscle actin density and reduced cell proliferation. UCB treatment in ventilated FGR lambs further decreased septal crest density and increased collagen deposition, however, it increased angiogenesis as evidenced by increased vascular endothelial growth factor (VEGF) expression and vessel density. This is the first time that a cell therapy has been investigated in the lungs of growth restricted animals. We show that the uterine environment can alter the response to both secondary stress (ventilation) and therapy (UCB). This study highlights the need for further research on the potential impact of novel therapies on a growth restricted offspring.

Keywords: growth restriction, ventilation induced lung injury, umbilical cord blood (UCB), treatment, animal model

INTRODUCTION

Fetal growth restriction (FGR) is a common complication of pregnancy, where a fetus fails to reach its expected growth potential, primarily due to placental insufficiency (1). FGR significantly increases the risk of morbidity and pulmonary conditions following preterm birth, with increased rates of bronchopulmonary dysplasia and pulmonary hypertension (2, 3). Despite the increased risk of pulmonary complications, lung pathology following FGR remains contentious. We and others have found comparable lung weight, structure, surfactant protein expression, and ventilation requirements compared to appropriately grown (AG) cohorts (4, 5). However, it is evident that early and late onset FGR have differential effects (6), and animal studies to date have primarily induced FGR during late gestation, and it is, thus, possible that crucial lung development has already occurred at this stage (7); whereas preclinical studies of long term growth restriction describe altered surfactant protein (8, 9) disrupted alveolarization, with thickened parenchyma (10) and large alveoli resulting in reduced alveolar and vascular density (11).

There is currently no cure or therapy for FGR. Current treatment of FGR primarily involves the adjustment of the delivery time, thus infants are often delivered preterm (<37 weeks gestation), particularly those with early-onset FGR (12). Prematurity itself is a significant risk factor for pulmonary morbidity and necessitates medical interventions such as mechanical ventilation. Whilst ventilation is usually essential for survival in such scenarios, it has the potential to exacerbate pathology in FGR lungs, particularly since lung development may already be adversely affected by the chronic hypoxemia caused by placental insufficiency (11). The resultant lung injury after birth is known as ventilation induced lung injury (VILI). VILI and elevated inflammation cause direct tissue injury and in turn, exacerbate lung inflammation. Long term ventilation can reduce alveoli number, disrupt vasculature and alveolar architecture (13–16), hampering lung mechanics and necessitating the further need for assisted ventilation. Current treatment focuses on ensuring the survival of the FGR infant while ameliorating the detrimental effects of FGR on the lungs.

Umbilical cord blood (UCB) cells have been highlighted as a potential treatment for infants born preterm, due to their potent anti-inflammatory properties and easy access (17). Preclinical studies using specific stem like cell populations present within UCB have shown promising anti-inflammatory and immune modulatory effects in VILI of preterm animals (15, 18). UCB provides a unique source of the functionally important stem like cells that may each play a modulatory role in preventing injury (19). UCB therapy has been examined for prevention and repair of brain injury (20, 21), and has also shown promise in clinical trials where administration improved motor and neurodevelopmental outcomes in children with cerebral palsy (22, 23). UCB is comprised of many cell types including cells that mediate hematopoiesis and vascular growth (24–27). UCB also show strong anti-inflammatory benefits, and they are a feasible postnatal treatment with low immunogenicity (25, 26, 28). Within the lung, UCB therapy is thought to reduce inflammation through paracrine effects. Accordingly, we used our established model of ovine fetal growth restriction to examine (i) the effects of preterm birth and ventilation on FGR lungs, and (ii) if UCB could be a potential new treatment for VILI in FGR and/or AG infants. To focus on acute inflammation and injury, this study examined the first 24 h postnatally in FGR and AG preterm lambs.

METHODOLOGY

Umbilical Cord Blood Collection

Umbilical cord blood (UCB) was collected from separate healthy term ovine pregnancies. UCB was collected during cesarean section under general anesthesia. Approximately 90 mL of UCB was collected from the umbilical veins into heparinized tubes. UCB was diluted 1:1 with phosphate buffered saline and centrifuged at 3,200 rpm at RT for 12 min with no brake. The buffy coat was isolated to obtain the mononuclear cells (MNCs) and red blood cell lysis of this fraction performed. Cells were counted using trypan blue exclusion and a hemocytometer, and cells were cryopreserved at ~25 million cells/ml in freeze media (10% DMSO, 40% FBS and 50% DMEM/F12) until required. A minimum of three cryopreserved UCB donors was pooled after thawing and before administration to reduce intra-sample UCB variation.

Fetal Surgery

Aseptic surgery was performed on anesthetized (sodium thiopentone 20 mL; Pentothal; Boehringer Ingelheim, Australia; maintenance inhaled isoflurane 2–5%) Border-Leicester pregnant ewes ($n = 17$) carrying twin-pregnancies at 88 days gestation (term is 150 days). Prophylactic antibiotics were administered via the maternal jugular vein, including 5 mL of Engemycin (Engemycin 100, Coopers, MSD Animal Health, New Zealand) and 1 g of ampicillin (Ampicyn 1 g, Mylan N.V., USA). Following a thorough cleaning of the surgical sites, the fetus was exposed via cesarean section. Marcain (5 mL, Marcain (0.5%) with Adrenaline, Aspen Pharmacare Australia NSW, Australia) was applied to all surgical sites prior to incision to provide analgesic coverage. Single umbilical artery ligation was performed by placing two silk ties tightly around one of the umbilical arteries, that causes chronic placental insufficiency and fetal growth restriction (FGR). In control twins, the umbilical cord was handled but not ligated. The fetus was returned to the uterus and abdominal incisions were repaired. A maternal jugular vein catheter was inserted for antibiotic administration. Following surgery ewes were randomly allocated to an experimental group (UVC $n = 6$ ewes, V $n = 5$ ewes or CELLS $n = 6$ ewes).

For 3 consecutive days after surgery, antibiotics [to the fetus (Ampicillin, 1 g via the amniotic catheter] and the ewe [Engemycin 5 mL intravenous (i.v.)] and analgesia

[Panadol (100 mg/mL, Apotex, NSW, Australia) suppository] were administered.

Experimental Design

The ewe and fetuses were monitored daily until 124 days of fetal gestation. At 124 and 125 days, ewes received 11.4 mg betamethasone intramuscularly (Celestone Chronodose, Schering Plow, Sydney, Australia). At 126 days, ewes ($n = 11$) and their fetuses ($n = 21$) in the ventilation groups (AG_V $n = 6$, FGR_V $n = 6$ and AG_{CELLS} $n = 6$, FGR_{CELLS}, $n = 5$) underwent an additional cesarean section or post-mortem (AG_{UVC} $n = 6$, FGR_{UVC} $n = 5$). At this time, there had been $n = 2$ *in utero* deaths in the FGR groups; $n = 1$ in the FGR_{UVC} group and $n = 1$ in the FGR_{CELLS} group, hence the reduced number in these two groups at this timepoint. Following maternal anesthesia (sodium thiopentone 20 mL; maintenance inhaled isoflurane 2–5%), the first lamb was exteriorized and intubated with an endotracheal tube (size 4.0 mm). Lung liquid was drained passively and a transcutaneous arterial oxygen saturation (SpO_2) probe (Masimo, Radical 4, CA, USA) was placed around the right forelimb of the lamb and the output digitally recorded.

The umbilical cord was then clamped and cut, the lambs were delivered, dried, weighed and placed on an infant warmer (Fisher and Paykel Healthcare, Auckland, New Zealand) for initiation of assisted ventilation. An umbilical vein and artery were immediately catheterized for maintenance of anesthesia and analgesia (Alfaxane i.v. 5 mg/kg/h; Jurox, East Tamaki, Auckland, New Zealand). Arterial pressure was digitally recorded in real-time (1 kHz, Powerlab; ADInstruments, Castle Hill, NSW, Australia). The lambs were anesthetized for the entirety of the experiment to prevent spontaneous breathing. Ventilation was commenced using positive pressure ventilation with PIP set at 30 cmH_2O and PEEP at 5 cmH_2O (Babylog 8000+, Dräger, Lübeck, Germany): inspiratory time was 0.4 s and expiratory time was 0.6 s. Lambs were ventilated with warmed, humidified gas with an initial fraction of inspired oxygen (F_iO_2) of 0.4 and subsequently adjusted to maintain SaO_2 between 90 and 95%. At 10 min, all lambs received surfactant (Curosurf, 100 mg/kg, Chiesi Farmaceutica, Italy). At 20 min, ventilation continued in volume guarantee mode set at 5–7 ml/kg, which is the tidal volume for lambs at this gestation (29). Physiological parameters pH and $PaCO_2$ were kept within normal limits (7.2–7.4 and 45–55 mmHg, respectively) by adjusting the ventilator rate and inspired O_2 levels. Lamb well-being was monitored throughout ventilation via assessment of the partial pressure of arterial oxygen (PaO_2) and carbon dioxide ($PaCO_2$), oxygen saturation (SaO_2), pH, hematocrit, glucose and lacate with regular blood gas samples (ABL 700 blood gas analyzer; Radiometer, Copenhagen, Denmark). Lambs were ventilated for 24 h.

For groups that received UCB (AG_{CELLS} $n = 6$ and FGR_{CELLS} $n = 5$), 25 million cells/kg was administered intravenously to lambs at 1 h after birth, control groups (AG_V $n = 5$ and FGR_V $n = 5$) were administered the equivalent volume of saline. UCB cells were quantified via cell counts of UCB mononuclear cells to establish an accurate dose prior to administration.

Post-mortem

At 24 h, ventilated lambs were euthanized with an overdose of 20 mL of phenobarbitone, whilst unventilated control groups were immediately euthanized at 125 ± 1 days gestation via an overdose of phenobarbitone. Lambs were weighed and lungs isolated for collection. The left bronchus was ligated before the left lung was removed distal to the ligature. The left lung was snap frozen in liquid nitrogen for RNA processing. The right whole lung was pressure fixed at 20 cmH_2O via the trachea with formalin. Nine sections (2 cm^3) of the lung were randomly selected from an area devoid of major airways from each lobe (upper, middle, lower) and processed for assessment of lung histology. Lung sections were embedded in paraffin, then cut into 5 μm sections and mounted on to Superfrost Plus slides for histological and immunohistochemical analysis.

Detecting Stem Cell Migration

To detect if UCB stem cells were present in the lungs of treated lambs, the UCB cells were tagged with carboxyfluorescein succinimidyl ester (CFSE) before administration (30). Cut lung sections were dewaxed and counter-stained in Hoechst (Invitrogen, USA) and coverslipped. Stem cell identification was conducted using fluorescent microscopy (Olympus BX-41, Japan).

Histological Analysis of Lung Morphology

Gross histological pathology and parenchymal elastin was detected via Hematoxylin and Eosin and Hart's elastin stains, respectively, as previously described (31) Masson's Trichrome was used to identify collagen fibers (32). Three sections (obtained as described above) were randomly selected for each histological assessment. Quantification of histology is outlined below.

Immunohistochemistry

Lung tissue was immunostained for Ki67, α-smooth muscle actin and CD45. Ki67 and α-smooth muscle actin immunostaining was carried out as previously described [(5, 33) see **Supplementary Table 1**]. For immunostaining of CD45, slides were heated in a 60°C oven for 2 h to remove excess wax, followed with histolene clearing and ethanol rehydrating steps. Antigen retrieval was performed by boiling tissue sections in 0.01 M Citrate buffer (pH 6.0) for 3 × 10 min bursts. Sections were then washed in phosphate buffer solution (PBS) before endogenous peroxidase in the tissue was blocked with 3% hydrogen peroxide for 10 min. Tissue sections were washed and then slides were blocked in Serum-Free Protein Block (DAKO) before incubation with the primary antibody CD45 (BD Pharmingen Rat Anti-Mouse, 1:500) for 60 min. Sections were washed in PBS and then incubated with biotinylated secondary antibody (Rabbit anti-mouse, 1:200) for 60 min followed with streptavidin horseradish peroxidase and developed with diaminobenzidine (DAB) and hydrogen peroxide. Sections were counterstained with hematoxylin and dehydrated with ethanol and histolene before mounting with a coverslip. All immunostains were performed in the presence of a negative control.

TABLE 1 | Total sample size, animal and lung weights and sex of fetuses and lambs.

	AG_{UVC}	FGR_{UVC}	AG_V	FGR_V	AG_{CELLS}	FGR_{CELLS}
n	6	5	6	6	6	5
Animal weight (kg)	3.56 ± 0.13	2.25 ± 0.17#	3.21 ± 0.17	2.46 ± 0.22#	3.40 ± 0.18	2.29 ± 0.17#
Lung corrected for body weight (g/kg)	35.94 ± 1.98	31.04 ± 3.07	29.33 ± 0.91	30.36 ± 3.22	27.32 ± 1.55	29.44 ± 1.90
Males, n (%)	5 (83)	2 (40)	2 (33.3)	2 (33.3)	5 (83)	2 (40)

AG, appropriately grown; UVC, unventilated control; FGR, growth restricted; V, ventilated; CELLS, animals treated with umbilical cord blood cells. #Indicates p < 0.05 for growth effects using a 2-way ANOVA.

Cytokine Array

To assess cytokine expression in the lungs, frozen lung tissue was weighed out in 50–100 mg quantities, for protein expression of pro-inflammatory and anti-inflammatory cytokines. The concentrations of *interferon gamma (IFNγ), interleukin (IL)-17A, IL-21, IL-8, IL-10 TNFα*, and *VEGF-A* in lung tissue lysate were measured using an ovine cytokine array (ovine QAO-CYT-1-1, RayBiotech, Georgia, USA).

Analysis

For histological and immunohistochemistry analysis, five random fields of view were taken of each section and analyzed by a single blinded observer (H.Y.). Images were non-overlapping and excluded large airways or vessels.

Lung morphology was assessed through quantification of tissue to airspace ratio and density of secondary septal crests as previously described (4). Elastin, collagen and αSMA density were assessed through Smart Segmentation on Image Pro Premier (Media Cybernetics, USA) (16). Elastin and collagen were then expressed as ratios of lung tissue. Manual point counting was utilized to assess Ki67 and CD45 to tissue ratios (16). Measurement of vascular vessel number was assessed using αSMA immunostained tissue by a single observer blinded to the experimental group (B.J.A.). Vessels were identified by positive staining and were only included when a full cross section of the vessel was visible in the field of view.

Data are expressed as mean ± standard error of the mean (SEM). Statistical analysis was performed with SPSS using a mixed model using growth and treatment as factors in all immunohistochemical and morphological assessments and growth, treatment and time in ventilation parameters. Where significant interactions were detected, differences were isolated with *post-hoc* Tukey's testing. Statistical significance was accepted as $P < 0.05$.

RESULTS

Lamb Characteristics

Lamb characteristics are presented in **Table 1**. Single umbilical artery ligation (SUAL) resulted in ~30% overall reduction in birth weight in FGR lambs. SUAL also resulted in the death of two fetuses, one in the UVC and one in the CELLS group. FGR_{UVC} weighed 37% $<AG_{UVC}$ ($P = 0.0001$), whilst FGR_V weights were 23% lower than AG_V ($P = 0.04$) and FGR_{CELLS} lambs weighed

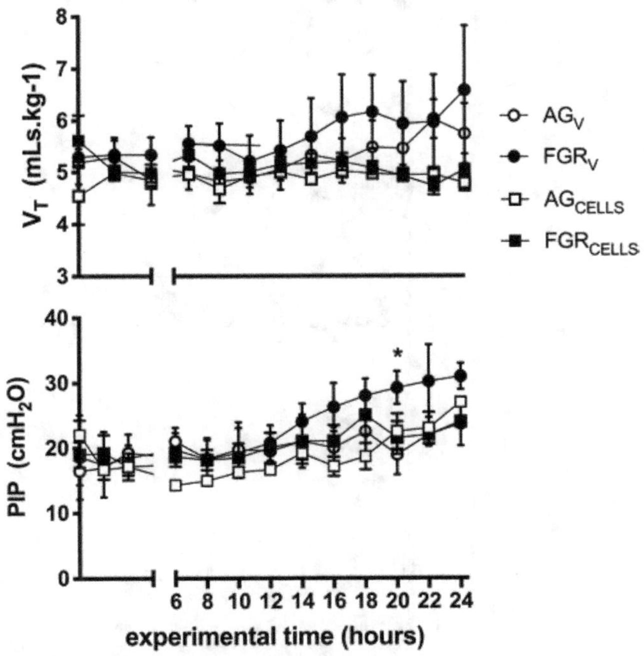

FIGURE 1 | Ventilation parameters. Mean ± SEM tidal volume V_T ($mLs.kg^{-1}$) and peak inspiratory pressure (PIP) in appropriately grown (AG_V, white circles, $n = 5$), growth restricted (FGR_V, black circles $n = 5$) and appropriately grown and growth restricted treated with umbilical cord blood cells (AG_{CELLS}, white squares $n = 6$; FGR_{CELLS}, black squares $n = 5$) over the experimental period (hours) *indicates significant differences ($p < 0.05$) across time.

32% $<AG_{CELLS}$ ($P = 0.01$, **Table 1**). Lung weight, corrected for body weight, was not different across groups.

Ventilation Parameters

There were no differences in tidal volumes (V_T, 5–6 mL/kg) between groups. Peak inspiratory pressure (PIP) required to achieve V_T was initially not different between groups, however PIPs were significantly ($P > 0.003$) increased at 20 h in FGR_V lambs compared to all groups (**Figure 1**). There was no effect of FGR or UCB on the requirement for PIP. Lung compliance was not different between groups (data not shown).

Stem Cell Migration

Lung tissue was examined for the presence of CFSE tagged UCB cells in all ventilated groups (**Figure 2**). Fluorescing cells were

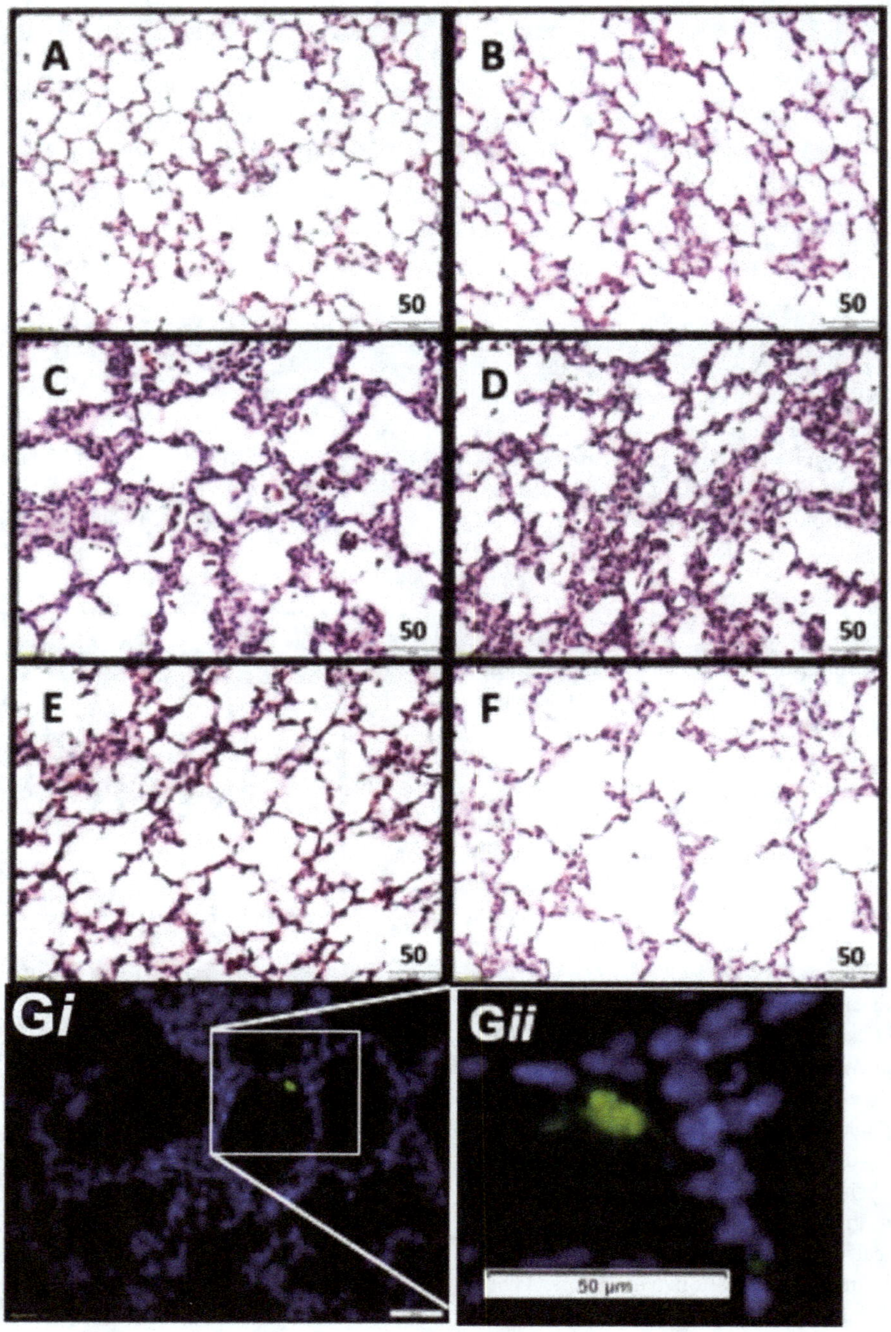

FIGURE 2 | Representative lung morphology images. Photomicrographs of Masson Trichrome stained sections in appropriately grown (**A** AG_{UVC}, **C** AG_{VENT}, **E** AG_{CELLS}) and growth restricted (**B** FGR_{UVC}, **D** FGR_{VENT}, **F** FGR_{CELLS}) animals. Fluorescent tagged cell in lung parenchyma UCB cells present within parenchymal lung tissue (blue) and a fluorescing UCB cell (green). Magnification ×400 (**G***i* and at higher magnification **G***ii*).

apparent in all cell treated animals, and were not present in saline controls (**Figure 2G**).

Lung Morphology

Two lungs were not appropriately fixed (one from FGR_{UVC} and one from FGR_{CELLS}) and were thus excluded from morphological and immunohistochemical analysis. Final sample size for morphological and immunohistochemical analysis is AG_{UVC} $n = 6$, AG_V $n = 6$, AG_{CELLS} $n = 6$, FGR_{UVC} $n = 4$, FGR_V $n = 6$ and FGR_{CELLS} $n = 4$.

Tissue to airspace ratio was not altered by FGR or ventilation (**Figure 3A**). Heterogeneous lung injury was observed in AG_V and FGR_V compared to their unventilated cohorts, with areas containing thickened blood-air barriers, contrasting against

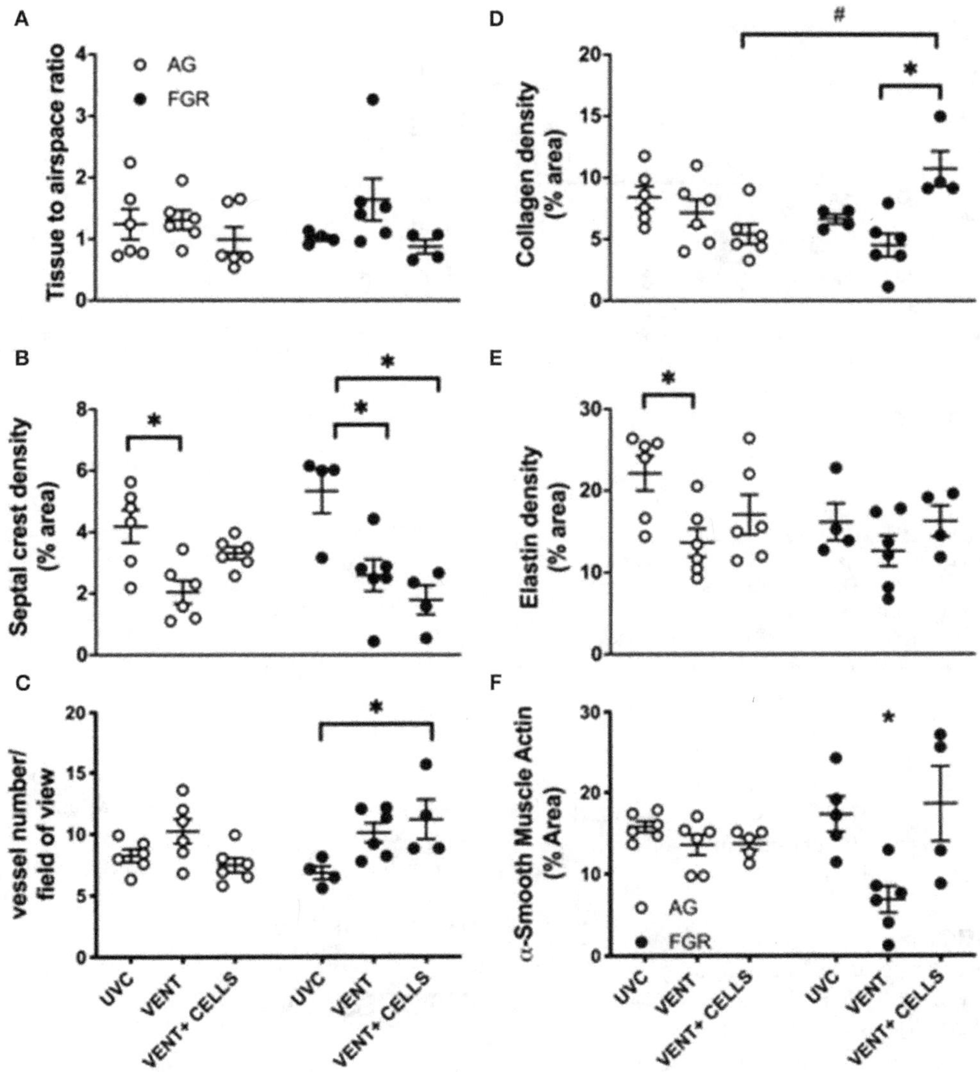

FIGURE 3 | Lung parenchymal and vascular structure. Data are mean ± SEM tissue airspace ratio **(A)**, secondary crest density **(B)**, arteriolar vessel wall number **(C)** and collagen **(D)** elastin **(E)** and α-smooth muscle actin **(F)** density (corrected for total tissue area) in appropriately grown (AG) and growth restricted (FGR) unventilated controls (AG_{UVC} and FGR_{UVC}, white circles), following ventilation (AG_{VENT} and FGR_{VENT}, black circles) and following ventilation and cell treatment (AG_{CELLS} and FGR_{CELLS}, gray circles). Data were compared using a two-way ANOVA. *Indicates $p < 0.05$ treatment effects and #indicates $p < 0.05$ growth effects using a two-way ANOVA.

other regions showing prominent airway enlargement. This heterogeneity was reduced with UCB (AG_{CELLS} and FGR_{CELLS}), although alveoli remained enlarged (**Figure 2**). Septal crest density was significantly reduced following ventilation compared to unventilated controls (**Figure 3B**) resulting in a 57.6% reduction in AG lambs (AG_{UVC} 4.2 ± 0.5 vs. AG_V 2.0 ± 0.4, $P = 0.0001$) and 44.6% reduction in FGR lambs (FGR_{UVC} 5.3 ± 0.7 vs. FGR_V 2.5 ± 0.5, $P = 0.002$, **Figure 3B**). Treatment with UCB restored septal crest density in AG (AG_{CELLS} 3.3 ± 0.2, $P = 0.02$) but not FGR lambs.

Vessel number, as assessed in α-smooth muscle actin-stained lungs (**Figure 3C**). was significantly increased in ventilated growth restricted lambs treated with UCB compared to unventilated, growth restricted lambs (FGR_{CELLS} 11.2 ± 1.6 vs. FGR_{UVC} 6.8 ± 0.5, $P = 0.04$). No differences in vessel density were observed across groups in the AG lambs.

Collagen density was not altered in either AG or FGR lambs following ventilation (**Figure 3D**). Treatment with UCB significantly increased collagen density in FGR_{CELLS} animals compared to FGR_V and AG_{CELLS} lambs (FGR_{CELLS} 10.7 ± 1.4% vs. AG_{CELLS} 5.3 ± 0.8% and FGR_V 4.5 ± 0.9%; $p > 0.02$).

Elastin density was significantly reduced in ventilated AG lambs compared to AG control lambs (AG_{UVC} 22.1 ± 2.2% vs. AG_V 13.6 ± 1.7%, $P < 0.05$). Elastin density was restored following treatment with UCB in AG lambs (**Figure 3E**). Elastin density was not different in FGR lambs either with ventilation or UCB treatment.

We assessed positively stained α-smooth muscle actin tissue to determine density (**Figure 3F**). Ventilation of FGR lambs

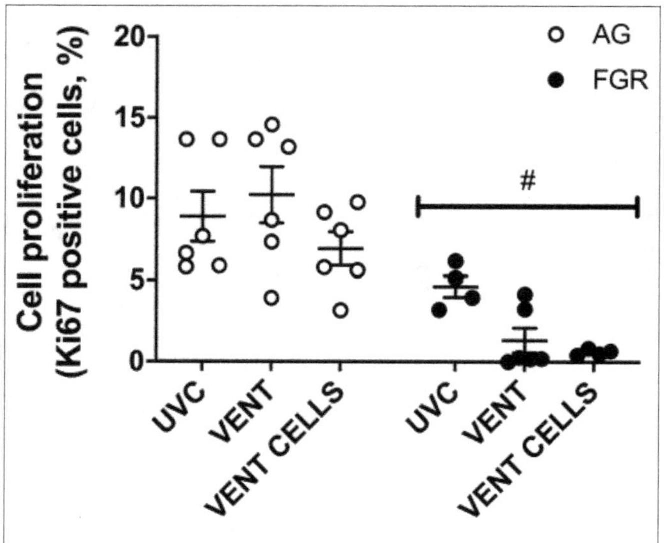

FIGURE 4 | Cell proliferation. Data are mean ± SEM Ki67 (cell proliferation marker) positive cells in appropriately grown (AG, white) and growth restricted (FGR, black) unventilated controls (AG_{UVC} and FGR_{UVC}), following ventilation (AG_{VENT} and FGR_{VENT}) and following ventilation and cell treatment (AG_{CELLS} and FGR_{CELLS}). Data were compared using a two-way ANOVA. #Indicates $p < 0.05$ treatment effects using a two-way ANOVA.

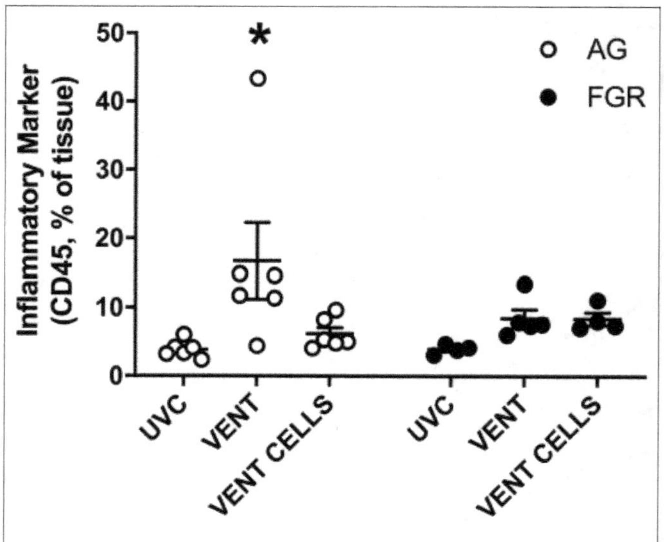

FIGURE 5 | Inflammation. Data are mean ± SEM CD45 (inflammation marker) positive cells in appropriately grown (AG, white) and growth restricted (FGR, black) unventilated controls (AG_{UVC} and FGR_{UVC}), following ventilation (AG_{VENT} and FGR_{VENT}) and following ventilation and cell treatment (AG_{CELLS} and FGR_{CELLS}). Data were compared using a two-way ANOVA. *Indicates $p < 0.05$ treatment effects using a two-way ANOVA.

significantly reduced α-smooth muscle actin density (FGR_V 6.8 ± 1.3% vs. FGR_{UVC} 17.3 ± 2.1%). Treatment with UCB reversed this finding (FGR_V 6.8 ± 1.3% vs. FGR_{CELLS} 18.6 ± 4.6%). α-smooth muscle actin density was not different in AG lambs either with ventilation or UCB treatment.

Cell Proliferation

Cell proliferation was assessed in lung parenchyma using the proliferation marker Ki67. Cell proliferation was significantly decreased ($P < 0.0001$, **Figure 4**) in FGR, compared to AG groups. Cell proliferation was significantly reduced by 80% in FGR_{VENT} compared to AG_{VENT}, and also decreased in FGR_{CELLS} compared to AG_{CELLS} (by 90%).

Inflammation

We used immunohistochemical analysis of CD45 to visually examine the infiltration of inflammatory cells into pulmonary tissue. Ventilation induced an inflammatory response in AG lambs (AG_{UVC} 3.9 ±.5 cells vs. AG_V 16.7 ± 5.5 cells, $P = 0.0079$). Inflammatory cell infiltration of the lungs was attenuated by treatment with UCB (**Figure 5**, $p < 0.05$) in AG lambs. Neither ventilation nor cell treatment induced a significant inflammatory response within the lungs of FGR lambs (FGR_{UVC} vs. FGR_V $p = 0.5$; FGR_V vs. FGR_{CELLS} $p = 0.9$).

A cytokine array was performed to further characterize the inflammatory profile within the lungs. Pro-inflammatory marker IL-8 was significantly increased in response to ventilation, in both AG and FGR lambs ($P < 0.05$), while treatment with UCB did not reduce IL-8 levels (**Figure 6A**). UCB treatment significantly increased IL-21 levels in FGR and AG lambs (**Figure 6E**). VEGF concentration was significantly increased in FGR lambs treated with UCB compared to both FGR_{UVC} ($P = 0.007$, **Figure 6E**) and FGR_V ($P = 0.04$) lambs. However, treatment with UCB cells significantly increase VEGF protein levels in FGR lambs compared to AG lambs treated with UCB cells (FGR_{CELLS} 16.6 ± 0.7 vs. AG_{CELLS} 9.9 ± 1.8, $P = 0.002$). There was no difference in TNFα, IL-17A, IL-10 or IFNγ levels between groups (**Figures 6B–D,F**, respectively).

DISCUSSION

Postnatally, FGR infants have increased risk of lung injury and bronchopulmonary dysplasia (BPD). Stem cell therapy has proven benefits to reduce VILI in preterm infants (34) as well as in reducing BPD incidence in preterm humans (33) and in animal models of neonatal lung injury (35). However, no previous studies have investigated if stem cell therapy is also beneficial for very low birthweight infants affected by growth restriction. In the current model, UCB therapy attenuated injury in AG but not FGR lambs. Our findings in appropriately grown lambs confirm previous studies showing improved lung structure following administration of placental stem-like cells, such as human amnion epithelial cells (34). Therefore, our current study increases the body of evidence for the use of UCB as an effective therapy for VILI in preterm infants who are appropriately grown. UCB treatment in FGR lambs increased pulmonary vascularization, but did not improve structural deficits in secondary septal crests, and increased collagen deposition, which is an early marker of fibrosis. Our research demonstrates that after 24 h of ventilation, UCB therapy shows differential effects in appropriately grown and growth restricted lambs, where protection from VILI was evident in AG lambs but not FGR lambs.

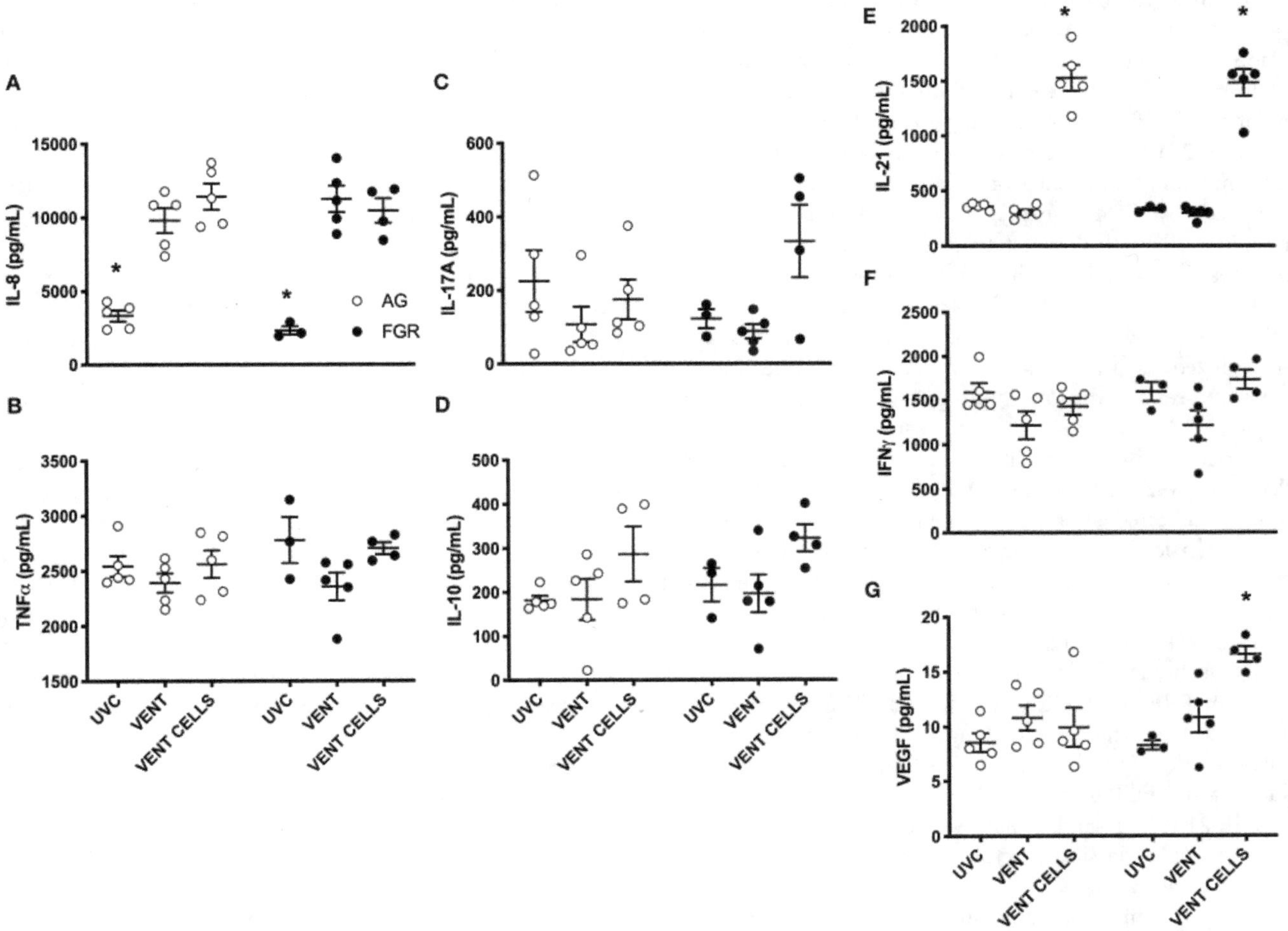

FIGURE 6 | Inflammatory proteins. Data are mean ± SEM interleukin *(IL)-8* **(A)**, tumor necrosis factor alpha *(TNFα)* **(B)**, *IL-17A* **(C)**, *IL-10* **(D)**, *IL-21* **(E)** interferon gamma *(IFN)* **(F)**, and vascular endothelial growth factor *(VEGF)* **(G)**, cytokine levels in appropriately grown (AG, white) and growth restricted (FGR, black) unventilated controls (AG_{UVC} and FGR_{UVC}), following ventilation (AG_{VENT} and FGR_{VENT}) and following ventilation and cell treatment (AG_{CELLS} and FGR_{CELLS}). *Indicates $p < 0.05$ treatment effects using a two-way ANOVA.

In the current study, we found little difference in the baseline lung morphology between the preterm unventilated FGR and AG fetuses, in line with previous observations from our group (4), although we induced early-onset placental insufficiency and FGR in this study, where we have previously examined late-onset (36). We hypothesized that longer exposure to placental insufficiency over a period of critical lung development would lead to the arrest of alveolar development as observed in other preclinical FGR studies (10, 11, 37). The latter being a probable mechanism for the increased risk of BPD (3) in this cohort. However, we did not see detectable differences in lung weights, when corrected for body weight, or baseline lung morphology in this study. Differences between the mode of inducing FGR and timing of compromise are most likely to contribute to differences in experimental outcomes. It is interesting to note that, despite a lack of gross or microscopic changes in lung morphology before ventilation, critical differences in response to ventilation were evident in the current study between AG and FGR lambs, suggesting sub-clinical alterations in lung development and/or biochemistry.

We have previously shown that AG and FGR newborns do not have significantly different ventilator requirements in the first 2 h of life (4, 38), however, in this study we extended these findings to show that, with a prolonged period of ventilation, FGR lambs begin to require a greater PIP to maintain V_T, suggesting stiffer and less compliant lungs, a change that was sub-clinical throughout our experiment period as shown by dynamic compliance. All our lambs received antenatal betamethasone, which enhances surfactant production (39) and pulmonary function (40), and temporarily preserves lung compliance (41, 42) however, this may have had decreased efficacy in FGR. The rise in PIP over time may be a precursor to worsening VILI, lung compliance and ventilatory requirements, and certainly suggests that a longer period (>24 h) of study is necessary to tease apart differences associated with FGR.

Mechanical trauma as occurs with assisted ventilation induces an acute inflammatory response that initiates the inflammatory cascade and stimulation of inflammatory cytokine production (14, 16, 35). This was confirmed in the current study with ventilation significantly increasing pro-inflammatory cytokine IL-8 in FGR and AG lambs. In keeping with pulmonary IL-8 upregulation, infiltration of immune cells into the lungs (as evident by $CD45^+$ expression) was also increased with ventilation, albeit this was statistically significant only in the AG lambs. Upregulation of inflammation following lung injury is well-described (4, 14, 16, 43, 44). Interestingly, IFNγ and TNFα were not altered in ventilated FGR or AG lambs. IFNγ is recognized as a key pro-inflammatory cytokine that has previously been shown to be up-regulated in response to lung injury (45). We did not see an up-regulation of IFNγ in the current study, this is likely due to the timing of lung collection, given that we measured inflammatory proteins in the lungs collected after 24 h of ventilation. IFNγ is seen to increase transiently in response to the initiation of ventilation with levels reducing over a period of hours-to-days after initial increase (46). TNFα is also found to be released in response to VILI in preterm neonates (45) however, pre-treatment with betamethasone, as was given in the current study, can prevent an increase in TNFα (47). UCB treatment in AG lambs attenuated immune cell infiltration into lungs but did not prevent the increase in IL-8 in either AG or FGR lambs. Moreover, UCB induced a 1.6-fold increase in lung IL-21 in AG and FGR lambs. IL-21 is a pro-inflammatory cytokine that promotes M2 "repair" to M1 "classically activated" macrophage phenotype, as well as increasing $CD4^+$ and $CD8^+$ T cell production (48), thus promoting inflammation. Persistence of inflammatory markers upregulated in response to mechanical ventilation in the current study are in contrast to previous reports where administration of placental stem cells increased expression of anti-inflammatory cytokines and reduced markers of lung inflammation following hyperoxic injury, thereby preventing downstream fibrosis and normalizing lung morphology (49). Differences between the findings here and those of previous studies for cell efficacy may reflect differences in the timing of tissue collection, mode of lung injury, the stage of lung development, or indeed the cells administered. It is perhaps too early to speculate whether the large increase in pulmonary IL-21 in response to UCB cells is a reparative or damaging effect, but it is increasingly well-understood that stem cells can modify a reparative response via immunomodulatory actions. This, however, is contingent on the inflammatory environment at the time of cell administration; stem cells introduced into a highly inflammatory host inhibit the protective capacity of stem cells (50), and can, in some instances, result in stem cells themselves becoming pro-inflammatory (51). This is a research area that requires further characterization, particularly for the vulnerable fragile preterm lungs.

Consistent with previous findings, we observed suppression of septal crests density following ventilation (16), and elastin distribution became diffuse along the alveolar wall; in AG lambs elastin density was significantly reduced and a similar (non-significant) trend was seen in lungs from FGR lambs. Ventilation in neonatal sheep and mice induces an upregulation of elastin production, but not the regulators of elastin assembly, leading to disordered accumulation of elastin along the alveolar walls (52). The qualitative changes we observed are likely a precursor to abnormal elastin deposition, highlighting the importance of treating in this acute period, before structural changes. Collagen, elastin and α-smooth muscle actin are essential structural components of the lung (53), and perturbations to the density and distribution of these factors will alter the mechanics of the lung. Twenty-four hours of ventilation in our preterm lambs decreased α-smooth muscle actin density in the FGR cohort compared to unventilated controls. Long-term (1 month) of ventilation increases α-smooth muscle actin (54), and thus we may have observed a transient decrease in this study, before a secondary compensatory increase. The mechanisms underlying the decreased α-smooth muscle actin in this current study are unknown, however, it is interesting to speculate on the possible role of nitric oxide (NO). In culture, increased NO reduces smooth muscle production, whilst inhibition of NO results in smooth muscle accumulation (55). It is well-accepted that growth restriction impairs NO handling (56, 57), and we have shown decreased content and altered distribution of the NO precursor, eNOS, following 2 h of ventilation (58). However, exposure to hyperoxia in the first day of life may increase local NO production due to impaired NO handling in FGR newborns, thereby resulting in inhibition of smooth muscle production.

Septal crest density is vital for increasing the surface area available for gas exchange. Ventilation induced a decrease in septal crest density in AG and FGR lambs, which is representative of simplification of the airways, and this is a hallmark of bronchopulmonary dysplasia (59). UCB was protective for septal crest density in the lungs of AG lambs, but not the FGR lambs. Despite this, we observed an improvement of injury heterogeneity in both AG and FGR lambs with treatment. Therefore, UCB may also promote, via paracrine mechanisms, surfactant production to reduce atelectasis.

Strikingly, there was an increase in the collagen to tissue ratio after UCB administration in FGR lambs. In previous studies, UCB-derived mesenchymal stem cells (MSCs) have increased fibroblast formation compared to those sourced from adipose tissue or bone marrow (13, 60). Despite this, no previous studies observed increased collagen; and UCB-MSCs or mononuclear cells administered to mice with VILI did not alter levels of TGF-β, a regulator of collagen production, or collagen content 14 days after cell administration (15, 50). However, to the authors' knowledge, there are no other studies specifically aimed at determining the efficacy of cell treatment in a growth restricted population. Whilst it is possible that the increase in collagen in FGR lambs in the current study is transient, given the relationship between collagen deposition and fibrotic disease, this relationship requires additional research.

Alveolar epithelial cells are a key source of increased cell proliferation following ventilation induced lung injury (61). Interestingly, cell proliferation was significantly increased in ventilated AG lambs but reduced in FGR ventilated lambs. FGR is linked with lower levels of growth factors and decreased pulmonary cell growth in culture (11). We have previously shown that glucocorticoids reduce cell proliferation, both in AG and FGR fetuses (38) but since all groups received betamethasone, this is unlikely to have caused the difference observed here. It is more likely that the growth restricted lung does not respond to stretch by inducing proliferation, a well-established mechanism in the lungs of AG infants. Indeed, another key stretch response, the baroreflex response, is significantly attenuated in growth restricted fetuses (62), suggesting a possible decreased responsivity to this critical form of stimulus. Overall, these unexpected findings re-emphasize that even though ventilator requirements and fetal histology was not different between groups, FGR lungs respond differently to ventilation compared to AG lungs, and these changes may underpin the increased vulnerability to injury and long-term morbidity in FGR offspring. UCB treatment did not improve cell proliferation in FGR lungs. The underlying physiology is unknown, however investigating which cells are proliferative in AG would be of interest.

Treatment with UCB in FGR ventilated lambs promoted blood vessel growth as evidenced by the increased VEGF and vessel number, a finding not seen in AG lambs. VEGF is a potent inducer of angiogenesis and decreased VEGF expression is seen in newborns with BPD. *In vitro*, both MSCs (63) and endothelial progenitor cells (64) promote angiogenesis, via increases in VEGF. It is possible that, given time, increased vascularization of the lung would promote restoration of alveolarization, given the known positive relationship between these two factors (65). It is interesting, but not immediately apparent, why VEGF was increased in FGR, but not AG ventilated lambs. It is known that hypoxia increases VEGF production, and placental insufficiency directly exposes the developing fetus to chronic hypoxemia, which may in turn, result in impaired or altered hypoxia sensing and handling, and response.

How stem cells exert a reparative benefit is still not fully understood, however several mechanisms are possible. They may migrate to areas of injury and release trophic factors to reduce inflammation and promote endogenous repair mechanisms or they may alter systemic immune-modulatory responses (66). We observed only small numbers of UCB cells within the lungs, suggesting that their main effect was not via cell engraftment, but rather a paracrine effect as expected. *In vitro*, MSCs demonstrated preferential migration to hyperoxia-injured lung tissue rather than control medium or healthy lung tissue (49), suggesting stem cells are specifically recruited to sites of injury. Intra-tracheal UCB administration provides direct access to the lung and may improve lung outcomes (35), however, given that intubation is increasingly infrequent in pediatrics (67), systemic administration of cells is more clinically relevant.

It is now well-established that a poor uterine environment has the potential to program disease in later life (68). Emerging evidence also suggests that subtle, sub-clinical alterations are present in the lung (69) at the time of birth, which not only changes the function of the organ but can also alter the response of the organs to additional insults. It is likely that the lung is similarly affected, where an altered response to injury in FGR as compared to AG offspring has been demonstrated in animal models (70) and humans (3). It follows that treatments also may have different therapeutic ranges in infants following a sub-optimal pregnancy, and therefore further research is required to determine how to best target therapies to this population.

Limitations

We administered the UCB cells at a dose of 25 million cells/kg, based on evidence that this level is neuroprotective, and gave this dose 1 h after birth. It is possible that this cell dose and timing is not optimal for treatment of the lungs of the FGR infant and highlights the need to consider the FGR population independent of AG preterm infants. As with many other therapeutics, the timing of stem cell administration is vital, and it is possible that delaying cell administration until after the primary inflammatory phase is more protective in the lung, as has been observed *in vitro* (51). Further studies should examine this possibility and also determine the effects of UCB on VILI, in AG and FGR animals, beyond the 24-h. This will offer a better understanding of how UCB may benefit functional and morphological outcomes and chronic lung disease. Finally, the FGR infant has multi-organ dysfunctions and, while we only examined lung outcomes in the current study, optimizing postnatal therapeutics for multiple organs, including the lung, brain and cardiovascular system, must be considered. Treatment strategies to improve neurological structure and function are now being examined, including cell therapies. The current study suggests that we need additional targeted research to determine the interaction between organ systems, possible developmental programming and postnatal treatments, such as cell therapies.

Conclusion

FGR newborns have an increased risk of bronchopulmonary dysplasia and, whilst there is currently no cure for FGR or lung disease in this vulnerable cohort, UCB stem cells have shown potential therapeutic benefits in preterm infants. Here we sought to determine if UCB cells would also be beneficial for growth restricted preterm newborns. Our results have demonstrated that UCB shows promising anti-inflammatory benefits for treating ventilation induced lung injury in appropriately grown newborn lambs. However, UCB treatment was not equally effective for FGR infants, where it promoted angiogenesis, did not reverse detrimental changes in lung structure, and increased collagen and its precursor αSMA, which may be injurious. Interestingly, the pulmonary response to cell administration was differentially regulated in AG and FGR lambs, wherein UCB increased VEGF and decreased cell proliferation in FGR lambs only, however, whether this would be beneficial or not for the future of the offspring is yet to be determined. Our study is the first to highlight that the FGR infant responds differently to cell therapy, and these results suggest that developmental programming *in utero* needs to be considered when giving postnatal treatments.

AUTHOR CONTRIBUTIONS

BA, AM, GP, and SM conceived and designed the analysis. BA, HY, AM, CM, MC-M, YP, AS, GJ, GP, and SM collected and contributed to the data. BA and HY performed the analysis and BA, HY, AM, CM, MC-M, YP, AS, GJ, GP, and SM wrote the paper.

ACKNOWLEDGMENTS

We would like to acknowledge the assistance of Ilias Nitsos, Tamara Yawno, and Michael Fahey who assisted with the animal studies.

REFERENCES

1. Morrison JL. Sheep models of intrauterine growth restriction: fetal adaptations and consequences. *Clin Exp Pharmacol Physiol.* (2008) 35:730–43. doi: 10.1111/j.1440-1681.2008.04975.x
2. Soudée S, Vuillemin L, Alberti C, Mohamed D, Becquet O, Farnoux C, et al. Fetal growth restriction is worse than extreme prematurity for the developing lung. *Neonatology.* (2014) 106:304–10. doi: 10.1159/000360842
3. Sasi A, Abraham V, Davies-Tuck M, Polglase GR, Jenkin G, Miller SL, et al. Impact of intrauterine growth restriction on preterm lung disease. *Acta Paediatr.* (2015) 104:e552–6. doi: 10.1111/apa.13220
4. Allison BJ, Hooper SB, Coia E, Zahra VA, Jenkin G, Malhotra A, et al. Ventilation-induced lung injury is not exacerbated by growth restriction in preterm lambs. *Am J Physiol Lung Cell Mol Physiol.* (2016) 310:L213–23. doi: 10.1152/ajplung.00328.2015
5. Joyce BJ, Louey S, Davey MG, Cock ML, Hooper SB, Harding R. Compromised respiratory function in postnatal lambs after placental insufficiency and intrauterine growth restriction. *Pediatr Res.* (2001) 50:641–9. doi: 10.1203/00006450-200111000-00018
6. Zana-Taieb E, Butruille L, Franco-Montoya ML, Lopez E, Vernier F, Grandvuillemin I, et al. Effect of two models of intrauterine growth restriction on alveolarization in rat lungs: morphometric and gene expression analysis. *PLoS ONE.* (2013) 8:e78326. doi: 10.1371/journal.pone.0078326
7. Alcorn DG, Adamson TM, Maloney JE, Robinson PM. A morphologic and morphometric analysis of fetal lung development in the sheep. *Anat Record.* (1981) 201:655–67. doi: 10.1002/ar.1092010410
8. Gagnon R, Langridge J, Inchley K, Murotsuki J, Possmayer F. Changes in surfactant-associated protein mRNA profile in growth-restricted fetal sheep. *Am J Physiol.* (1999) 276:L459–65. doi: 10.1152/ajplung.1999.276.3.L459
9. Orgeig S, Crittenden TA, Marchant C, McMillen IC, Morrison JL. Intrauterine growth restriction delays surfactant protein maturation in the sheep fetus. *Am J Physiol Lung Cell Mol Physiol.* (2010) 298:L575–83. doi: 10.1152/ajplung.00226.2009
10. Maritz GS, Cock ML, Louey S, Joyce BJ, Albuquerque CA, Harding R. Effects of fetal growth restriction on lung development before and after birth: a morphometric analysis. *Pediatr Pulmonol.* (2001) 32:201–10. doi: 10.1002/ppul.1109
11. Rozance PJ, Seedorf GJ, Brown A, Roe G, O'Meara MC, Gien J, et al. Intrauterine growth restriction decreases pulmonary alveolar and vessel growth and causes pulmonary artery endothelial cell dysfunction *in vitro* in fetal sheep. *Am J Physiol Lung Cell Mol Physiol.* (2011) 301:L860–71. doi: 10.1152/ajplung.00197.2011
12. Figueras F, Gratacos E. Stage-based approach to the management of fetal growth restriction. *Prenat Diagn.* (2014) 34:655–9. doi: 10.1002/pd.4412
13. Chang YS, Oh W, Choi SJ, Sung DK, Kim SY, Choi EY, et al. Human umbilical cord blood-derived mesenchymal stem cells attenuate hyperoxia-induced lung injury in neonatal rats. *Cell Transplant.* (2009) 18:869–86. doi: 10.3727/096368909X471189
14. Hodges RJ, Jenkin G, Hooper SB, Allison B, Lim R, Dickinson H, et al. Human amnion epithelial cells reduce ventilation-induced preterm lung injury in fetal sheep. *Am J Obstetr Gynecol.* (2012) 206:448.e8–15. doi: 10.1016/j.ajog.2012.02.038
15. Monz D, Tutdibi E, Mildau C, Shen J, Kasoha M, Laschke MW, et al. Human umbilical cord blood mononuclear cells in a double-hit model of bronchopulmonary dysplasia in neonatal mice. *PLoS ONE.* (2013) 8:e74740. doi: 10.1371/journal.pone.0074740
16. Allison BJ, Crossley KJ, Flecknoe SJ, Davis PG, Morley CJ, Harding R, et al. Ventilation of the very immature lung *in utero* induces injury and BPD-Like changes in lung structure in fetal sheep. *Pediatr Res.* (2008) 64:387–92. doi: 10.1203/PDR.0b013e318181e05e
17. Castillo-Melendez M, Yawno T, Jenkin G, Miller SL. Stem cell therapy to protect and repair the developing brain: a review of mechanisms of action of cord blood and amnion epithelial derived cells. *Front Neurosci.* (2013) 7:194. doi: 10.3389/fnins.2013.00194
18. Liu L, Mao Q, Chu S, Mounayar M, Abdi R, Fodor W, et al. De Paepe: intranasal versus intraperitoneal delivery of human umbilical cord tissue-derived cultured mesenchymal stromal cells in a murine model of neonatal lung injury. *Am J Pathol.* (2014) 184:3344–58. doi: 10.1016/j.ajpath.2014.08.010
19. Secco M, Zucconi E, Vieira NM, Fogaça LLQ, Cerqueira A, Carvalho MDF, et al. Multipotent stem cells from umbilical cord: cord is richer than blood! *Stem Cells.* (2008) 26:146–50. doi: 10.1634/stemcells.2007-0381
20. Li J, Yawno T, SutherlAE, Gurung S, Paton M, McDonald C, et al. Preterm umbilical cord blood derived mesenchymal stem/stromal cells protect preterm white matter brain development against hypoxia-ischemia. *Exp Neurol.* (2018) 308:120–31. doi: 10.1016/j.expneurol.2018.07.006
21. Paton MCB, McDonald CA, Allison BJ, Fahey MC, Jenkin G, Miller SL. Perinatal brain injury as a consequence of preterm birth and intrauterine inflammation: designing targeted stem cell therapies. *Front Neurosci.* (2017) 11:200. doi: 10.3389/fnins.2017.00200
22. Min K, Song J, Kang JY, Ko J, Ryu JS, Kang MS, et al. Umbilical cord blood therapy potentiated with erythropoietin for children with cerebral palsy: a Double-blind, randomized, placebo-Controlled trial. *Stem Cells.* (2013) 31:581–91. doi: 10.1002/stem.1304
23. Novak I, Walker K, Hunt RW, Wallace EM, Fahey M, Badawi N. Concise review: stem cell interventions for people with cerebral palsy: systematic review with meta-analysis. *Stem Cells Transl Med.* (2016) 5:1014–25. doi: 10.5966/sctm.2015-0372
24. Erices A, Conget P, Minguell JJ. Mesenchymal progenitor cells in human umbilical cord blood. *British Journal of Haematology.* (2000) 109:235–42. doi: 10.1046/j.1365-2141.2000.01986.x
25. Cairo MS, Wagner JE. Placental and/or umbilical cord blood: an alternative source of hematopoietic stem cells for transplantation. *Blood.* (1997) 90:4665–78. doi: 10.1182/blood.V90.12.4665
26. Phuc PV, Ngoc VB, Lam DH, Tam NT, Viet PQ, Ngoc PK. Isolation of three important types of stem cells from the same samples of banked umbilical cord blood. *Cell Tissue Bank.* (2012) 13:341–51. doi: 10.1007/s10561-011-9262-4
27. Lee MW, Jang IK, Yoo KH, Sung KW, Koo HH. Stem and progenitor cells in human umbilical cord blood. *Int J Hematol.* (2010) 92:45–51. doi: 10.1007/s12185-010-0619-4
28. Wagner JE, Barker JN, DeFor TE, Baker KS, Blazar BR, Eide C, et al. Transplantation of unrelated donor umbilical cord blood in 102 patients with malignant and nonmalignant diseases: influence of CD34 cell dose and HLA disparity on treatment-related mortality and survival. *Blood.* (2002) 100:1611–8. doi: 10.1182/blood-2002-01-0294
29. Polglase GR, Morley CJ, Crossley KJ, Dargaville P, Harding R, Morgan DL, et al. Positive end-expiratory pressure differentially alters pulmonary hemodynamics and oxygenation in ventilated, very premature lambs.

J Appl Physiol. (2005) 99:1453–61. doi: 10.1152/japplphysiol.00055.2005
30. Yawno T, Sabaretnam T, Li J, McDonald C, Lim R, Jenkin G, et al. Human amnion epithelial cells protect against white matter brain injury after repeated endotoxin exposure in the preterm ovine fetus. *Cell Transplant.* (2017) 26:541–53. doi: 10.3727/096368916X693572
31. Joyce BJ, Wallace MJ, Pierce RA, Harding R, Hooper SB. Sustained changes in lung expansion alter tropoelastin mRNA levels and elastin content in fetal sheep lungs. *Am J Physiol Lung Cell Mol Physiol.* (2003) 284:L643–9. doi: 10.1152/ajplung.00090.2002
32. Tian J, Tian S, Gridley DS. Comparison of acute proton, photon, and low-dose priming effects on genes associated with extracellular matrix and adhesion molecules in the lungs. *Fibrogenesis Tissue Repair.* (2013) 6:4. doi: 10.1186/1755-1536-6-4
33. Chang YS, Ahn SY, Yoo HS, Sung SI, Choi SJ, Oh WI, et al. Mesenchymal stem cells for bronchopulmonary dysplasia: phase 1 dose-escalation clinical trial. *J Pediatr.* (2014) 164:966–72 e6. doi: 10.1016/j.jpeds.2013.12.011
34. Zhu D, Tan J, Maleken AS, Muljadi R, Chan ST, Lau SN, et al. Human amnion cells reverse acute and chronic pulmonary damage in experimental neonatal lung injury. *Stem Cell Res Ther.* (2017) 8:257. doi: 10.1186/s13287-017-0689-9
35. Vosdoganes P, Hodges RJ, Lim R, Westover AJ, Acharya RY, Wallace EM, et al. Moss. Human amnion epithelial cells as a treatment for inflammation-induced fetal lung injury in sheep. *Am J Obstetr Gynecol.* (2011) 205:156.e26–33. doi: 10.1016/j.ajog.2011.03.054
36. Alves de Alencar Rocha AK, Allison BJ, Yawno T, Polglase GR, Sutherland AE, Malhotra A, et al. Early- versus late-onset fetal growth restriction differentially affects the development of the fetal sheep brain. *Dev Neurosci.* (2017) 39:141–55. doi: 10.1159/000456542
37. Joss-Moore LA, Wang Y, Yu X, Campbell MS, Callaway CW, McKnight RA, et al. IUGR decreases elastin mRNA expression in the developing rat lung and alters elastin content and lung compliance in the mature rat lung. *Physiol Genom.* (2011) 43:499–505. doi: 10.1152/physiolgenomics.00183.2010
38. Sutherland AE, Crossley K, Allison B, Jenkin G, Wallace E, Miller S. The effects of intrauterine growth restriction and antenatal glucocorticoids on ovine fetal lung development. *Pediatr Res.* (2012) 71:689–96. doi: 10.1038/pr.2012.19
39. Flecknoe SJ, Bol RE, Wallace MJ, Harding R, Hooper SB. Regulation of alveolar epithelial cell phenotypes in fetal sheep: roles of cortisol and lung expansion. *Am J Physiol Lung Cell Mol Physiol.* (2004) 287:L1207–14. doi: 10.1152/ajplung.00375.2003
40. Jobe AH, Nitsos I, Pillow JJ, Polglase GR, Kallapur SG, Newnham JP. Betamethasone dose and formulation for induced lung maturation in fetal sheep. *Am J Obstetr Gynecol.* (2009) 201:611.e1–7. doi: 10.1016/j.ajog.2009.07.014
41. Krause MF, Jakel C, Haberstroh J, Schulte-Monting J, Leititis JU, Orlowska-Volk M. Orlowska-Volk: alveolar recruitment promotes homogeneous surfactant distribution in a piglet model of lung injury. *Pediatr Res.* (2001) 50:34–43. doi: 10.1203/00006450-200107000-00009
42. Ueda T, Ikegami M, Rider ED, Jobe AH. Distribution of surfactant and ventilation in surfactant-treated preterm lambs. *J Appl Physiol.* (1994) 76:45–55. doi: 10.1152/jappl.1994.76.1.45
43. Hillman NH, Moss TJM, Kallapur SG, Bachurski C, Pillow JJ, Polglase GR, et al. Brief, large tidal volume ventilation initiates lung injury and a systemic response in fetal sheep. *Am J Respir Crit Care Med.* (2007) 176:575–81. doi: 10.1164/rccm.200701-051OC
44. Vosdoganes P, Lim R, Koulaeva E, Chan ST, Acharya R, Moss TJ, et al. Human amnion epithelial cells modulate hyperoxia-induced neonatal lung injury in mice. *Cytotherapy.* (2013) 15:1021–9. doi: 10.1016/j.jcyt.2013.03.004
45. Tremblay L, Valenza F, Ribeiro SP, Li J, Slutsky AS. Injurious ventilatory strategies increase cytokines and c-fos m-RNA expression in an isolated rat lung model. *J Clin Invest.* (1997) 99:944–52. doi: 10.1172/JCI119259
46. Hikino S, Ohga S, Kinjo T, Kusuda T, Ochiai M, Inoue H, et al. Tracheal aspirate gene expression in preterm newborns and development of bronchopulmonary dysplasia. *Pediatr Int.* (2012) 54:208–14. doi: 10.1111/j.1442-200X.2011.03510.x
47. Pugin J, Dunn I, Jolliet P, Tassaux D, Magnenat JL, Nicod LP, et al. Activation of human macrophages by mechanical ventilation *in vitro*. *Am J Physiol.* (1998) 275(6 Pt 1):L1040–50. doi: 10.1152/ajplung.1998.275.6.L1040
48. Pelletier M, Bouchard A, Girard D. *In vivo* and *in vitro* roles of IL-21 in inflammation. *J Immunol.* (2004) 173:7521–30. doi: 10.4049/jimmunol.173.12.7521
49. van Haaften T, Byrne R, Bonnet S, Rochefort GY, Akabutu J, Bouchentouf M, et al. Airway delivery of mesenchymal stem cells prevents arrested alveolar growth in neonatal lung injury in rats. *Am J Respir Crit Care Med.* (2009) 180:1131–42. doi: 10.1164/rccm.200902-0179OC
50. Chang YS, Choi SJ, Sung DK, Kim SY, Oh W, Yang YS, et al. Intratracheal transplantation of human umbilical cord blood-derived mesenchymal stem cells dose-dependently attenuates hyperoxia-induced lung injury in neonatal rats. *Cell Transplant.* (2011) 20:1843–54. doi: 10.3727/096368911X565038a
51. Hemeda H, Jakob M, Ludwig AK, Giebel B, Lang S, Brandau S. Interferon-gamma and tumor necrosis factor-alpha differentially affect cytokine expression and migration properties of mesenchymal stem cells. *Stem Cells Dev.* (2010) 19:693–706. doi: 10.1089/scd.2009.0365
52. Bland RD, Ertsey R, Mokres LM, Xu L, Jacobson BE, Jiang S, et al. Mechanical ventilation uncouples synthesis and assembly of elastin and increases apoptosis in lungs of newborn mice. Prelude to defective alveolar septation during lung development? *Lung Cell Mol Physiol.* (2008) 294:L3–14. doi: 10.1152/ajplung.00362.2007
53. Dunsmore SE, Rannels DE. Extracellular matrix biology in the lung. *Am J Physiol.* (1996) 270(1 Pt 1):L3–27. doi: 10.1152/ajplung.1996.270.1.L3
54. Pierce RA, Albertine KH, Starcher BC, Bohnsack JF, Carlton DP, Bland RD. Chronic lung injury in preterm lambs: disordered pulmonary elastin deposition. *Am J Physiol.* (1997) 272(3 Pt 1):L452–60. doi: 10.1152/ajplung.1997.272.3.L452
55. Rudic RD, Shesely EG, Maeda N, Smithies O, Segal SS, Sessa WC. Direct evidence for the importance of endothelium-derived nitric oxide in vascular remodeling. *J Clin Invest.* (1998) 101:731–6. doi: 10.1172/JCI1699
56. Allison BJ, Kaandorp JJ, Kane AD, Camm EJ, Lusby C, Cross CM, et al. Divergence of mechanistic pathways mediating cardiovascular aging and developmental programming of cardiovascular disease. *FASEB J.* (2016) 30:1968–75. doi: 10.1096/fj.201500057
57. Brain KL, Allison BJ, Niu Y, Cross CM, Itani N, Kane AD, et al. Induction of controlled hypoxic pregnancy in large mammalian species. *Physiol Rep.* (2015) 3:e12614. doi: 10.14814/phy2.12614
58. Polglase GR, Allison BJ, Coia E, Li A, Jenkin G, Malhotra A, et al. Altered cardiovascular function at birth in growth-restricted preterm lambs. *Pediatr Res.* (2016) 80:538–46. doi: 10.1038/pr.2016.104
59. Coalson JJ. Pathology of new bronchopulmonary dysplasia. *Semin Neonatol.* (2003) 8:73–81. doi: 10.1016/S1084-2756(02)00193-8
60. Kern S, Eichler H, Stoeve J, Klüter H, Bieback K. Comparative analysis of mesenchymal stem cells from bone marrow, umbilical cord blood, or adipose tissue. *Stem Cells.* (2006) 24:1294–301. doi: 10.1634/stemcells.2005-0342
61. Chess P, Benson R, Maniscalco W, Wright T, O'Reilly MA, Johnston C. Murine mechanical ventilation stimulates alveolar epithelial cell proliferation. *Exp Lung Res.* (2010) 36:331–41. doi: 10.3109/01902141003632332
62. Murotsuki J, Challis JR, Han VK, Fraher LJ, Gagnon R. Chronic fetal placental embolization and hypoxemia cause hypertension and myocardial hypertrophy in fetal sheep. *Am J Physiol.* (1997) 272(1 Pt 2):R201–7. doi: 10.1152/ajpregu.1997.272.1.R201
63. Chang YS, Choi SJ, Ahn SY, Sung DK, Sung SI, Yoo HS, et al. Timing of umbilical cord blood derived mesenchymal stem cells transplantation determines therapeutic efficacy in the neonatal hyperoxic lung injury. *PLoS ONE.* (2013) 8:e52419. doi: 10.1371/journal.pone.0052419
64. Wang W, Zhu X, Du X, Xu A, Yuan X, Zhan Y, et al. MiR-150 promotes angiogensis and proliferation of endothelial progenitor cells in deep venous thrombosis by targeting SRCIN1. *Microvasc Res.* (2018) 123:35–41. doi: 10.1016/j.mvr.2018.10.003
65. Gao Y, Cornfield DN, Stenmark KR, Thebaud B, Abman SH, Raj JU. Unique aspects of the developing lung circulation: structural development and regulation of vasomotor tone. *Pulm Circ.* (2016) 6:407–25. doi: 10.1086/688890
66. McDonald CA, Penny TR, Paton MCB, SutherlAE, Nekkanti L, Yawno T, et al. Effects of umbilical cord blood cells, and subtypes, to reduce neuroinflammation following perinatal hypoxic-ischemic brain injury. *J*

Neuroinflammation. (2018) 15:47. doi: 10.1186/s12974-018-1089-5

67. Marx A, Arnemann C, Horton RL, Amon K, Joseph N, Carlson J. Decreasing neonatal intubation rates: trends at a community hospital. *J Neonatal Nursing.* (2016) 22:231–35. doi: 10.1016/j.jnn.2016.04.006
68. Barker DJ, Osmond C, Kajantie E, Eriksson JG. Growth and chronic disease: findings in the helsinki birth cohort. *Ann Hum Biol.* (2009) 36:445–58. doi: 10.1080/03014460902980295
69. Sehgal A, Gwini SM, Menahem S, Allison BJ, Miller SL, Polglase GR. Preterm growth restriction and bronchopulmonary dysplasia: the vascular hypothesis and related physiology. *J Physiol.* (2018) 597:1209–20. doi: 10.1113/JP276040
70. Gortner L, Monz D, Mildau C, Shen J, Kasoha M, Laschke MW, et al. Bronchopulmonary dysplasia in a double-hit mouse model induced by intrauterine hypoxia and postnatal hyperoxia: closer to clinical features? *Ann Anat.* (2013) 195:351–8. doi: 10.1016/j.aanat.2013.02.010

8

Knowledge Gaps and Emerging Research Areas in Intrauterine Growth Restriction-Associated Brain Injury

Bobbi Fleiss[1,2,3], Flora Wong[4,5,6], Fiona Brownfoot[7], Isabelle K. Shearer[1], Olivier Baud[2,8], David W. Walker[1], Pierre Gressens[2,3,9] and Mary Tolcos[1]*

[1] School of Health and Biomedical Sciences, RMIT University, Bundoora, VIC, Australia, [2] NeuroDiderot, INSERM, Université Paris Diderot, Sorbonne Paris Cité, Paris, France, [3] Centre for the Developing Brain, School of Biomedical Engineering and Imaging Sciences, King's College London, St Thomas' Hospital, London, United Kingdom, [4] The Ritchie Centre, Hudson Institute of Medical Research, Clayton, VIC, Australia, [5] Department of Paediatrics, Monash University, Clayton, VIC, Australia, [6] Monash Newborn, Monash Children's Hospital, Clayton, VIC, Australia, [7] Translational Obstetrics Group, Department of Obstetrics and Gynaecology, Mercy Hospital for Women, University of Melbourne, Heidelberg, VIC, Australia, [8] Division of Neonatal Intensive Care, University Hospitals of Geneva, Children's Hospital, University of Geneva, Geneva, Switzerland, [9] PremUP, Paris, France

***Correspondence:**
Bobbi Fleiss
bobbi.fleiss@rmit.edu.au

Intrauterine growth restriction (IUGR) is a complex global healthcare issue. Concerted research and clinical efforts have improved our knowledge of the neurodevelopmental sequelae of IUGR which has raised the profile of this complex problem. Nevertheless, there is still a lack of therapies to prevent the substantial rates of fetal demise or the constellation of permanent neurological deficits that arise from IUGR. The purpose of this article is to highlight the clinical and translational gaps in our knowledge that hamper our collective efforts to improve the neurological sequelae of IUGR. Also, we draw attention to cutting-edge tools and techniques that can provide novel insights into this disorder, and technologies that offer the potential for better drug design and delivery. We cover topics including: how we can improve our use of crib-side monitoring options, what we still need to know about inflammation in IUGR, the necessity for more human post-mortem studies, lessons from improved integrated histology-imaging analyses regarding the cell-specific nature of magnetic resonance imaging (MRI) signals, options to improve risk stratification with genomic analysis, and treatments mediated by nanoparticle delivery which are designed to modify specific cell functions.

Keywords: growth restriction, neurobiology and brain physiology, brain development, neuroprotection, neuroinflammation

INTRODUCTION

Intrauterine (or fetal) growth restriction (IUGR, FGR) is caused by a heterogeneous set of maternal and fetal clinical pathologies. Stillbirth, neonatal mortality and poor neurological, and cardiovascular outcomes are all too common consequences of IUGR. We do not have the clinical tests to reliably predict the onset of IUGR, or even to reliably detect it, when present in late gestation. A diagnosis of IUGR is simply the indication that the infant has a birth weight below their genetically predetermined potential, with no etiological meaning. Our understanding of the clinical progression of IUGR including the poor neurodevelopmental outcomes has increased due to improved imaging techniques, such as Doppler velocimetry and magnetic resonance imaging (MRI). Nevertheless, as a research community, we are still striving to understand the pathological mechanisms leading to the various subtypes of IUGR (discussed below). Increase of this knowledge is crucial for tailoring therapies to prevent or treat IUGR and, in particular to reduce brain injury. Highlighting the need for a continuing collective research efforts is that, depending on the specific definition of IUGR applied (discussed below), the incidence of IUGR is between 3 and 9% of pregnancies in high resource settings, but horrifically, in low-resource settings, the rates are as high as 30% of pregnancies (1).

The purpose of our review, written in a narrative form [as defined in McGaghie (2)], is to highlight the gaps in our clinical and translational knowledge, and the weaknesses of our research methods that hamper our collective efforts to improve the neurological outcomes of those infants diagnosed with IUGR. Our opinions and interests are diverse—as authors we include clinicians working as obstetricians, neonatologists, and neonatal neurologists, plus researchers with expertise in fetal physiology and developmental neurobiology. We will focus on new cutting-edge tools and techniques that might provide novel insights into this disorder of fetal growth, and on technologies that offer the potential for better drug design and delivery. We will cover topics including maximizing the benefit of data from scarce human post-mortem tissues, lessons from advanced histological analyses regarding the cell-specific nature of MRI signals, options to improve risk stratification with genomic analysis, and new treatments based on delivery of nanoparticles designed to modify cell-specific functions.

WHAT IS IUGR?

The issue of an optimal definition for IUGR has been called "one of the most common, controversial, and complex problems in obstetrics" (3). Simply, IUGR is usually recognized when an infant appears to have failed to grow to its expected size—based on it genetically pre-determined potential. Most surprisingly though, there is no universally applied definition of what threshold of body weight clearly defines an infant as IUGR, with birth weights at or below the 10th or the 3rd centile, and concomitant changes in placental blood flow and gestational age all taken into account with varying frequencies across health care centers even within countries. An advance in bringing a universally recognized definition to the field was made with the recent publication of a Delphi procedure resulting in an agreed definition of IUGR (4). However, although a Delphi procedure is a well-established method for finding consensus, only 45 participants from across the entire world took part; 54% of these being from Europe, encompassing 37 member states with various population risk factors and health care paradigms. In addition, Asia and Australia were grouped as a single entity with only 10 opinions received from these diverse areas of the world. The Delphi procedure presented clinical variables and outcomes already known to be associated with IUGR and asked the participants to rank or stratify the importance of these. The end result was that somatic growth indices, umbilical artery pulsatility index, and absent end-diastolic flow were the favored diagnostic criteria. At this point we would like to highlight there is no pathophysiological meaning within the term IUGR (or FGR) as IUGR ultimately is a symptom, like the diagnosis of microcephaly (i.e., brain growth at or below two standard deviations from the mean). The term IUGR (or FGR) is as useful for understanding the disorder as if we used the term PRBS (poorly regulated blood sugar) in place of diabetes. The Delphi procedure offers no clarification on whether it is possible to stratify patients based on the underlying cause of their IUGR, although admittedly, this was not its purpose. However, we need to revaluate the criteria currently used to determine IUGR, (e.g., somatic growth, umbilical blood flow) some of which might well-reflect compensation and adaptation to an underlying, unidentified causal mechanism. Additional measurements could include blood-based biochemical measures of inflammation, placentally-derived biomarkers, postnatal blood pressure and urine parameters, and additional biometrics such as skin folds, and skeletal phenotype. Meta-analysis of clinical data banks, together with studies on stored chorionic villi and maternal blood retained after routine clinical testing, and (albeit, complicated) the recruitment of further large prospective cohorts—could provide us with biochemical parameters that closely reflect the underlying causes of reduced fetal growth, and how these stratify with risk across the lifespan.

How we name a disease has a significant bearing on how we then think about it, and ultimately, how we model and aim to treat it, so these issues of universal nomenclature are important; see commentaries by Dammann et al. (5), and McIntyre et al. (6) for the importance of classifying known causes, and not symptomatic outcomes. A recent summary of the definition(s) of IUGR as they have evolved over the past 30 years highlights three facts: (1) that a significant number of clinical studies on IUGR (11%) gave no definition of IUGR; (2) that ultrasound measurements of fetal biometrics, but not Doppler measurements of placental and/or fetal brain blood flows, have been increasingly used to define IUGR, and; (3) that overall the primary, consistently used characteristic of IUGR diagnosis is birth weight (7). This last observation highlights that we are missing opportunities to identify the early prenatal events that lead to IUGR, and therefore of developing our approaches to increase the efficacy of interventions, and the opportunity to prevent, rather than repair brain damage and therefore to improve neurological outcomes for these infants via early identification. A further confounder in diagnosing IUGR is the lack of accurate gestational dating, as in many countries (including the USA) routine ultrasound dating scans are not available and estimates based on last menstrual period are generally unreliable.

Maternal and fetal genetic factors are responsible for >50% of the variance in birth weight (8). As such, is it critical to separate healthy infants that are small for gestational age (SGA) due to inherent genetic factors from those with reduced growth that are at risk of sustaining neurological injury and metabolic dysfunction. Personalized growth charts, based on maternal and fetal characteristics (such as age, body weight, fetal sex, and ethnicity), have improved our ability to differentiate IUGR and SGA infants [for a commentary see (9)]. While correcting for maternal parameters seems appropriate, perhaps correcting for ethnicity might normalize a socially disadvantaged group with higher rates of growth restriction and poor obstetric outcome. This was perhaps best reflected in INTERGORWTH 21 which recruited over 20,000 pregnant women from numerous countries around the world in regions where the health and nutrition of the mother were met and antenatal care was adequate, and they demonstrated that the growth parameters were similar regardless of ethnicity.

IUGR is also classified as symmetric or asymmetric IUGR (**Figure 2**), dependent on the ratio of the head circumference to the abdominal circumference, which is increased in asymmetric IUGR. This categorization is based on the idea of brain sparing arising (typically) from late-onset IUGR. Early-onset IUGR (before 32 weeks post-conceptional age [PCA]) is more often associated with the symmetrical form of IUGR, and late-onset IUGR (after 31 + 6 weeks PCA) is more often associated with asymmetric IUGR. For further details on brain sparing and a discussion on the consequences and relationship between adaptive to maladaptive (compensatory vs. decompensatory) processes, see the section on "Causes of IUGR," below. There is also a third phenotype of IUGR reflecting the accumulated effects of early *and* late IUGR risk factors (10). This mixed phenotype is observed predominantly in pregnancies complicated by peri-conceptual malnutrition, and then by placental dysfunction later in pregnancy. These infants are suggested to present with symmetric growth, but with severe signs of malnutrition, such as high numbers of scapula skin folds (10).

WHAT ARE THE OUTCOMES ASSOCIATED WITH IUGR?

IUGR fetuses are at increased risk of stillbirth, fetal compromise, early neonatal death, and neonatal morbidity (11). A vast literature including many works from Winder et al. has demonstrated that the availability of physiological resources that support growth *in utero*, which include not only maternal nutritional status (12) but also placental size, shape, and metabolic efficiency, have effects that continue to have an impact on health throughout childhood and adult life (13, 14). Indeed, IUGR-born infants are prone to a range of health problems, including increased risk of cardiovascular diseases and neurodevelopmental disorders (15, 16).

It has been difficult to compile outcome data from the many studies on IUGR, because in addition to the fact that IUGR includes an inconsistent, heterogeneous set of clinical characteristics and underlying etiologies, postnatal data reporting includes further inconsistencies in patient selection and outcome parameters. To enable future trials to measure similar meaningful outcomes, the Core Outcome Set for GROwth restriction: deVeloping Endpoints (COSGROVE) consortium is developing two core outcome sets—one for prevention and the other for treatment of IUGR (17). These guidelines will ensure the collection and reporting of a minimum dataset, agreed by stakeholder consensus that will reduce inconsistencies in the reporting of outcomes across relevant trials. For comprehensive reviews on IUGR-related brain injury, including specifics related to the type and severity of IUGR and outcomes, we refer the reader to Miller et al. (18), Tolcos et al. (19), and Gilchrist et al. (20). Over all, infants that were born IUGR have a significantly increased risk of motor and sensory neurodevelopmental deficits, cognitive and learning impairments, and cerebral palsy (see papers above). In particular, in near-term and term infants the rates of cerebral palsy are higher in IUGR infants (16.5%) than the rates in infants exposed to birth asphyxia (8.5%) or inflammation (4.8%) (21). A common comorbidity of IUGR is preterm birth, and this confounds our understanding of the specific effects of IUGR on brain development and function (discussed below). In addition, the risk of delivering an IUGR baby is higher for woman with chronic hypertension, pre-eclampsia, low socioeconomic status, overt diabetes, anemia, gestational diabetes mellitus, low pre-pregnancy body mass index, or hypothyroidism (22). Whether each of these risk factors leads to a specific phenotype of outcome for the IUGR infant is still a matter that requires considerable study. A number of these risk factors and their causal role in IUGR is discussed further below.

WHAT ARE THE CAUSES OF IUGR?

The primary cause of IUGR is widely considered to be placental insufficiency; i.e., inability of the placenta to adequately support fetal growth. However, the causes of placental insufficiency are many and over-lapping, and include constricted spiral arteries and increased coagulation leading to fetal hypoxia (as in maternal hypertension), and inappropriate substrate availability due to maternal under-nutrition or over-nutrition (22, 23) (see **Figure 1**). For the purposes of this review we won't discuss in detail the relationship between IUGR and maternal drug use (alcohol, tobacco, cocaine etc) or the association with infectious agents, the so-called "TORCH" infections; Toxoplasmosis, Other (syphilis, hepatitis B, varicella-zoster virus, human immunodeficiency virus [HIV], parvovirus B19, enteroviruses, lymphocytic choriomeningitic virus etc.), Rubella, Cytomegalovirus, and Herpes simplex virus. However, these infections and exposure to environmental toxins often lead to a complex constellation of outcomes (microcephaly, facial abnormalities, intracranial calcifications, rash, jaundice, hepatosplenomegaly, elevated transaminase concentrations, and thrombocytopenia) which, although low in incidence in high-income settings (24), are significant in low resource settings (25).

Late vs. Early Onset IUGR and the "*Head-Sparing*" Effect

In addition to linking IUGR to specific pathological processes, as discussed above we also classify IUGR as symmetric or asymmetric (**Figure 2**), dependent on the ratio of the head circumference to the abdominal circumference of the infant. Asymmetric IUGR is the result of "brain sparing," a process

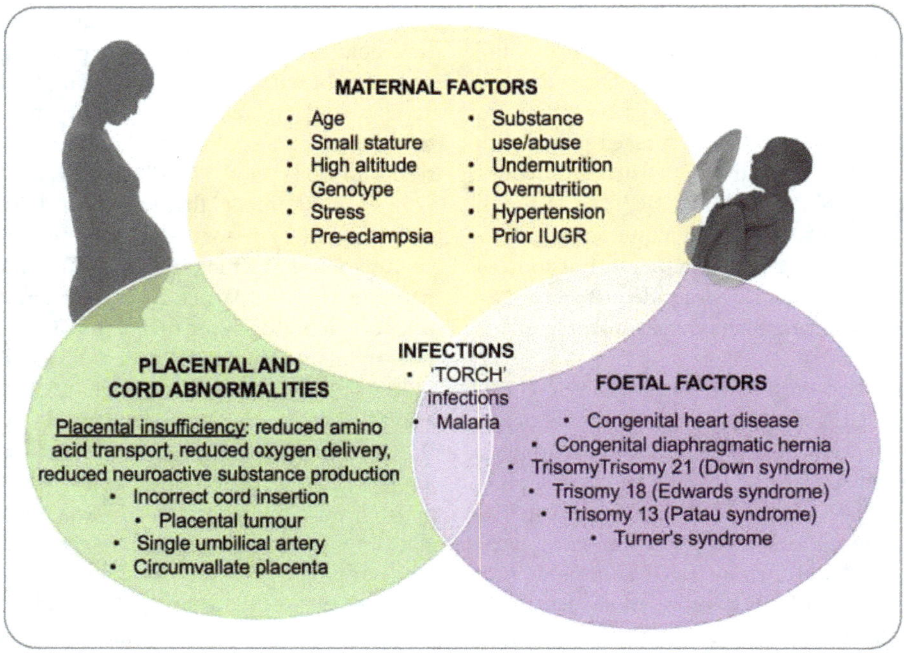

FIGURE 1 | Outline of the causes of IUGR including contributions from maternal, placental and umbilical cord, and fetal dysfunction or injury. Adapted from Vijayaselvi and Cherian (22) and Gaccioli and Lager (23).

whereby brain growth is less affected than body growth due to the redistribution of cardiac output. While brain sparing does not completely prevent the damaging effects of IUGR on brain development (26, 27), it is nonetheless associated with better neurological outcomes than when brain sparing does not occur (28). It is also worth noting that mortality is higher in IUGR with symmetric growth even after adjusting for possible cofounding factors (26). Brain sparing can be detected prenatally based on the Doppler pulsatility index (PI) in the middle cerebral artery (MCA); PI is reduced by the decreased cerebral resistance which allows a greater fraction of the cardiac output to perfuse the brain. However, this compensatory process of blood distribution can become "decompensatory" because the increase of brain blood flow and blood volume themselves become damaging (29). Understanding when and how the alteration of relative cerebral blood flow is switched from a compensatory to decompensatory response is clearly important for devising the most appropriate interventions and therapies. It is worth noting that brain sparing does not reduce the consequences of IUGR on later health, such as increased adiposity, diabetes, and cardiovascular risks, etc [reviewed in Sehgal et al. (30) and Devaskar and Chu (31)].

Maternal risk factors, especially diabetes, high body-mass-index and hypertension, are relevant risk factors for IUGR across both high- and low-income settings. This blurring of income-related demarcations is driven in part by changes in diet and lifestyle, such as adoption of a "western-style" diet and changes in the nature of "work" with more people employed in sedentary activities in urban centers across continents. An illustration of this is the increased risk for an IUGR infant when a woman is diabetic; in Africa the rate of diabetes in adults 25–64 years of age is at 15%, in India 9%, and in Australia 5% (WHO, heath-topics, 2018). An increased body-mass-index is also a major risk factor for gestational diabetes that also associates with poor fetal outcomes. The effects of diabetes on the placenta occur irrespective of the cause of diabetes and the careful management of blood sugar, and include thickening of the trophoblast basement membrane (32), which impairs oxygen and nutrient delivery. Diabetes is associated with a higher release of placental cytokines such as leptin, tumor necrosis factor-α (TNF-α), and Interleukin-6 (IL-6) [see Pantham et al. (33)]. Overnutrition in the (apparent) absence of co-morbidities is also associated with poor placental development/function and poor fetal outcomes [recently reviewed in Howell and Powell (34)], and this has also been demonstrated in experimental models, including sheep, mouse, rat, and rabbit (35–37).

An important link between maternal overnutrition, poor placental development, and poor brain development is inflammation. Obesity is a known driver of systemic inflammation and neuroinflammation (see microglial section, below) (38), and a precise regulation of the maternal and fetal immune system is required for proper placental function and fetal brain development. Of note, adipose tissue produces adipokines, including the pro-inflammatory factors TNF-*a*, IL-6, and MCP1 (macrophage chemotactic protein 1 also known as CCL2). This is considered to explain (at least, in part) why maternal obesity is associated with higher levels of circulating inflammatory mediators during pregnancy and dysregulated placental nutrient transport (39, 40); such systemic and placental inflammatory effects can be reproduced by over-nutrition in pregnant sheep, leading to IUGR (41, 42).

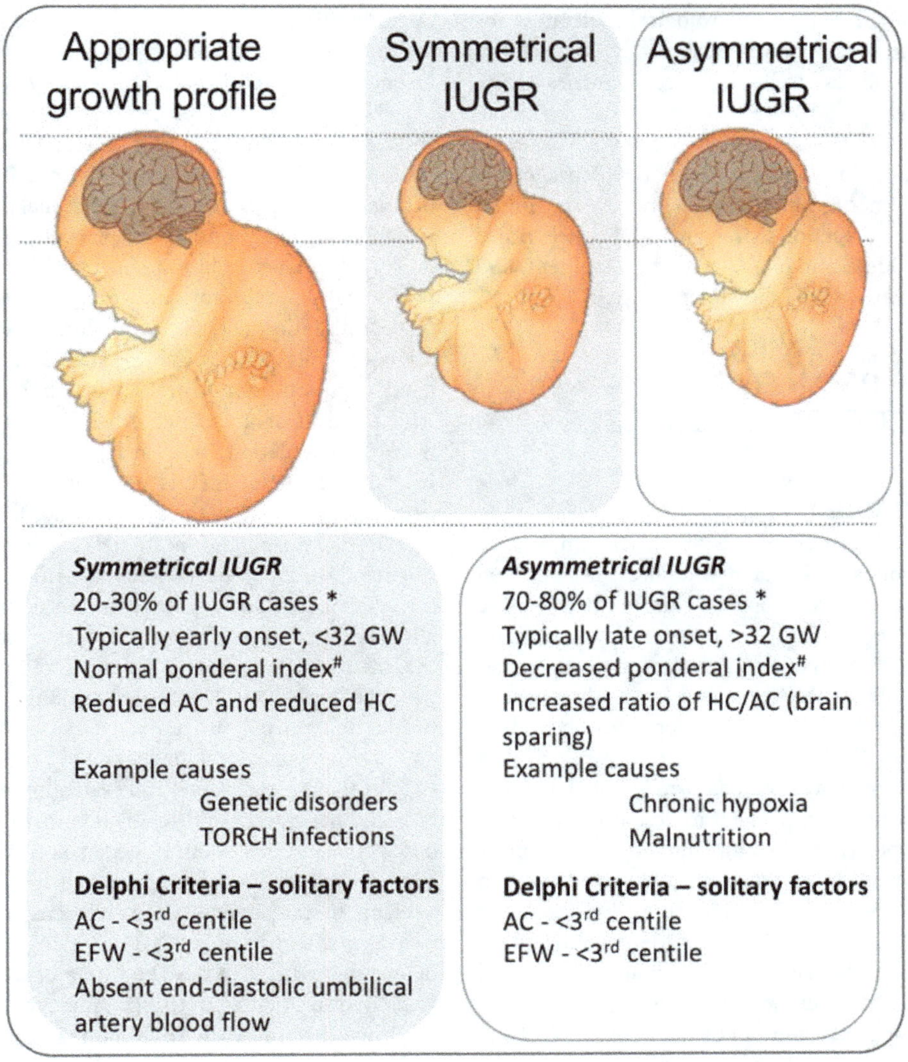

FIGURE 2 | Representation of the physical presentation of symmetrical and asymmetrical IUGR and a short list of clinical characteristics and causes. * note that incidence data are from high-resource settings. A third phenotype is proposed in low-resource settings, that includes characteristics of malnutrition and late gestation placental insufficiency (10), not shown. # Ponderal index, (birth weight (g)/length(cm)^3 × 100). HC, head circumference. AC, Abdominal circumference. GW, gestational weeks. AC, abdominal circumference. EFW, Estimated fetal weight. Delphi criteria from Gordijn et al. (4).

Preeclampsia increases the risks for IUGR 4-fold and is a leading cause of maternal and fetal death. Preeclampsia is a condition of vascular endothelial dysfunction and vasospasm that occurs after 20 weeks of gestation that has its origins in inadequate trophoblastic invasion of the uterine vascular bed, in particular, of the spiral arteries. World-wide, preeclampsia occurs in 8–10% of pregnancies and this rate is consistent across high, middle-, and low-income settings. The factors associated with the onset of preeclampsia include pregnancy at a young or advanced age, high maternal body-mass-index and psychosocial stress. Preeclampsia is usually associated with IUGR, but early onset preeclampsia may be associated with an enlarged placenta and over-large birth weight. While reports show there are differences in placental function and biomarkers between IUGR and preeclampsia, there is overlap between the outcome in these disorders and understanding the similarities and differences will be useful for managing maternal and fetal risk (43–47).

In low resource settings malnutrition is a leading causal factor in IUGR, and all too often these IUGR infants are also delivered preterm adding to the burden of mortality and neurodevelopmental injury (48, 49). Malnutrition is linked not only to economic factors, but also to cultural and social norms that include young maternal age, and repeated and closely spaced pregnancies. UNICEF estimates that in the most developed countries 7% of babies are of low birth weight (encompassing prematurity and IUGR predominantly), whereas in less developed, and the least developed countries, rates of low birth weight deliveries increase to 16.5 and 18.6%, respectively, representing more than 22 million babies annually. Although great improvements in health and well-being are being made, especially as part of the Millennium Development Goals, specific focus on how to overcome poor neurological outcomes for the infants born to these mothers is still greatly needed. For more details on IUGR in less well-developed countries please refer to these references (1, 10, 48–52). Trials of nutritional supplements (micronutrient-supplemented protein, balanced calorie supplements etc.) in women with an IUGR pregnancy identified in the 2nd trimester have failed to improve outcomes, and overall the literature supports pre- and peri-conceptional nutrition as a major determinant of fetal development and pregnancy outcome [reviewed in Liberato et al. (53)].

WHAT ARE THE PRIMARY NEUROPATHOLOGICAL PROCESSES IN IUGR?

Placental Dysfunction

Early-onset IUGR is associated with high impedance uteroplacental perfusion and elevated umbilical artery blood flow resistance as measured by Doppler ultrasound [reviewed in detail by Dall'Asta et al. (54)]. Late-onset IUGR is more common, occurring in 70–80% of IUGR cases and the diagnosis and monitoring of late-onset IUGR has been recently reviewed by Figueras et al. (55). Overt placental pathology may be mild, or even absent in late-onset IUGR, and the Doppler parameters of umbilical artery blood flow may even be normal, but changes in brain blood flow dynamics, such as fetal middle cerebral artery impedance, may be reported indicating compensatory changes to cardiac output indicative of established IUGR. In addition to changes in uterine artery blood flow indicating high vascular resistance, placental studies reveal the important contribution of placental infarcts, and changes in placental amino acid and micro-nutrient transporters, and pathways for growth factor production, further support the concept of "functional" placental insufficiency of IUGR (56, 57). Based on these human studies, animal models of IUGR have been created that recapitulate aspects of the human condition (discussed below), and by and large demonstrate the link between the deprivation of oxygen, glucose, amino acid, and growth factors to the slowing of fetal growth. In addition to this it is now apparent that the abnormal change in placental metabolism results in increased production of reactive oxygen species (ROS), aberrant activation of the complement cascade, re-programming of microglial phenotype (see below), and changes in the trajectory of brain maturation that include dysregulated neural cell proliferation, slower maturation of oligodendrocytes resulting in hypomyelination, and increased programmed (apoptotic) cell death (58–61). We refer the reader to publications describing the mechanisms underpinning the neuropathology of IUGR for more details on these processes (19, 62, 63).

In addition to the somewhat obvious link between the placenta as a source of cytotoxicity, there is the possibility that growth promoting cytokines and neurotrophic growth factors are altered with placental insufficiency. In addition to somatic growth factors such as IGF1, the placenta is a source of pregnene and androgen steroids that directly, or via metabolites such as allopregnanolone, promote, and protect fetal brain development by promoting fetal sleep and quiescence [(64);and references within (65)]. It has been hypothesized the allopregnanolone is an endogenous neuroprotectant, via its effect of global inhibition of CNS activity, that protects against antenatal brain injury (66–68).This field of steroid research has given rise to the notion that there is a "placenta-brain axis" that reflects the co-ordinate development of the fetal adrenal gland, liver, and steroid metabolizing functions of the placenta (69, 70). Neurosteroids derived from progesterone such as allopregnanolone interact with GABA-A receptors and increase central nervous system (CNS) inhibition (71, 72). In uncomplicated pregnancies there are high levels of neurosteroids such as allopregnanolone in the fetal brain immediately before birth, but these levels fall rapidly with removal of the placenta because they are cleared quickly from the circulation, and have a half-life of only minutes (73). In the placenta of infants born preterm the activity of these neurosteroidogenic pathways is reduced, raising the possibility that the prenatal and postnatal paucity of allopregnanolone might affect brain development in these infants (74). In the serum of pregnant women carrying an IUGR fetus, levels of allopregnanolone are lower (75), and in animal models of IUGR the neurosteroid systems (genes and proteins) are lower in the fetal brain (76, 77). Direct inhibition of allopregnanolone production during development causes brain injury (78, 79) and lasting behavioral deficits (80). It is thus reasonable to suggest that progesterone, and even allopregnanolone, should be replaced in preterm and IUGR infants to improve neurological outcomes (81). For example, Ganaxolone is a synthetic analog of allopregnanolone that has a long half-life, has shown promise as a seizure therapy in adults and children refractory to anti-seizure treatments, and in animal studies does not alter fetal viability, neonatal growth, and is without teratogenic or genotoxic effects [reviewed in Hirst et al. (81)]. Ganaxolone therapy should (like all drugs) be trialed in large animal models (powered for sex and with long term outcome) of the various types of IUGR that can now be modeled—for example, by delayed onset chronic hypoxia such as the single artery ligation (SUAL) sheep model (82); early onset placental insufficiency in piglets—(60); maternal overnutrition before and during pregnancy in the sheep—(83). An important layer of safety data that needs to be obtained is the specific interaction that early treatment with ganaxolone might have on the developmental switch of GABA receptors from excitatory to inhibitory (84). This event is predicted to be before 26 weeks' gestation in humans and it might be expected that before this time that ganaxolone would induce, not supress, neuronal activity.

Of the amino acids transported and metabolized by the placenta, tryptophan has a special significance (85). It is an essential amino acid, but protein synthesis accounts for only a minor part of its fate, the greater part being committed to the kynurenine and serotonin pathways. Conversion of tryptophan to kynurenine via indoleamine 2,3-dioxygenase (IDO) in early pregnancy may be important for immune suppression and acceptance of the conceptus as an allograft (86). Later in pregnancy the synthesis of kynurenine may be more important because it is the precursor of kynurenic acid, a physiological glutamate receptor antagonist, which acts as a neuroprotectant (87). Both gene and protein expression of IDO and tryptophan 2,3-dioxygenase (the second enzyme in the kynurenine to tryptophan conversion) are significantly lower in IUGR-affected placentas compared with controls [reviewed by, (88)]. IDO is an oxygenase, and its activity is downregulated in reduced oxygen conditions; demonstrated in *ex vivo* first and third trimester human placental explants exposed to lower oxygen (5–8% O_2) or higher oxygen (20% O_2) conditions. Exposure to lower oxygen levels reduced IDO mRNA and protein expression, and other kynurenine pathway enzymes and kynurenine output was also significantly reduced (88). Inflammatory mediators, such as TNF-α, IL-1β, and interferon-gamma, induce IDO expression thereby increasing tryptophan degradation to kynurenine, but with the result that pro-oxidant (e.g., 3OH-anthranilic acid) and glutamate agonist metabolites (e.g., quinolinic acid) are produced (85). The impact of IUGR on the placental metabolism of tryptophan is not fully understood, but it can be seen from the above that placental insufficiency could have a significant impact on the fetal brain via alterations in the placental degradation of tryptophan.

Tryptophan is also the precursor for the synthesis of serotonin (5-HT). Abnormal levels of brain 5HT have been linked to neurodevelopmental disorders such as autism spectrum disorder (ASD) (89), but when these abnormalities arise in humans (i.e., antenatally or postnatally?) is unclear. There is evidence from mouse pregnancies that placental 5-HT has an important role in early fetal brain development, in that the 5-HT needed for early forebrain development initially comes from the placenta (90). In early neurodevelopment 5-HT functions to regulate a number of key processes, including cell proliferation and neuronal differentiation, migration, and synaptogenesis (89), and experiments in the mouse clearly show the free entry of 5-HT into the immature brain. However, by late gestation, there is a decrease of placental 5-HT synthesis in humans and mice as the raphe nuclei in the midbrain become competent and 5HT axons reach the forebrain (90). This co-ordinate change of 5-HT synthesis between the placenta and brain really does suggest the presence of a "placenta-brain axis" which should be investigated more fully in experimental settings using where IUGR, placental insufficiency, and preterm birth can be modeled in animals with more relevance to human pregnancy. Specifically, an issue with traditional mouse studies is that the fetus is delivered at a stage of brain development equivalent to the start of the second trimester in the human; this makes studies of the last trimester fetal-placental axis impossible. However, peripherally synthesized 5-HT does not freely cross the blood-brain barrier in more fully developed (i.e., adult) brains (91). Goeden et al. (92) have also demonstrated the effects of mild maternal inflammation on placental tryptophan catabolism to 5-HT. Their findings suggest that maternal inflammation during human pregnancy may lead to increased 5-HT synthesis in the placenta and output to the fetus, resulting in abnormal serotonergic axon outgrowth into the developing forebrain.

It is therefore evident that chronic placental hypoxia and inflammation affect the catabolism of tryptophan in the placenta. It is suggested that IDO may act as a "sink" for superoxide, since IDO is known to utilize the superoxide anion as well as molecular oxygen for its oxygenase activity (93). A decrease in IDO expression as a result of hypoxia may therefore lead to decreased clearance of superoxide and an inflammatory response, potentially increasing placental 5-HT synthesis, with consequences for brain growth (94). Alternatively, decreased kynurenine synthesis as a result of hypoxia may shift the tryptophan catabolism pathway in favor of 5-HT synthesis. Clearly, the full effects of IUGR and placental hypoxia on placental tryptophan catabolism are largely unknown but likely to be important for setting the chemical environment in the IUGR brain, and determining vulnerability to damage arising from hypoxia, oxidative stress, or inflammation.

Inflammation and Neuroinflammation

The term inflammation is used to describe the production of cytokines, chemokines, reactive oxygen species, and secondary messengers, together with the paracrine and autocrine effects of these factors. In the CNS, microglia and astrocytes are the primary drivers of inflammation, i.e., neuroinflammation. Both systemic inflammation and neuroinflammation play a central role in the pathophysiology of various forms of perinatal brain damage, as shown by observations from both animal models and the human neonate (95–97). The levels of circulating cytokines in neonates born after IUGR are significantly increased on postnatal days 7 and 14 compared to levels measured in neonates without IUGR (98–100). This postnatal systemic pro-inflammatory state following IUGR could be, at least in part, responsible for the frank brain damage and neurodevelopmental impairments detected in childhood in these individuals. Indeed, at the heart of the vulnerability of the immature brain lies the systemic up-regulation of pro-inflammatory cytokines and the diffuse activation of cerebral microglia, the mediators of brain inflammation (95). The activation of microglia and astrocytes occurs via inflammatory signals coming from the systemic circulation via receptors on endothelial cells and the vagal nerve, and also by local pathogen- and damage-associated proteins (PAMPS and DAMPS, respectively) [reviewed in Carty and Bowie (101)]. In the context of IUGR, and in the absence of obvious pathogens, inflammation can come from at least two sources: (i) inflammation propagating from the placenta owing to the release of DAMPS due to tissue injury (see paragraph below), aberrant macrophage activation (102), and idiopathic villitis (103), and; (ii) from direct effects of hypoxia or other nutrient deprivation or intoxication on the brain (39–42).

Brain cell death, as a predicted consequence of hypoxia and other deprivations on the brain, would cause the release of DAMPS, such as HMGB1 (high mobility group box 1) that activate immune cells including microglia. Neuroinflammation, mediated by microglia, perturbs normal brain development directly by causing injury to cells such as maturing oligodendrocytes. In addition, an important set of developmental processes fulfilled by microglia is left undone when microglia are recruited to a neuroinflammatory response and this also damages the developing brain (see developmental dysfunction, below for further information on the role of microglia). A study of gene expression in microglia and oligodendrocytes in a model of protein restriction-induced IUGR has revealed a striking induction of inflammation-related genes in microglia accompanying the reduction in oligodendrocyte maturation and connectivity and functional deficits (59). This was the first comprehensive study to link protein-restriction with neuroinflammatory-associated brain injury, and in the future, we will look for similarities in related animal models, and undertake human post-mortem studies to look for these dysregulated pathways. We also point the reader toward two excellent reviews on the role of microglia/neuroinflammation in IUGR, one written by a team of experts in pre-clinical modeling and brain injury including observations of microglia and macro-gliosis in various animal models, Wixey et al. (104), and one from the perspective of experienced reproductive immunologists with a focus on maternal immune activation as a driver of microglial activation, Prins et al. (105).

It is worth noting that neuroinflammation (i.e., activated microglia) typically carries assumptions of completely maladaptive or damaging processes. However, less well-understood processes of protection, repair and regeneration are also mediated by micro- and macro-glia, which occur at specific times after injury or insult (106–109). Although there has not been sufficient study of microglial phenotypes in clinical or preclinical IUGR models, more knowledge on microglial activation (phenotypes and temporal regulation) will likely help the development of drugs and treatments that exploit and expand the reparative effects of microglia, while decreasing the negative effects of these cells. Harnessing microglia to regenerate the brain is an approach being applied in the field of multiple sclerosis and adult neurodegeneration (110–112), and it clearly has a place in neonatal neurology.

Developmental Disturbance

The trajectory of brain development is altered by the presence of damaging stimuli, but also by the loss of cells, processes and factors that are important for brain building. As mentioned above, the causes and effects of IUGR include processes of inflammation, placental growth factor deprivation and hypoxia, which together affect the trophic actions of secreted factors such as serotonin, allopregnanolone, tryptophan, and IGF1/2. In addition, we wish to highlight that the "distraction" of microglia away from their normal physiological role in promoting proliferation, pathfinding, myelination and synaptogenesis will cause significant damage to the developmental trajectory of the brain [reviewed extensively in Prins et al. (105), Hagberg et al. (113), Pierre et al. (114) and Tay et al. (115)]

MANAGING THE RISKS OF CONTINUING PREGNANCY VS. PRETERM BIRTH—THE PRENATAL CARE TEAM

As there are currently no effective medical interventions for IUGR, management consists of close surveillance aimed at determining the most appropriate time for delivery. The definition of "most appropriate time" is a question for which the prenatal team has few specific criteria, and balancing the risks of prematurity with the consequences of IUGR (including, stillbirth) remains a contentious issue. Clinical trials to determine the optimal time of delivery have focused on survival and immediate perinatal outcomes, and often lack long-term follow up or an exploration of what features of delivery result in optimal long-term outcomes and reduced neurodevelopmental complications. Recent randomized controlled trials (e.g., Growth Restriction Intervention Trial [GRIT]; Trial of Randomized Umbilical and Fetal Flow in Europe [TRUFFLE]) have helped to shed light on delivery parameters of IUGR babies that lead to improved long-term outcomes. Both studies had a primary outcome of neurodevelopmental delay at 2 years of age.

The GRIT study randomized women at 24–36 weeks PCA to early or delayed delivery and included patients when the clinician was in equipoise about whether they needed delivery. "A priori" parameters set to determine when patients would be delivered were not used in this study. This agnostic approach can be seen as a benefit, as retrospective analysis could shed light on novel parameters common to infants who did well, but it is also difficult, as the motivation for the clinician's decisions are not easy to describe or document, and may not have been adequately captured in the analysis. There was generally only a 4-day delivery interval delay between randomizing the participants to immediate vs. delayed delivery. The 2- and 7 year follow-ups did not show a difference in neurodevelopmental outcome between groups (discussed further below)

The TRUFFLE trial was performed to examine whether parameters set "a priori" for delivery are effective in optimizing delivery outcomes. Participants with IUGR diagnosed at 26–32 weeks PCA with an elevated umbilical artery pulsatility index were randomized to delivery based on: (1) reduced cardiotocography fetal heart rate short-term variation (STV-CTG); or (2) early ductus venosus (DV) changes via doppler; or (3) late ductus venosus changes. They found that more infants randomly assigned to delivery based on late changes in the ductus venosus (95%) were free of neurological impairment compared to those assigned to cardiotocography (85%), but this was accompanied by a non-significant increase in perinatal and infant mortality. They therefore concluded that delivery based on late changes in DV flow might reduce long-term neuro-impairment. When the actual criteria for delivery in these cohorts was dissected it became clear that the majority of patients in the delivery for DV changes were being delivered based on the safety net criteria of spontaneous decelerations in the fetal heart rate. When the two cohorts being delivered for DV changes were combined the neurodevelopmental outcomes at 2 years of age were more favorable compared to those delivered based on STV CTG changes. Therefore, optimal neurodevelopmental outcomes may result if delivery of very preterm patients is restricted until late changes arise in the DV with a caveat of delivery whenever the CTG is abnormal (116, 117).

Severe growth restriction at term is also associated with poor neurodevelopmental outcomes (118). The Disproportionate Intrauterine Growth Intervention Trial At Term (DIGITAT) assessed the impact of immediate delivery vs. expectant management in patients with growth-restricted fetuses at term. The follow-up at 2 years of age demonstrated similar neurodevelopmental gains. However, when assessed by gestation at birth, those in the lowest 2.3 percentile had significantly more neurodevelopmental compromise on an "ages and stages" questionnaire compared to those with a higher birth weight centile. Indeed, 43% of babies born with a birth weight centile below 2.3 had an abnormality on the their "ages and stages" questionnaire compared to 29% of those born at <10th centile and 13% of those with a birth weight greater than the 10th centile. This is consistent with a number of cohort studies demonstrating that low birth weight resulted in increased learning difficulties, defects in speech, neurological deficits, and behavioral problems (119).

BRAIN INJURY IN THE PRETERM BORN IUGR INFANT—THE POSTNATAL CARE TEAM

The incidence of spontaneous preterm birth in pregnancies with severe IUGR is 2 to 3-fold greater than the incidence of pregnancies with appropriate fetal growth (120). In addition, antenatal care focuses heavily on fetal growth monitoring in order to identify pregnancies with poor growth that may benefit from a timely, planned preterm delivery to improve outcomes. However, the contribution of antenatal compromise vs. the postnatal complication of being born preterm, or potential interactions between the two, in contributing to the neurodevelopmental sequelae of IUGR is still unclear. This is important for the clinical decision on when to deliver, when IUGR is diagnosed antenatally.

In a large cohort study comparing more than 1,400 preterm IUGR infants with age-matched AGA controls from 25 to 32 weeks PCA, the incidence of severe intraventricular hemorrhage (IVH) in each gestational age group was similar, but prematurely born IUGR neonates had increased morbidity and mortality (121). On the other hand, preterm birth has been suggested to override the effects of IUGR *per se* on neurological outcomes (122, 123), with the impact most marked for births at the earlier gestational ages. In early-onset IUGR, the gestational age at delivery shows a consistent independent relationship with parameters of motor development with a maximum impact for infants delivered before 28 weeks PCA (124–126), independent of the severity of attrition of growth and the degree of cardiovascular and biophysical deterioration. In the GRIT study which randomly allocated women to early or delayed delivery in the presence of IUGR, and when the obstetrician was unsure whether to deliver, 98% of these patients (n = 376) completed a 2 year follow-up, revealing that the rate of cerebral palsy was greater for patients delivered prior to 31 weeks PCA, and prematurity-related complications were important contributors to this risk (127). Notably, the relationship between gestational age, IUGR and motor deficits suggests the impact of IUGR becomes more apparent with delivery at a later gestation (128). The large prospective EPIPAGE (Etude EPIdémiologique sur les Petits Ages Gestationnels, epidemiologic study of early gestation ages) study (>5,000 births) examined neurological outcomes in school-age children that were born AGA or IUGR (<10th centile for birth weight) at 24–28 weeks or 29–32 weeks PCA, and found similar cognitive deficits in AGA and IUGR infants born at 24–28 weeks PCA, but much less in AGA infants born at 29–32 weeks (129). This clearly indicates the importance of *in utero* brain maturation up to at least 32 weeks PCA. The rate of neurocognitive deficits in the moderately preterm infants with IUGR was around 40% and was identical to the incidence of neurocognitive deficits in extremely preterm infants (129), indicating that the impact of intra-uterine and extra-uterine adverse conditions may be similar on the developing brain in early third trimester. However, a limitation of the EPIPAGE study was stratification of infants by birth weight alone, with no supporting evidence for IUGR.

Consistent with these findings, another study using neuroimaging showed that at 6 years of age, both extremely preterm infants (born before 28 weeks) and moderately preterm IUGR infants (born after 28 weeks), had decreased brain connectivity (measured using MRI fractional anisotropy) when compared with moderately preterm AGA controls, which in turn is associated with poorer socio-cognitive performance (130). IUGR infants born moderately preterm and assessed at term equivalent age also demonstrated reduced cerebral cortex gray matter volume and lower scores in attention-interaction availability, compared to appropriately grown preterm infants (131). Again, these observations support the importance of *in utero* brain maturation.

Interestingly, the rates of several prematurity-associated neonatal diseases in IUGR vs. AGA infants also vary with the gestational age at birth. In preterm infants born at or before 28 weeks PCA, the rates of IVH, respiratory distress syndrome and necrotizing enterocolitis are largely unaffected by IUGR. From then on, all adverse outcomes including IVH increase in IUGR compared with AGA premature infants, suggesting a need for closer surveillance for IUGR in the moderate and late preterm infants (118, 132). Such findings are of concern since late preterm births account for the vast majority of preterm births. Studies on infants born at later preterm to term gestational ages suggest that impaired fetal growth increases the risk for low intellectual performance (16, 133, 134). Comparing monozygotic twin pairs born after 32 weeks PCA, the growth-restricted twin is at increased risk for low cognitive performance at school age or in adulthood compared to the appropriately grown twin (135). In addition, a further study in twins has quantified the effects of low birth weight, showing that a 500 g increase in (term) birth weight results in a 2% increase in total brain volume, gray matter volume and white matter volume, and a 2-point increase in IQ (136).

In summary, the gestational age at delivery has a remarkable impact for IUGR infants who are born extremely preterm, such that the prematurity-related complications "override" the effects of IUGR on neurodevelopmental outcome. For the moderately late preterm infants, the independent impacts of IUGR and prematurity on neurodevelopmental outcome becomes more apparent. Altogether, these studies highlight that we need more information on when to deliver IUGR babies, and the criteria on which to base this decision.

CLINICAL TRIALS AND PRESUMPTIVE THERAPIES

We wish to acknowledge the enormous contributions of researchers and clinicians in bringing therapies to clinical trials and generating the preclinical data to support these transitions, although the purpose of this article is not to review all of these. We will highlight some trials and their outcomes as, while we have no conclusively effective therapies as yet, we can learn a great deal about improving patient stratification and the efficacy in drugs with shared mechanisms of actions. For example, a recent double-blind randomized study using dydrogesterone, a synthetic progestogen, has reported increased birth weight, and decreased MCA resistance index in idiopathic IUGR (137), supporting the therapeutic use of progesterone replacement suggested in preclinical studies in guinea pigs (138). Specifically, in this human trial weight increased by ~50% in the treatment arm, vs. 23% in the control arm. Although these effects are promising, this was a single center, small study (89 participants), recruiting early and late IUGR (range 28–35 weeks of gestation) with no postnatal follow-up, thus further work remains to be done. The action of dydrogesterone includes effects that altogether increase myometrial perfusion and immunomodulation by increasing progesterone-induced blocking factor (PIBF) levels (139). PIBF is secreted by peripheral lymphocytes from healthy pregnant women, and it has important immunomodulatory functions that appear to protect fetuses from resorption and therefore plays a role in the maintenance of pregnancy, most likely by inhibiting NK lymphocytes and producing a dominant TH_2 cytokine response (140); hence, many poor pregnancy outcomes including miscarriage and preterm birth are linked to low PIBF levels. Manipulation and control of PIGF levels in pregnancy is therefore a priority for researchers.

The STRIDER-UK study (multicentre, randomized, double-blind, 156 participants) tested the use of sildenafil in women with severe early-onset IUGR and found that treatment did not prolong pregnancy or cause any adverse effects, but did not improve pregnancy outcomes (141). However, this study is part of a more extensive international study, and in isolation, it does not have the power to adequately assess outcomes in this very high-risk cohort (45% of recruited infants in this study died) (142). A meta-analysis (nine studies, total of 576 treated patients) has shown that arginine supplementation increases gestational length and birth weight in IUGR pregnancies, except for infants born preterm (<32 weeks PCA) with severe IUGR (143); there were no reported side effects. The proposed mechanisms of action of arginine include the increased production of placental insulin that acts as a fetal trophic factor.

Creatine may also be a potential treatment for IUGR (144, 145), with recent studies showing a positive correlation of birth weight to placental creatine load (146), and the discovery that the human placenta expresses the enzymes to synthesize and transport creatine (147). Creatine is an energy substrate which protects ATP turnover during periods of oxidative stress (148) and as such may be a potential prophylactic treatment for IUGR outcomes (144, 145). Creatine readily crosses the placenta in humans and some other omnivores (but not in sheep, an herbivore), suggesting that maternal creatine supplementation could be used to increase placental creatine transfer and promote fetal growth in a hypoxic uterine environment. Supporting data include a number of pre-clinical studies (149–151). Whilst there has been extensive animal research suggesting creatine's potential to protect the fetus against periods of oxygen deprivation in several animal models, and there is a strong rationale for moving toward clinical trials for maternal creatine supplementation to reduce or prevent IUGR, no intervention studies have yet been undertaken in pregnant women. IUGR is also proposed to be a disorder of insulin-like growth factor-1 (IGF-1) deprivation (discussed below). Of particular note is an extensive preclinical study of prenatal IGF-1 treatment in a sheep model of IUGR (41 controls, 66 IUGR + saline, 28 IUGR + IGF-1, powered for sex-specific analysis and long term follow-up) which show that prenatal IGF-1 treatment improves prenatal and postnatal indices of growth and biochemical dysfunction in IUGR (152, 153).

OVERCOMING THE HURDLES TO PROGRESS

Early Markers for IUGR Screening: A Challenge Faced by Researchers and Clinicians

Less than 30% of infants with a birth weight <10th percentile are detected during pregnancy (154, 155). Infants born after undiagnosed IUGR have 2–9 times higher risk of perinatal death and severe neurological complications to those diagnosed prenatally (156–158).

The current, commonly used antenatal assessment of IUGR is examination of the symphysiofundal height, and this has a sensitivity of just 17% and a positive predictive value of 20% (159). Once a red flag has been raised, even selective ultrasound and universal ultrasound perform poorly with a sensitively of 20 and 57%, respectively (160). This perhaps reflects the larger caliber vessels and reduced downstream resistance of the late preterm placenta that means that the umbilical artery Doppler parameters are rarely abnormal; indeed, most adverse events in late pregnancy occur in fetuses with normal Doppler readings (161). However, as mentioned above, FGR babies assessed at term age will often demonstrate abnormal middle cerebral artery (MCA) blood flow represented by a reduced MCA pulsatility index (PI) due to "brain sparing." A more sensitive and specific measure of fetal well-being may be the cerebral-placental PI ratio, which is calculated as the MCA PI divided by umbilical artery PI. This parameter has improved the sensitivity for detecting babies at risk of adverse perinatal outcome including perinatal mortality, admission to NICU, low 5-min Apgar score and cesarean for fetal distress (26, 162, 163).

Given the importance of placental insufficiency for the origin of IUGR, blood-based markers in the mother that relate to early-onset placental insufficiency are logical starting points for identifying biomarkers that detect IUGR. Biomarkers are molecules, genes, or a particular combination of these by which a pathological or physiological process is identified. Recent reports of biomarkers in maternal blood related to early-onset placental insufficiency include pregnancy-associated plasma protein-A (PAPP-A), alpha-fetoprotein (AFP), inhibin A, placental growth factor (PlGF), uric acid, and free beta- or total human chorionic gonadotropin (102, 164). For example, a 2 to 3-fold increase in late-onset IUGR is noted in women who were found to have elevated first trimester PAPP-A and elevated second trimester AFP (165). Combining maternal risk factors, biochemical markers such as ADAM12 (A Disintegrin and Metalloprotease-12) and placental protein-13, plus abnormal uterine artery waveforms for the prediction of late-onset IUGR (with a false positive rate of 5%), provides a sensitivity of 61% for IUGR at <37 weeks but unfortunately only 32% for IUGR at >37 weeks (166).

The use of these putative biomarkers (and the development of new biomarkers) is constrained by the absence of robust baseline data on their expression and function. We could overcome these problems with population profiling and further basic research into the mechanisms underlying typical placental development and function. Biomarkers for identification and stratification could improve outcomes even with current clinical practices, and are likely to have two additional benefits: firstly, prenatal treatment options [e.g., intra-amniotic IGF-1–(153)] are showing great promise, and biomarkers would identify those needing therapy; and secondly, by avoiding treatment of healthy babies and the risk of complications arising from newly developed prenatal therapies.

In utero assessment of brain structure and metabolism is now possible, and these techniques have been applied to cohorts of IUGR infants (167). These studies aim to understand the underlying pathology, but also to determine biomarkers as indicators of pathology and outcome. For example, in 19 IUGR and 25 non-complicated pregnancies, T2-weighted MRI allowed for the assessment of neuropathology and magnetic resonance spectroscopy allowed for analysis of indices of cell membrane and myelin formation (choline), glycolytic enzyme activity as an indicator of cerebral hypoxia (lactate), and for cerebral mitochondrial function (NAA) (167). Of the 15 infants with complete data sets in the IUGR arm, three died *in utero*, and only two had an uncomplicated neonatal course. However, MRI was not sensitive enough to detect injury in any of the 15 IUGR infants *before delivery* (median scan age of 27 + 6 weeks PCA). Interestingly, fetal brain lactate levels were elevated in three control infants with normal progress of growth, birth and outcomes. Increased brain lactate has previously been considered a hallmark of hypoxic changes, but lactate may also play a role as an energy source in the developing brain (168). The authors suggest that the altered magnetic resonance spectroscopy parameters represent changes in mitochondrial metabolic status, and these warrants further study in a preclinical model as a novel therapeutic approach. This study is a valuable example of how these still tricky and expensive prenatal screening techniques could be applied to larger cohorts, but whether this effort can provide invaluable data on the mechanism of damàge and criteria for risk stratification will require further research.

Circulatory biomarkers based on the detection of microRNAs (miRs), mitochondrial DNA (mDNA), cell-free RNA (cfRNA), and exosomes could also have diagnostic value, but remain to be fully validated. Two recent studies demonstrate how these new analytic approaches provide early diagnostic biomarkers for preterm birth and preeclampsia. Firstly (169), demonstrated that a panel of seven cfRNAs present in the maternal blood had utility in predicting preterm birth with an AUC (area under the curve) of 0.81. Similarly, Jelliffe-Pawlowski et al. (170) used a 25-target screen of serum proteins that, together with maternal risk factors, predicted preterm birth with an AUC of 0.806. Both studies might be said to be limited by low patient numbers and a lack of ethnic diversity in the patient groups, but this multi-marker approach seems to increase sensitivity and specificity compared to previous mono-marker approaches, and improvements (decrease) in the time needed to perform such analyses means that effective bedside screening is becoming a reality.

A further elaboration on the multi-marker approach is the application of personalized risk-based screening methods that combines maternal factors and biomarkers, as in the combined use of uterine artery Doppler, maternal risk factors, and serum biomarkers. This approach, taken as part of a study nested in clinical trial for pre-term preeclampsia (ASPRE, Aspirin for Evidence-Based Preeclampsia Prevention) (171), showed clearly that prospective screening for preterm preeclampsia by means of the FMF (Fetal Medicine Foundation) algorithm, which combines maternal factors and biomarkers at 11–13 weeks' gestation, was better at predicting disease risk than current biometric criteria.

A Holistic vs. Mechanistic View of Modeling IUGR—How to Improve the Validity of Our Models

An important question when modeling any disease or disorder is whether it is necessary for the phenotype (in this case a reduction in body and brain weight) to be the same as observed clinically if we don't know that the mechanism of injury has been faithfully reproduced. Also, how much importance should we place on the phenotype (body and brain weight) being matched if we have to apply an injury/perturbation (in type or magnitude) that is not clinically relevant? In the case of IUGR there has been a proliferation of animal models that produce fetal growth restriction, but often by means that have limited clinical reality; e.g., abrupt and late onset reductions of uterine or umbilical blood flows. These procedures do produce hypoxia-induced cell death, and various complex inflammatory processes that help us to understand and look for effects in IUGR infants, but they are of limited use in understanding how IUGR and placental dysfunction actually arise in human pregnancy. Perhaps, with our increasingly detailed knowledge of how and when placental dysfunction in IUGR occurs (88, 172, 173), we could aim to model these specific changes, and this would be valuable in the collective move toward developing therapies that can be applied early in pregnancy. We will below describe some of the common approaches to modeling IUGR and some suggestions for how these could be altered to add to our collective data on how to prevent IUGR, and treat or repair the damage caused by IUGR.

Surgical interventions that reduce perfusion of the maternal or fetal side of the placenta: The seminal study demonstrating that poor placental growth itself causes attrition of fetal growth is that of Wigglesworth (174). Since that time there has been a proliferation of models of IUGR, predominantly focused on fetal/neonatal weight and based on the conceptual paradigm that it is utero-placental perfusion that determines placental function, which in turn determines fetal growth and the vulnerability of the fetal brain to damage. These models of IUGR include (but are not limited to): acute onset hypoxia/ischemia (uterine artery ligation), progressive onset hypoxia/ischemia (uterine artery restriction); and placental damage/reduction (inert microsphere injection, partial placentotomy). However, these approaches offers little consideration to the idea that the fetus(es), or the feto-placental compartment might themselves be the source of physiological changes that cause the typical uterine hyperaemia and the appropriate increase of utero-placental perfusion with increasing gestation. Evidence of this type (and almost forgotten) was acquired nearly 50 years ago by Christopher Bell in guinea pigs who showed that progesterone produced by the placenta causes a loss of constrictor adrenergic nerves in uterine blood vessels, and simultaneously induces synthesis of a vasodilator mechanism not present in the non-pregnant uterine vasculature (175, 176). Hence, there is a good reason to think that a cause of IUGR is the *failure* of the placenta to adequately modify the uterine circulation to support time-dependent fetal growth. As such, more work needs to be done on the differences in feto-placental signaling as a driver for poor utero-placental vascular development across gestation.

In all experimental studies to date, the attention is almost always directed to the fetal effects, with few observations made of maternal or placental physiology, especially the clinical conditions usually associated with IUGR, such as uterine artery and myometrial remodeling, immune regulation of trophoblast implantation, placental metabolism *per se*, and the causes of placenta infarction and abruption, etc. A chief mechanism by which we should validate animal models of IUGR should be to measure uterine blood flow, as is done clinically. Admittedly, historically this was not easy to do in rodents, although it is increasingly possible due to advancements such as ultrafast doppler. We now have the ability to measure these clinical indices and to associate them with fetal outcomes as we attempt to better understand this relationship.

Poor placental structure and function—from the beginning: Placental insufficiency is a process that evidence suggests is present from the earliest stages of trophoblast invasion, supported by the observation of abnormal levels of inflammatory and placental factors from the 1st trimester with poor pregnancy outcomes [(47) and reviewed in Kane et al. (177)]. From the time of trophoblast invasion into the endometrium, the uterus undergoes phenomenal modification (178, 179), increasing in weight and internal volume by ~16- and 500-fold, respectively, together with major re-modeling of the uterine vasculature (as discussed above) to create a low resistance, non-reactive vascular bed. It is perhaps not surprising that these features have received less attention as determinants of IUGR because, except for non-human primates, these key features of pregnancy are not present in the commonly used laboratory animals. However, comparative studies of more unusual species, like the Spiny Mouse (*Accomys caihrinus*) reveal that unlike in the conventional rodent that there is a large vascular contribution to the fetal membranes originating from the umbilical vessels close to the fetal surface of the placenta (unpublished observations). As such, studying basic process of placentation in small species such as these may be a useful start to developing models of early-onset placental dysfunction that mimics what is seen clinically (57, 152, 180). Non-traditional species such as the spiny mouse, gerbil, and guinea pig studied from the time of conception offer advantages such as a relatively long gestation (from 39 to ~67 days), and the birth of offspring where development of the major organ systems is largely complete at the time of birth. For the spiny mouse in particular, an additional advantage is that the fetal adrenal gland produces dehydroepiandosterone and cortisol (181–183), with evidence of the presence of a feto-placental unit as in humans, and not present in other rodent-like animals, or sheep.

A clear example of how a candidate mechanism has been effectively applied to model IUGR is the knockout of IGF2 production in the mouse placenta. Levels of the IGF proteins are often reduced and IGF1 binding proteins increased in the placentas of IUGR human pregnancies (184), although this is not consistently found (185). The regulation of IGF signaling is a complex balance between the IGFs and their binding partners that regulate bioavailability during pregnancy, including in IUGR [reviewed in Martin-Estal et al. (186)]. Mice born from dams with a placenta-specific IGF2 gene knock out (KO) have clearly reduced body weight, brain injury, and lasting cognitive and metabolic phenotypes with postnatal development. The mating of the IGF2 placenta-specific KO mice with the endothelial NOS (eNOS) KO mice provides an interesting example of the cross-talk between (putative) pathological mechanisms. As expected, the phenotype of these two KOs was additive (more severe IUGR), but the diminished placental nutrient transport typically observed in the eNOS KO mice was not seen in the IGF2-eNOS double crossed mice (187). The basis of the application of the eNOS KO mice to IUGR research is that the absence of eNOS reduces the capacity of the maternal vascular to accommodate the changes in blood flow necessary for adequate placentation, and that the dams are hypertensive (including with proteinuria) as observed in women with pre-eclampsia, a risk factor for IUGR. Thus, it was concluded that a "multiplicity of dysfunction" probably underlies IUGR in women, so the multiple facets of vascular dysfunction in this mouse line would be useful to assess placental hypoxia with free radical formation, reduced placental nutrient transport capacity, and reduced fetal growth (188).

Assessment of the epigenetic landscape of the eNOS and IGF2 genes from IUGR placental tissues shows that epigenetic modifications are present and might be drivers of gene dysregulation (189). However IGF2 gene expression changes and methylation changes of IGF2 are not consistently reported in clinical studies, One of the negative clinical studies found neither gene or methylation changes the cohort was older mothers (39–40 years of age), although changes in placental methylation are only detectable with the techniques used when substantial differences are present (173). Alternatively, this negative study is evidence that methylation and gene expression changes in IGF2 are not present in the first trimester but evolve over time, and so this important study that warrants repeating with larger and more diverse cohorts.

Immunological dysfunction: There is clear evidence that the immune system in women with an IUGR pregnancy differs compared to those without IUGR (190). This study found that peripheral monocytes in women with an IUGR pregnancy had a more classically anti-inflammatory profile than monocytes from women with an uncompromised pregnancy. In addition, when peripheral blood mononuclear cells from women with IUGR and normal pregnancies were stimulated with trophoblast antigen (191), a greater pro-inflammatory reaction occurred in women with an IUGR pregnancy. When these dysfunctional processes first arise in pregnancy, and their impact on early placentation, would be interesting to pursue further, albeit requiring large cohorts of prospectively recruited, not-yet-pregnant women—a difficult task, but one with important public health outcomes. This information would then be possible to overlay into more specifically focussed animal models.

As pointed out by Sir Peter Medawar many years ago (192) it is clear that immune modulation is a fundamental response to conception that allows implantation and persistence of the fetus as a foreign allograft, and a response likely to be shared by humans and laboratory animals. It is a process that involves a phenotypic transformation of decidual macrophages and natural killer cells that occurs in parallel with remodeling of the vasculature adjacent to the implantation site. As such, it is possible that these shared features could be used to drive spontaneous cases of IUGR in non-human pregnancies. Indeed, some cross-breeding of mice of mixed genetic background has been found to produce IUGR of varying degrees, together with, as for most clinical situations, other complications of implantation, uterine re-modeling, and pathophysiology suggesting preeclampsia in the dam (193, 194). These "immune" models have been shown to have similarities pathological changes as occurs in the human IUGR placenta in the trophoblast remodeling protein Formyl peptide receptor-2 [FPR2; (195)], and a dysfunction of decidual arteriolar remodeling (196) such as that associated with pre-eclampsia and IUGR (197). Thus, we may have experimental models at hand which will aid in the understanding of the origin of IUGR together with the other obstetric problems that usually accompany it. A strength of this approach is that each of the parents and the offspring are immunologically competent, and it is only the combination of the fetal and maternal tissues that is abnormal. This model will require further assessment of fetal brain phenotypes to support the similarities in placental immune dysfunction to the human, but it promises to be valuable to assess therapies to minimize the neonatal morbidities that IUGR produces.

Finally, we would like to highlight the comments made by Saleem et al. from Karachi, Pakistan that "Concerted efforts should be made to gather indigenous data about the risk factors of IUGR that are more pertinent to our population. Evidence-based recommendations deduced from such data sets are more likely to be successful and valid" (198). Although they were addressing the need for improved medical services, we think this comment also points to the need for improvements in preclinical modeling to be "*population specific.*" This specificity must take into account not just high vs. low income, but etiologies and conditions specific to local care centers, and this is where in-depth epidemiology needs to take a more prominent role in guiding preclinical research.

Human Neuropathological Studies and How They Need to Play a Bigger Role in the Study of IUGR

The emergence of modern medicine was firmly based on pathology and post-mortem examinations, and while never being able to identify mechanisms of disease or injury *per se*, have been invaluable as the basis for setting diagnostic criteria and the effectiveness of treatments and interventions. The expectations of many that modern imaging, genetics, and -omics would make pathology obsolete has been a significant error of twenty-first-century science, and in neonatology it was high-quality neuropathology studies by groups in Portland (OR, USA), Paris (France), and Boston (MA, USA) (199–201) that were persuasive in changing our understanding of the genesis of perinatal brain injury over the past 20 years. Specifically, these foundational studies provide the basis for interpreting MRI studies, and for designing improved animal models to test neuroprotective strategies. This is important because most IUGR babies survive, and the injuries present in very severe IUGR fetuses may not be representative of the major population of IUGR infants.

It is indeed worth highlighting a number of human studies; this is not exhaustive but is intended to allow us to remark on what we have learnt, and what we need to add to the field. Studies from Samuelsen et al. (202) show a reduction in the numbers of cells in the brains of IUGR infants; these infants displayed brain sparing (relative increase in brain weight to body weight) but still had significantly lower brain weights. In this study, control fetuses acquired an average of 173 million cells per day from mid-gestation to term, and the IUGR fetuses acquired only 86 million new cells per day. Samuelsen et al's exhaustive cell counting assessment [reviewed in, Larsen (203)] supports the findings of two studies from over 30 years ago which used a lower total DNA content to infer a reduction in cell numbers (50, 204). Samuelsen's conjectures that his data supports the hypothesis that the reduction in head circumference in IUGR is due to reduced proliferation rather than cell death is provocative, but needs to be confirmed by objective assessment of cell death and proliferation.

Another set of studies includes a concerted effort by researchers based primarily at the Mater Hospitals in Brisbane, Australia, that included 37 asymmetric IUGR cases (weight <3rd centile) identified from a series of 225 stillbirths (205). This first study, over 20 years old now, critically demonstrated the importance of cell death, and to a lesser extent astrogliosis, in the IUGR brain. It is worth noting that although the analysis was limited to hematoxylin and eosin assessment of cell death, and in some cases glial fibrillary acidic protein for astrocytosis, that even with the expertise of a neuropathologist no injury was found in 5 of the 37 brains. Of these 5 "uninjured" IUGR brains, four were from infants below 26 weeks PCA—does this suggest an important window for treatment specificity? Striking limitations of this study are that there was no breakdown of the specific gestational ages of the infants, no body or brain weight data, and no case-by-case description of the findings, making it very difficult to draw further conclusions. These authors overcame many of these limitations in a more recent publication (206) using brains from the first cohorts and sourced from a further 305 stillbirths where they assessed cell death with three separate markers. This more recent study clearly showed that third trimester stillborn fetuses with both IUGR (weight <3rd centile) and placental infarction (<5% of total placental villus surface) had neuronal apoptotic changes in regions including the pons and the frontal and temporal cortex. These studies involved the use of controls that were stillborn but had neither IUGR nor placental infarction. Staining for micro- or macrogliosis or proliferation was not included, unfortunately.

The Value of Continuous Neuro-Monitoring to Understand Risk for the IUGR Infant

Much has already been reported on the neuroimaging findings of IUGR infants and their relationships to neurodevelopmental delay. However, neuroimaging such as MRI can only be done at specific time-points and is not applicable as continuous neuro-monitoring to reveal temporal changes with impact on clinical conditions and to guide management.

Cerebral Haemodynamic Measurements in the IUGR Fetus

With advancing fetal hypoxia and compromise, the cerebral haemodynamic response involves two components—firstly an initial stage of increased cerebral blood flow aimed at protecting the brain (brain sparing), followed by a second decompensatory stage that is associated with brain injury, and probably due to the increased cerebral blood volume (207). At the early stages (i.e., brain sparing) blood flow (CBF) of the frontal lobes is increased, perhaps with the effect of protecting higher cognitive functions, but under chronic and more severe circumstances this change is lost and CBF is diverted to deeper (more essential?) structures such as the basal ganglia and the brainstem (29). Also, in the IUGR fetus there appears to be a loss of cerebral vasoreactivity; using prenatal Doppler sonography, a subset of IUGR fetuses did not show the expected rise in cerebral resistance in response to maternal hyperoxygenation, suggestive of impaired cerebrovascular regulation. Indeed, these "non-responders" had a higher risk of being delivered for fetal distress, indicating that they were more compromised (208).

It is interesting that there is an increased incidence of stroke in adults born with low birth weight. The association between low birth weight and adult stroke was most pronounced for individuals with relatively increased head size, suggestive of *in utero* conditions that induce brain sparing (13). It is very plausible that these mechanisms of increased adult stroke are due to vascular remodeling secondary to the shear stress and wall tension, leading to structural changes in the vascular wall (209). Thus. understanding IUGR-associated cerebral haemodynamic changes has implications for improving brain health even in adults.

Cotside Cerebral Haemodynamic Measurements: Cerebral Blood Flow and Oxygenation

Studies in IUGR infants have made the following important observations:

- increased CBF on the first day of life (210);
- reduced cerebrovascular resistance and persistent dilatation of the cerebral arteries (211, 212);
- higher regional cerebral oxygen saturation and reduced cerebral oxygen extraction within the first 24 h (213) and up to 3 days of age (214); and,
- cerebral haemodynamic parameters normalize within a few days of birth (210, 211, 213).

To date there is little postnatal research investigating the relationship between cerebral hemodynamics after birth and neurological injury in IUGR infants; this is an area of need as there is evidence to indicate that the altered cerebral hemodynamics that exist in the IUGR fetus persist postnatally. Notably, cerebral oxygenation has been shown to predict neurodevelopmental outcome in preterm infants (215). Moreover, fluctuations of cerebral oxygenation and oxygen extraction have also been related to the occurrence of intracranial hemorrhage in preterm infants (216, 217). Finally, if CBF remains elevated when the neonate is no longer exposed to a hypoxic environment, the increased CBF could cause hyperoxia within the fragile brain and contribute to further neurological damage (218).

Cotside Cerebral Haemodynamic Measurements: Cerebral Autoregulation

Autoregulation is the ability of the cerebral vasculature to maintain reasonably constant CBF despite fluctuations in cerebral perfusion pressure which are mainly affected by changes in systemic blood pressure, and it is likely that autoregulation is impaired in sick preterm neonates and this contributes to the cerebral ischaemic and haemorrhagic injury (219). As IUGR fetuses are often delivered preterm, and due to the vascular structural and functional changes set in place by the "brain sparing" response to IUGR, these infants are theoretically at risk of impaired autoregulation, resulting in cerebral hypo- or hyperperfusion when systemic blood pressure fluctuates. In case of prolonged brain sparing due to chronic hypoxaemia, maximal cerebral vessel dilatation may have already been reached and may persist after birth, which would further limit protective autoregulatory responses. In addition, IUGR neonates appear to have higher blood pressures compared to their AGA peers (30, 220), theoretically contributing to risk of cerebral hyperperfusion and hemorrhage in the presence of a pressure-passive cerebral circulation; indeed, this has been shown in IUGR lambs where, compromised structural integrity of the cerebral microvasculature leading to cerebral hemorrhage has been demonstrated (82). Despite its clinical significance, to date no study has investigated cerebral autoregulation in human IUGR neonates.

Cotside Electroencephalographic (EEG) Monitoring

Cerebral electrographic activity can serve as an indicator of neuronal integrity, organization, and the differentiation and maturation of brain networks in term and preterm newborns (221). In acute brain insult, electroencephalographic (EEG) activity shows various degrees of depression, and its severity parallels the magnitude of the brain lesion. These "acute-stage" abnormalities gradually improve with time and are replaced by "chronic-stage" abnormalities such as dysmaturity and disorganization of the EEG pattern (222). In the weeks following preterm birth, IUGR infants reportedly have altered EEG and amplitude integrated EEG, which has been correlated with poor neuromotor development (223, 224). In contrast, another study found that the subset of stable preterm IUGR with good clinical indices had more mature EEG patterns compared to the AGA peers (225), and similarly, preterm IUGR infants had accelerated EEG power spectrum maturation compared to preterm AGA controls at 1 month post-term equivalent age (226). However, no differences were observed at 6 months' post-term age between preterm IUGR and AGA infants, or in comparison to a term AGA group, suggesting such changes may resolve with time (226). Notably, using visual evoked potentials as an indicator of brain myelination in preterm infants born at <33 weeks of gestation age, shorter visual evoked potential latency, suggestive of increased myelination, was found at 6 months post-term age in IUGR infants who had fetal Doppler parameters showing brain sparing (227). The shorter latency was no longer detected at 12 months of post-term age and visual functioning was not affected when followed up at 11 years of age (228). These findings suggested transient accelerated neurophysiological maturation in the IUGR infant brain, possibly as an adaptive process to the severe fetal growth restriction. Overall, it appears there are temporal EEG characteristics in IUGR infants which may relate to their neurodevelopmental outcome. However, EEG data on preterm infants with IUGR are few, as are studies that link EEG parameters with MRI-derived tractography. Early and prolonged continuous recording in larger populations would be required to clarify the prognostic value of EEG in IUGR infants.

INNOVATIONS FOR USE IN IUGR RESEARCH:

Nanomedicine Approaches

Engineered nanomaterials offer therapeutic options as diverse as implantable monitoring devices, drug delivery scaffolds, and wound dressings. An excellent review on nanomaterials for perinatal applications was recently published (229), but we will highlight ways in which these approaches could be employed to improve infant neurological outcomes in the context of IUGR. The greatest need for the IUGR fetus is safe, effective therapies that can be delivered as early as possible in gestation and without the need for preterm delivery. As such, we should turn our attention to nanomedicine approaches if these can be maternally delivered and directly affect the function of the placenta. Nanoparticles delivered intravenously can cross the placenta, and are found in the fetus, including in the non-human primate [see Menezes et al. (230)]. They can also be found in the fetus when administered intranasally to pregnant rats (231). A recent study monitored the "protein corona" of polystyrene nanoparticles, which is the spontaneously adsorbed protein on the nanoparticle surface when the nanoparticles were exposed to maternal plasma. They found that the protein corona formed by maternal serum included vesicular transport proteins such as clathrin, tubulin, actin, and Ras. As such, rather than pose any barrier to transmigration, maternal serum proteins increase the transport of the polystyrene nanoparticles across the *ex vivo* placenta (232). However, in the pregnant rat, inhaled silver nanoparticles caused increased fetal resorption and increased expression of placental inflammatory markers (231). Although this silver nanoparticle study suggests caution in the application of nanoparticles, we can overcome these problems via our ability to modulate the size, physical composition, charge, and delivery method of nanoparticles. Of note, another recent study has shown success in reducing fetal inflammation and neonatal brain injury in a mouse model which mimics exposure to inflammation in the preterm infant. Specifically, polyamidoamine dendrimers were used to carry the anti-oxidant n-acetylcysteine into the blood of the dam (233). This dendrimer treatment was associated with improvements in inflammatory and neuropathology indices in the fetal compartments. It is important to note that these polyamidoamine dendrimers did not need to pass to the fetus to be neuroprotective and thus, this maternal-placental delivery reduces any potential of off-target, damaging effects of stray nanoparticles in the fetus.

Work from our lab has taken the approach of targeting one cell type—microglia—rather than being compartment-specific (234). Microglia are regularly found to mediate injury in neurological paradigms. The microglia-specific nanoparticles in our work are comprised of DNA, further demonstrating the flexibility in the design possibilities of nanoparticles. However, we do not yet know if these DNA nanoparticles cross the placenta, and what specific aspect of microglial activation would be the most appropriate to target in IUGR. There is a lack of knowledge of nanoparticle biodistribution in non-human primates, or other species with more human-like placental structures, such as the spiny mouse (235). More studies using IUGR models developed in species with a more human-like placental structure would be valuable steps toward uncovering the potential of nanoparticles to deliver anti-oxidants, vasodilators, or growth factors to specifically target pathological processes in the placenta.

Altogether these tools and approaches show that we have made the technological advances and have the monitoring skills with which to move forward to design targeted therapies for the placenta and the fetus to overcome the damage associated with IUGR.

Using Advanced Imaging and Histology Techniques

We have a poor understanding of the direct correspondence between medical imaging outputs and tissue microstructure. This lack of knowledge is due to differences in scale and resolution between medical imaging modalities and traditional neuropathology techniques that have been further frustrated with complexities of image registration (236). A lack of knowledge of the actual biological substrate of imaging outputs frustrates our ability to understand the specific nature of changes occurring in the IUGR infant brain, as the most severely affected infants do not survive, as discussed above. Improvements in histological techniques, specifically the use of optically clear histology, is allowing us to overcome some of these hurdles (237), but obviously not in living tissue. Optically clear histology allows whole brains from small experimental animals, and sections of human post-mortem tissue, to be made optically clear and stained with multiple specific markers of various cell types. This advance allows us to visualize the 3D organization of tissue microstructure in tissue sections large enough to be studied beforehand with MRI techniques, and then to co-register the imaging and histological data. This approach has been applied to the developing mouse brain to provide data on what types of cells or cell compartments contribute to specific imaging signals (238). A finding from this study worth noting is a positive correlation between mean MRI diffusivity and cell density, which is unexpected based on the current assumption that cells provide an impediment to the diffusion of water molecules in tissue (238). This and other findings suggest that a great deal of work in human post-mortem tissues is required to ensure that our assumptions of the microstructural correlates of human imaging in the literature are robust (239, 240).

The current gold standard for functional brain imaging is blood–oxygen dependent (BOLD) signals measured using MRI (241), but this technique is costly and practically difficult to use in infants. An easier to implement optical imaging alternative is functional near-infrared spectroscopy (fNIRS), which also measures the level of blood oxygenation and can be applied on neonates or young children through the skull but with spatial resolution measured in mm (242). The next level of technological development is functional ultrasound (fUS) neuroimaging that provides high sensitivity imaging, with a resolution of $\sim$100 μm, and can identify cerebral blood volume changes in the whole brain without contrast agents. The fUS image is based on the phenomenon of neurovascular coupling, about which little is known in the developing brain [see, (243, 244) for recent animal studies] and the ability to measure cerebral blood volume changes with high sensitivity, which is an attribute of fUS (245). Non-invasive fUS imaging of brain activity in humans is possible through the fontanel of human neonates at the bedside. In combination with surface EEG recordings in preterm babies, fUS allowed for the estimation of cerebral blood volume variations to measure the spatiotemporal dynamics of epileptic seizures (246). The sensitivity of fUS, such as measuring small diameter blood flow even in rodents with millisecond temporal resolution, should allow it to become a useful and valuable tool to understand the effects of IUGR on the brain in clinical and in preclinical settings. We have applied fUS to study the brains of rats in a paradigm of protein restriction-induced IUGR and found that it identified connectivity deficits (59), and was able to validate improvements in connectivity associated with neuroprotection. For further comprehensive information on the applications of fUS, please see the recent review by Deffieux et al. (247).

Genomic Analysis as a Means to Diagnose, Stratify Risk and Understand Disease Mechanisms

Genomic screening offers the promise of early and specific diagnosis, risk stratification and personalized therapeutic deployment. There are inherent ethical issues with genetic screening that are in no way limited to the field of IUGR. These include incidental findings of unknown significance and the more complex issue of the rights of the child, and specifically the child's right "not to know." Violations of the child's rights may relate to the discovery of gene variants that have no bearing on fetal development or childhood health, but which alter adult disease risk. Although generally these problems are overcome with targeted analysis, variants with impact at multiple stages of life make this problem harder to manage. For a lively discussion on bioethics related to prenatal genome sequencing we refer the reader to these references (248–250).

Despite these concerns, non-invasive prenatal screening (NIPS) for fetal aneuploidies using cell-free DNA has been widely adopted in clinical practice due to its improved accuracy compared to traditional screening approaches (251). NIPS approaches can include whole genome sequencing techniques with high sensitivity and specificity even with very low sample input (252). The benefits of whole-genome sequencing include the identification of micro-deletions that would be missed by karyotyping. These micro-deletions are relevant to human growth and have identified some genetic causes of IUGR (253). It might not be necessary to sequence the genome to identify disease risk but to examine single nucleotide polymorphisms (SNPs). SNP analysis is increasingly accessible with sequencing, and whole-genome SNP arrays can be processed within 3 days (254). This short time frame means that the data can affect prenatal diagnostic decisions, and in the future, may guide treatment decisions. An approach to risk stratification has been tested in the related field of preterm birth, identifying an unbiased association of SNPs with white matter imaging phenotype. This approach has successfully identified several SNPs that associate with a clinical white matter phenotype in preterm infants—namely, specific SNPs within the genes for *FADS2* (Fatty Acid Desaturase 2) (255), *PPARG* (Peroxisome proliferator-activated receptor gamma) (256), and *DLG4* (discs large homolog 4, the gene Post-Synaptic Protein-95) (257). Although these SNPs provide a biomarker for infant outcome, they are also under further investigation to understand the mechanistic link between these genes variants and brain development.

What is lacking in the field of IUGR to date is the application of these genomics approaches in massive populations to identify variants denoting risk of obstetric and (neuro)developmental outcomes. In the fields of Alzheimer's disease and cancer, it has taken the study of many thousands of patients (and their tumors) to identify risk phenotypes that are now used to drive drug discovery efforts and to identify targets for personalized drug therapy, and these approaches have been effective in public health (258). Altogether, dramatic improvements in technology open avenues for understanding three important aspects of IUGR—diagnosis, risk stratification, and mechanisms of disease. The logistical and monetary support to bring together a vast number of patients across multiple centers, and the bioinformatics needed to understand these processes, are now within reach if we apply the lessons from genetics studies of adult diseases.

CONCLUSION

IUGR remains a complex health care issue across the globe. Concerted research and clinical effort have raised the profile of this complex problem and improved our knowledge of the neurodevelopmental sequelae of IUGR. What we cannot yet offer in the field of IUGR is an animal model that recapitulates the underlying pathophysiology of IUGR, primarily because we do not yet know the etiology (probably, more than one etiology) underlying the various sub-groups of IUGR. Valuable post-mortem studies, imaging studies using newly optimized *in utero* fetal and placental imaging, and pooling our research data across models to find common elements, will be key to overcoming this hurdle. Optimized fetal and placental imaging will also be important future methods of early diagnosis and risk stratification. These will enable us to treat the IUGR infant *in utero* with the goal of preventing brain injury rather than attempting postnatal repair or regeneration. We do not yet understand the role of neuroinflammation in the human IUGR infant, and as such cannot determine if the multitude of immunomodulatory drugs being fast-tracked in fields such as multiple sclerosis and Alzheimer's disease apply to the IUGR infant. The role of neuroinflammation can be studied by bringing together multiple models capturing many facets of IUGR-related neurodevelopmental injury, and more post-mortem studies. We are also limited in our ability to target drugs to either the placenta or the fetus, but these issues will be overcome by advances in materials bioengineering, and proof-of-concept drugs and tools entering the fields of adult medicine. Given the vast numbers of infants born IUGR due to preventable causes such as malnutrition, malaria, HIV infection, and even psychosocial stress such as domestic abuse, we already have a mandate to reduce its impact across the world. Initiatives such as the Millennium Development Goals are making significant improvements in these areas but require our further support.

AUTHOR CONTRIBUTIONS

All authors listed have made a substantial, direct and intellectual contribution to the work, and approved it for publication.

REFERENCES

1. Lee AC, Kozuki N, Cousens S, Stevens GA, Blencowe H, Silveira MF, et al. Estimates of burden and consequences of infants born small for gestational age in low and middle income countries with INTERGROWTH-21(st) standard: analysis of CHERG datasets. *BMJ.* (2017) 358:j3677. doi: 10.1136/bmj.j3677
2. Mcgaghie WC. Varieties of integrative scholarship: why rules of evidence, criteria, and standards matter. *Acad Med.* (2015) 90:294–302. doi: 10.1097/ACM.0000000000000585
3. Unterscheider J, Daly S, Geary MP, Kennelly MM, Mcauliffe FM, O'donoghue K, et al. Optimizing the definition of intrauterine growth restriction: the multicenter prospective PORTO study editorial comment. *Obst Gynecol Surv.* (2013) 68:549–51. doi: 10.1097/OGX.0b013e3182a0597f
4. Gordijn SJ, Beune IM, Thilaganathan B, Papageorghiou A, Baschat AA, Baker PN, et al. Consensus definition of fetal growth restriction: a Delphi procedure. *Ultrasound Obstetr Gynecol.* (2016) 48:333–9. doi: 10.1002/uog.15884
5. Dammann O, Ferriero D, Gressens P. Neonatal encephalopathy or hypoxic-ischemic encephalopathy? *Appropr Terminol. Matters Pediatr Res.* (2011) 70:1–2. doi: 10.1203/PDR.0b013e318223f38d
6. Mcintyre S, Badawi N, Blair E, Nelson KB. Does aetiology of neonatal encephalopathy and hypoxic-ischaemic encephalopathy influence the outcome of treatment? *Dev Med Child Neurol.* (2015) 57 (Suppl 3):2–7. doi: 10.1111/dmcn.12725
7. Beune IM, Pels A, Gordijn SJ, Ganzevoort W. Definitions of fetal growth restriction in existing literature over time. *Ultrasound Obstet Gynecol.* (2018). doi: 10.1002/uog.19189. [Epub ahead of print].
8. Lunde A, Melve KK, Gjessing HK, Skjaerven R, Irgens LM. Genetic and environmental influences on birth weight, birth length, head circumference, and gestational age by use of population-based parent-offspring data. *Am J Epidemiol.* (2007) 165:734–41. doi: 10.1093/aje/kwk107
9. Gardosi J. Customized charts and their role in identifying pregnancies at risk because of fetal growth restriction. *J Obstet Gynaecol Can.* (2014) 36:408–15. doi: 10.1016/S1701-2163(15)30587-9
10. Sharma D, Shastri S, Sharma P. Intrauterine growth restriction: antenatal and postnatal aspects. *Clin Med Insights Pediatr.* (2016) 10:67–83. doi: 10.4137/CMPed.S40070
11. Unterscheider J, O'donoghue K, Daly S, Geary MP, Kennelly MM, Mcauliffe FM, et al. Fetal growth restriction and the risk of perinatal mortality-case studies from the multicentre PORTO study. *BMC Pregnancy Childbirth.* (2014) 14:63. doi: 10.1186/1471-2393-14-63
12. Winder NR, Krishnaveni GV, Veena SR, Hill JC, Karat CL, Thornburg KL, et al. Mother's lifetime nutrition and the size, shape and efficiency of the placenta. *Placenta.* (2011) 32:806–10. doi: 10.1016/j.placenta.2011.09.001
13. Martyn CN, Barker DJ, Osmond C. Mothers' pelvic size, fetal growth, and death from stroke and coronary heart disease in men in the UK. *Lancet.* (1996) 348:1264–8. doi: 10.1016/S0140-6736(96)04257-2
14. Barker DJ, Osmond C, Thornburg KL, Kajantie E, Eriksson JG. The lifespan of men and the shape of their placental surface at birth. *Placenta.* (2011) 32:783–7. doi: 10.1016/j.placenta.2011.07.031
15. Barker DJ, Osmond C, Golding J, Kuh D, Wadsworth ME. Growth in utero, blood pressure in childhood and adult life, and mortality from cardiovascular disease. *BMJ.* (1989) 298:564–7. doi: 10.1136/bmj.298.6673.564
16. Leitner Y, Fattal-Valevski A, Geva R, Eshel R, Toledano-Alhadef H, Rotstein M, et al. Neurodevelopmental outcome of children with intrauterine growth retardation: a longitudinal, 10-year prospective study. *J Child Neurol.* (2007) 22:580–7. doi: 10.1177/0883073807302605
17. Healy P, Gordijn S, Ganzevoort W, Beune I, Baschat A, Khalil A, et al. Core outcome set for growth restriction: developing endpoints (COSGROVE). *Trials.* (2018) 19:451. doi: 10.1186/s13063-018-2819-9
18. Miller SL, Huppi PS, Mallard C. The consequences of fetal growth restriction on brain structure and neurodevelopmental outcome. *J Physiol.* (2016) 594:807–23. doi: 10.1113/JP271402

19. Tolcos M, Petratos S, Hirst JJ, Wong F, Spencer SJ, Azhan A, et al. Blocked, delayed, or obstructed: what causes poor white matter development in intrauterine growth restricted infants? *Prog Neurobiol.* (2017) 154:62–77. doi: 10.1016/j.pneurobio.2017.03.009
20. Gilchrist C, Cumberland A, Walker D, Tolcos M. Intrauterine growth restriction and development of the hippocampus: implications for learning and memory in children and adolescents. *Lancet Child Adolesc Health.* (2018) 2:755–64. doi: 10.1016/S2352-4642(18)30245-1
21. Mcintyre S, Blair E, Badawi N, Keogh J, Nelson KB. Antecedents of cerebral palsy and perinatal death in term and late preterm singletons. *Obstet Gynecol.* (2013) 122:869–77. doi: 10.1097/AOG.0b013e3182a265ab
22. Vijayaselvi R, Cherian A. Risk assessment of intrauterine growth restriction. *Curr Med Issues.* (2017) 15:262–6. doi: 10.4103/cmi.cmi_76_17
23. Gaccioli F, Lager S. Placental nutrient transport and intrauterine growth restriction. *Front Physiol.* (2016) 7:40. doi: 10.3389/fphys.2016.00040
24. Khan NA, Kazzi SN. Yield and costs of screening growth-retarded infants for torch infections. *Am J Perinatol.* (2000) 17:131–5. doi: 10.1055/s-2000-9288
25. Accrombessi M, Zeitlin J, Massougbodji A, Cot M, Briand V. What do we know about risk factors for fetal growth restriction in africa at the time of sustainable development goals? A scoping review. *Paediatr Perinat Epidemiol.* (2018) 32:184–96. doi: 10.1111/ppe.12433
26. Flood K, Unterscheider J, Daly S, Geary MP, Kennelly MM, Mcauliffe FM, et al. The role of brain sparing in the prediction of adverse outcomes in intrauterine growth restriction: results of the multicenter PORTO Study. *Am J Obstet Gynecol.* (2014) 211:288 e281–285. doi: 10.1016/j.ajog.2014.05.008
27. Beukers F, Aarnoudse-Moens CSH, Van Weissenbruch MM, Ganzevoort W, Van Goudoever JB, Van Wassenaer-Leemhuis AG. Fetal growth restriction with brain sparing: neurocognitive and behavioral outcomes at 12 years of age. *J Pediatr.* (2017) 188:103–9.e102. doi: 10.1016/j.jpeds.2017.06.003
28. Scherjon S, Briet J, Oosting H, Kok J. The discrepancy between maturation of visual-evoked potentials and cognitive outcome at five years in very preterm infants with and without hemodynamic signs of fetal brain-sparing. *Pediatrics.* (2000) 105:385–91. doi: 10.1542/peds.105.2.385
29. Hernandez-Andrade E, Figueroa-Diesel H, Jansson T, Rangel-Nava H, Gratacos E. Changes in regional fetal cerebral blood flow perfusion in relation to hemodynamic deterioration in severely growth-restricted fetuses. *Ultrasound Obstet Gynecol.* (2008) 32:71–6. doi: 10.1002/uog.5377
30. Sehgal A, Doctor T, Menahem S. Cardiac function and arterial biophysical properties in small for gestational age infants: postnatal manifestations of fetal programming. *J Pediatr.* (2013) 163:1296–300. doi: 10.1016/j.jpeds.2013.06.030
31. Devaskar SU, Chu A. Intrauterine growth restriction: hungry for an answer. *Physiology.* (2016) 31:131–46. doi: 10.1152/physiol.00033.2015
32. Younes B, Baez-Giangreco A, Al-Nuaim L, Al-Hakeem A, Abu Talib Z. Basement membrane thickening in the placentae from diabetic women. *Pathol Int.* (1996) 46:100–4. doi: 10.1111/j.1440-1827.1996.tb03585.x
33. Pantham P, Aye IL, Powell TL. Inflammation in maternal obesity and gestational diabetes mellitus. *Placenta.* (2015) 36:709–15. doi: 10.1016/j.placenta.2015.04.006
34. Howell KR, Powell TL. Effects of maternal obesity on placental function and fetal development. *Reproduction.* (2017) 153:R97–108. doi: 10.1530/REP-16-0495
35. Nivoit P, Morens C, Van Assche FA, Jansen E, Poston L, Remacle C, et al. Established diet-induced obesity in female rats leads to offspring hyperphagia, adiposity and insulin resistance. *Diabetologia.* (2009) 52:1133–42. doi: 10.1007/s00125-009-1316-9
36. Picone O, Laigre P, Fortun-Lamothe L, Archilla C, Peynot N, Ponter AA, et al. Hyperlipidic hypercholesterolemic diet in prepubertal rabbits affects gene expression in the embryo, restricts fetal growth and increases offspring susceptibility to obesity. *Theriogenology.* (2011) 75:287–99. doi: 10.1016/j.theriogenology.2010.08.015
37. Carr DJ, Aitken RP, Milne JS, David AL, Wallace JM. Fetoplacental biometry and umbilical artery Doppler velocimetry in the overnourished adolescent model of fetal growth restriction. *Am J Obstet Gynecol.* (2012) 207:141 e146–e115. doi: 10.1016/j.ajog.2012.05.008
38. Cai D. Neuroinflammation and neurodegeneration in overnutrition-induced diseases. *Trends Endocrinol Metab.* (2013) 24:40–7. doi: 10.1016/j.tem.2012.11.003
39. Challier JC, Basu S, Bintein T, Minium J, Hotmire K, Catalano PM, et al. Obesity in pregnancy stimulates macrophage accumulation and inflammation in the placenta. *Placenta.* (2008) 29:274–81. doi: 10.1016/j.placenta.2007.12.010
40. Sureshchandra S, Marshall NE, Wilson RM, Barr T, Rais M, Purnell JQ, et al. Inflammatory determinants of pregravid obesity in placenta and peripheral blood. *Front Physiol.* (2018) 9:1089. doi: 10.3389/fphys.2018.01089
41. Zhu MJ, Du M, Nathanielsz PW, Ford SP. Maternal obesity up-regulates inflammatory signaling pathways and enhances cytokine expression in the mid-gestation sheep placenta. *Placenta.* (2010) 31:387–91. doi: 10.1016/j.placenta.2010.02.002
42. Yan X, Huang Y, Wang H, Du M, Hess BW, Ford SP, et al. Maternal obesity induces sustained inflammation in both fetal and offspring large intestine of sheep. *Inflamm Bowel Dis.* (2011) 17:1513–22. doi: 10.1002/ibd.21539
43. Crocker IP, Cooper S, Ong SC, Baker PN. Differences in apoptotic susceptibility of cytotrophoblasts and syncytiotrophoblasts in normal pregnancy to those complicated with preeclampsia and intrauterine growth restriction. *Am J Pathol.* (2003) 162:637–43. doi: 10.1016/S0002-9440(10)63857-6
44. Mcelrath TF, Allred EN, Leviton A. Placental pathology and neonatal outcome among growth-restricted fetuses in pregnancies complicated by preeclampsia, idiopathic growth restriction, and intrauterine inflammation. *Am J Obstetr Gynecol.* (2003) 189:S220. doi: 10.1016/j.ajog.2003.10.595
45. Mayhew TM, Wijesekara J, Baker PN, Ong SS. Morphometric evidence that villous development and fetoplacental angiogenesis are compromised by intrauterine growth restriction but not by pre-eclampsia. *Placenta.* (2004) 25:829–33. doi: 10.1016/j.placenta.2004.04.011
46. Mcelrath TF, Fichorova RN, Allred EN, Hecht JL, Ismail MA, Yuan H, et al. Blood protein profiles of infants born before 28 weeks differ by pregnancy complication. *Am J Obstet Gynecol.* (2011) 204:418 e411-418 e412. doi: 10.1016/j.ajog.2010.12.010
47. Odibo AO, Zhong Y, Longtine M, Tuuli M, Odibo L, Cahill AG, et al. First-trimester serum analytes, biophysical tests and the association with pathological morphometry in the placenta of pregnancies with preeclampsia and fetal growth restriction. *Placenta.* (2011) 32:333–8. doi: 10.1016/j.placenta.2011.01.016
48. Mavalankar DV, Gray RH, Trivedi CR, Parikh VC. Risk factors for small for gestational age births in Ahmedabad, India. *J Trop Pediatr.* (1994) 40:285–90. doi: 10.1093/tropej/40.5.285
49. Mumbare SS, Maindarkar G, Darade R, Yenge S, Tolani MK, Patole K. Maternal risk factors associated with term low birth weight neonates: a matched-pair case control study. *Indian Pediatr.* (2012) 49:25–8. doi: 10.1007/s13312-012-0010-z
50. Winick M, Rosso P. The effect of severe early malnutrition on cellular growth of human brain. *Pediatr Res.* (1969) 3:181–4. doi: 10.1203/00006450-196903000-00010
51. Moormann AM, Sullivan AD, Rochford RA, Chensue SW, Bock PJ, Nyirenda T, et al. Malaria and pregnancy: placental cytokine expression and its relationship to intrauterine growth retardation. *J Infect Dis.* (1999) 180:1987–93. doi: 10.1086/315135
52. Boeuf P, Tan A, Romagosa C, Radford J, Mwapasa V, Molyneux ME, et al. Placental hypoxia during placental malaria. *J Infect Dis.* (2008) 197:757–65. doi: 10.1086/526521
53. Liberato SC, Singh G, Mulholland K. Effects of protein energy supplementation during pregnancy on fetal growth: a review of the literature focusing on contextual factors. *Food Nutr Res.* (2013) 57. doi: 10.3402/fnr.v57i0.20499
54. Dall'asta A, Brunelli V, Prefumo F, Frusca T, Lees CC. Early onset fetal growth restriction. *Matern Health Neonatol Perinatol.* (2017) 3:2. doi: 10.1186/s40748-016-0041-x
55. Figueras F, Caradeux J, Crispi F, Eixarch E, Peguero A, Gratacos E. Diagnosis and surveillance of late-onset fetal growth restriction. *Am J Obstet Gynecol.* (2018) 218:S790–802 e791. doi: 10.1016/j.ajog.2017.12.003
56. Avagliano L, Garo C, Marconi AM. Placental amino acids transport in intrauterine growth restriction. *J Pregnancy.* (2012) 2012:972562. doi: 10.1155/2012/972562

57. Chen YY, Gupta MB, Grattton R, Powell TL, Jansson T. Down-regulation of placental folate transporters in intrauterine growth restriction. *J Nutr Biochem.* (2018) 59:136–41. doi: 10.1016/j.jnutbio.2018.06.003
58. Miller SL, Yawno T, Alers NO, Castillo-Melendez M, Supramaniam VG, Vanzyl N, et al. Antenatal antioxidant treatment with melatonin to decrease newborn neurodevelopmental deficits and brain injury caused by fetal growth restriction. *J Pineal Res.* (2014) 56:283–94. doi: 10.1111/jpi.12121
59. Rideau Batista Novais A, Pham H, Van De Looij Y, Bernal M, Mairesse J, Zana-Taieb E, et al. Transcriptomic regulations in oligodendroglial and microglial cells related to brain damage following fetal growth restriction. *Glia.* (2016) 64:2306–20. doi: 10.1002/glia.23079
60. Kalanjati VP, Wixey JA, Miller SM, Colditz PB, Bjorkman ST. GABAA receptor expression and white matter disruption in intrauterine growth restricted piglets. *Int J Dev Neurosci.* (2017) 59:1–9. doi: 10.1016/j.ijdevneu.2017.02.004
61. Tolcos M, Mcdougall A, Shields A, Chung Y, O'dowd R, Turnley A, et al. Intrauterine growth restriction affects cerebellar granule cells in the developing guinea pig brain. *Dev Neurosci.* (2018) 40:162–74. doi: 10.1159/000487797
62. Ke X, Lei Q, James SJ, Kelleher SL, Melnyk S, Jernigan S, et al. Uteroplacental insufficiency affects epigenetic determinants of chromatin structure in brains of neonatal and juvenile IUGR rats. *Physiol Genomics.* (2006) 25:16–28. doi: 10.1152/physiolgenomics.00093.2005
63. Zinni M, Colella M, Batista Novais AR, Baud O, Mairesse J. Modulating the oxytocin system during the perinatal period: a new strategy for neuroprotection of the immature brain? *Front Neurol.* (2018) 9:229. doi: 10.3389/fneur.2018.00229
64. Dombroski RA, Casey ML, Macdonald PC. 5-Alpha-dihydroprogesterone formation in human placenta from 5alpha-pregnan-3beta/alpha-ol-20-ones and 5-pregnan-3beta-yl-20-one sulfate. *J Steroid Biochem Mol Biol.* (1997) 63:155–63. doi: 10.1016/S0960-0760(97)00058-7
65. Hirst JJ, Palliser HK, Yates DM, Yawno T, Walker DW. Neurosteroids in the fetus and neonate: potential protective role in compromised pregnancies. *Neurochem Int.* (2008) 52:602–10. doi: 10.1016/j.neuint.2007.07.018
66. Hirst JJ, Yawno T, Nguyen P, Walker DW. Stress in pregnancy activates neurosteroid production in the fetal brain. *Neuroendocrinology.* (2006) 84:264–74. doi: 10.1159/000097990
67. Yawno T, Yan EB, Walker DW, Hirst JJ. Inhibition of neurosteroid synthesis increases asphyxia-induced brain injury in the late gestation fetal sheep. *Neuroscience.* (2007) 146:1726–33. doi: 10.1016/j.neuroscience.2007.03.023
68. Fleiss B, Parkington HC, Coleman HA, Dickinson H, Yawno T, Castillo-Melendez M, et al. Effect of maternal administration of allopregnanolone before birth asphyxia on neonatal hippocampal function in the spiny mouse. *Brain Res.* (2012) 1433:9–19. doi: 10.1016/j.brainres.2011.11.035
69. Wood CE. Estrogen/hypothalamus-pituitary-adrenal axis interactions in the fetus: the interplay between placenta and fetal brain. *J Soc Gynecol Invest.* (2005) 12:67–76. doi: 10.1016/j.jsgi.2004.10.011
70. Hirst JJ, Cumberland AL, Shaw JC, Bennett GA, Kelleher MA, Walker DW, et al. Loss of neurosteroid-mediated protection following stress during fetal life. *J Steroid Biochem Mol Biol.* (2016) 160:181–8. doi: 10.1016/j.jsbmb.2015.09.012
71. Belelli D, Lambert JJ. Neurosteroids: endogenous regulators of the GABA(A) receptor. *Nat Rev Neurosci.* (2005) 6:565–75. doi: 10.1038/nrn1703
72. Schumacher M, Mattern C, Ghoumari A, Oudinet JP, Liere P, Labombarda F, et al. Revisiting the roles of progesterone and allopregnanolone in the nervous system: resurgence of the progesterone receptors. *Prog Neurobiol.* (2014) 113:6–39. doi: 10.1016/j.pneurobio.2013.09.004
73. Johansson IM, Birzniece V, Lindblad C, Olsson T, Backstrom T. Allopregnanolone inhibits learning in the Morris water maze. *Brain Res.* (2002) 934:125–31. doi: 10.1016/S0006-8993(02)02414-9
74. Vu TT, Hirst JJ, Stark M, Wright IM, Palliser HK, Hodyl N, et al. Changes in human placental 5alpha-reductase isoenzyme expression with advancing gestation: effects of fetal sex and glucocorticoid exposure. *Reprod Fertil Dev.* (2009) 21:599–607. doi: 10.1071/RD08224
75. Pecks U, Rath W, Kleine-Eggebrecht N, Maass N, Voigt F, Goecke TW, et al. Maternal serum lipid, estradiol, and progesterone levels in pregnancy, and the impact of placental and hepatic pathologies. *Geburtshilfe Frauenheilkd.* (2016) 76:799–808. doi: 10.1055/s-0042-107078
76. Westcott KT, Hirst JJ, Ciurej I, Walker DW, Wlodek ME. Brain allopregnanolone in the fetal and postnatal rat in response to uteroplacental insufficiency. *Neuroendocrinology.* (2008) 88:287–92. doi: 10.1159/000139771
77. Kelleher MA, Palliser HK, Walker DW, Hirst JJ. Sex-dependent effect of a low neurosteroid environment and intrauterine growth restriction on foetal guinea pig brain development. *J Endocrinol.* (2011) 208:301–9. doi: 10.1677/JOE-10-0248
78. Yawno T, Hirst JJ, Castillo-Melendez M, Walker DW. Role of neurosteroids in regulating cell death and proliferation in the late gestation fetal brain. *Neuroscience.* (2009) 163:838–47. doi: 10.1016/j.neuroscience.2009.07.009
79. Cumberland AL, Palliser HK, Walker DW, Hirst JJ. Cerebellar changes in guinea pig offspring following suppression of neurosteroid synthesis during late gestation. *Cerebellum.* (2017) 16:306–13. doi: 10.1007/s12311-016-0802-0
80. Cumberland AL, Palliser HK, Crombie GK, Walker DW, Hirst JJ. Increased anxiety-like phenotype in female guinea pigs following reduced neurosteroid exposure in utero. *Int J Dev Neurosci.* (2017) 58:50–8. doi: 10.1016/j.ijdevneu.2017.02.001
81. Hirst JJ, Kelleher MA, Walker DW, Palliser HK. Neuroactive steroids in pregnancy: key regulatory and protective roles in the foetal brain. *J Steroid Biochem Mol Biol.* (2014) 139:144–53. doi: 10.1016/j.jsbmb.2013.04.002
82. Castillo-Melendez M, Yawno T, Allison BJ, Jenkin G, Wallace EM, Miller SL. Cerebrovascular adaptations to chronic hypoxia in the growth restricted lamb. *Int J Dev Neurosci.* (2015) 45:55–65. doi: 10.1016/j.ijdevneu.2015.01.004
83. Wallace JM, Bourke DA, Aitken RP, Palmer RM, Da Silva P, Cruickshank MA. Relationship between nutritionally-mediated placental growth restriction and fetal growth, body composition and endocrine status during late gestation in adolescent sheep. *Placenta.* (2000) 21:100–8. doi: 10.1053/plac.1999.0440
84. Ben-Ari Y, Khalilov I, Kahle KT, Cherubini E. The GABA excitatory/inhibitory shift in brain maturation and neurological disorders. *Neuroscientist.* (2012) 18:467–86. doi: 10.1177/1073858412438697
85. Badawy AA. Tryptophan metabolism, disposition and utilization in pregnancy. *Biosci Rep.* (2015) 35:e00261. doi: 10.1042/BSR20150197
86. Badawy AA, Namboodiri AM, Moffett JR. The end of the road for the tryptophan depletion concept in pregnancy and infection. *Clin Sci.* (2016) 130:1327–33. doi: 10.1042/CS20160153
87. Schwarcz R, Bruno JP, Muchowski PJ, Wu HQ. Kynurenines in the mammalian brain: when physiology meets pathology. *Nat Rev Neurosci.* (2012) 13:465–77. doi: 10.1038/nrn3257
88. Murthi P, Wallace EM, Walker DW. Altered placental tryptophan metabolic pathway in human fetal growth restriction. *Placenta.* (2017) 52:62–70. doi: 10.1016/j.placenta.2017.02.013
89. Whitaker-Azmitia PM. Behavioral and cellular consequences of increasing serotonergic activity during brain development: a role in autism? *Int J Dev Neurosci.* (2005) 23:75–83. doi: 10.1016/j.ijdevneu.2004.07.022
90. Bonnin A, Goeden N, Chen K, Wilson ML, King J, Shih JC, et al. A transient placental source of serotonin for the fetal forebrain. *Nature.* (2011) 472:347–50. doi: 10.1038/nature09972
91. Jacobs BL, Azmitia EC. Structure and function of the brain serotonin system. *Physiol Rev.* (1992) 72:165–229. doi: 10.1152/physrev.1992.72.1.165
92. Goeden N, Velasquez J, Arnold KA, Chan Y, Lund BT, Anderson GM, et al. Maternal inflammation disrupts fetal neurodevelopment via increased placental output of serotonin to the fetal brain. *J Neurosci.* (2016) 36:6041–9. doi: 10.1523/JNEUROSCI.2534-15.2016
93. Hayaishi O, Hirata F, Ohnishi T, Henry JP, Rosenthal I, Katoh A. Indoleamine 2,3-dioxygenase: incorporation of 18O2– and 18O2 into the reaction products. *J Biol Chem.* (1977) 252:3548–50.
94. Azmitia EC. Modern views on an ancient chemical: serotonin effects on cell proliferation, maturation, and apoptosis. *Brain Res Bull.* (2001) 56:413–24. doi: 10.1016/S0361-9230(01)00614-1
95. Hagberg H, Mallard C. Effect of inflammation on central nervous system development and vulnerability. *Curr Opin Neurol.* (2005) 18:117–23. doi: 10.1097/01.wco.0000162851.44897.8f
96. Van Steenwinckel J, Schang AL, Sigaut S, Chhor V, Degos V, Hagberg H, et al. Brain damage of the preterm infant: new insights into

the role of inflammation. *Biochem Soc Trans.* (2014) 42:557–63. doi: 10.1042/BST20130284

97. Lai JCY, Rocha-Ferreira E, Ek CJ, Wang X, Hagberg H, Mallard C. Immune responses in perinatal brain injury. *Brain Behav Immun.* (2017) 63:210–23. doi: 10.1016/j.bbi.2016.10.022
98. Leviton A, Fichorova RN, O'shea TM, Kuban K, Paneth N, Dammann O, et al. Two-hit model of brain damage in the very preterm newborn: small for gestational age and postnatal systemic inflammation. *Pediatr Res.* (2013) 73:362–70. doi: 10.1038/pr.2012.188
99. Mcelrath TF, Allred EN, Van Marter L, Fichorova RN, Leviton A, Investigators ES. Perinatal systemic inflammatory responses of growth-restricted preterm newborns. *Acta Paediatr.* (2013) 102:e439–442. doi: 10.1111/apa.12339
100. Leviton A, Allred EN, Fichorova RN, Kuban KC, O'shea TM, Dammann O, et al. Antecedents of inflammation biomarkers in preterm newborns on days 21 and 28. *Acta Paediatr.* (2016) 105:274–80. doi: 10.1111/apa.13286
101. Carty M, Bowie AG. Evaluating the role of Toll-like receptors in diseases of the central nervous system. *Biochem Pharmacol.* (2011) 81:825–37. doi: 10.1016/j.bcp.2011.01.003
102. Girard S, Heazell AE, Derricott H, Allan SM, Sibley CP, Abrahams VM, et al. Circulating cytokines and alarmins associated with placental inflammation in high-risk pregnancies. *Am J Reprod Immunol.* (2014) 72:422–34. doi: 10.1111/aji.12274
103. Derricott H, Heazell AEP, Greenwood SL, Jones RL. A novel in vitro model of villitis of unknown etiology demonstrates altered placental hormone and cytokine profile. *Am J Reprod Immunol.* 2017 78:e12725. doi: 10.1111/aji.12725
104. Wixey JA, Chand KK, Colditz PB, Bjorkman ST. Review: neuroinflammation in intrauterine growth restriction. *Placenta.* (2017) 54:117–24. doi: 10.1016/j.placenta.2016.11.012
105. Prins JR, Eskandar S, Eggen BJL, Scherjon SA. Microglia, the missing link in maternal immune activation and fetal neurodevelopment; and a possible link in preeclampsia and disturbed neurodevelopment? *J Reprod Immunol.* (2018) 126:18–22. doi: 10.1016/j.jri.2018.01.004
106. Faustino JV, Wang X, Johnson CE, Klibanov A, Derugin N, Wendland MF, et al. Microglial cells contribute to endogenous brain defenses after acute neonatal focal stroke. *J Neurosci.* (2011) 31:12992–3001. doi: 10.1523/JNEUROSCI.2102-11.2011
107. Hamelin L, Lagarde J, Dorothee G, Leroy C, Labit M, Comley RA, et al. Early and protective microglial activation in Alzheimer's disease: a prospective study using 18F-DPA-714 PET imaging. *Brain.* (2016) 139:1252–64. doi: 10.1093/brain/aww017
108. Hanlon LA, Huh JW, Raghupathi R. Minocycline transiently reduces microglia/macrophage activation but exacerbates cognitive deficits following repetitive traumatic brain injury in the neonatal rat. *J Neuropathol Exp Neurol.* (2016) 75:214–26. doi: 10.1093/jnen/nlv021
109. Kumar A, Alvarez-Croda DM, Stoica BA, Faden AI, Loane DJ. Microglial/macrophage polarization dynamics following traumatic brain injury. *J Neurotrauma.* (2016) 33:1732–50. doi: 10.1089/neu.2015.4268
110. Mikita J, Dubourdieu-Cassagno N, Deloire MS, Vekris A, Biran M, Raffard G, et al. Altered M1/M2 activation patterns of monocytes in severe relapsing experimental rat model of multiple sclerosis. Amelioration of clinical status by M2 activated monocyte administration. *Mult Scler.* (2011) 17:2–15. doi: 10.1177/1352458510379243
111. Miron VE, Boyd A, Zhao JW, Yuen TJ, Ruckh JM, Shadrach JL, et al. M2 microglia and macrophages drive oligodendrocyte differentiation during CNS remyelination. *Nat Neurosci.* (2013) 16:1211–8. doi: 10.1038/nn.3469
112. Song GJ, Suk K. Pharmacological modulation of functional phenotypes of microglia in neurodegenerative diseases. *Front Aging Neurosci.* (2017) 9:139. doi: 10.3389/fnagi.2017.00139
113. Hagberg H, Mallard C, Ferriero DM, Vannucci SJ, Levison SW, Vexler ZS, et al. The role of inflammation in perinatal brain injury. *Nat Rev Neurol.* (2015) 11:192–208. doi: 10.1038/nrneurol.2015.13
114. Pierre WC, Smith PLP, Londono I, Chemtob S, Mallard C, Lodygensky GA. Neonatal microglia: the cornerstone of brain fate. *Brain Behav Immun.* (2017) 59:333–45. doi: 10.1016/j.bbi.2016.08.018
115. Tay TL, Savage JC, Hui CW, Bisht K, Tremblay ME. Microglia across the lifespan: from origin to function in brain development, plasticity and cognition. *J Physiol.* (2017) 595:1929–45. doi: 10.1113/JP272134
116. Bilardo CM, Hecher K, Visser GHA, Papageorghiou AT, Marlow N, Thilaganathan B, et al. Severe fetal growth restriction at 26-32 weeks: key messages from the TRUFFLE study. *Ultrasound Obstet Gynecol.* (2017) 50:285–90. doi: 10.1002/uog.18815
117. Visser GHA, Bilardo CM, Derks JB, Ferrazzi E, Fratelli N, Frusca T, et al. Fetal monitoring indications for delivery and 2-year outcome in 310 infants with fetal growth restriction delivered before 32 weeks' gestation in the TRUFFLE study. *Ultrasound Obstet Gynecol.* (2017) 50:347–52. doi: 10.1002/uog.17361
118. Gilbert WM, Danielsen B. Pregnancy outcomes associated with intrauterine growth restriction. *Am J Obstet Gynecol.* (2003) 188:1596–9; discussion 1599–601. doi: 10.1067/mob.2003.384
119. Van Wyk L, Boers KE, Van Der Post JA, Van Pampus MG, Van Wassenaer AG, Van Baar AL, et al. Effects on (neuro)developmental and behavioral outcome at 2 years of age of induced labor compared with expectant management in intrauterine growth-restricted infants: long-term outcomes of the DIGITAT trial. *Am J Obstet Gynecol.* (2012) 206:406 e401–407. doi: 10.1016/j.ajog.2012.02.003
120. Lackman F, Capewell V, Richardson B, Dasilva O, Gagnon R. The risks of spontaneous preterm delivery and perinatal mortality in relation to size at birth according to fetal versus neonatal growth standards. *Am J Obstet Gynecol.* (2001) 184:946–53. doi: 10.1067/mob.2001.111719
121. Garite TJ, Clark R, Thorp JA. Intrauterine growth restriction increases morbidity and mortality among premature neonates. *Am J Obstet Gynecol.* (2004) 191:481–7. doi: 10.1016/j.ajog.2004.01.036
122. Gortner L, Van Husen M, Thyen U, Gembruch U, Friedrich HJ, Landmann E. Outcome in preterm small for gestational age infants compared to appropriate for gestational age preterms at the age of 2 years: a prospective study. *Eur J Obstet Gynecol Reprod Biol.* (2003) 110 (Suppl 1):S93–7. doi: 10.1016/S0301-2115(03)00178-7
123. Yanney M, Marlow N. Paediatric consequences of fetal growth restriction. *Semin Fetal Neonatal Med.* (2004) 9:411–8. doi: 10.1016/j.siny.2004.03.005
124. Sung IK, Vohr B, Oh W. Growth and neurodevelopmental outcome of very low birth weight infants with intrauterine growth retardation: comparison with control subjects matched by birth weight and gestational age. *J Pediatr.* (1993) 123:618–24. doi: 10.1016/S0022-3476(05)80965-5
125. Shand AW, Hornbuckle J, Nathan E, Dickinson JE, French NP. Small for gestational age preterm infants and relationship of abnormal umbilical artery Doppler blood flow to perinatal mortality and neurodevelopmental outcomes. *Aust N Z J Obstet Gynaecol.* (2009) 49:52–8. doi: 10.1111/j.1479-828X.2008.00941.x
126. Padilla N, Perapoch J, Carrascosa A, Acosta-Rojas R, Botet F, Gratacos E. Twelve-month neurodevelopmental outcome in preterm infants with and without intrauterine growth restriction. *Acta Paediatr.* (2010) 99:1498–503. doi: 10.1111/j.1651-2227.2010.01848.x
127. Thornton JG, Hornbuckle J, Vail A, Spiegelhalter DJ, Levene M, Group GS. Infant wellbeing at 2 years of age in the Growth Restriction Intervention Trial (GRIT): multicentred randomised controlled trial. *Lancet.* (2004) 364:513–20. doi: 10.1016/S0140-6736(04)16809-8
128. Walker DM, Marlow N, Upstone L, Gross H, Hornbuckle J, Vail A, et al. The growth restriction intervention trial: long-term outcomes in a randomized trial of timing of delivery in fetal growth restriction. *Am J Obstet Gynecol.* (2011) 204:34 e31–39. doi: 10.1016/j.ajog.2010.09.019
129. Guellec I, Lapillonne A, Renolleau S, Charlaluk ML, Roze JC, Marret S, et al. Neurologic outcomes at school age in very preterm infants born with severe or mild growth restriction. *Pediatrics.* (2011) 127:e883–891. doi: 10.1542/peds.2010-2442
130. Fischi-Gomez E, Vasung L, Meskaldji DE, Lazeyras F, Borradori-Tolsa C, Hagmann P, et al. Structural brain connectivity in school-age preterm infants provides evidence for impaired networks relevant for higher order cognitive skills and social cognition. *Cereb Cortex.* (2015) 25:2793–805. doi: 10.1093/cercor/bhu073
131. Tolsa CB, Zimine S, Warfield SK, Freschi M, Sancho Rossignol A, Lazeyras F, et al. Early alteration of structural and functional brain development in premature infants born with intrauterine growth restriction. *Pediatr Res.* (2004) 56:132–8. doi: 10.1203/01.PDR.0000128983.54614.7E

132. Ortigosa Rocha C, Bittar RE, Zugaib M. Neonatal outcomes of late-preterm birth associated or not with intrauterine growth restriction. *Obstet Gynecol Int.* (2010) 2010:231842. doi: 10.1155/2010/231842
133. Geva R, Eshel R, Leitner Y, Valevski AF, Harel S. Neuropsychological outcome of children with intrauterine growth restriction: a 9-year prospective study. *Pediatrics.* (2006) 118:91–100. doi: 10.1542/peds.2005-2343
134. Figueras F, Oros D, Cruz-Martinez R, Padilla N, Hernandez-Andrade E, Botet F, et al. Neurobehavior in term, small-for-gestational age infants with normal placental function. *Pediatrics.* (2009) 124:e934–41. doi: 10.1542/peds.2008-3346
135. Edmonds CJ, Isaacs EB, Cole TJ, Rogers MH, Lanigan J, Singhal A, et al. The effect of intrauterine growth on verbal IQ scores in childhood: a study of monozygotic twins. *Pediatrics.* (2010) 126:e1095–101. doi: 10.1542/peds.2008-3684
136. Raznahan A, Greenstein D, Lee NR, Clasen LS, Giedd JN. Prenatal growth in humans and postnatal brain maturation into late adolescence. *Proc Natl Acad Sci USA.* (2012) 109:11366–71. doi: 10.1073/pnas.1203350109
137. Zarean E, Mostajeran F, Dayani Z. Effect of dydrogesterone on the outcome of idiopathic intrauterine growth restriction: a double-blind clinical trial study. *Adv Biomed Res.* (2018) 7:93. doi: 10.4103/abr.abr_250_16
138. Palliser HK, Bennett GA, Kelleher MA, Cumberland AL, Walker DW, Hirst JJ. Models of perinatal compromises in the guinea pig: their use in showing the role of neurosteroids in pregnancy and the newborn. *Prenatal Postnatal Determ Dev.* (2016) 109:221–43. doi: 10.1007/978-1-4939-3014-2_11
139. Kalinka J, Szekeres-Bartho J. The impact of dydrogesterone supplementation on hormonal profile and progesterone-induced blocking factor concentrations in women with threatened abortion. *Am J Reprod Immunol.* (2005) 53:166–71. doi: 10.1111/j.1600-0897.2005.00261.x
140. Polgar B, Nagy E, Miko E, Varga P, Szekeres-Bartho J. Urinary progesterone-induced blocking factor concentration is related to pregnancy outcome. *Biol Reprod.* (2004) 71:1699–705. doi: 10.1095/biolreprod.104.030437
141. Sharp A, Cornforth C, Jackson R, Harrold J, Turner MA, Kenny LC, et al. Maternal sildenafil for severe fetal growth restriction (STRIDER): a multicentre, randomised, placebo-controlled, double-blind trial. *Lancet Child Adolesc Health.* (2018) 2:93–102. doi: 10.1016/S2352-4642(17)30173-6
142. Smith GCS. The STRIDER trial: one step forward, one step back. *Lancet Child Adolesc Health.* (2018) 2:80–1. doi: 10.1016/S2352-4642(17)30176-1
143. Chen J, Gong X, Chen P, Luo K, Zhang X. Effect of L-arginine and sildenafil citrate on intrauterine growth restriction fetuses: a meta-analysis. *BMC Pregnancy Childbirth.* (2016) 16:225. doi: 10.1186/s12884-016-1009-6
144. Dickinson H, Ellery S, Ireland Z, Larosa D, Snow R, Walker DW. Creatine supplementation during pregnancy: summary of experimental studies suggesting a treatment to improve fetal and neonatal morbidity and reduce mortality in high-risk human pregnancy. *BMC Pregnancy Childbirth.* (2014) 14:150. doi: 10.1186/1471-2393-14-150
145. Ellery SJ, Dickinson H, Mckenzie M, Walker DW. Dietary interventions designed to protect the perinatal brain from hypoxic-ischemic encephalopathy–Creatine prophylaxis and the need for multi-organ protection. *Neurochem Int.* (2016) 95:15–23. doi: 10.1016/j.neuint.2015.11.002
146. Dickinson H, Davies-Tuck M, Ellery SJ, Grieger JA, Wallace EM, Snow RJ, et al. Maternal creatine in pregnancy: a retrospective cohort study. *BJOG.* (2016) 123:1830–8. doi: 10.1111/1471-0528.14237
147. Ellery SJ, Della Gatta PA, Bruce CR, Kowalski GM, Davies-Tuck M, Mockler JC, et al. Creatine biosynthesis and transport by the term human placenta. *Placenta.* (2017) 52:86–93. doi: 10.1016/j.placenta.2017.02.020
148. Wallimann T, Tokarska-Schlattner M, Schlattner U. The creatine kinase system and pleiotropic effects of creatine. *Amino Acids.* (2011) 40:1271–96. doi: 10.1007/s00726-011-0877-3
149. Adcock KH, Nedelcu J, Loenneker T, Martin E, Wallimann T, Wagner BP. Neuroprotection of creatine supplementation in neonatal rats with transient cerebral hypoxia-ischemia. *Dev Neurosci.* (2002) 24:382–8. doi: 10.1159/000069043
150. Ireland Z, Dickinson H, Snow R, Walker DW. Maternal creatine: does it reach the fetus and improve survival after an acute hypoxic episode in the spiny mouse (Acomys cahirinus)? *Am J Obstet Gynecol.* (2008) 198:431 e1–6. doi: 10.1016/j.ajog.2007.10.790
151. Ireland Z, Castillo-Melendez M, Dickinson H, Snow R, Walker DW. A maternal diet supplemented with creatine from mid-pregnancy protects the newborn spiny mouse brain from birth hypoxia. *Neuroscience.* (2011) 194:372–9. doi: 10.1016/j.neuroscience.2011.05.012
152. Wali JA, De Boo HA, Derraik JG, Phua HH, Oliver MH, Bloomfield FH, et al. Weekly intra-amniotic IGF-1 treatment increases growth of growth-restricted ovine fetuses and up-regulates placental amino acid transporters. *PLoS ONE.* (2012) 7:e37899. doi: 10.1371/journal.pone.0037899
153. Spiroski AM, Oliver MH, Jaquiery AL, Prickett TCR, Espiner EA, Harding JE, et al. Postnatal effects of intrauterine treatment of the growth-restricted ovine fetus with intra-amniotic insulin-like growth factor-1. *J Physiol.* (2018) 596:5925–45. doi: 10.1113/JP274999
154. Verlijsdonk JW, Winkens B, Boers K, Scherjon S, Roumen F. Suspected versus non-suspected small-for-gestational age fetuses at term: perinatal outcomes. *J Matern Fetal Neonatal Med.* (2012) 25:938–43. doi: 10.3109/14767058.2011.600793
155. Fratelli N, Valcamonico A, Prefumo F, Pagani G, Guarneri T, Frusca T. Effects of antenatal recognition and follow-up on perinatal outcomes in small-for-gestational age infants delivered after 36 weeks. *Acta Obstet Gynecol Scand.* (2013) 92:223–9. doi: 10.1111/aogs.12020
156. Richardus JH, Graafmans WC, Verloove-Vanhorick SP, Mackenbach JP, Euronatal International Audit Panel, Euronatal Working Group. Differences in perinatal mortality and suboptimal care between 10 European regions: results of an international audit. *BJOG.* (2003) 110:97–105. doi: 10.1046/j.1471-0528.2003.02053.x
157. Evers AC, Nikkels PG, Brouwers HA, Boon J, Van Egmond-Linden A, Hart C, et al. Substandard care in antepartum term stillbirths: prospective cohort study. *Acta Obstet Gynecol Scand.* (2011) 90:1416–22. doi: 10.1111/j.1600-0412.2011.01251.x
158. Gardosi J, Madurasinghe V, Williams M, Malik A, Francis A. Maternal and fetal risk factors for stillbirth: population based study. *BMJ.* (2013) 346:f108. doi: 10.1136/bmj.f108
159. Sparks TN, Cheng YW, Mclaughlin B, Esakoff TF, Caughey AB. Fundal height: a useful screening tool for fetal growth? *J Matern Fetal Neonatal Med.* (2011) 24:708–12. doi: 10.3109/14767058.2010.516285
160. Sovio U, White IR, Dacey A, Pasupathy D, Smith GCS. Screening for fetal growth restriction with universal third trimester ultrasonography in nulliparous women in the Pregnancy Outcome Prediction (POP) study: a prospective cohort study. *Lancet.* (2015) 386:2089–97. doi: 10.1016/S0140-6736(15)00131-2
161. Baschat AA. Fetal growth restriction - from observation to intervention. *J Perinat Med.* (2010) 38:239–46. doi: 10.1515/jpm.2010.041
162. Cruz-Martinez R, Figueras F, Hernandez-Andrade E, Oros D, Gratacos E. Fetal brain Doppler to predict cesarean delivery for nonreassuring fetal status in term small-for-gestational-age fetuses. *Obstet Gynecol.* (2011) 117:618–26. doi: 10.1097/AOG.0b013e31820b0884
163. Oros D, Figueras F, Cruz-Martinez R, Meler E, Munmany M, Gratacos E. Longitudinal changes in uterine, umbilical and fetal cerebral Doppler indices in late-onset small-for-gestational age fetuses. *Ultrasound Obstet Gynecol.* (2011) 37:191–5. doi: 10.1002/uog.7738
164. Lausman A, Kingdom J, Maternal Fetal Medicine Committee. Intrauterine growth restriction: screening, diagnosis, and management. *J Obstet Gynaecol Can.* (2013) 35:741–8. doi: 10.1016/S1701-2163(15)30865-3
165. Morris RK, Cnossen JS, Langejans M, Robson SC, Kleijnen J, Ter Riet G, et al. Serum screening with Down's syndrome markers to predict pre-eclampsia and small for gestational age: systematic review and meta-analysis. *BMC Pregnancy Childbirth.* (2008) 8:33. doi: 10.1186/1471-2393-8-33
166. Karagiannis G, Akolekar R, Sarquis R, Wright D, Nicolaides KH. Prediction of small-for-gestation neonates from biophysical and biochemical markers at 11-13 weeks. *Fetal Diagn Ther.* (2011) 29:148–54. doi: 10.1159/000321694
167. Story L, Hutter J, Zhang T, Shennan AH, Rutherford M. The use of antenatal fetal magnetic resonance imaging in the assessment of patients at high risk of preterm birth. *Eur J Obstet Gynecol Reprod Biol.* (2018) 222:134–41. doi: 10.1016/j.ejogrb.2018.01.014
168. Baud O, Fayol L, Gressens P, Pellerin L, Magistretti P, Evrard P, et al. Perinatal and early postnatal changes in the expression of monocarboxylate

transporters MCT1 and MCT2 in the rat forebrain. *J Compar Neurol.* (2003) 465:445–54. doi: 10.1002/cne.10853

169. Ngo TTM, Moufarrej MN, Rasmussen MH, Camunas-Soler J, Pan W, Okamoto J, et al. Noninvasive blood tests for fetal development predict gestational age and preterm delivery. *Science.* (2018) 360:1133–6. doi: 10.1126/science.aar3819
170. Jelliffe-Pawlowski LL, Rand L, Bedell B, Baer RJ, Oltman SP, Norton ME, et al. Prediction of preterm birth with and without preeclampsia using mid-pregnancy immune and growth-related molecular factors and maternal characteristics. *J Perinatol.* (2018) 38:963–72. doi: 10.1038/s41372-018-0112-0
171. Poon LC, Rolnik DL, Tan MY, Delgado JL, Tsokaki T, Akolekar R, et al. ASPRE trial: incidence of preterm pre-eclampsia in patients fulfilling ACOG and NICE criteria according to risk by FMF algorithm. *Ultrasound Obstet Gynecol.* (2018) 51:738–42. doi: 10.1002/uog.19019
172. Mills TA, Wareing M, Bugg GJ, Greenwood SL, Baker PN. Chorionic plate artery function and Doppler indices in normal pregnancy and intrauterine growth restriction. *Eur J Clin Invest.* (2005) 35:758–64. doi: 10.1111/j.1365-2362.2005.01577.x
173. Leeuwerke M, Eilander MS, Pruis MG, Lendvai A, Erwich JJ, Scherjon SA, et al. DNA methylation and expression patterns of selected genes in first-trimester placental tissue from pregnancies with small-for-gestational-age infants at birth. *Biol Reprod.* (2016) 94:37. doi: 10.1095/biolreprod.115.131698
174. Wigglesworth JS. Experimental growth retardation in the foetal rat. *J Pathol Bacteriol.* (1964) 88:1–13. doi: 10.1002/path.1700880102
175. Bell C, Brown MJ. Arteriographic evidence for a cholinergic dilator mechanism in uterine hyperaemia of pregnancy in the guinea-pig. *J Reprod Fertil.* (1971) 27:59–65. doi: 10.1530/jrf.0.0270059
176. Bell C, Malcolm SJ. Observations on the loss of catecholamine fluorescence from intrauterine adrenergic nerves during pregnancy in the guinea-pig. *J Reprod Fertil.* (1978) 53:51–8. doi: 10.1530/jrf.0.0530051
177. Kane SC, Costa FDS, Brennecke S. First trimester biomarkers in the prediction of later pregnancy complications. *BioMed Res. Int.* (2014) 2014:807196. doi: 10.1155/2014/807196
178. Myatt L. Control of vascular resistance in the human placenta. *Placenta.* (1992) 13:329–41. doi: 10.1016/0143-4004(92)90057-Z
179. Regnault TR, Galan HL, Parker TA, Anthony RV. Placental development in normal and compromised pregnancies– a review. *Placenta.* (2002) 23 (Suppl. A):S119–29. doi: 10.1053/plac.2002.0792
180. Chan SY, Hancox LA, Martin-Santos A, Loubiere LS, Walter MN, Gonzalez AM, et al. MCT8 expression in human fetal cerebral cortex is reduced in severe intrauterine growth restriction. *J Endocrinol.* (2014) 220:85–95. doi: 10.1530/JOE-13-0400
181. Dickinson H, Walker DW, Cullen-Mcewen L, Wintour EM, Moritz K. The spiny mouse (Acomys cahirinus) completes nephrogenesis before birth. *Am J Physiol Renal Physiol.* (2005) 289:F273–9. doi: 10.1152/ajprenal.00400.2004
182. Quinn TA, Ratnayake U, Dickinson H, Nguyen TH, Mcintosh M, Castillo-Melendez M, et al. Ontogeny of the adrenal gland in the spiny mouse, with particular reference to production of the steroids cortisol and dehydroepiandrosterone. *Endocrinology.* (2013) 154:1190–201. doi: 10.1210/en.2012-1953
183. Quinn TA, Ratnayake U, Dickinson H, Castillo-Melendez M, Walker DW. Ontogenetic change in the regional distribution of dehydroepiandrosterone-synthesizing enzyme and the glucocorticoid receptor in the brain of the spiny mouse (*Acomys cahirinus*). *Dev Neurosci.* (2016) 38:54–73. doi: 10.1159/000438986
184. Nawathe AR, Christian M, Kim SH, Johnson M, Savvidou MD, Terzidou V. Insulin-like growth factor axis in pregnancies affected by fetal growth disorders. *Clin Epigenet.* (2016) 8:11. doi: 10.1186/s13148-016-0178-5
185. Abu-Amero SN, Ali Z, Bennett P, Vaughan JI, Moore GE. Expression of the insulin-like growth factors and their receptors in term placentas: a comparison between normal and IUGR births. *Mol Reprod Dev.* (1998) 49:229–35. doi: 10.1002/(SICI)1098-2795(199803)49:3<229::AID-MRD2>3.0.CO;2-Q
186. Martin-Estal I, De La Garza RG, Castilla-Cortazar I. Intrauterine growth retardation (IUGR) as a novel condition of insulin-like growth factor-1 (IGF-1) deficiency. *Rev Physiol Biochem Pharmacol.* (2016) 170:1–35. doi: 10.1007/112_2015_5001
187. Dilworth MR, Kusinski LC, Baker BC, Renshall LJ, Baker PN, Greenwood SL, et al. Crossing mice deficient in eNOS with placental-specific Igf2 knockout mice: a new model of fetal growth restriction. *Placenta.* (2012) 33:1052–4. doi: 10.1016/j.placenta.2012.09.012
188. Kusinski LC, Stanley JL, Dilworth MR, Hirt CJ, Andersson IJ, Renshall LJ, et al. eNOS knockout mouse as a model of fetal growth restriction with an impaired uterine artery function and placental transport phenotype. *Am J Physiol Regul Integr Comp Physiol.* (2012) 303:R86–93. doi: 10.1152/ajpregu.00600.2011
189. Krause BJ, Costello PM, Munoz-Urrutia E, Lillycrop KA, Hanson MA, Casanello P. Role of DNA methyltransferase 1 on the altered eNOS expression in human umbilical endothelium from intrauterine growth restricted fetuses. *Epigenetics.* (2013) 8:944–52. doi: 10.4161/epi.25579
190. Alahakoon TI, Medbury H, Williams H, Fewings N, Wang XM, Lee VW. Distribution of monocyte subsets and polarization in preeclampsia and intrauterine fetal growth restriction. *J Obstet Gynaecol Res.* (2018) 44:2135–48. doi: 10.1111/jog.13770
191. Raghupathy R, Al-Azemi M, Azizieh F. Intrauterine growth restriction: cytokine profiles of trophoblast antigen-stimulated maternal lymphocytes. *Clin Dev Immunol.* (2012) 2012:734865. doi: 10.1155/2012/734865
192. Medawar P. *An Unsolved Problem of Biology*. London: Published for the College by Lewis, H K (1952).
193. Girardi G, Yarilin D, Thurman JM, Holers VM, Salmon JE. Complement activation induces dysregulation of angiogenic factors and causes fetal rejection and growth restriction. *J Exp Med.* (2006) 203:2165–75. doi: 10.1084/jem.20061022
194. Mckelvey KJ, Yenson VM, Ashton AW, Morris JM, Mccracken SA. Embryonic/fetal mortality and intrauterine growth restriction is not exclusive to the CBA/J sub-strain in the CBA x DBA model. *Sci Rep.* (2016) 6:35138. doi: 10.1038/srep35138
195. Lappas M, Mccracken S, Mckelvey K, Lim R, James J, Roberts CT, et al. Formyl peptide receptor-2 is decreased in foetal growth restriction and contributes to placental dysfunction. *Mol Hum Reprod.* (2018) 24:94–109. doi: 10.1093/molehr/gax067
196. Dixon ME, Chien EK, Osol G, Callas PW, Bonney EA. Failure of decidual arteriolar remodeling in the CBA/J x DBA/2 murine model of recurrent pregnancy loss is linked to increased expression of tissue inhibitor of metalloproteinase 2 (TIMP-2). *Am J Obstet Gynecol.* (2006) 194:113–9. doi: 10.1016/j.ajog.2005.06.063
197. Labarrere CA, Dicarlo HL, Bammerlin E, Hardin JW, Kim YM, Chaemsaithong P, et al. Failure of physiologic transformation of spiral arteries, endothelial and trophoblast cell activation, and acute atherosis in the basal plate of the placenta. *Am J Obstet Gynecol.* (2017) 216:287.e281–287.e216. doi: 10.1016/j.ajog.2016.12.029
198. Saleem T, Sajjad N, Fatima S, Habib N, Ali SR, Qadir M. Intrauterine growth retardation–small events, big consequences. *Ital J Pediatr.* (2011) 37:41. doi: 10.1186/1824-7288-37-41
199. Back SA, Luo NL, Borenstein NS, Levine JM, Volpe JJ, Kinney HC. Late oligodendrocyte progenitors coincide with the developmental window of vulnerability for human perinatal white matter injury. *J Neurosci.* (2001) 21:1302–12. doi: 10.1523/JNEUROSCI.21-04-01302.2001
200. Billiards SS, Haynes RL, Folkerth RD, Borenstein NS, Trachtenberg FL, Rowitch DH, et al. Myelin abnormalities without oligodendrocyte loss in periventricular leukomalacia. *Brain Pathol.* (2008) 18:153–63. doi: 10.1111/j.1750-3639.2007.00107.x
201. Verney C, Pogledic I, Biran V, Adle-Biassette H, Fallet-Bianco C, Gressens P. Microglial reaction in axonal crossroads is a hallmark of noncystic periventricular white matter injury in very preterm infants. *J Neuropathol Exp Neurol.* (2012) 71:251–64. doi: 10.1097/NEN.0b013e3182496429
202. Samuelsen GB, Pakkenberg B, Bogdanovic N, Gundersen HJ, Larsen JF, Graem N, et al. Severe cell reduction in the future brain cortex in human growth-restricted fetuses and infants. *Am J Obstet Gynecol.* (2007) 197:56 e51–57. doi: 10.1016/j.ajog.2007.02.011

203. Larsen KB. Using the optical fractionator to estimate total cell numbers in the normal and abnormal developing human forebrain. *Front Neuroanat.* (2017) 11:112. doi: 10.3389/fnana.2017.00112
204. Chase HP, Welch NN, Dabiere CS, Vasan NS, Butterfield LJ. Alterations in human brain biochemistry following intrauterine growth retardation. *Pediatrics.* (1972) 50:403–11.
205. Burke CJ, Tannenberg AE, Payton DJ. Ischaemic cerebral injury, intrauterine growth retardation, and placental infarction. *Dev Med Child Neurol.* (1997) 39:726–30. doi: 10.1111/j.1469-8749.1997.tb07373.x
206. Burke C, Gobe G. Pontosubicular apoptosis ("necrosis") in human neonates with intrauterine growth retardation and placental infarction. *Virchows Arch.* (2005) 446:640–5. doi: 10.1007/s00428-005-1251-1
207. Hernandez-Andrade E, Serralde JA, Cruz-Martinez R. Can anomalies of fetal brain circulation be useful in the management of growth restricted fetuses? *Prenat Diagn.* (2012) 32:103–12. doi: 10.1002/pd.2913
208. Arduini D, Rizzo G, Romanini C, Mancuso S. Fetal haemodynamic response to acute maternal hyperoxygenation as predictor of fetal distress in intrauterine growth retardation. *BMJ.* (1989) 298:1561–2. doi: 10.1136/bmj.298.6687.1561
209. Langille BL. Arterial remodeling: relation to hemodynamics. *Can J Physiol Pharmacol.* (1996) 74:834–41. doi: 10.1139/y96-082
210. Baenziger O, Jaggi JL, Mueller AC, Morales CG, Lipp HP, Lipp AE, et al. Cerebral blood flow in preterm infants affected by sex, mechanical ventilation, and intrauterine growth. *Pediatr Neurol.* (1994) 11:319–24. doi: 10.1016/0887-8994(94)90009-4
211. Van Bel F, Van De Bor M, Stijnen T, Ruys JH. Decreased cerebrovascular resistance in small for gestational age infants. *Eur J Obstet Gynecol Reprod Biol.* (1986) 23:137–44. doi: 10.1016/0028-2243(86)90141-3
212. Nishimaki S, Shima Y, Yoda H, Kawakami T, Akamatsu H. Blood flow velocities in the cerebral arteries and descending aorta in small-for-dates infants. *Pediatr Radiol.* (1993) 23:575–7. doi: 10.1007/BF02014966
213. Ishii H, Takami T, Fujioka T, Mizukaki N, Kondo A, Sunohara D, et al. Comparison of changes in cerebral and systemic perfusion between appropriate- and small-for-gestational-age infants during the first three days after birth. *Brain Dev.* (2014) 36:380–7. doi: 10.1016/j.braindev.2013.06.006
214. Cohen E, Baerts W, Alderliesten T, Derks J, Lemmers P, Van Bel F. Growth restriction and gender influence cerebral oxygenation in preterm neonates. *Arch Dis Child Fetal Neonatal Ed.* (2016) 101:F156–61. doi: 10.1136/archdischild-2015-308843
215. Alderliesten T, Lemmers PM, Van Haastert IC, De Vries LS, Bonestroo HJ, Baerts W, et al. Hypotension in preterm neonates: low blood pressure alone does not affect neurodevelopmental outcome. *J Pediatr.* (2014) 164:986–91. doi: 10.1016/j.jpeds.2013.12.042
216. Alderliesten T, Lemmers PM, Smarius JJ, Van De Vosse RE, Baerts W, Van Bel F. Cerebral oxygenation, extraction, and autoregulation in very preterm infants who develop peri-intraventricular hemorrhage. *J Pediatr.* (2013) 162:698–704 e692. doi: 10.1016/j.jpeds.2012.09.038
217. Noori S, Mccoy M, Anderson MP, Ramji F, Seri I. Changes in cardiac function and cerebral blood flow in relation to peri/intraventricular hemorrhage in extremely preterm infants. *J Pediatr.* (2014) 164:264–270 e1–3. doi: 10.1016/j.jpeds.2013.09.045
218. Gerstner B, Desilva TM, Genz K, Armstrong A, Brehmer F, Neve RL, et al. Hyperoxia causes maturation-dependent cell death in the developing white matter. *J Neurosci.* (2008) 28:1236–45. doi: 10.1523/JNEUROSCI.3213-07.2008
219. Brew N, Walker D, Wong FY. Cerebral vascular regulation and brain injury in preterm infants. *Am J Physiol Regul Integr Comp Physiol.* (2014) 306:R773–86. doi: 10.1152/ajpregu.00487.2013
220. Sehgal A, Doctor T, Menahem S. Cardiac function and arterial indices in infants born small for gestational age: analysis by speckle tracking. *Acta Paediatr.* (2014) 103:e49–54. doi: 10.1111/apa.12465
221. Watanabe K, Hayakawa F, Okumura A. Neonatal EEG: a powerful tool in the assessment of brain damage in preterm infants. *Brain Dev.* (1999) 21:361–72. doi: 10.1016/S0387-7604(99)00034-0
222. Klebermass K, Olischar M, Waldhoer T, Fuiko R, Pollak A, Weninger M. Amplitude-integrated EEG pattern predicts further outcome in preterm infants. *Pediatr Res.* (2011) 70:102–8. doi: 10.1203/PDR.0b013e31821ba200
223. Yerushalmy-Feler A, Marom R, Peylan T, Korn A, Haham A, Mandel D, et al. Electroencephalographic characteristics in preterm infants born with intrauterine growth restriction. *J Pediatr.* (2014) 164:756–761 e751. doi: 10.1016/j.jpeds.2013.12.030
224. Schwindt E, Thaller C, Czaba-Hnizdo C, Giordano V, Olischar M, Waldhoer T, et al. Being born small for gestational age influences amplitude-integrated electroencephalography and later outcome in preterm infants. *Neonatology.* (2015) 108:81–7. doi: 10.1159/000382013
225. Benavente-Fernandez I, Lubian-Lopez SP, Zafra-Rodriguez P, Alonso-Ojembarrena A, Segado-Arenas A, Lechuga-Sancho AM. Amplitude-integrated, EEG and brain sparing in preterm small-for-gestational-age infants *J Clin Neurophysiol.* (2017) 34:456–60. doi: 10.1097/WNP.0000000000000399
226. Cohen E, Wong FY, Wallace EM, Mockler JC, Odoi A, Hollis S, et al. EEG power spectrum maturation in preterm fetal growth restricted infants. *Brain Res.* (2018) 1678:180–6. doi: 10.1016/j.brainres.2017.10.010
227. Scherjon SA, Oosting H, De Visser BW, De Wilde T, Zondervan HA, Kok JH. Fetal brain sparing is associated with accelerated shortening of visual evoked potential latencies during early infancy. *Am J Obstet Gynecol.* (1996) 175:1569–75. doi: 10.1016/S0002-9378(96)70108-4
228. Kok JH, Prick L, Merckel E, Everhard Y, Verkerk GJ, Scherjon SA. Visual function at 11 years of age in preterm-born children with and without fetal brain sparing. *Pediatrics.* (2007) 119:e1342–1350. doi: 10.1542/peds.2005-2857
229. Fournier SB, D'errico JN, Stapleton PA. Engineered nanomaterial applications in perinatal therapeutics. *Pharmacol Res.* (2018) 130:36–43. doi: 10.1016/j.phrs.2018.02.027
230. Menezes V, Malek A, Keelan JA. Nanoparticulate drug delivery in pregnancy: placental passage and fetal exposure. *Curr Pharm Biotechnol.* (2011) 12:731–42. doi: 10.2174/138920111795471010
231. Campagnolo L, Massimiani M, Vecchione L, Piccirilli D, Toschi N, Magrini A, et al. Silver nanoparticles inhaled during pregnancy reach and affect the placenta and the foetus. *Nanotoxicology.* (2017) 11:687–98. doi: 10.1080/17435390.2017.1343875
232. Gruber M, Birner-Grünberger R, Wadsack C. Altered kinetics of nanoparticles in the presence of plasma proteins at the human placental barrier. an *ex-vivo* placental perfusion and proteomics approach. *Placenta.* (2017) 57:294–5. doi: 10.1016/j.placenta.2017.07.224
233. Lei J, Rosenzweig JM, Mishra MK, Alshehri W, Brancusi F, Mclane M, et al. Maternal dendrimer-based therapy for inflammation-induced preterm birth and perinatal brain injury. *Sci Rep.* (2017) 7:6106. doi: 10.1038/s41598-017-06113-2
234. Van Steenwinckel J, Schang A-L, Krishnan ML, Degos V, Delahaye-Duriez A, Bokobza C, et al. Loss of the Wnt/β-catenin pathway in microglia of the developing brain drives proinflammatory activation leading to white matter injury. *bioRXiv* [Preprint]. (2018). doi: 10.1101/334359
235. O'connell BA, Moritz KM, Walker DW, Dickinson H. Sexually dimorphic placental development throughout gestation in the spiny mouse (*Acomys cahirinus*). *Placenta.* (2013) 34:119–26. doi: 10.1016/j.placenta.2012.11.009
236. Singh M, Rajagopalan A, Kim TS, Hwang D, Chui H, Zhang XL, et al. Co-registration of *in-vivo* human MRI brain images to postmortem histological microscopic images. *Int J Imaging Syst Technol.* (2008) 18:325–35. doi: 10.1002/ima.20168
237. Chung K, Wallace J, Kim SY, Kalyanasundaram S, Andalman AS, Davidson TJ, et al. Structural and molecular interrogation of intact biological systems. *Nature.* (2013) 497:332–7. doi: 10.1038/nature12107
238. Stolp HB, Ball G, So PW, Tournier JD, Jones M, Thornton C, et al. Voxel-wise comparisons of cellular microstructure and diffusion-MRI in mouse hippocampus using 3D Bridging of Optically-clear histology with Neuroimaging Data (3D-BOND). *Sci Rep.* (2018) 8:4011. doi: 10.1038/s41598-018-22295-9
239. Ball G, Srinivasan L, Aljabar P, Counsell SJ, Durighel G, Hajnal JV, et al. Development of cortical microstructure in the preterm human brain. *Proc Natl Acad Sci USA.* (2013) 110:9541–6. doi: 10.1073/pnas.1301652110
240. Kelly CE, Thompson DK, Chen J, Leemans A, Adamson CL, Inder TE, et al. Axon density and axon orientation dispersion in children born preterm. *Hum Brain Mapp.* (2016) 37:3080–102. doi: 10.1002/hbm.23227

241. Gore JC. Principles and practice of functional MRI of the human brain. *J Clin Invest.* (2003) 112:4–9. doi: 10.1172/JCI200319010
242. Meek J. Basic principles of optical imaging and application to the study of infant development. *Dev Sci.* (2002) 5:371–80. doi: 10.1111/1467-7687.00376
243. Nakamura S, Walker DW, Wong FY. Cerebral haemodynamic response to somatosensory stimulation in neonatal lambs. *J Physiol.* (2017) 595:6007–21. doi: 10.1113/JP274244
244. Nakamura S, Walker DW, Wong FY. Cerebral haemodynamic response to somatosensory stimulation in near-term fetal sheep. *J Physiol.* (2017) 595:1289–303. doi: 10.1113/JP273163
245. Mace E, Montaldo G, Cohen I, Baulac M, Fink M, Tanter M. Functional ultrasound imaging of the brain. *Nat Methods.* (2011) 8:662–4. doi: 10.1038/nmeth.1641
246. Demene C, Baranger J, Bernal M, Delanoe C, Auvin S, Biran V, et al. Functional ultrasound imaging of brain activity in human newborns. *Sci Transl Med.* (2017) 9:eaah6756. doi: 10.1126/scitranslmed.aah6756
247. Deffieux T, Demene C, Pernot M, Tanter M. Functional ultrasound neuroimaging: a review of the preclinical and clinical state of the art. *Curr Opin Neurobiol.* (2018) 50:128–35. doi: 10.1016/j.conb.2018.02.001
248. Berkman BE, Bayefsky M. Prenatal whole genome sequencing: an argument for professional self-regulation. *Am J Bioeth.* (2017) 17:26–8. doi: 10.1080/15265161.2016.1251653
249. Chen SC, Wasserman DT. A framework for unrestricted prenatal whole-genome sequencing: respecting and enhancing the autonomy of prospective parents. *Am J Bioeth.* (2017) 17:3–18. doi: 10.1080/15265161.2016.1251632
250. Rhodes R. Resisting paternalism in prenatal whole-genome sequencing. *Am J Bioeth.* (2017) 17:35–7. doi: 10.1080/15265161.2016.1251662
251. Norton ME, Jacobsson B, Swamy GK, Laurent LC, Ranzini AC, Brar H, et al. Cell-free DNA analysis for noninvasive examination of trisomy. *N Engl J Med.* (2015) 372:1589–97. doi: 10.1056/NEJMoa1407349
252. Artieri CG, Haverty C, Evans EA, Goldberg JD, Haque IS, Yaron Y, et al. Noninvasive prenatal screening at low fetal fraction: comparing whole-genome sequencing and single-nucleotide polymorphism methods. *Prenat Diagn.* (2017) 37:482–90. doi: 10.1002/pd.5036
253. Luo S, Fu C, Zhang S, Wang J, Fan X, Luo J, et al. Application of SNP-array technology in the genetic analysis of pediatric patients with growth retardation. *Zhonghua Yi Xue Yi Chuan Xue Za Zhi.* (2017) 34:321–6. doi: 10.3760/cma.j.issn.1003-9406.2017.03.002
254. Srebniak M, Boter M, Oudesluijs G, Joosten M, Govaerts L, Van Opstal D, et al. Application of SNP array for rapid prenatal diagnosis: implementation, genetic counselling and diagnostic flow. *Eur J Hum Genet.* (2011) 19:1230–7. doi: 10.1038/ejhg.2011.119
255. Krishnan ML, Wang Z, Silver M, Boardman JP, Ball G, Counsell SJ, et al. Possible relationship between common genetic variation and white matter development in a pilot study of preterm infants. *Brain Behav.* (2016) 6:e00434. doi: 10.1002/brb3.434
256. Krishnan ML, Wang Z, Aljabar P, Ball G, Mirza G, Saxena A, et al. Machine learning shows association between genetic variability in PPARG and cerebral connectivity in preterm infants. *Proc Natl Acad Sci USA.* (2017) 114:13744–9. doi: 10.1073/pnas.1704907114
257. Krishnan ML, Van Steenwinckel J, Schang AL, Yan J, Arnadottir J, Le Charpentier T, et al. Integrative genomics of microglia implicates DLG4 (PSD95) in the white matter development of preterm infants. *Nat Commun.* (2017) 8:428. doi: 10.1038/s41467-017-00422-w
258. Freudenberg-Hua Y, Li W, Davies P. The role of genetics in advancing precision medicine for alzheimer's disease-a narrative review. *Front Med.* (2018) 5:108. doi: 10.3389/fmed.2018.00108

9

More Maternal Vascular Malperfusion and Chorioamnionitis in Placentas after Expectant Management vs. Immediate Delivery in Fetal Growth Restriction at (Near) Term: A Further Analysis of the DIGITAT Trial

Marjon E. Feenstra[1†], Mirthe H. Schoots[2†], Torsten Plösch[1], Jelmer R. Prins[1], Sicco A. Scherjon[1], Albertus Timmer[2], Harry van Goor[2] and Sanne J. Gordijn[1]*

[1] *Department of Obstetrics and Gynecology, University Medical Center Groningen, University of Groningen, Groningen, Netherlands,*
[2] *Department of Pathology and Medical Biology, University Medical Center Groningen, University of Groningen, Groningen, Netherlands*

Correspondence:
Sanne J. Gordijn
s.j.gordijn@umcg.nl

† These authors have contributed equally to this work as first authors

Objective: Management of late fetal growth restriction (FGR) is limited to adequate fetal monitoring and optimal timing of delivery. The *Disproportionate Intrauterine Growth Intervention Trial At Term* (DIGITAT) trial compared induction of labor with expectant management in pregnancies at (near) term complicated by suspected FGR. Findings of the DIGITAT trial were that expectant monitoring prolonged pregnancy for 10 days and increased birth weight with only 130 grams. This resulted in more infants born below the 2.3rd percentile compared to induction of labor, respectively, 12.5% in induction of labor and 30.6% in expectant monitoring group. The main placental lesions associated with FGR are maternal vascular malperfusion, fetal vascular malperfusion, and villitis of unknown etiology. We investigated whether placentas of pregnancies complicated with FGR in the expectant monitoring group reveal more and more severe pathology due to pregnancy prolongation.

Material and methods: The DIGITAT trial was a multicenter, randomized controlled trial with suspected FGR beyond 36 + 0 weeks. We now analyzed all available cases ($n = 191$) for placental pathology. The macroscopic details were collected and histological slides were recorded and classified by a single perinatal pathologist, blinded for pregnancy details and outcome. The different placental lesions were scored based on the latest international criteria for placental lesions as defined in the Amsterdam Placental Workshop Group Consensus Statement.

Results: The presence of maternal vascular malperfusion and chorioamnionitis were higher in the expectant management group ($p < 0.05$ and $p < 0.01$, respectively). No differences in placental weight and maturation of the placenta between the induction of labor and the expectant management group were seen. Fetal vascular malperfusion, villitis of unknown etiology and nucleated red blood cell count did not differ between the groups.

Conclusion: Expectant management of late FGR is associated with increased maternal vascular malperfusion and chorioamnionitis. This may have implications for fetal and neonatal outcome, such as programming in the developing child influencing health outcomes later in life.

Keywords: fetal growth restriction, placental pathology, DIGITAT trial, maternal vascular malperfusion, chorioamnionitis

INTRODUCTION

Fetal growth restriction (FGR) is a condition in pregnancy in which the fetus fails to reach its growth potential. FGR affects up to 15% of all pregnancies (1, 2) and is not only associated with mortality, but also with long term morbidity (3–5). Appropriate placental nutrient and oxygen supply is essential for normal fetal growth. The origin of placental insufficiency is multifactorial (6, 7). Several types of lesions can be found in placentas of pregnancies complicated by FGR (7–9). The main placental lesions found in FGR placentas are maternal vascular malperfusion, fetal vascular malperfusion, and villitis of unknown etiology (9). Elevated nucleated red blood cells are considered as an indication of fetal hypoxia (10, 11). Other rare findings in placentas of FGR complicated pregnancies include chronic histiocytic intervillositis and massive perivillous fibrinoid deposition (12, 13).

Until now, adequate fetal monitoring and optimal timing of delivery are the only possible interventions for FGR as other therapeutic options are lacking (14). Timing of delivery in case of FGR is balanced between (relative) prematurity on the one side and prolonged undernutrition/hypoxia on the other side. The DIGITAT study investigated whether timely delivery in (near) term FGR would result in better outcomes. The primary analysis (36 + 0 till 41 + 0 weeks of gestation) showed equivalence in composite neonatal outcome between expectant monitoring and induction of labor (15, 16). Sub analysis revealed that the optimal time to minimize neonatal consequences is delivery around 38 weeks of gestation, when benefits of a planned delivery outweigh consequences of prolongation of pregnancy, as this is associated with a longer exposure to a malnourished environment (17). The DIGITAT trial found that expectant monitoring resulted in a pregnancy prolongation of a further 10 days compared to those in the immediate induction group. This was associated with an increase of only 130 grams in the birth weight of those expectantly managed and a higher proportion of infants born below the 2.3 percentile (30.6% compared to 12.5% in the immediate induction of labor group).

In this study we investigate whether placentas of pregnancies complicated with FGR at (near) term show specific features due to prolongation of pregnancy. The aim of this study is to assess the structural impact on the placenta when pregnancy is prolonged in FGR at term.

MATERIALS AND METHODS

DIGITAT-Original Study Design

The *Disproportionate Intrauterine Growth Intervention Trial At Term* (DIGITAT) trial was a multicenter, randomized controlled trial of women pregnant with a singleton fetus with suspected FGR from 36 + 0 till 41 + 0 weeks of gestation onwards. Details of the DIGITAT trial protocol have been described elsewhere (15). In brief, consenting and eligible women were randomized to either expectant monitoring or induction of labor. The expectant monitoring group was monitored until the onset of spontaneous delivery or when for other reasons than suspected FGR an indication for delivery became apparent. In the induction of labor group delivery was induced within 48 h after randomization (17, 18).

Data Collection of Further Analysis (Current Study)

All participating hospitals in the DIGITAT trial were asked to evaluate whether the placentas of their trial participants had been examined by a local pathologist. If so, all available material such as pathology reports, histologic slides, and tissue blocks were collected and re-analyzed. The analyses included details of the macroscopic description of the placental disk, membranes and umbilical cord as described in the placental pathology report.

Furthermore, the histologic slides, routinely stained with Hematoxylin and Eosin (H&E) were revised, scored and classified to latest international criteria (9) by a single perinatal pathologist (MS), who was blinded for pregnancy details and outcome.

Placental Histology

The various placental lesions were evaluated based on the latest international criteria for placental lesions as described in the Amsterdam Placental Workshop Group Consensus Statement (9). Lesions evaluated were placental pathology consistent with maternal vascular malperfusion (MVM), fetal vascular malperfusion (FVM), chorioamnionitis (CA), villitis of unknown etiology (VUE), elevated nucleated red blood cell count (NRBC), chronic histiocytic intervillositis (CHI), and massive perivillous fibrin deposition (MPVFD). Also, if available, placental weight, placental weight percentile, birth weight placenta weight ratio (BWPW) (19), umbilical cord length and coiling index were included in the analyzes. The coiling index was calculated by dividing the number of whole coils by the umbilical cord length in centimeters. A normal coiling index is considered to be between 0.1 and 0.3. Due to the retrospective nature of this analysis unfortunately no other placental characteristic data (like the extension of infarction) were available.

Statistical Analysis

SPSS 24.0 software for Windows (SPSS Inc. Chicago, IL) was used for the statistical analyses. Continued variables were evaluated with a two-tailed unpaired T-test and binary or categorical variables were evaluated with a Fisher Exact Test. Statistical significance was assumed at $p < 0.05$.

RESULTS

A total of 191 cases were available for review of placental pathology, respectively, 97 (321 in the original DIGITAT trail) participants in the induction of labor group and 94 (329 in original DIGITAT trail) participants in the expectant monitoring group.

In contrast to the original DIGITAT study the baseline characteristics of the two groups were statistically different for parity, maternal smoking and BMI (**Table 1**). Similar to the original DIGITAT study gestational hypertension was significantly higher in the expectant monitoring group. In the DIGITAT trial pre-eclampsia was more prominent in the expectant monitoring group than in the induction of labor group, but in our cohort of this re-analysis no significant difference was seen in the presence of pre-eclampsia.

Most women in the current analysis met the DIGITAT study criteria of FGR by combinations of inclusion criteria, usually by a fetal abdominal circumference (AC) below the 10th percentile (respectively $n = 74$ in induction of labor and $n = 77$ in expectant monitoring) and/or an estimated fetal weight (EFW) below the 10th percentile (respectively $n = 92$ in the induction of labor and $n = 72$ in the expectant monitoring). Furthermore, a decline in AC growth was also a criterium for study inclusion (not as a single criterium, but in combination with either AC or EFW below p10) and was differently observed between the groups, with a higher presence in the expectant monitoring group (induction of labor was $n = 14$ and expectant monitoring $n = 24$; $p < 0.05$) (**Table 1**).

In the expectant monitoring group in 51 of the 94 cases labor was induced due to either maternal indication (8), fetal indication (20), combined maternal and fetal indication (4), or rupture of membranes (2) (**Table 1**).

In the current analysis, women in the expectant monitoring group had a longer gestational age (8 days), compared to the induction of labor group ($p < 0.01$). This is slightly less prolongation than in the original DIGITAT study in which pregnancy was prolonged by 10 days. Birth weight in the study population of this sub analysis was not significantly different between the groups. However, there was a difference of 60 grams between the expectant management and induction of labor, which means a weight gain of 60 grams in the achieved 8 days of pregnancy prolongation. This is also slightly less than in the original DIGITAT study (with 130 grams weight gain in 10 days) (**Table 1**). The average neonatal stay in hospital was approximately 8 days in both groups. A few cases needed admission to the neonatal intensive care unit, significantly more in the expectant monitoring group ($p < 0.05$). The length of stay in the neonatal intensive care unit was approximately 6 days for both groups. There were no neonatal deaths reported in both groups.

Placental Characteristics

In **Table 2** placental characteristics are described of both the induction of labor group and the expectant monitoring group. No differences in placental weight, umbilical cord length, coiling index and BWPW ratio were found between the two groups.

Placental Histology

The findings of placental histology in both groups are described in **Table 3**. Maturation of the placenta was similar in both groups. Maternal vascular malperfusion (MVM) was significantly higher in the expectant monitoring group compared to the induction of labor group ($p < 0.05$). Fetal vascular malperfusion (FVM) was similar in both groups. In placentas from the expectant monitoring group we found a significantly higher incidence of chorioamnionitis (CA) ($p < 0.01$). The presence of villitis of unknown etiology (VUE) and the nucleated red blood cell count (NRBC) was similar in both groups. Rare placental findings like chronic histiocytic intervillositis (CHI) and massive perivillous fibrinoid deposition (MPFD) were seen in a few cases ($n = 2$ for CHI in the induction group and 0 in the expectant monitoring group; $n = 4$ and $n = 1$ for MPFD in the induction group and expectant monitoring group, respectively).

DISCUSSION

In this sub analysis of the DIGITAT study we found that maternal vascular malperfusion (MVM) occurred significantly more often in the expectant monitoring group in comparison to the induction of labor group ($p < 0.05$) in (near) term FGR. Moreover, participants in the expectant monitoring group had a significantly higher incidence of chorioamnionitis (CA) ($p < 0.01$). The DIGITAT trial previously showed no differences in composite neonatal outcome between expectant monitoring and induction of labor, however, it was seen that the average weight gain was only 130 grams in 10 days delivery delay, which resulted in more babies born with a birth weight below the p2.3. The follow up study of the original DIGITAT trial at 2 years of age showed that babies born with a birth weight below p2.3 scored lower at the ages and stages questionnaire (ASQ) for developmental disorders.

MVM occurs early in pregnancy and is likely due to maladaptation of the spiral arteries. It develops over time when gestation prolongs (21, 22). By inadequate remodeling of spiral arteries a high resistance flow induces shear stress and damage to parenchyma, like infarctions, and differences in oxygen tension leading to oxidative stress and free radical damage (12, 22–25). The higher prevalence of MVM in the expectant monitoring group could be caused by a prolonged time of hypoxia caused by inadequate maternal vascularization. This could further lead to increase in cellular stress, e.g., oxidative stress and endoplasmic reticulum (ER) stress. This may ultimately lead to an increase in the occurrence of FGR and development of preeclampsia (23–26).

To support this theory of prolonged exposure to a pathologic environment, a significant higher prevalence of the development of gestational hypertension in the expectant monitoring group was seen. MVM has been described to be causal in gestational hypertension and preeclampsia (20, 27). This finding further strengthens the clinical experience that expectant monitoring or prolongation of pregnancy in FGR at (near) term is not without

TABLE 1 | Demographic and baseline characteristics of the selected randomized participants for this analysis of placental pathology in FGR at term.

Baseline characteristics	Induction of labor ($n = 97$)	Expectant monitoring ($n = 94$)	Sig.
Nulliparous (%)	48	37	$p = 0.013$
Maternal age (years)	28.07 ± 5.58	27.65 ± 5.41	$p = 0.500$
BMI at study entry (kg/m^2)	24.31 ± 6.09	23.18 ± 4.82	$p = 0.024$
Maternal smoking	58	39	$p = 0.010$
Gestational hypertension	7	13	$p = 0.035$
Pre-eclampsia	6	9	$p = 0.150$
INCLUSION CRITERIA			
Fetal abdominal circumference <10th percentile	76	82	$p = 0.211$
Estimated fetal weight <10th percentile	95	76	$p = 0.224$
Deceleration of fetal abdominal circumference curve	14	26	$p = 0.038$
MODE OF DELIVERY			
Induced labor	95	51	$p = 0.001$
Vaginal delivery	43	39	$p = 0.100$
Vaginal instrumental	33	34	$p = 0.352$
Cesarean section	24	27	$p = 0.248$
NEONATAL CHARACTERISTICS			
Gestational age at birth (days)	264 ± 7.71	272 ± 9.27	$p = 0.010$
Birth weight (grams)	2242.23 ± 285	2303.10 ± 365	$p = 0.065$
Length of neonatal stay in hospital (days)	8.9 ± 7.00	9.1 ± 8.41	$p = 0.690$
Admission to the neonatal intensive care unit (NICU)	2	5	$p = 0.020$

Data is presented as proportion, unless stated otherwise in the table. Significance is presented as p-value, a $p < 0.05$ is assumed significant.

TABLE 2 | Comparison of placental characteristics between the induction of labor and expectant monitoring group in FGR at term.

Placental characteristics	Induction of labor ($n = 97$)	Expectant monitoring ($n = 94$)	Sig.
Placental weight (grams)	371.49 ± 15.50	361.40 ± 15.54	$p = 0.707$
Umbilical cord length (cm)	35.44 ± 1.92	35.36 ± 1.93	$p = 0.789$
Coiling index	0.35 ± 0.189	0.30 ± 0.216	$p = 0.483$
Birth Weight to Placental Weight ratio (BWPW)	6.29 ± 1.336	6.71 ± 1.787	$p = 0.284$

Data is presented as mean. Significance is presented as p-value, a $p < 0.05$ is assumed significant. No statistical differences were found in placental characteristics.

TABLE 3 | The comparison of placental pathology between induction of labor and expectant monitoring in FGR at term.

Placental histology	Induction of labor ($n = 97$)	Expectant monitoring ($n = 94$)	Sig.
Maturation matching gestational age (MAT)	89	82	$p = 0.701$
Maternal vascular malperfusion (MVM)	9	17	$p = 0.049$
Fetal vascular malperfusion (FVM)	10	16	$p = 0.069$
Chorioamnionitis (CA)	13	32	$p = 0.010$
Villitis of unknown etiology (VUE)	29	30	$p = 0.507$
Elevated nucleated Red Blood Cell Count (NRBC)	2	3	$p = 0.485$
Chronic histiocytic intervillositis (CHI)	2	0	$p = 0.257$
Massive perivillous fibrinoid deposition (MPFD)	4	1	$p = 0.194$

Data is presented as proportion in the table. Significance is presented as p-value, a $p < 0.05$ is considered significant.

risks especially for the mother (28), even though on short term no differences were seen in neonatal outcome. A study from Parra-Saavedra et al. implies in a group of late onset Small-for-Gestational Age (SGA) that placental under perfusion (PUP) can also lead to higher neonatal morbidity; in this study in 77/84 placentas maternal vascular supply was—as in our study-compromised (29). Furthermore, similar to the original study, in this sub-study a large group of women had labor induced although being allocated to the expectant monitoring group (51/94: 66%), indicating that the difference between the groups in MVM is in fact an underestimation of what would really happen when delivery was awaited.

The histologic diagnosis of chorioamnionitis (CA) is made when an inflammatory infiltrate is seen in the chorioamniotic membranes. At term CA is most frequently induced by inflammation and cellular stress, in the absence of a microorganism (30). During labor the uteroplacental blood flow is compromised leading to hypoxia of the placenta and its membranes. This leads to an increase in pro-inflammatory markers in the placenta. In fact, labor at term has been associated with infiltration of inflammatory cells in the placenta and higher plasma levels of pro-inflammatory chemokines and cytokines, such as Interleukin 6 (IL-6), Interleukin 8 (IL-8), and Tumor Necrosis Factor alpha (TNF-alpha) (30–32). Hypothetically, the inflammatory response in the chorioamniotic membranes and cervix could be the result of an increase in pro-inflammatory cytokines caused by cellular stress, e.g., oxidative stress and ER stress (23, 24, 33, 34).

Furthermore, even though in the expectant monitoring group labor was often induced, significantly more spontaneous deliveries took place in the expectant monitoring group. Recent studies showed a higher incidence of histological chorioamnionitis in spontaneous labor compared to, respectively, induced labor, or cesarean section (33, 35). This could be an additional explanation for the significantly higher incidence of chorioamnionitis in the expectant monitoring group.

In our analysis, we observed a higher prevalence of CA in the expectant monitoring group. As described above, this is conceivably explained by increase of pro-inflammatory cytokines due to the prolonged hypoxic environment.

The incidence of fetal vascular malperfusion (FVM) was not significantly different although a higher number of cases were seen in the expectant monitoring group in comparison with induction of labor.

Like MVM, FVM has been associated with fetal growth restriction (FGR) due to decreased availability of functional parenchyma (36). The etiology of FVM is however multifactorial and not specifically related to FGR. FVM has been associated with multiple factors as placental (for example umbilical cord pathology), maternal (for example preeclampsia), and fetal (for example cardiac malformations) etiologies (6, 37, 38). Also, intra-amniotic infection with a fetal response (vasculitis) and chronic villitis of unknown etiology (VUE) are known associations (39).

In our study, villitis of unknown etiology (VUE) occurred in approximately 30% of all cases, distributed equally between both randomized groups. In existing literature, a broad range of incidences of VUE is described, partly because the definition has not been uniform and also due to differences in sampling of placental parenchyma (40–43). With an equal distribution between our groups, we conclude that prolonged pregnancy in the expectant monitoring group is not associated with an increased prevalence of VUE.

At term, normally only a small number of circulating nucleated red blood cells (NRBCs) are seen in the fetal circulation, if any (11). In response to fetal hypoxia the NRBC count increases (10, 11). In our study, only a few cases showed elevated NRBCs, suggesting that fetal monitoring to prevent fetal hypoxia has been adequate in the two randomized groups as no differences were seen in number of cases with elevated NRBCs.

In addition to the placental lesions described above, we also investigated the presence of chronic histiocytic intervillositis (CHI), massive perivillous fibrinoid deposition (MPFD), and maternal floor infarction (MFI). These are rare placental lesions, associated with (severe) FGR, with high recurrence risks (12, 13, 44–47). In our analyses, we found 2 cases of CHI in the induction of labor group and none in the expectant monitoring group. Five cases of MPFD were encountered, four of which in the induction of labor group and one in the expectant monitoring group. No cases with maternal floor infarction (MFI) were found in the total study population. No significant differences were seen between the induction of labor group and the expectant monitoring group for CHI and MPFD.

We did not find any differences in placental weight or birth weight to placental weight ratio (BWPW ratio) (**Table 2**). It has been described that placental weight from fetuses with FGR is significantly lower than placentas from fetuses with a normal birth weight and that the BWPW ratio is higher, although in fact fetal weight per placental unit is high and the placenta performed well in that sense. A low BWPW ration (a relatively low fetal weight per placental unit) has also been described in relation to adverse outcome (19). Given the fact that pregnancy prolongation resulted in only little weight gain and placental weights were not different the BWPW ratio was, as expected lower (although not significant) in the induction group (8, 48, 49).

CONCLUSION

Placental pathology in FGR encompasses a broad group of diagnoses, not exclusive for FGR. Our study shows that expectant monitoring is associated with a higher incidence of maternal vascular malperfusion (MVM) and chorioamnionitis (CA), whilst fetal vascular malperfusion, severe acute fetal hypoxia and villitis of unknown etiology are similar in both groups. This study further strengthens the results from a previous sub-analysis that prolongation of gestation has no additional benefits and even increases the prevalence of MVM and CA in FGR; both placental findings are associated with an increase in children born with severe growth restriction and are possibly associated with unfavorable outcome at later ages.

Strengths and Limitations of the Study

The strengths of this study are a dedicated, uniform examination of the placentas, done by one perinatal pathologist unaware of clinical details, by the latest criteria, in a large number of placentas from pregnancies complicated with FGR. In this sub-study prolongation of pregnancy is 2 days less than the original DIGITAT study and the weight gain in that period is on average less per day (13 grams per day in the original study vs. 7.5 grams in this study). This combined with the fact that more inclusions showed a decline in AC growth than the original study and finally that more inductions in the expectant management group of this analysis (66%) occurred than in the original study (25.5%) indicates that there is probably an inclusion bias with the more severe cases included in the study. We however believe that this inclusion bias does not undermine the results of this study. In the induction group there may also be a similar trend in sending more placenta's of clinically severe cases to the pathologist than the clinically less severe cases. A limitation of this study is that only 29% cases of the original DIGITAT trial were included, due to the availability of placental histological samples, which were collected from all participating hospitals in the Netherlands. We believe it is of great importance to analyze the placenta histopathology for understanding the underlying pathophysiology, especially in cases of FGR in which a common mechanism is placental insufficiency. All in all, we found that expectant management of late FGR is associated with increased maternal vascular malperfusion and chorioamnionitis. Further studies on the clinical implications of these findings are warranted.

AUTHOR CONTRIBUTIONS

MF, MS, JP, TP, SS, AT, HvG, and SG contributed to the design and implementation of the research, to the analysis of the results, and to the writing of the manuscript.

REFERENCES

1. Cuffe JSM, Holland O, Salomon C, Rice GE, Perkins AV. Review: placental derived biomarkers of pregnancy disorders. *Placenta.* (2017) 54:104–10. doi: 10.1016/j.placenta.2017.01.119
2. Gordijn SJ, Beune IM, Thilaganathan B, Papageorghiou A, Baschat AA, Baker PN, et al. Consensus definition of fetal growth restriction: a Delphi procedure. *Ultrasound Obstet Gynecol.* (2016) 48:333–9. doi: 10.1002/uog.15884
3. Barker DJ, Osmond C, Law CM. The intrauterine and early postnatal origins of cardiovascular disease and chronic bronchitis. *J Epidemiol Community Health.* (1989) 43:237–40. doi: 10.1136/jech.43.3.237
4. De Jong M, Cranendonk A, Van Weissenbruch MM. Components of the metabolic syndrome in early childhood in very-low-birth-weight infants and term small and appropriate for gestational age infants. *Pediatr Res.* (2015) 78:457–61. doi: 10.1038/pr.2015.118
5. Drillten CM. A longitudinal study of the growth and development of prematurely and maturely born children. *Arch Dis Child.* (1961) 36:233–40. doi: 10.1136/adc.36.187.233
6. Mifsud W, Sebire NJ. Placental pathology in early-onset and late-onset fetal growth restriction. *Fetal Diagn Ther.* (2014) 36:117–28. doi: 10.1159/000359969
7. Salafia CM, Charles AK, Maas EM. Placenta and fetal growth restriction. *Clin Obstet Gynecol.* (2006) 49:236–56. doi: 10.1097/00003081-200606000-00007
8. Vedmedovska N, Rezeberga D, Teibe U, Melderis I, Donders GGG. Placental pathology in fetal growth restriction. *Eur J Obstet Gynecol Reprod Biol.* (2011) 155:36–40. doi: 10.1016/j.ejogrb.2010.11.017
9. Khong TY, Mooney EE, Ariel I, Balmus NCM, Boyd TK, Brundler MA, et al. Sampling and definitions of placental lesions Amsterdam placental workshop group consensus statement. *Arch Pathol Lab Med.* (2016) 140:698–713. doi: 10.5858/arpa.2015-0225-CC
10. Redline RW. Elevated circulating fetal nucleated red blood cells and placental pathology in term infants who develop cerebral palsy. *Hum Pathol.* (2008) 39:1378–84. doi: 10.1016/j.humpath.2008.01.017
11. Hermansen MC. Nucleated red blood cells in the fetus and newborn. *Arch Dis Child Fetal Neonatal Ed.* (2001) 84:F211–5. doi: 10.1136/fn.84.3.F211
12. Katzman PJ, Genest DR. Maternal floor infarction and massive perivillous fibrin deposition: histological definitions, association with intrauterine fetal growth restriction, and risk of recurrence. *Pediatr Dev Pathol.* (2002) 5:159–64. doi: 10.1007/s10024001-0195-y
13. Parant O, Capdet J, Kessler S, Aziza J, Berrebi A. Chronic intervillositis of unknown etiology (CIUE): relation between placental lesions and perinatal outcome. *Eur J Obstet Gynecol Reprod Biol.* (2009) 143:9–13. doi: 10.1016/j.ejogrb.2008.06.012
14. Pels A, Kenny LC, Alfirevic Z, Baker PN, von Dadelszen P, Gluud C, et al. STRIDER (Sildenafil TheRapy in dismal prognosis early onset fetal growth restriction): an international consortium of randomised placebo-controlled trials. *BMC Pregnancy Childbirth.* (2017) 17:440. doi: 10.1186/s12884-017-1594-z
15. Boers KE, Bijlenga D, Mol BWJ, LeCessie S, Birnie E, van Pampus MG, et al. Disproportionate intrauterine growth intervention trial at term: DIGITAT. *BMC Pregnancy Childbirth.* (2007) 7:12. doi: 10.1186/1471-2393-7-12
16. Boers KE, Vijgen SMC, Bijlenga D, Van Der Post JAM, Bekedam DJ, Kwee A, et al. Induction versus expectant monitoring for intrauterine growth restriction at term: randomised equivalence trial (DIGITAT). *Br Med J.* (2011) 342:35. doi: 10.1136/bmj.c7087
17. Boers KE, Van Wyk L, Van Der Post JAM, Kwee A, Van Pampus MG, Spaanderdam MEA, et al. Neonatal morbidity after induction vs expectant monitoring in intrauterine growth restriction at term: a subanalysis of the DIGITAT RCT. *Obstet Gynecol Surv.* (2012) 67:389–91. doi: 10.1097/01.ogx.0000418566.91278.43
18. Tajik P, Van Wyk L, Boers KE, Le Cessie S, Zafarmand MH, Roumen F, et al. Which intrauterine growth restricted fetuses at term benefit from early labour induction? A secondary analysis of the DIGITAT randomised trial. *Eur J Obstet Gynecol Reprod Biol.* (2014) 172:20–5. doi: 10.1016/j.ejogrb.2013.10.014
19. Salavati N, Gordijn SJ, Sovio U, Zill-E-Huma R, Gebril A, Charnock-Jones DS, et al. Birth weight to placenta weight ratio and its relationship to ultrasonic measurements, maternal and neonatal morbidity: a prospective cohort study of nulliparous women. *Placenta.* (2017) 63:45–52. doi: 10.1016/j.placenta.2017.11.008
20. Kovo M, Bar J, Schreiber L, Shargorodsky M. The relationship between hypertensive disorders in pregnancy and placental maternal and fetal vascular circulation. *J Am Soc Hypertens.* (2017) 11:724–9. doi: 10.1016/j.jash.2017.09.001
21. Ernst LM. Maternal vascular malperfusion of the placental bed. *Apmis.* (2018) 126:551–60. doi: 10.1111/apm.12833
22. Parks WT. Placental hypoxia: the lesions of maternal malperfusion. *Semin Perinatol.* (2015) 39:9–19. doi: 10.1053/j.semperi.2014.10.003
23. Burton GJ, Yung HW, Cindrova-Davies T, Charnock-Jones DS. Placental endoplasmic reticulum stress and oxidative stress in the pathophysiology of unexplained intrauterine growth restriction and early onset preeclampsia. *Placenta.* (2009) 30:43–8. doi: 10.1016/j.placenta.2008.11.003
24. Burton GJ, Jauniaux E. Oxidative stress. *Best Pract Res Clin Obstet Gynaecol.* (2011) 25:287–99. doi: 10.1016/j.bpobgyn.2010.10.016
25. Schoots MH, Gordijn SJ, Scherjon SA, van Goor H, Hillebrands JL. Oxidative stress in placental pathology. *Placenta.* (2018) 69:153–61. doi: 10.1016/j.placenta.2018.03.003
26. Hempstock J, Jauniaux E, Greenwold N, Burton GJ. The contribution of placental oxidative stress to early pregnancy failure. *Hum Pathol.* (2003) 34:1265–75. doi: 10.1016/j.humpath.2003.08.006
27. Scifres CM, Parks WT, Feghali M, Caritis SN, Catov JM. Placental maternal vascular malperfusion and adverse pregnancy outcomes in gestational diabetes mellitus. *Placenta.* (2017) 49:10–5. doi: 10.1016/j.placenta.2016.11.004
28. Koopmans CM, Bijlenga D, Groen H, Vijgen SM, Aarnoudse JG, Bekedam DJ, et al. Induction of labour versus expectant monitoring for gestational hypertension or mild pre-eclampsia after 36 weeks' gestation (HYPITAT): a multicentre, open-label randomised controlled trial. *Lancet.* (2009) 374:979–88. doi: 10.1016/S0140-6736(09)60736-4
29. Parra-Saavedra M, Simeone S, Triunfo S, Crovetto F, Botet F, Gratacos E, et al. Correlation between histological signs of placental underperfusion and perinatal morbidity in late-onset small-for-gestational-age fetuses. *Ultrasound Obstet Gynecol.* (2015) 45:149–55. doi: 10.1002/uog.13415
30. Roberts DJ, Celi AC, Riley LE, Onderdonk AB, Boyd TK, Johnson LC, et al. Acute histologic chorioamnionitis at term: nearly always noninfectious. *PLoS ONE.* (2012) 7:e31819. doi: 10.1371/journal.pone.0031819
31. Challis, J. R., Lockwood, C. J., Myatt, L., Norman, J. E., Strauss J. F. III., and Petraglia, F. (2009). Inflammation in Pregnancy. *Reproductive Sci.* 16, 206–15. doi: 10.1177/1933719108329095
32. Cierny JT, Unal ER, Flood P, Rhee KY, Praktish A, Olson TH, et al. Maternal inflammatory markers and term labor performance. *Am J Obstet Gynecol.* (2014) 210:447.e1–e6. doi: 10.1016/j.ajog.2013.11.038
33. Park HS, Romero R, Lee SM, Park CW, Jun JK, Yoon BH. Histologic chorioamnionitis is more common after spontaneous labor than after induced labor at term. *Placenta.* (2010) 31:792–5. doi: 10.1016/j.placenta.2010.06.013
34. Kim CJ, Romero R, Chaemsiathong P, Chaiyasitt N, Yoon BH, Kim YM. Acute chorioamniotis and funisitis: definition, pathologic features

and clinical significance. *Am J Obstet Gynecol.* (2016) 213:S29–52. doi: 10.1016/j.ajog.2015.08.040

35. Torricelli M, Voltolini C, Conti N, Vellucci FL, Orlandini C, Bocchi C, et al. Histologic chorioamnionitis at term: implications for the progress of labor and neonatal wellbeing. *J Matern Neonatal Med.* (2013) 26:188–92. doi: 10.3109/14767058.2012.722724
36. Heider A. Fetal vascular malperfusion. *Arch Pathol Lab Med.* (2017) 141:1484–9. doi: 10.5858/arpa.2017-0212-RA
37. Saleemuddin A, Tantbirojn P, Sirois K, Crum CP, Boyd TK, Tworoger S, et al. Obstetric and perinatal complications in placentas with fetal thrombotic vasculopathy. *Pediatr Dev Pathol.* (2010) 13:459–64. doi: 10.2350/10-01-0774-OA.1
38. Kovo M, Schreiber L, Elyashiv O, Ben-Haroush A, Abraham G, Bar J. Pregnancy outcome and placental findings in pregnancies complicated by fetal growth restriction with and without preeclampsia. *Reprod Sci.* (2015) 22:316–21. doi: 10.1177/1933719114542024
39. Kovo M, Schreiber L, Ben-Haroush A, Cohen G, Weiner E, Golan A, et al. The placental factor in early- and late-onset normotensive fetal growth restriction. *Placenta.* (2013) 34:320–4. doi: 10.1016/j.placenta.2012.11.010
40. Labarrere CA, Hardin JW, Haas DM, Kassab GS. Chronic villitis of unknown etiology and massive chronic intervillositis have similar immune cell composition. *Placenta.* (2015) 36:681–6. doi: 10.1016/j.placenta.2015.03.008
41. Becroft DM, Thompson JM, Mitchell EA. Placental villitis of unknown origin: epidemiologic associations. *Am J Obstet Gynecol.* (2005) 192:264–71. doi: 10.1016/j.ajog.2004.06.062
42. Iskender C, Zergeroglu S, Kaymak O, Çelen S, Danisman N. Villitis of unknown aetiology: clinical implications in preterm population. *J Obstet Gynaecol.* (2016) 36:192–5. doi: 10.3109/01443615.2015.1036410
43. Derricott H, Jones RL, Heazell AEP. Investigating the association of villitis of unknown etiology with stillbirth and fetal growth restriction - a systematic review. *Placenta.* (2013) 34:856–62. doi: 10.1016/j.placenta.2013.07.003
44. Koby L, Keating S, Malinowski AK, D'Souza R. Chronic histiocytic intervillositis – clinical, biochemical and radiological findings: an observational study. *Placenta.* (2018) 64:1–6. doi: 10.1016/j.placenta.2018.02.002
45. Marchaudon V, Devisme L, Petit S, Ansart-Franquet H, Vaast P, Subtil D. Chronic histiocytic intervillositis of unknown etiology: clinical features in a consecutive series of 69 cases. *Placenta.* (2011) 32:140–5. doi: 10.1016/j.placenta.2010.11.021
46. Bos M, Nikkels PGJ, Cohen D, Schoones JW, Bloemenkamp KWM, Bruijn JA, et al. Towards standardized criteria for diagnosing chronic intervillositis of unknown etiology: a systematic review. *Placenta.* (2018) 61:80–8. doi: 10.1016/j.placenta.2017.11.012
47. Devisme L, Chauvière C, Franquet-Ansart H, Chudzinski A, Stichelbout M, Houfflin-Debarge V, et al. Perinatal outcome of placental massive perivillous fibrin deposition: a case-control study. *Prenat Diagn.* (2017) 37:323–8. doi: 10.1002/pd.5013
48. Ogunyemi D, Murillo M, Jackson U, Hunter N, Alperson B. The relationship between placental histopathology findings and perinatal outcome in preterm infants. *J Matern Neonatal Med.* (2003) 13:102–9. doi: 10.1080/jmf.13.2.102.109
49. Korteweg FJ, Erwich JJHM, Holm JP, Ravisé JM, Van Der Meer J, Veeger NJGM, et al. Diverse placental pathologies as the main causes of fetal death. *Obstet Gynecol.* (2009) 114:809–17. doi: 10.1097/AOG.0b013e3181b72ebe

10

Cardiovascular Programming during and after Diabetic Pregnancy: Role of Placental Dysfunction and IUGR

*Immaculate M. Langmia[1,2,3], Kristin Kräker[1,2,4,5,6], Sara E. Weiss[1,2,4], Nadine Haase[1,2,4,5,6], Till Schütte[2,6,7], Florian Herse[1,2,5] and Ralf Dechend[1,2,4,6,8]**

[1] Experimental and Clinical Research Center, A Joint Cooperation Between the Max-Delbrueck Center for Molecular Medicine and the Charité Universitätsmedizin Berlin, Berlin, Germany, [2] Berlin Institute of Health (BIH), Berlin, Germany, [3] Alexander von Humboldt Foundation, Bonn, Germany, [4] Charité–Universitätsmedizin Berlin, Corporate member of Freie Universität Berlin, Berlin Institute of Health, Humboldt-Universität zu Berlin, Berlin, Germany, [5] Max-Delbrueck Center for Molecular Medicine in the Helmholtz Association, Berlin, Germany, [6] DZHK (German Centre for Cardiovascular Research), Partner Site Berlin, Berlin, Germany, [7] Center for Cardiovascular Research, Institute of Pharmacology, Charité -Universitätsmedizin Berlin, Berlin, Germany, [8] HELIOS-Klinikum, Berlin, Germany

Correspondence:
Ralf Dechend
ralf.dechend@charite.de

Intrauterine growth restriction (IUGR) is a condition whereby a fetus is unable to achieve its genetically determined potential size. IUGR is a global health challenge due to high mortality and morbidity amongst affected neonates. It is a multifactorial condition caused by maternal, fetal, placental, and genetic confounders. Babies born of diabetic pregnancies are usually large for gestational age but under certain conditions whereby prolonged uncontrolled hyperglycemia leads to placental dysfunction, the outcome of the pregnancy is an intrauterine growth restricted fetus with clinical features of malnutrition. Placental dysfunction leads to undernutrition and hypoxia, which triggers gene modification in the developing fetus due to fetal adaptation to adverse *utero* environmental conditions. Thus, *in utero* gene modification results in future cardiovascular programming in postnatal and adult life. Ongoing research aims to broaden our understanding of the molecular mechanisms and pathological pathways involved in fetal programming due to IUGR. There is a need for the development of effective preventive and therapeutic strategies for the management of growth-restricted infants. Information on the mechanisms involved with *in utero* epigenetic modification leading to development of cardiovascular disease in adult life will increase our understanding and allow the identification of susceptible individuals as well as the design of targeted prevention strategies. This article aims to systematically review the latest molecular mechanisms involved in the pathogenesis of IUGR in cardiovascular programming. Animal models of IUGR that used nutrient restriction and hypoxia to mimic the clinical conditions in humans of reduced flow of nutrients and oxygen to the fetus will be discussed in terms of cardiac remodeling and epigenetic programming of cardiovascular disease. Experimental evidence of long-term fetal programming due to IUGR will also be included.

Keywords: diabetes, placental dysfunction, gene modification, intra uterine growth restriction, cardiovascular programming

FETAL CARDIOVASCULAR PROGRAMMING IN CONDITIONS OF PLACENTAL DYSFUNCTION AND IUGR

Cardiovascular disease (CVD) is the main cause of mortality and morbidity in the twenty-first century (1–3). According to the World Health Organization (WHO), coronary heart disease and stroke accounted for ~15.2 million deaths in 2016 globally. Previously, CVD was assumed to be caused by a series of events that occur after birth, such as a person's lifestyle, age, and other disease conditions. In other words, postnatal gene-environment interactions are important factors promoting CVD, but recently we began to understand that *in utero* environmental changes that occur in the first few months of prenatal development epigenetically program the fetus for development of CVD in adulthood (4–6). Therefore, apart from postnatal gene-environment interaction, information on *in utero* gene-environment interactions is needed to improve our understanding of CVD.

The placenta performs many functions ranging from growth of the fetus, prevention of fetal rejection by maternal immune system, as well as the transport/exchange of gases, nutrients, and waste products between mother and fetus (7). In addition, the placenta is involved in metabolism and production of many hormones that play vital roles in the maintenance of pregnancy (7). In a normal pregnancy the placental weight and birth weight are highly correlated (8). In adverse situations where the maternal-fetal circulation is altered due to disease conditions such as diabetes, the development of the placenta also changes (9). The determining factor in placental dysfunction is the extent of exposure to hyperglycemia during fetal and placental development (10). Depending on the degree of hyperglycemia, the growth of the placenta and the fetus can be severely affected (10). Long-term uncontrolled hyperglycemia can lead to placental vascular dysfunction in women suffering from diabetes (10). Endothelial dysfunction was observed in hyperglycemic human umbilical vein cells (HUVEC) compared to control cells (11). According to studies by Starikov et al. pre-gestational diabetes led to placentas that were small for gestational age in 20% of pregnancies and placentas that were large for gestational age in 30% of cases (9). In conditions where maternal hyperglycemia is not controlled, it results in histological changes of the placental tissues (10, 12). Placentas from mothers with diabetes display different histological features such as immature villous, increased number of fetal capillaries, and fibrinoid necrosis of the placental villi (7). Prolonged maternal insults such as hyperglycemia, dyslipidemia, and hyperinsulinemia may exceed the placental capacity to adapt and respond leading to placental dysfunction and adverse fetal outcome such as in IUGR (13, 14). Placental dysfunction is the most common cause of asymmetrical intrauterine growth restriction (15–17). Uteroplacental malperfusion, decidual vasculopathy, placental infarct, and maternal vasculopathy were observed in women with diabetes (12) and are associated with reduced fetal growth and adverse outcome (17, 18). Abnormal placental vascular development decreases normal placental blood supply, leading to reduced oxygen (hypoxia) and nutrient delivery (undernutrition) to the fetus and a subsequent IUGR fetus (16, 17). As a result of reduced oxygen and nutrition, the fetus redistributes its cardiac output to increase oxygen and nutrient supply to the brain, which is referred to as brain sparing (19). This prenatal cerebral circulatory adaptation has been associated with long-term behavioral problems in schoolchildren who were growth-restricted at birth. These difficulties include problems in memory, cognition, motor skills, and neuropsychological malfunction (20). IUGR offspring experience the highest rate of coronary heart disease, myocardial dysfunction, type 2 diabetes, hypertension, and stroke as adults (21, 22). The underlying molecular mechanisms leading to fetal susceptibility to adult disease are still under investigation. Interestingly, we now know that clinical symptoms of cardiovascular disease may not appear until adult life (4). In 1989, David Barker demonstrated this aspect amongst individuals with low birth weight, showing a direct association between low birth weight and CVD in adulthood. This study demonstrated that the incidence of ischemic heart disease and death were three times higher among men with low birth weight compared to men with high birth weight (5). Epidemiological investigations of adults born at the time of the Dutch famine between 1944 and 1945 revealed an association between maternal starvation and a low infant birth weight with a high incidence of hypertension and coronary heart disease in these adults (23). Furthermore, Painter et al. reported the incidence of early onset coronary heart disease among persons conceived during the Dutch famine (24). In that regard, Barker's findings led to the concept of fetal adaptation to prenatal environmental changes and vulnerability to chronic diseases in adult life, a concept known as "fetal programming." In 2003, the concept of "Developmental origins of health and disease (DOHaD)" was published (25). DOHaD describes the scenario whereby *in utero* maternal insults result in structural and functional changes in fetal organs extending in postnatal life and increasing susceptibility of chronic disease in adulthood. Fetal programming of other organs such as the brain (19), lungs (26), and hypothalamic-pituitary-adrenal (HPA) axis have been greatly studied, however the heart is also very important and few studies have investigated fetal programming of the heart as summarized below (27).

FETAL PROGRAMMING OF THE HEART IN IUGR

The heart is the first organ to develop and function during embryogenesis (28). Fetal organs that develop early are more vulnerable to changes of the *in utero* environment than organs that develop later (29). There is a direct correlation between the amount of oxygen and nutrient supply to the fetus and cardiomyocytes development and function (29). Chronic hyperglycemia causes placental vascular dysfunction, which leads to reduced nutrient and oxygen supply to the fetus resulting in IUGR (10). Neonates exposed to IUGR present significant changes in cardiac morphology and subclinical myocardial dysfunction at birth (29). As such, in placental dysfunction due to maternal diabetes involving undernutrition and hypoxia, the developing myocardium undergoes structural and functional changes referred to as cardiac remodeling (30). In 1982, Hochman and Bulkley were the first to use the term "remodeling" to describe the substitution of infarcted tissue with scar tissue in a model of myocardial infarction (31). Later, in the year 2000, an international forum defined cardiac remodeling as molecular, cellular, and interstitial changes that manifest clinically as changes in size, shape, and function of the heart resulting from cardiac load and injury (30). Therefore, the clinical phenotype is a consequence of genomic changes that occur due to *in utero* gene environment interaction. Few clinical studies and experimental animal models have investigated the impact of IUGR on cardiac remodeling as discussed below.

IMPACT OF PLACENTAL DYSFUNCTION ON CARDIAC STRUCTURE AND FUNCTION

Epidemiological studies have shown changes in the structure and function of the heart in IUGR infants and neonates (29, 32). Clinical investigations have reported that postnatal catch-up growth in IUGR infants can result in abnormal cardiac function (33–35). Cardiovascular evaluation using echocardiographic assessment of IUGR fetuses revealed cardiac hypertrophy characterized by globular cardiac shape, higher intraventricular septum thickness, and increased pressure overload leading to both systolic and diastolic dysfunction (36–38). Primary cardiac and vascular changes observed at birth in IUGR fetus can persist from a few months up to a few years of age (35, 37).

Recently, clinical investigations have shown evidence of cardiac remodeling in IUGR offspring (32). For example, high systolic blood pressure and smaller aortic diameter (ascending aorta; IUGR:24.4 $\pm$ 1.5 mm, Control: 26.3 $\pm$ 2.2 mm, $P < 0.05$) were observed 20 years later in young adults (age 22–25 years) who were born growth restricted due to placental dysfunction (32). Compared to healthy controls, the diameter of the ascending aorta was smaller in IUGR subjects and a high aortic pressure augmentation index was observed (32). Electrocardiography (ECG) measurement revealed electrical remodeling in preadolescence who were born with IUGR (39). These studies evaluated signs of ventricular electrical remodeling in subjects with IUGR compared to controls by assessing changes in ventricular depolarization and repolarization using the QRS complex and *T*-wave, respectively (39). The classical frontal QRS-T angle was significantly narrower in IUGR preadolescents compared to control subjects (39). They also reported wider angles between the depolarization dominant vector and the frontal XY body plane in preterm-IUGR subjects, resulting in significantly wider angles between depolarization and repolarization vectors (39). The studies concluded that ventricular electrical remodeling observed in the pre-adolescent subjects might predispose to cardiovascular disease in later life (39). Electrical remodeling is induced by functional (altered electrical activation) and structural stressors (such as in hypertrophy and heart failure). These electrophysiological changes generate a substrate that is vulnerable to malignant ventricular arrhythmias. Cardiac remodeling and dysfunction increases with greater severity of IUGR (33, 40). The above-mentioned studies show evidence of cardiac remodeling in neonates, pre-adolescents, and young adults who were born with IUGR (41–44). These findings are supported by animal models; IUGR programming resulted in myocardial remodeling, reduced systolic and diastolic function and premature aging of the heart in growth restricted baboons (45). These structural and functional changes of the heart can be associated to changes in fetal cardiac gene expression that have occurred because of fetal adaptations to intrauterine environmental changes (46). These *in utero* changes, which result in reduced nutrition and oxygen, are due to placental dysfunction caused by maternal insults such as maternal vasculopathy in a diabetic pregnancy (46).

DIFFERENTIAL EXPRESSION OF CARDIAC GENES LEADING TO DYSFUNCTIONAL HEART IN IUGR

Pre-gestational and gestational diabetes have been associated with maternal vasculopathy which can be caused by long-term poor glycemic control (12). Fetal growth in diabetic pregnancy might be affected in two different ways; maternal hyperglycemia stimulates fetal overgrowth and maternal vasculopathy may be associated with placental dysfunction leading to a reduced nutrient and oxygen supply and subsequent IUGR (12). The majority of animal models use either maternal undernutrition and/or hypoxia to mimic IUGR (6, 47, 48). Hypoxia, undernutrition, or both interventions induce cardiac remodeling in adult rats (47). IUGR models have linked cardiac remodeling with changes in fetal gene expression. Several genes that play key roles in cardiac development have been studied in detail. One prominent example is the hypoxia-inducible factor 1 (HIF-1), which is required for normal growth of the myocardium and coronary blood vessels in conditions of low oxygen (49, 50). High levels of HIF-1 were reported in fetal rodent hearts exposed to hypoxia (49, 50). Abnormal cardiogenesis was seen in HIF-1 alpha-deficient mice (51). Therefore, elevated expression of *HIF1* and its downstream genes is essential for fetal adaptation and proper cardiac development in conditions of placental dysfunction in which oxygen supply to the fetus is relatively low (51–55). In a guinea pig model of maternal nutrient restriction, hearts of growth restricted offspring revealed increased expression of Poly [ADP-ribose] polymerase 1 (*PARP1*) gene and a reduction in cardiomyocyte number as well as hypertrophy (56). Another interesting class of genes associated with cardiac remodeling are the cardioprotective genes such as heat shock protein 70 (*HSP70*) and protein kinase C epsilon (*PKCε*) (57). Male rats exposed to hypoxia had increased expression of HSP70 and ischemic injury (48, 58–60). In addition, hypoxia in rat hearts resulted in a significant increase in *PKCε* expression and increased susceptibility to ischemia and perfusion injury in a sex-dependent manner (61). Furthermore, the mammalian target of the rapamycin complex 1 (mTORC1) pathway has also been associated with cardiac remodeling in IUGR mice, and prenatal *mTORC1* inhibition caused a reduction in cardiomyocyte number in adult hearts compared to controls

(62). In a rabbit model, IUGR was associated with cardiac mitochondrial Complex II dysfunction and an increase in Sirtuin 3 expression (63). In a rat model, maternal diabetes was associated with increased expression of forkhead box protein O1 (*FOXO1)* and its target genes in the heart of the offspring (64). Under conditions of undernutrition and hypoxia, changes that occur to enable the growing fetus to adapt and survive the inadequate substrate supply results in programming of fetal cardiac genes (4, 6, 65–67).

ROLE OF EPIGENETICS IN CARDIAC PROGRAMMING

Researchers have been investigating the mechanisms by which IUGR caused changes in fetal cardiac genes. Epigenetic regulation is one principle underlying molecular mechanism that causes differential gene expression in IUGR fetuses compared to normally grown fetuses. Epigenetic activities can alter gene expression throughout an individual's lifetime; thus, the function of the corresponding protein products as well as the organs involved are affected. Gene modifications occur in response to environmental changes, and genes are switched on and off via epigenetic mechanisms. Epigenetic alterations could be altered by lifestyle (for example overnutrition or undernutrition) or possibly by using treatments strategies postnatally (68). Hence, it is proposed that epigenetic mechanisms are important for understanding pathophysiology as well as potential targets for diagnosis and treatment of cardiovascular diseases (69, 70). Epigenetic regulation occurs by DNA methylation, histone modification, or regulation of genes by non-coding RNAs (ncRNAs) such as small microRNA and long non-coding RNA (71). So far, DNA methylation and histone acetylation are the most studied epigenetic mechanisms and clinical evidence of epigenetic programming is reported in adult patients with various cardiovascular diseases as reviewed by Muka et al. (72). Other studies have investigated the posttranscriptional regulatory role of non-coding RNA in relation to cardiovascular disease susceptibility in adult cardiac patients (73–75). We will focus on DNA methylation in IUGR leading to cardiovascular disease.

DNA METHYLATION MECHANISMS IN IUGR LEADING TO DEVELOPMENT OF CARDIOVASCULAR DISEASE

DNA methylation is the covalent addition of methyl groups to the C5 position of cytosine in dinucleotide CpG islands (76). CpG islands are regions with a high frequency of CpG sites where a cytosine nucleotide is followed by a guanine nucleotide. Methylation of CpG sites is catalyzed by DNA methyl transferases (DNMTs), such as DNMT1, DNMT3a, and DNMT3b. Very few studies have examined DNA methylation mechanisms in IUGR leading to cardiovascular remodeling or cardiac dysfunction. In a UK cohort of 144 children, investigators used umbilical cord blood to examine the relationship between prenatal antisense non-coding RNA in the INK4 locus (*ANRIL)* promoter DNA methylation and risk markers of coronary heart disease (76). Hypermethylation at CpG5 of the *ANRIL* promoter was associated with increased childhood pulse wave velocity, indicating increased arterial stiffness and a risk of coronary heart disease in these children at 9 years old (76). The *ANRIL* promoter is present on chromosome 2p21 which is considered a strong candidate for coronary heart disease in adult patients (77). Methylation of *ANRIL* and other genes on this chromosome might contribute to the prolonged cardiovascular programming in coronary disease patients. However, it is difficult to conclude the epigenetic contribution unless studies involving long-term follow-up of IUGR individuals are performed. Several studies have investigated epigenetic disturbances of nitric oxide synthase (NOS), which may predispose individuals to cardiovascular disease by modulating endothelial dysfunction (78–80). Human endothelial cells isolated from umbilical arteries and veins of IUGR fetuses were analyzed for a DNA methylation pattern in the promoter region of the endothelial nitric oxide synthase 3 (*eNOS3*) and arginine-2 (*ARG2*) genes. Compared to control cells, differential DNA methylation at the CpG-352 site of *NOS3* gene promoter of IUGR-endothelial cells was observed (80). Differential *eNOS* expression could be normalized by simply silencing the DNA methylation machinery (80). Hypoxia downregulates *eNOS* gene expression and activity, resulting in a reduced production of nitric oxide and endothelial dysfunction (78). Endothelial dysfunction is a very early stage in the development of atherosclerosis, which appears prior to the existence of atherosclerotic plaques or cardiovascular outcomes (81–84). This favors the concept that an epigenetic marker detectable as early as during prenatal and early postnatal developmental periods might be capable of identifying persons at risk of endothelial-related cardiovascular end organ damage. Furthermore, it has been shown that hypoxia-related IUGR changes the methylation pattern and expression of the *PKCε* gene in rat hearts, causing ischemic injuries in offspring (85). Hypoxia causes increased production of reactive oxygen species (ROS) which induces epigenetic repression of the PKCε gene leading to susceptibility of the heart to ischemic injury in the offspring (85). Hypermethylation patterns were observed within the promoter region of the *PKCε* gene in IUGR male rat hearts compared to controls (85). *PKCε* promoter hypermethylation was associated with a corresponding down regulation of *PKCε* gene expression in the heart of male rats but not in females. Activation of the *PKCε* gene in the heart restored hypoxia-induced cardiac vulnerability to ischemic injury in male rats (85). The transcription factor, early growth response factor (Egr-1), is involved in the regulation of *PKCe* promoter activity (86) since it binds to the *PKCε* promoter region, increasing its activity. Further studies showed that the absence of methylation in females was due to high levels of estrogen receptors in the female rat heart. Estrogen receptors bind to the regulatory gene Egr-1 and inhibit *PKCε* promoter methylation activity (86). Therefore, compared to males, the female hearts are protected against hypoxia-induced ischemic injury due to high levels of estrogen. These data help to explain the differences in the prevalence of CVD between men and women and gives a molecular mechanism for the role of sex hormone

(87). Postmenopausal women seem to lose this hormonally-induced cardioprotective ability and as such, hormone therapy is suggested as one of the remedies for prevention of cardiovascular disease in this group of women (88). However, large studies do not favor hormone replacement therapy for prevention of cardiovascular disease since it also has side effects such as increased risk for breast cancer and pulmonary embolism (88). For IUGR epigenetically programmed hearts, the best preventive strategy would be the use of epigenetic therapies (drugs) that aim to reverse fetal heart programming in early postnatal life (89). Postnatal drugs are capable of altering the epigenetic modifications that occurred during prenatal life as a result of fetal adaptations to changes in the intrauterine environment (89). Animal models and human studies of IUGR revealed epigenetic changes in 10 genes which result in a predisposition to type 2 diabetes as reviewed in detail by Liguori et al. (90). These epigenetic mechanisms may further contribute to the high prevalence of cardiovascular disease in type 2 diabetes patients (90). Another gene involved in growth and development of the fetal heart is insulin-like growth factor *(IGF)*. Upregulation of cardiac IGF receptor is associated with an increase in ventricular mass in a sheep model of nutrient restriction (91). Moreover, epigenetic mechanisms in the renin angiotensin system are linked to cardiovascular programming. Animal models revealed epigenetic modification of the renin-angiotensin system in fetal programming of hypertension (92, 93). Significantly lower renal expression of angiotensin II type 2 receptor, impairment of renal development and elevation of blood pressure were observed (93). Maternal insults during pregnancy induce placental dysfunction, leading to IUGR (**Figure 1**) (10). So far, it is well established that IUGR leads to cardiac remodeling via epigenetic modulation of cardiac genes which play important roles in cardiac development and function. However, many epigenetic pathways are still to be elucidated.

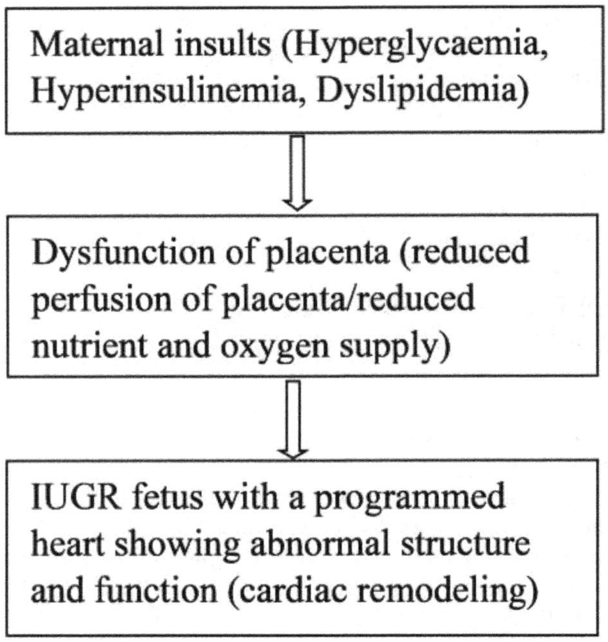

FIGURE 1 | Maternal insults result in placental dysfunction, IUGR, and cardiac remodeling.

DISCUSSION AND FUTURE PERSPECTIVE

Placental dysfunction due to maternal insults can result in IUGR, which result in an altered fetal epigenome leading to cardiac remodeling and subclinical symptoms of cardiovascular phenotypes in offspring. It is well-proven that IUGR leads to cardiac remodeling, likewise evidence linking altered genome expression and cardiovascular disease in IUGR has been published (85, 86, 91, 94). However, research involving epigenetic mechanisms of cardiovascular programming in growth restricted fetuses has just commenced. To date, most research has focused on fetal programming leading to CVD-related risk factors such as a predisposition to metabolic syndrome (95–97). Although such studies improve our understanding of how to prevent cardiovascular disease in carriers of cardiovascular risk factors, it is important to fully understand the epigenetic mechanisms acting directly on cardiovascular structure and function in IUGR offspring. It seems IUGR results in DNA methylation in a tissue-specific manner; thus, understanding the epigenetic mechanisms in various tissues that have direct impact on the cardiac system will be beneficial (98). The greatest task is to uncover the specific pathways of prenatal methylation of gene expression, as it is vital to the development and function of heart tissues, and to be able to link these pathways to specific cardiac diseases. Even though one can find DNA methylation in interesting CpG island in clinical samples obtained from affected IUGR offspring, it is also difficult to conclude a causal link between these epigenetic modifications and the various heart diseases. However, animal models may help to improve our understanding. Another challenge is linking affected pathways based on the severity of the IUGR since the extent of cardiac remodeling is based on the severity of IUGR (40). Epidemiological time point experiments have been performed to widen our understanding on the role of IUGR in fetal vulnerability to cardiovascular disease (33–35); however, there is need for longitudinal studies involving long-term follow-up of affected IUGR offspring. The use of epigenetic therapies in treatment of CVD is promising but it is still at its early experimental stage. In other diseases such as cancer, systemic lupus erythematosus, acute myeloid leukemia, and Alzheimer's disease, many epigenetic-related therapeutic agents are being tested for their possible use in clinical practice, but many are still awaiting approval to begin clinical trials or to receive approval by the FDA (99–102). In terms of DNA methylation mechanisms, therapeutic agents such as inhibitors of DNA methyl transferase (DNMT), hormonal therapy, and certain dietary compounds have been suggested for treatment of cardiovascular disease (89). Early prediction of cardiovascular disease might reduce risk as well as improve follow-up and treatment of susceptible patients. Effective biomarkers of risk are needed for development of

CVD prevention strategies (103). Epigenetic biomarkers could be useful for early prediction of high-risk individuals (103).

Growth restricted newborns are at high risk of respiratory distress syndrome, retinopathy of prematurity, and long-term complications such as metabolic syndrome and cardiovascular disease (104, 105). Therefore, it is vital to identify and follow those who are likely to be affected. Studies also show that an inheritable altered fetal cardiac genome can be transferred from one generation to another, which is referred to as transgenerational programing of the cardiac system (106). "Healthy aging starts with a healthy pregnancy," summarizes very beautifully this important concept and was first introduced in an editorial of Scioscia (107). A timely diagnosis of IUGR pregnancies and application of various therapeutic measures to treat and monitor affected neonates will help to reduce cardiac problems in future generations.

AUTHOR CONTRIBUTIONS

RD and IL conceived the presented idea. IL wrote the first draft of the manuscript. KK, SW, NH, TS, FH, and RD contributed to the manuscript revision, read and approved the submitted version.

REFERENCES

1. Ofori SN, Odia OJ. Risk assessment in the prevention of cardiovascular disease in low-resource settings. *Ind Heart J.* (2016) 68:391–8. doi: 10.1016/j.ihj.2015.07.004
2. Hariram V, Arramraju SK. Assessment of cardiovascular risk in low resource settings "So much to do - So little done". *Ind Heart J.* (2016) 68:260–2. doi: 10.1016/j.ihj.2015.07.046
3. Sanchis-Gomar F, Perez-Quilis C, Leischik R, Lucia A. Epidemiology of coronary heart disease and acute coronary syndrome. *Ann Transl Med.* (2016) 4:256. doi: 10.21037/atm.2016.06.33
4. Barker DJ. *In utero* programming of cardiovascular disease. *Theriogenology.* (2000) 53:555–74. doi: 10.1016/S0093-691X(99)00258-7
5. Barker DJ, Winter PD, Osmond C, Margetts B, Simmonds SJ. Weight in infancy and death from ischaemic heart disease. *Lancet.* (1989) 2:577–80. doi: 10.1016/S0140-6736(89)90710-1
6. Beauchamp B, Thrush AB, Quizi J, Antoun G, McIntosh N, Al-Dirbashi OY, et al. Undernutrition during pregnancy in mice leads to dysfunctional cardiac muscle respiration in adult offspring. *Biosci Rep.* (2015) 35:e00200. doi: 10.1042/BSR20150007
7. Gude NM, Roberts CT, Kalionis B, King RG. Growth and function of the normal human placenta. *Thromb Res.* (2004) 114:397–407. doi: 10.1016/j.thromres.2004.06.038
8. Roland MC, Friis CM, Voldner N, Godang K, Bollerslev J, Haugen G, et al. Fetal growth versus birthweight: the role of placenta versus other determinants. *PLos ONE.* (2012) 7:e39324. doi: 10.1371/journal.pone.0039324
9. Starikov R, Inman K, Chen K, Lopes V, Coviello E, Pinar H, et al. Comparison of placental findings in type 1 and type 2 diabetic pregnancies. *Placenta.* (2014) 35:1001–6. doi: 10.1016/j.placenta.2014.10.008
10. Leach L, Taylor A, Sciota F. Vascular dysfunction in the diabetic placenta: causes and consequences. *J Anatomy.* (2009) 215:69–76. doi: 10.1111/j.1469-7580.2009.01098.x
11. Patel H, Chen J, Das KC, Kavdia M. Hyperglycemia induces differential change in oxidative stress at gene expression and functional levels in HUVEC and HMVEC. *Cardiovasc Diabetol.* (2013) 12:142. doi: 10.1186/1475-2840-12-142
12. Huynh J, Yamada J, Beauharnais C, Wenger JB, Thadhani RI, Wexler D, et al. Type 1, type 2 and gestational diabetes mellitus differentially impact placental pathologic characteristics of uteroplacental malperfusion. *Placenta.* (2015) 36:1161–6. doi: 10.1016/j.placenta.2015.08.004
13. Gabbay-Benziv R, Baschat AA. Gestational diabetes as one of the "great obstetrical syndromes"-the maternal, placental, and fetal dialog. *Best Pract Res Clin Obstet Gynaecol.* (2015) 29:150–5. doi: 10.1016/j.bpobgyn.2014.04.025
14. Golic M, Stojanovska V, Bendix I, Wehner A, Herse F, Haase N, et al. Diabetes mellitus in pregnancy leads to growth restriction and epigenetic modification of the Srebf2 gene in rat fetuses. *Hypertension.* (2018) 71:911–20. doi: 10.1161/HYPERTENSIONAHA.117.10782
15. Gagnon R. Placental insufficiency and its consequences. *Eur J Obstetr Gynecol Reprod Biol.* (2003) 110(Suppl. 1):S99–107. doi: 10.1016/S0301-2115(03)00179-9
16. Dicke JM. Placenta: chronicle of intrauterine growth restriction. *F1000 Med Rep.* (2010) 2:69. doi: 10.3410/M2-69
17. Silver RM. Examining the link between placental pathology, growth restriction, and stillbirth. *Best Pract Res Clin Obstet Gynaecol.* (2018) 49:89–102. doi: 10.1016/j.bpobgyn.2018.03.004
18. Mifsud W, Sebire NJ. Placental pathology in early-onset and late-onset fetal growth restriction. *Fetal Diagn Ther.* (2014) 36:117–28. doi: 10.1159/000359969
19. Cohen E, Baerts W, van Bel F. Brain-sparing in intrauterine growth restriction: considerations for the neonatologist. *Neonatology.* (2015) 108:269–76. doi: 10.1159/000438451
20. Miller SL, Huppi PS, Mallard C. The consequences of fetal growth restriction on brain structure and neurodevelopmental outcome. *J Physiol.* (2016) 594:807–23. doi: 10.1113/JP271402
21. Lal MK, Manktelow BN, Draper ES, Field DJ. Chronic lung disease of prematurity and intrauterine growth retardation: a population-based study. *Pediatrics.* (2003) 111:483–7. doi: 10.1542/peds.111.3.483
22. Danhaive O, Margossian R, Geva T, Kourembanas S. Pulmonary hypertension and right ventricular dysfunction in growth-restricted, extremely low birth weight neonates. *J Perinatol.* (2005) 25:495–99. doi: 10.1038/sj.jp.7211299
23. Stein AD, Zybert PA, van der Pal-de Bruin K, Lumey LH. Exposure to famine during gestation, size at birth, and blood pressure at age 59 y: evidence from the Dutch Famine. *Eur J Epidemiol.* (2006) 21:759–65. doi: 10.1007/s10654-006-9065-2
24. Painter RC, de Rooij SR, Bossuyt PM, Simmers TA, Osmond C, Barker DJ, et al. Early onset of coronary artery disease after prenatal exposure to the Dutch famine. *Am J Clin Nutr.* (2006) 84:322–7; quiz 466–327. doi: 10.1093/ajcn/84.1.322
25. Gillman MW, Barker D, Bier D, Cagampang F, Challis J, Fall C, et al. Meeting report on the 3rd International Congress on Developmental Origins of Health and Disease (DOHaD). *Pediatr Res.* (2007) 61(5 Pt 1):625–9. doi: 10.1203/pdr.0b013e3180459fcd
26. Mestan KK, Steinhorn RH. Fetal origins of neonatal lung disease: understanding the pathogenesis of bronchopulmonary dysplasia. *Am J Physiol Lung Cell Mol Physiol.* (2011) 301:L858–9. doi: 10.1152/ajplung.00314.2011
27. Kapoor A, Dunn E, Kostaki A, Andrews MH, Matthews SG. Fetal programming of hypothalamo-pituitary-adrenal function: prenatal stress and glucocorticoids. *J Physiol.* (2006) 572(Pt 1):31–44. doi: 10.1113/jphysiol.2006.105254
28. Burton GJ, Jauniaux E. Development of the human placenta and fetal heart: synergic or independent? *Front Physiol.* (2018) 9:373. doi: 10.3389/fphys.2018.00373
29. Fouzas S, Karatza AA, Davlouros PA, Chrysis D, Alexopoulos D, Mantagos S, et al. Neonatal cardiac dysfunction in intrauterine growth restriction. *Pediatr Res.* (2014) 75:651–7. doi: 10.1038/pr.2014.22
30. Cohn JN, Ferrari R, Sharpe N. Cardiac remodeling–concepts and clinical implications: a consensus paper from an international forum on cardiac remodeling. Behalf of an International Forum on Cardiac Remodeling. *J Am Coll Cardiol.* (2000) 35:569–82. doi: 10.1016/S0735-1097(99)00630-0

31. Hochman JS, Bulkley BH. Expansion of acute myocardial infarction: an experimental study. *Circulation*. (1982) 65:1446–50. doi: 10.1161/01.CIR.65.7.1446
32. Bjarnegard N, Morsing E, Cinthio M, Lanne T, Brodszki J. Cardiovascular function in adulthood following intrauterine growth restriction with abnormal fetal blood flow. *Ultrasound Obstet Gynecol*. (2013) 41:177–84. doi: 10.1002/uog.12314
33. Crispi F, Hernandez-Andrade E, Pelsers MM, Plasencia W, Benavides-Serralde JA, Eixarch E, et al. Cardiac dysfunction and cell damage across clinical stages of severity in growth-restricted fetuses. *Am J Obstetr Gynecol*. (2008) 199:254.e1–8. doi: 10.1016/j.ajog.2008.06.056
34. Kaijser M, Bonamy AK, Akre O, Cnattingius S, Granath F, Norman M, et al. Perinatal risk factors for ischemic heart disease: disentangling the roles of birth weight and preterm birth. *Circulation*. (2008) 117:405–10. doi: 10.1161/CIRCULATIONAHA.107.710715
35. Crispi F, Bijnens B, Figueras F, Bartrons J, Eixarch E, Le Noble F, et al. Fetal growth restriction results in remodeled and less efficient hearts in children. *Circulation*. (2010) 121:2427–36. doi: 10.1161/CIRCULATIONAHA.110.937995
36. Leipälä JA, Boldt T, Turpeinen U, Vuolteenaho O, Fellman V. Cardiac hypertrophy and altered hemodynamic adaptation in growth-restricted preterm infants. *Pediatr Res*. (2003) 53:989–93. doi: 10.1203/01.PDR.0000061564.86797.78
37. Cruz-Lemini M, Crispi F, Valenzuela-Alcaraz B, Figueras F, Sitges M, Bijnens B, et al. Fetal cardiovascular remodeling persists at 6 months in infants with intrauterine growth restriction. *Ultrasound Obstet Gynecol*. (2016) 48:349–56. doi: 10.1002/uog.15767
38. Azevedo PS, Polegato BF, Minicucci MF, Paiva SAR, Zornoff LAM. Cardiac remodeling: concepts, clinical impact, pathophysiological mechanisms and pharmacologic treatment. *Arq Bras Cardiol*. (2016) 106:62–9. doi: 10.5935/abc.20160005
39. Ortigosa N, Rodriguez-Lopez M, Bailon R, Sarvari SI, Sitges M, Gratacos E, et al. Heart morphology differences induced by intrauterine growth restriction and preterm birth measured on the ECG at preadolescent age. *J Electrocardiol*. (2016) 49:401–9. doi: 10.1016/j.jelectrocard.2016.03.011
40. Akazawa Y, Hachiya A, Yamazaki S, Kawasaki Y, Nakamura C, Takeuchi Y, et al. Cardiovascular remodeling and dysfunction across a range of growth restriction severity in small for gestational age infants- implications for fetal programming. *Circ J*. (2016) 80:2212–20. doi: 10.1253/circj.CJ-16-0352
41. Menendez-Castro C, Rascher W, Hartner A. Intrauterine growth restriction - impact on cardiovascular diseases later in life. *Mol Cell Pediatr*. (2018) 5:4. doi: 10.1186/s40348-018-0082-5
42. Jendryczko A, Poreba R. [Effect of fetal and neonatal growth on the occurrence of some diseases in adults]. *Ginekol Polska*. (1996) 67:34–6.
43. Crispi F, Bijnens B, Sepulveda-Swatson E, Cruz-Lemini M, Rojas-Benavente J, Gonzalez-Tendero A, et al. Postsystolic shortening by myocardial deformation imaging as a sign of cardiac adaptation to pressure overload in fetal growth restriction. *Circu Cardiovasc Imaging*. (2014) 7:781–7. doi: 10.1161/CIRCIMAGING.113.001490
44. Cruz-Lemini M, Crispi F, Valenzuela-Alcaraz B, Figueras F, Gomez O, Sitges M, et al. A fetal cardiovascular score to predict infant hypertension and arterial remodeling in intrauterine growth restriction. *Am J Obstetr Gynecol*. (2014) 210: 552.e1–552.e22. doi: 10.1016/j.ajog.2013.12.031
45. Kuo AH, Li C, Huber HF, Clarke GD, Nathanielsz PW. Intrauterine growth restriction results in persistent vascular mismatch in adulthood. *J Physiol*. (2017) 596:5777–90. doi: 10.1113/JP275139
46. Scifres CM, Parks WT, Feghali M, Caritis SN, Catov JM. Placental maternal vascular malperfusion and adverse pregnancy outcomes in gestational diabetes mellitus. *Placenta*. (2017) 49:10–5. doi: 10.1016/j.placenta.2016.11.004
47. Xu Y, Williams SJ, O'Brien D, Davidge ST. Hypoxia or nutrient restriction during pregnancy in rats leads to progressive cardiac remodeling and impairs postischemic recovery in adult male offspring. *FASEB J*. (2006) 20:1251–3. doi: 10.1096/fj.05-4917fje
48. Li G, Xiao Y, Estrella JL, Ducsay CA, Gilbert RD, Zhang L. Effect of fetal hypoxia on heart susceptibility to ischemia and reperfusion injury in the adult rat. *J Soc Gynecol Invest*. (2003) 10:265–74. doi: 10.1016/S1071-55760300074-1
49. Bae S, Xiao Y, Li G, Casiano CA, Zhang L. Effect of maternal chronic hypoxic exposure during gestation on apoptosis in fetal rat heart. *Am J Physiol Heart Circul Physiol*. (2003) 285:H983–90. doi: 10.1152/ajpheart.00005.2003
50. Sugishita Y, Leifer DW, Agani F, Watanabe M, Fisher SA. Hypoxia-responsive signaling regulates the apoptosis-dependent remodeling of the embryonic avian cardiac outflow tract. *Dev Biol*. (2004) 273:285–96. doi: 10.1016/j.ydbio.2004.05.036
51. Compernolle V, Brusselmans K, Franco D, Moorman A, Dewerchin M, Collen D, et al. Cardia bifida, defective heart development and abnormal neural crest migration in embryos lacking hypoxia-inducible factor-1alpha. *Cardiovasc Res*. (2003) 60:569–79. doi: 10.1016/j.cardiores.2003.07.003
52. Wenger RH, Gassmann M. Oxygen(es) and the hypoxia-inducible factor-1. *Biol Chem*. (1997) 378:609–16.
53. Gordan JD, Simon MC. Hypoxia-inducible factors: central regulators of the tumor phenotype. *Curr Opin Genet Dev*. (2007) 17:71–7. doi: 10.1016/j.gde.2006.12.006
54. Maloyan A, Eli-Berchoer L, Semenza GL, Gerstenblith G, Stern MD, Horowitz M. HIF-1alpha-targeted pathways are activated by heat acclimation and contribute to acclimation-ischemic cross-tolerance in the heart. *Physiol Genom*. (2005) 23:79–88. doi: 10.1152/physiolgenomics.00279.2004
55. Ladoux A, Frelin C. Cardiac expressions of HIF-1 alpha and HLF/EPAS, two basic loop helix/PAS domain transcription factors involved in adaptative responses to hypoxic stresses. *Biochem Biophys Res Commun*. (1997) 240:552–6. doi: 10.1006/bbrc.1997.7708
56. Masoumy EP, Sawyer AA, Sharma S, Patel JA, Gordon PMK, Regnault TRH, et al. The lifelong impact of fetal growth restriction on cardiac development. *Pediatr Res*. (2018) 84:537–44. doi: 10.1038/s41390-018-0069-x
57. Snoeckx LH, Cornelussen RN, Van Nieuwenhoven FA, Reneman RS, Van Der Vusse GJ. Heat shock proteins and cardiovascular pathophysiology. *Physiol Rev*. (2001) 81:1461–97. doi: 10.1152/physrev.2001.81.4.1461
58. Saurin AT, Pennington DJ, Raat NJ, Latchman DS, Owen MJ, Marber MS. Targeted disruption of the protein kinase C epsilon gene abolishes the infarct size reduction that follows ischaemic preconditioning of isolated buffer-perfused mouse hearts. *Cardiovasc Res*. (2002) 55:672–80. doi: 10.1016/S0008-6363(02)00325-5
59. Inagaki K, Begley R, Ikeno F, Mochly-Rosen D. Cardioprotection by epsilon-protein kinase C activation from ischemia: continuous delivery and antiarrhythmic effect of an epsilon-protein kinase C-activating peptide. *Circulation*. (2005) 111:44–50. doi: 10.1161/01.CIR.0000151614.22282.F1
60. Inagaki K, Churchill E, Mochly-Rosen D. Epsilon protein kinase C as a potential therapeutic target for the ischemic heart. *Cardiovasc Res*. (2006) 70:222–30. doi: 10.1016/j.cardiores.2006.02.015
61. Xue Q, Zhang L. Prenatal hypoxia causes a sex-dependent increase in heart susceptibility to ischemia and reperfusion injury in adult male offspring: role of protein kinase C epsilon. *J Pharmacol Exp Ther*. (2009) 330:624–32. doi: 10.1124/jpet.109.153239
62. Hennig M, Fiedler S, Jux C, Thierfelder L, Drenckhahn JD. Prenatal mechanistic target of rapamycin complex 1 (m TORC1) inhibition by rapamycin treatment of pregnant mice causes intrauterine growth restriction and alters postnatal cardiac growth, morphology, and function. *J Am Heart Assoc*. (2017) 6:e005506. doi: 10.1161/JAHA.117.005506
63. Guitart-Mampel M, Gonzalez-Tendero A, Niñerola S, Morén C, Catalán-Garcia M, González-Casacuberta I, et al. Cardiac and placental mitochondrial characterization in a rabbit model of intrauterine growth restriction. *Biochim Biophys Acta (BBA) Gen Subj*. (2018) 1862:1157–67. doi: 10.1016/j.bbagen.2018.02.006
64. Musikant D, Sato H, Capobianco E, White V, Jawerbaum A, Higa R. Altered FOXO1 activation in the programming of cardiovascular alterations by maternal diabetes. *Mol Cell Endocrinol*. (2018) 479:78–86. doi: 10.1016/j.mce.2018.09.003
65. Thompson JA, Piorkowska K, Gagnon R, Richardson BS, Regnault TR. Increased collagen deposition in the heart of chronically hypoxic ovine fetuses. *J Dev Origins Health Dis*. (2013) 4:470–8. doi: 10.1017/S2040174413000299
66. Barker DJ, Osmond C, Law CM. The intrauterine and early postnatal origins of cardiovascular disease and chronic bronchitis. *J Epidemiol Commun Health*. (1989) 43:237–40. doi: 10.1136/jech.43.3.237

67. Bassareo PP, Marras AR, Cugusi L, Zedda AM, Mercuro G. The reasons why cardiologists should consider prematurity at birth and intrauterine growth retardation among risk factors. *J Cardiovasc Med.* (2016) 17:323–9. doi: 10.2459/JCM.0000000000000338
68. Li CC, Maloney CA, Cropley JE, Suter CM. Epigenetic programming by maternal nutrition: shaping future generations. *Epigenomics.* (2010) 2:539–49. doi: 10.2217/epi.10.33
69. Schleithoff C, Voelter-Mahlknecht S, Dahmke IN, Mahlknecht U. On the epigenetics of vascular regulation and disease. *Clin Epigenetics.* (2012) 4:7. doi: 10.1186/1868-7083-4-7
70. Kim M, Long TI, Arakawa K, Wang R, Yu MC, Laird PW. DNA methylation as a biomarker for cardiovascular disease risk. *PLoS ONE.* (2010) 5:e9692. doi: 10.1371/journal.pone.0009692
71. Handy DE, Castro R, Loscalzo J. Epigenetic modifications: basic mechanisms and role in cardiovascular disease. *Circulation.* (2011) 123:2145–56. doi: 10.1161/CIRCULATIONAHA.110.956839
72. Muka T, Koromani F, Portilla E, O'Connor A, Bramer WM, Troup J, et al. The role of epigenetic modifications in cardiovascular disease: a systematic review. *Int J Cardiol.* (2016) 212:174–83. doi: 10.1016/j.ijcard.2016.03.062
73. Gangwar RS, Rajagopalan S, Natarajan R, Deiuliis JA. Noncoding RNAs in cardiovascular disease: pathological relevance and emerging role as biomarkers and therapeutics. *Am J Hypertension.* (2018) 31:150–65. doi: 10.1093/ajh/hpx197
74. Gurha P. MicroRNAs in cardiovascular disease. *Curr Opin Cardiol.* (2016) 31:249–54. doi: 10.1097/HCO.0000000000000280
75. Joladarashi D, Thandavarayan RA, Babu SS, Krishnamurthy P. Small engine, big power: microRNAs as regulators of cardiac diseases and regeneration. *Int J Mol Sci.* (2014) 15:15891–911. doi: 10.3390/ijms150915891
76. Murray R, Bryant J, Titcombe P, Barton SJ, Inskip H, Harvey NC, et al. DNA methylation at birth within the promoter of ANRIL predicts markers of cardiovascular risk at 9 years. *Clin Epigenet.* (2016) 8:90. doi: 10.1186/s13148-016-0259-5
77. Zhuang J, Peng W, Li H, Wang W, Wei Y, Li W, et al. Methylation of p15(INK4b) and Expression of ANRIL on Chromosome 9p21 Are Associated with Coronary Artery Disease. *PLoS ONE.* (2012) 7:e47193. doi: 10.1371/journal.pone.0047193
78. Widmer RJ, Lerman A. Endothelial dysfunction and cardiovascular disease. *Global Cardiol Sci Pract.* (2014) 2014:291–308. doi: 10.5339/gcsp.2014.43
79. Barthelmes J, Nägele MP, Ludovici V, Ruschitzka F, Sudano I, Flammer AJ. Endothelial dysfunction in cardiovascular disease and Flammer syndrome—similarities and differences. *EPMA J.* (2017) 8:99–109. doi: 10.1007/s13167-017-0099-1
80. Krause BJ, Costello PM, Munoz-Urrutia E, Lillycrop KA, Hanson MA, et al. Role of DNA methyltransferase 1 on the altered eNOS expression in human umbilical endothelium from intrauterine growth restricted fetuses. *Epigenetics.* (2013) 8:944–52. doi: 10.4161/epi.25579
81. Mudau M, Genis A, Lochner A, Strijdom H. Endothelial dysfunction: the early predictor of atherosclerosis. *Cardiovasc J Afr.* (2012) 23:222–31. doi: 10.5830/CVJA-2011-068
82. Gimbrone MA, García-Cardeña G. Endothelial cell dysfunction and the pathobiology of atherosclerosis. *Circul Res.* (2016) 118:620–36. doi: 10.1161/CIRCRESAHA.115.306301
83. Park K-H, Park WJ. Endothelial dysfunction: clinical implications in cardiovascular disease and therapeutic approaches. *J Korean Med Sci.* (2015) 30:1213–25. doi: 10.3346/jkms.2015.30.9.1213
84. Celermajer DS, Sorensen KE, Gooch VM, Spiegelhalter DJ, Miller OI, Sullivan ID, et al. Non-invasive detection of endothelial dysfunction in children and adults at risk of atherosclerosis. *Lancet.* (1992) 340:1111–5. doi: 10.1016/0140-6736(92)93147-F
85. Patterson AJ, Xiao D, Xiong F, Dixon B, Zhang L. Hypoxia-derived oxidative stress mediates epigenetic repression of PKCepsilon gene in foetal rat hearts. *Cardiovasc Res.* (2012) 93:302–10. doi: 10.1093/cvr/cvr322
86. Chen M, Xiong F, Zhang L. Promoter methylation of Egr-1 site contributes to fetal hypoxia-mediated PKCε gene repression in the developing heart. *Am J Physiol Regul Integrat Compar Physiol.* (2013) 304:R683–9. doi: 10.1152/ajpregu.00461.2012
87. Pilote L, Dasgupta K, Guru V, Humphries KH, McGrath J, Norris C, et al. A comprehensive view of sex-specific issues related to cardiovascular disease. *CMAJ Can Med Assoc J.* (2007) 176:S1–44. doi: 10.1503/cmaj.051455
88. Rossouw JE, Anderson GL, Prentice RL, LaCroix AZ, Kooperberg C, Stefanick ML, et al. Risks and benefits of estrogen plus progestin in healthy postmenopausal women: principal results From the Women's Health Initiative randomized controlled trial. *JAMA.* (2002) 288:321–33. doi: 10.1001/jama.288.3.321
89. Schiano C, Vietri MT, Grimaldi V, Picascia A, De Pascale MR, Napoli C. Epigenetic-related therapeutic challenges in cardiovascular disease. *Trends Pharmacol Sci.* (2015) 36:226–35. doi: 10.1016/j.tips.2015.02.005
90. Liguori A, Puglianiello A, Germani D, Deodati A, Peschiaroli E, Cianfarani S. Epigenetic changes predisposing to type 2 diabetes in intrauterine growth retardation. *Front Endocrinol.* (2010) 1:5. doi: 10.3389/fendo.2010.00005
91. Dong F, Ford SP, Fang CX, Nijland MJ, Nathanielsz PW, Ren J. Maternal nutrient restriction during early to mid gestation up-regulates cardiac insulin-like growth factor (IGF) receptors associated with enlarged ventricular size in fetal sheep. *Growth Horm IGF Res.* (2005) 15:291–9. doi: 10.1016/j.ghir.2005.05.003
92. Bogdarina I, Welham S, King PJ, Burns SP, Clark AJL. Epigenetic modification of the renin-angiotensin system in the fetal programming of hypertension. *Circul Res.* (2007) 100:520–6. doi: 10.1161/01.RES.0000258855.60637.58
93. McMullen S, Gardner DS, Langley-Evans SC. Prenatal programming of angiotensin II type 2 receptor expression in the rat. *Br J Nutr.* (2004) 91:133–40. doi: 10.1079/BJN20031029
94. Patterson AJ, Zhang L. Hypoxia and fetal heart development. *Curr Mol Med.* (2010) 10:653–66. doi: 10.2174/156652410792630643
95. Smith CJ, Ryckman KK. Epigenetic and developmental influences on the risk of obesity, diabetes, and metabolic syndrome. *Diabetes Metab Syndr Obes.* (2015) 8:295–302. doi: 10.2147/DMSO.S61296
96. Kampmann U, Madsen LR, Skajaa GO, Iversen DS, Moeller N, Ovesen P. Gestational diabetes: a clinical update. *World J Diabetes.* (2015) 6:1065–72. doi: 10.4239/wjd.v6.i8.1065
97. Kawasaki M, Arata N, Miyazaki C, Mori R, Kikuchi T, Ogawa Y, et al. Obesity and abnormal glucose tolerance in offspring of diabetic mothers: a systematic review and meta-analysis. *PLoS ONE.* (2018) 13:e0190676. doi: 10.1371/journal.pone.0190676
98. Ma B, Wilker EH, Willis-Owen SAG, Byun H-M, Wong KCC, Motta V, et al. Predicting DNA methylation level across human tissues. *Nucleic Acids Res.* (2014) 42:3515–28. doi: 10.1093/nar/gkt1380
99. Wang Z, Chang C, Peng M, Lu Q. Translating epigenetics into clinic: focus on lupus. *Clin Epigenet.* (2017) 9:78. doi: 10.1186/s13148-017-0378-7
100. Mazzone R, Zwergel C, Mai A, Valente S. Epi-drugs in combination with immunotherapy: a new avenue to improve anticancer efficacy. *Clin Epigenet.* (2017) 9:59. doi: 10.1186/s13148-017-0358-y
101. Yun S, Vincelette ND, Abraham I, Robertson KD, Fernandez-Zapico ME, Patnaik MM. Targeting epigenetic pathways in acute myeloid leukemia and myelodysplastic syndrome: a systematic review of hypomethylating agents trials. *Clin Epigenet.* (2016) 8:68. doi: 10.1186/s13148-016-0233-2
102. Cuadrado-Tejedor M, Garcia-Barroso C, Sanzhez-Arias J, Mederos S, Rabal O, Ugarte A, et al. Concomitant histone deacetylase and phosphodiesterase 5 inhibition synergistically prevents the disruption in synaptic plasticity and it reverses cognitive impairment in a mouse model of Alzheimer's disease. *Clin Epigenet.* (2015) 7:108. doi: 10.1186/s13148-015-0142-9
103. Cardona-Monzonís A, Beltrán-García J, Ibañez-Cabellos JS, Pérez-Machado G, Malkani K, Sanchis-Gomar F, et al. Epigenetic biomarkers in cardiovascular disease. *J Lab Precis Med.* (2018) 3:24. doi: 10.21037/jlpm.2018.02.04
104. Salam RA, Das JK, Bhutta ZA. Impact of intrauterine growth restriction on long-term health. *Curr Opin Clin Nutr Metab Care.* (2014) 17:249–54. doi: 10.1097/MCO.0000000000000051
105. Longo S, Bollani L, Decembrino L, Di Comite A, Angelini M, Stronati M. Short-term and long-term sequelae in

intrauterine growth retardation (IUGR). *J Matern Fetal Neonatal Med.* (2013) 26:222–5. doi: 10.3109/14767058.2012.715006

106. Master JS, Thouas GA, Harvey AJ, Sheedy JR, Hannan NJ, Gardner DK, et al. Fathers that are born small program alterations in the next-generation preimplantation rat embryos. *J Nutr.* (2015) 145:876–83. doi: 10.3945/jn.114.205724

107. Scioscia M. Relevant fetal epigenetic modifications result from a diabetic intrauterine environment: healthy aging starts with a healthy pregnancy. *Hypertension.* (2018) 71:822–3. doi: 10.1161/HYPERTENSIONAHA.118.10868

11

Nutritional Intervention for Developmental Brain Damage: Effects of Lactoferrin Supplementation in Hypocaloric Induced Intrauterine Growth Restriction Rat Pups

*Yohan van de Looij[1,2†], Camille Larpin[1†], Jan-Harry Cabungcal[3], Eduardo F. Sanches[1], Audrey Toulotte[1], Kim Q. Do[3] and Stéphane V. Sizonenko[1]**

[1] Division of Child Development and Growth, Department of Pediatrics, School of Medicine, University of Geneva, Geneva, Switzerland, [2] Laboratory for Functional and Metabolic Imaging, Ecole Polytechnique Fédérale de Lausanne, Lausanne, Switzerland, [3] Department of Psychiatry, Centre for Psychiatric Neuroscience, Lausanne University Hospital, Lausanne, Switzerland

***Correspondence:**
Stéphane V. Sizonenko
stephane.sizonenko@unige.ch

† These authors have contributed equally to this work

Introduction: Intrauterine Growth Restriction (IUGR) refers to an impaired development of the fetus and hence results in adverse neurodevelopmental and psychiatric consequences later in life. Lactoferrin (Lf) is a glycoprotein present in milk that has already shown neuroprotective effects through its anti-inflammatory and antioxidant properties on impaired developing brains. The aim of this study was to characterize a rat model of IUGR and assess the neuroprotective effect of a nutritional supplementation with bovine Lf during pregnancy and lactation on this model.

Methods: A model of 50% gestational caloric restriction (CR) was used. Three groups were designed, and pregnant rats had either *ad libitum* access to food (control group, CTL) or 50% of the controls' intake (restricted group, IUGR). The diet was isocaloric and supplemented with bovine Lf for the caloric restricted dams (restricted-Lf, IUGR_Lf). At postnatal day 7 and 21, advanced *ex-vivo* diffusion MRI techniques at 9.4T were used to investigate brain cortical and white matter microstructure. Further, genes and proteins involved in structure (synaptophysin, MBP), microglia (Iba-1), metabolism (MCT2, βCaMKII) and apoptosis (Bcl-2) were analyzed in the cortex and striatum. In the cortex, the number of parvalbumin immunoreactive interneurons and their perineuronal nets were quantified. Behavioral tests were performed at P31.

Results: Effects of the CR were significant in the cortex and striatum with reduction of synaptophysin (marker of synaptogenesis) at P7 and MBP (marker of myelin) at P21 in the cortex. Indeed, MCT2 (energy metabolism), Bcl-2 (anti-apoptotic protein) and βCaMKII (synapse activity) expressions were reduced in IUGR groups at P7. In the striatum NG2 (marker of oligodendrocyte precursor cells) and Bcl-2 at P7 as well as βCaMKII at P21 were decreased following IUGR and restored by Lf. Cortical microstructure was impaired following CR with partial effect of Lf. Lf prevented oxidative stress induced parvalbumin interneurons impairments whereas striatum and external capsule showed alterations in microstructure depicted by diffusion MRI, which were also partially reversed by Lf.

Discussion and Conclusion: The model of 50% caloric restriction induced mild impairment partially reversed by nutritional intervention using Lf during pregnancy and lactation.

Keywords: intrauterine growth restriction, caloric restriction, lactoferrin, neuroprotection, magnetic resonance imaging

HIGHLIGHTS

- Moderate undernutrition induced IUGR demonstrated mild cerebral impairment.
- Cerebral impairment is characterized by white and gray matters damage depicted by MRI.
- Oral Lf supplementation showed partial neuroprotection following caloric restriction during gestation.
- It represents a promising approach to reduce developmental diseases in IUGR and preterm infants.

INTRODUCTION

The definition of intrauterine growth retardation (IUGR) given by world health organization in 1995 was "An infant suffering from IUGR is defined as being below the 10% percentile of the recommended gender-specific birthweight for gestational age reference curves." It is one of the main causes of developmental brain damage with possible long life neurodevelopmental disabilities. If IUGR is an important public health concern worldwide, the rate of IUGR in the developing countries is about six times higher than in developed countries with at least 30 million IUGR infants per year. Poor antenatal and postnatal nutrition further prevents infants from attaining their full developmental potential. IUGR adults show a higher risk of altered cognitive and executive function and emotion control. The often-associated morbidities of IUGR, prematurity and poor postnatal growth represent a major risk for poor development of affective cognition and psychiatric disorders (1–3).

Lactoferrin (Lf), an iron-binding glycoprotein is involved in the intestinal iron uptake and regulates immune response with anti-inflammatory as well as antioxidant property (4, 5). In humans, higher concentration of Lf is found in the colostrum but Lf level decreases through lactation period (6). After oral administration, Lf is regulated through binding sites on brain endothelial cells allowing the passage from blood to tissues including the brain (7). Lf has been shown to down-regulate inflammation in lipopolysaccharides injury models (8). Importantly, Lf nutritional supplement in preterm shows significant reduction in late-onset sepsis and necrotizing enterocolitis (9). Our previous studies explored the effect of Lf on various animal models of perinatal brain injuries. Hypoxic-Ischemic post-natal day 3 (P3) pup rats demonstrated recovery with maternal Lf supplementation during lactation (10), characterized by a reduced cortical loss and an altered white matter recovery. Furthermore, inflammatory and apoptotic gene expressions were also reduced (10). Following lipopolysaccharides injection at P3, Lf administration during lactation reduced ventriculomegaly as well as impaired microstructure and white matter alterations (11). Finally, in a model of dexamethasone induced IUGR mimicking maternal stress and fetal growth restriction, the abnormal levels of brain metabolites as well as major neurotrophic factor (BDNF) were restored with Lf (12). Taken together, these findings suggest that Lf, with its anti-inflammatory and antioxidant properties, has great potential to reduce brain injury, improve cerebral development and prevent noxious programming due to adverse pre and postnatal conditions.

As such, the aim of this study was to evaluate structural and functional cerebral impairments in gestational caloric restriction induced IUGR as well as the potential neuroprotective effect of Lf supplementation. Effects of caloric restriction were assessed with advanced diffusion magnetic resonance imaging techniques [diffusion tensor imaging (DTI) as well as neurite orientation dispersion and density imaging (NODDI)] in conjunction with protein and gene expressions and behavioral tests.

MATERIALS AND METHODS

Animal Preparation

All experimental protocols have been previously approved by the Animal Research Ethics of Geneva, Switzerland (#GE7115). Nulliparous Wistar female (225–250 g) and Wistar male (250–275 g) rats (Charles River Laboratories, France) were used for breeding. During gestation, they had either *ad libitum* access to food: Control group (CTL) or access to 50% of the controls' intake: Restricted group (IUGR). Bovine lactoferrin (Lf) (Taradon laboratory, Tubize, Belgium) at an expected dose of 1g/kg/day according to daily intake of food by gestating and lactating dams, was added to the diet as a supplementation also during gestation and lactation for the Restricted-Lactoferrin group (IUGR_Lf). From the day before the parturition and during the whole lactation, all dams had *ad libitum* access to food, with either Lf enriched (1 g/kg/day) or isocaloric diet. Standard animal housing conditions according to the animal facility of the CMU, University of Geneva, were applied with free access to water. At birth, rat pups were culled or boarded out to another dam of the same group in order to control litter size to 10 to 12 pups per dam until weaning day. Dam and pup weight gain were measured daily until weaning and once a week until P42.

The number of pups per group is mentioned by experiment separately. The number of dams used in the study was: 6 controls, 10 IUGR and 9 IUGR_Lf.

Brain Collection for *ex-vivo* MRI and Immunofluorescence

After intraperitoneal injection of pentobarbital (50 μg/kg), rat pups were intra-cardially perfused with 0.9% NaCl and 4% paraformaldehyde solution at postnatal day 7 (P7) and 21 (P21). Brains were removed and immersed in 4% paraformaldehyde overnight for post fixation.

Magnetic Resonance (MR) Experiments

All MR experiments were performed on an actively-shielded 9.4T/31 cm magnet (Varian/Magnex) equipped with 12-cm gradient coils (400 mT/m, 120 μs). *Ex-vivo* MRI was performed on P7 (CTL; $n = 6$, IUGR; $n = 6$, and IUGR_Lf; $n = 6$) and P21 (CTL; $n = 7$, IUGR; $n = 4$, and IUGR_Lf; $n = 4$) fixed brains with a 2.5 mm diameter birdcage coil. A multi-b-value shell protocol was acquired using a spin-echo sequence with a field-of-view equal to 21 × 16 mm^2 and a matrix size of 128 × 92. Twelve slices of 0.6 mm thickness were acquired with 3 averages and TE/TR = 45/2,000 ms. Ninety-six diffusion weighted images were acquired including 15 b_0 images and 81 images separated in 3 non-collinear shells with a uniform distribution in each shell. Distribution of number of directions and *b*-value were as follow: 21 directions at a *b*-value of 1,750 s/mm^2, 30 directions at a *b*-value of 3,400 s/mm^2 and 30 directions at a *b*-value of 5,100 s/mm^2. NODDI toolbox (13) was used to fit the acquired data. Regions of interest were delineated in cortex (Cx), external capsule (EC), and striatum (St). DTI derived parameters [Axial diffusivity (AD), Radial diffusivity (RD), Mean diffusivity (MD) and Fractional anisotropy (FA)] as well as NODDI derived parameters [intra-neurite volume faction (f_{icvf}), isotropic volume fraction (f_{iso}) and orientation dispersion index (ODI)] were averaged in the different regions assessed as previously used in animal models of perinatal brain injuries (11, 14).

Tissue Collection for Protein and Gene Expression

Rat pups were euthanized by decapitation at P7 and P21. Pups were anesthetized with pentobarbital (50 μg/kg) prior to decapitation. Brains were quickly removed, dissected on ice and frozen instantly in liquid nitrogen. Two structures were dissected: cortex (Cx) and striatum (S). The samples were stored at −80°C until analyses.

Immunoblotting

Brain tissues from P7 (CTL; $n = 6$, IUGR; $n = 6$ and IUGR_Lf; $n = 7$) and P21 (CTL; $n = 10$, IUGR; $n = 14$ and IUGR_Lf; $n = 13$) rats were homogenized by sonication in RIPA buffer (Cell Signaling, 9806S), and the protein concentration was assessed using a Bradford assay. Proteins (25 μg) were separated by SDS-PAGE, transferred to a nitrocellulose membrane and analyzed by immunoblotting. All antibodies (**Table 1**) were diluted in blocking buffer containing 0.1% casein (Sigma-Aldrich, C8654). Antibodies were diluted in the concentrations suggested on the data sheet by the manufacturer (**Table 1**). After incubation of the primary antibodies, the following secondary antibodies were applied: goat anti-mouse IgG (H+L) conjugated with Dylight™ 680 (#5470, Cell Signaling Technology), goat anti-rabbit IgG conjugated with IRDye 800 (926-32210, LI-COR) and donkey anti-goat IgG conjugated with IRDye 680 (926-68074, LI-COR). The Odyssey Infra-red Imaging system (LI-COR) was used to visualize the protein bands. The densitometry was assessed by normalizing the optical density of each sample with respect to actin expression (mouse monoclonal anti-actin from Millipore, MAB1501), using Image Studio Lite ver.5.2 software. The results are expressed as a percentage of values obtained either for the control or for the restricted rat pups (100%) using actin as a standard.

Real-Time Quantitative PCR (RT-qPCR)

The extraction of the total mRNA was done using the RNase Mini Kit (Qiagen, 74104) following the manufacturer's instructions (**Table 2**). On P7 collected brains, 3 μg mRNA from the three regions of interest at P7 (CTL; $n = 6$, IUGR; $n = 6$ and IUGR_Lf; $n = 6$) and P21 (CTL; $n = 6$, IUGR; $n = 8$ and IUGR_Lf; $n = 8$) were reverse transcripted to cDNA using 400 units of Moloney murine leukemia virus reverse transcriptase (Invitrogen, 28025-013), 20 units of recombinant RNAsin (Promega, N2515), 0.5 μg of random hexamers (ThermoFischer Scientific, #S0142), 2 mmol/L dNTP (Invitrogen, 10297018), and 40 mmol/L of dithiothreitol (Invitrogen, 18080093). Real-time quantitative PCR was performed with the PowerUp SYBR Green Master Mix (Applied Biosystems, A25742) and using an StepOnePlus™ Real-Time PCR System (Applied Biosystems). Gene expressions were normalized using the housekeeping ribosomal gene RPS29. The results were calculated using the Livak approach and are expressed in arbitrary units (A.U) (12).

Quantification of Mitochondrial Oxidative Damage and Parvalbumin Immunoreactive Interneurons

Coronal frozen sections (40 μm) were used to investigate the anterior cingulate cortex (ACC), a region in the prefrontal cortex known to be sensitive to stress. Triple immunolabeling for labeling DNA oxidative damage, parvalbumin (PV), and perineuronal nets (PNNs) was performed as followed. An antibody against 8-oxo-2′-deoxyguanosine (8-oxo-dG), a product of DNA oxidation, was used as DNA oxidative marker, while the PNNs were labeled with the lectin *Wisteria floribunda Agglutinin* (WFA), which binds the N-acetylgalactosamines in chondroitin sulfate proteoglycans (15, 16). Brain sections containing the anterior ACC were first incubated with PBS + Triton 0.3% +sodium azide (1 g/L) containing 2–3% normal horse serum, then placed for 48 h in a solution with a mouse monoclonal anti-8-oxodG (1:400; AMS Biotechnology, Switzerland) and a rabbit polyclonal anti-parvalbumin (PV) (1:2,500; Swant Inc., Switzerland) primary antibody together with the biotin-conjugated WFA (1:2,000; Sigma, Switzerland). Sections were then washed, incubated with fluorescent secondary antibody conjugates: goat anti-mouse Alexa 488 (1:300; Life

TABLE 1 | Primary antibodies for immunoblotting including catalog numbers, companies, and dilutions.

Abbreviations	Primary antibodies	Catalog number/Company	Dilution
Actin	Anti-actin antibody clone C4	MAB1501/Millipore	1/1,000
CD68	Rabbit polyclonal anti-CD68	250594/Abbiotec™	1/500
DCX	Rabbit polyclonal anti-DCX	ab18723/Abcam	1/1,000
GFAP	Mouse monoclonal anti-GFAP	G6171/Sigma-Aldrich	1/1,000
Iba-1	Goat polyclonal anti-Iba1	ab5076/Abcam	1/1,000
MBP	Mouse monoclonal anti-MBP	ab62631/Abcam	1/1,000
NeuN	Mouse monoclonal anti-NeuN	MAB377/Millipore	1/1,000
NG2	Rabbit polyclonal anti-NG2	ab129051/Abcam	1/1,000
Synaptophysin	Mouse monoclonal anti-synaptophysin	ab8049/Abcam	1/500
βCaMKII	Rabbit polyclonal anti-CAMKII beta	ab34703/Abcam	1/1,000
DMT1	Rabbit polyclonal anti-DMT1	ab140977/Abcam	1/1,000
GLT1	Guinea pig polyclonal anti- GLT1	AB1783/Millipore	1/500
Leptin receptor	Rabbit polyclonal anti-Leptin Receptor	ab5593/Abcam	1/1,000
MCT2	Rabbit polyclonal anti-MCT2	AB3542/Millipore	1/1,000
NMDAR	Rabbit polyclonal anti-NMDA R2A	ab14596/Abcam	1/1,000
IGF 2	Rabbit polyclonal anti-IGF2	ab9574/Abcam	0.2 μg/mL
TrkB	Rabbit polyclonal anti-TrkB	ab18987/Abcam	1/1,000
Fractin	Rabbit polyclonal anti-Fractin	AB3150/Millipore	1/1,000

TABLE 2 | PCR primers for quantitative real-time PCR.

Primer	Forward	Reverse
Bax	5′-TGGAGCTGCAGAGGATGATTG-3′	5′-GCTGCCACACGGAAGAAGAC-3′
Bcl-2	5′-TGGGATGCCTTTGTGGAACT-3′	5′-GAGACAGCCAGGAGAAATCAAAC-3′
BDNF	5′-AAAAAGTTCCACCAGGTGAGAAGA-3′	5′-GCAACCGAAGTATGAAATAACCATAG-3′
RPS29	5′-GCCAGGGTTCTCGCTCTTG-3′	5′-GGCACATGTTCAGCCCGTAT-3′

Technologies, USA), goat anti-rabbit CY3 (1:300; Chemicon International, USA) and streptavidin 405 conjugate (1:300; Millipore Corporation, USA). Sections were visualized and processed with a Zeiss confocal microscope equipped with ×20 and ×40 Plan-NEOFLUAR objectives. All peripherals were controlled with LSM 710 Quasar software (Carl Zeiss AG, Switzerland). With the triple immunolabeling of 8-oxodG, PV, and WFA, Z-stacks of 12 images with ×20 objective (with a 1.8 μm interval) were scanned (1,024 × 1,024 pixels). Images were filtered with a Gaussian filter to remove background noise and sharpen cell profile contour. Only the inner 9 images of Z-stacks were used for the analyses. The stack images were merged in a tif file with Imaris. Analyses were performed in a delineated region of interest (ROI) comprising the ACC (mainly cg1 and small portion of cg2) by an observer unaware of the experimental groups. To quantify the overall 8-oxo-dG, the staining intensity and number of labeled voxels within the ROI were measured. For PV-IR cell count, PV cell bodies were counted and their mean intensity of labeling (arbitrary unit) also obtained. To analyze the number of PV+ cells surrounded by WFA labeled PNN (WFA+ PV), we used the same "spots module" used to count PV+ cells to assign spot markings on the profile-labeled voxels that fall within a given size. Briefly, the channels for PV and WFA immunolabeling were chosen, and the profile size criterion (>8 and >5 mm, respectively) was defined to quantify stained profiles above these given sizes. The procedure was visually monitored/verified before proceeding. Spots generated for PV that contacted/overlapped with spots generated for WFA (PNN) were considered as those PVI surrounded by PNN (WFA-positive PVI).

Behavioral Tests

Behavioral tests were performed from P31 to P41. Detailed protocol can be found in (17).$

The Elevated Plus Maze (EPM)

The test assesses anxiety-like behavior (17). Rats were placed in the central area, head facing one of the enclosed arms. Number of entries in the open or closed arms, time spent on each arm, head-dipping and rearing were recorded over 5 min to investigate anxiety-like state. The ratio based on the time spent in the closed arms and the time spent in the open spaces (open arms and center of the apparatus) was calculated by time in open space divided by time in closed arms (18).

The Open Field (OF)

Motor activity, exploratory drive, and anxiety state were assessed in this test in a circular arena (100 cm diameter) divided in 21 areas. The latency to leave the central circular area, the number of areas crossing and rearing were recorded for 5 min (17).

The Novel Object Recognition (NOR)

The novel object recognition (NOR) test was performed in the open field arena during two consecutive days. In the first day, each rat was confronted with two identical objects (A and A′) placed 20 cm apart from the walls of the apparatus. The time exploring each object was recorded for 4 min. In the second day, long-term memory was tested by exposing each animal to two objects in the same open field apparatus: one of the objects used in the first day, considered as the familiar object (A) and a novel (and distinct from A or A′) object (B). Object exploration time for each object was measured and a discriminative index (DI) was calculated by exploration time on object B minus exploration time on object A divided by total exploration time on both objects (19).

The Beam Walking (BW)

The beam walking (BW) test was composed of training phase and testing phase. In the first day, rats were trained (three trials) to traverse a wooden beam (width 2 cm, length 100 cm, elevated 70 cm above the floor). They were placed on one side and encouraged to walk to reach a black box on the other side of the beam. In the next day (24 h later) animals were exposed to the same beam and number of hind paw slips were counted as an index of locomotor deficits (17).

The Morris Water Maze (MWM)

The Morris water maze (MWM) was done for 6 days (5 days of training and 1 day of test—namely Probe Trial) consecutively in a black tank (200 diameters) filled with water (45 cm depth) at 21 ± 2°C. A black platform (diameter 10 cm) was placed at 2 cm under water level and remained hidden at the same location for the 5 training days. Rats underwent four trials with 10 min inter-trial interval per day and entered the pool facing the wall following a randomized sequence of the four starting points (North, East, South, and West). Latency to find the platform was measured up to 60 s and was considered as a learning indication. If the animal failed in finding the platform within the 60 s, it was conducted to the platform by the experimenter and left during 10–15 s for exploring the room clues. On the 6th day, the probe test trial day, the platform was removed and latency to cross the platform zone and time spent in the platform quadrant were assessed.

Statistics

For statistical analysis, a one-way ANOVA test followed by Tukey *post hoc* was done for normally distributed data. A Kruskal–Wallis test followed by a Mann–Whitney test ($P < \alpha$/number of tests) was done in case of non-normal distribution. Finally, the mean number of PV+ cells, WFA+PVI, and the overall 8-oxo-dG labeling intensity were compared between the three experimental groups and analyze with ANOVA test followed by a Dunnett test. Significance level was considered when $P < 0.05$ after rectification of *P*-values by Bonferroni correction. All data are presented as mean ± SEM except DTI and NODDI derived parameters as well as PV and WFA cells results expressed as mean ± SD.

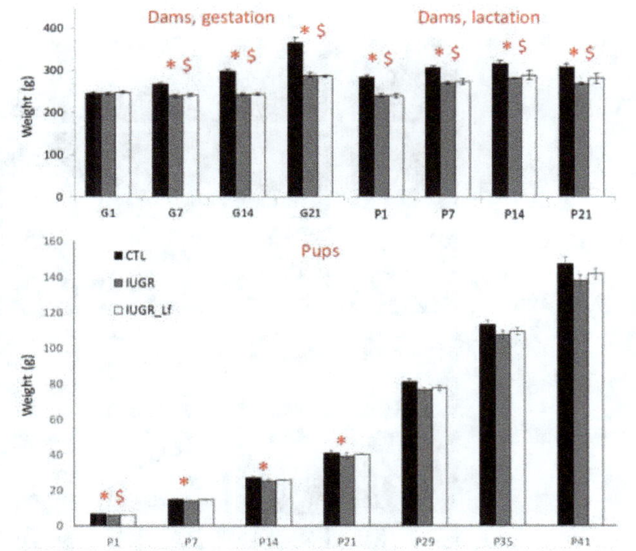

FIGURE 1 | High: dam weight monitoring through gestation (G1 to G21) and lactation until weaning (P1 to P21). Low: rat pups weight monitoring from post-natal day 1 to 41 (P1 to P41). Results are mean ± SEM. $P < 0.05$ *CTL vs. IUGR, $CTL vs. IUGR_Lf.

RESULTS

Caloric Restriction Effects on Maternal and Offspring Weights

In order to evaluate the impact of a 50% caloric restriction on dams, weights were measured daily during both gestation and lactation (**Figure 1**). Maternal body weights were significantly decreased in IUGR and IUGR_Lf groups compared to CTL group. The difference persisted postnatally until weaning. While IUGR and IUGR_Lf gained only 17% of initial weight at gestational day 21 (G21), whereas CTL dams gained 50% of initial weight. No significant effect of Lf supplementation was perceived on the IUGR_Lf dams compared to the IUGR ones. However, IUGR_Lf dam body weights were no longer statistically different from the control groups at the third week of lactation.

At P1 (**Figure 1**), IUGR and IUGR_Lf pups were lighter than CTL pups. At P7 and 14, only IUGR pup weights were different from CTL group. From P21, pups grew with no significant difference among them.

Microstructural Integrity

To allow the assessment of cerebral microstructure, diffusivity (Mean, MD; Axial, AD and Radial, AD), fractional anisotropy (FA) and direction encoded color maps (DEC), intra-neurite volume fraction (f_{icvf}), cerebrospinal volume fraction (f_{iso}) and orientation dispersion index (ODI) maps acquired at P7 and P21 on a 9.4T scanners are presented in **Figure 2**. High Signal-to-noise ratio and very good resolution were obtained leading

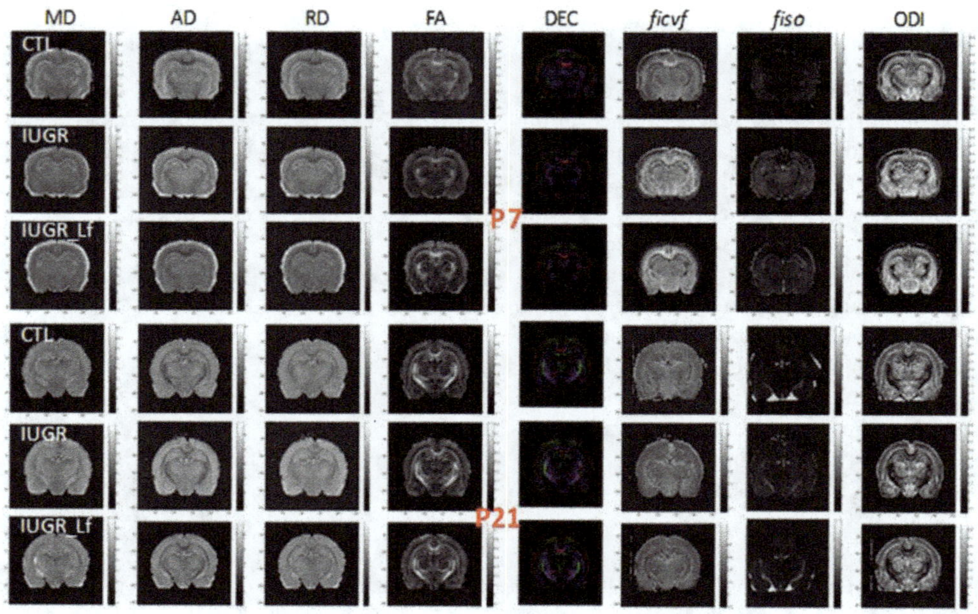

FIGURE 2 | Diffusivity (Mean, MD; Axial, AD; Radial, RD), fractional anisotropy (FA) and direction encoded color (DEC) maps, intra-neurite volume fraction (f_{icvf}), cerebrospinal volume fraction (f_{iso}), and orientation dispersion index (ODI) maps at P7 and P21 for each group.

to accurate measurement of the DTI and NODDI derived parameters (20).

Cortical Microstructure

Cortical DTI and NODDI derived parameters assessing cortical microstructure integrity, were obtained by diffusion MR imaging (**Figure 3**). IUGR and CTL derived parameters were not different from each other at P7, but IUGR_Lf parameters were different compared to the IUGR group: Indeed, a significant decrease in radial (RD) and mean diffusivity (MD), and also increased fractional anisotropy (FA) and intraneurite volume fraction (f_{icvf}) were observed with Lf. At P21, caloric restriction induced significant increase of RD, MD and f_{iso}, this last parameter was not restored by Lf.

In the cortex, most of the cell markers were not modified (**Figure 4**). At P7, only synaptophysin expression was significantly decreased in the IUGR group compared to CTL, showing a potential delay in synaptogenesis (**Figure 4**) but expression was similar between IUGR and IUGR_Lf cortices (**Figure 4**). At P21, only MBP expression was different among the groups (**Figure 4**). This marker of myelin formation and compaction was significantly decreased in the IUGR group. In the IUGR_Lf group, MBP expression was not statistically different from both IUGR and CTL groups (**Figure 4**). Also, Iba-1 expression was increased in IUGR pups, suggesting an impact on microglia. However, no alteration in CD68 expression, as marker of reactive microglia, expressions in the IUGR_Lf group were not different from the IUGR group at both ages (**Figure 4**).

Key receptors, transporters and kinases taking part in the global cerebral metabolism were quantified (**Figure 5**). At P7, MCT2 cortical expression was significantly decreased in the IUGR group (**Figure 5**), probably as a consequence of disrupted energy metabolism. Also, at P7, a trend was visible with an increased expression of leptin receptor in IUGR pups when compared to CTL pups ($P = 0.055$). βCaMKII, a major kinase in pre- and postsynaptic mechanisms and related to synaptic plasticity, was statistically less expressed in P7 IUGR pups, and showed a trend to be more expressed in IUGR_Lf animals (**Figure 5**, $P = 0.086$). No statistical difference was observed in the IUGR_Lf group (**Figure 5**). Protein and gene expressions involved in growth, differentiation and survival, as well as in apoptotic pathways were analyzed by immunoblotting and RT-qPCR. Cortical mRNA levels of BDNF showed a trend ($P = 0.068$) to be decreased (**Figure 5**) and the Bcl-2 mRNA level was significantly decreased in the P7 IUGR group (**Figure 5**), whereas no statistical difference with IUGR_Lf was observed (**Figure 5**) compared to CTL. Fractin expression, known to attest caspase 3 activity, was not statistically different among the groups (**Figure 5**).

At P21, we assessed whether a hypocaloric induced IUGR would induce oxidative stress in the brain of rat pups, leading to impairment of the cortical parvalbumin (PV) expressing neurons, known to play a critical role in cognition. A significantly higher 8-oxo-dG [marker for DNA oxidative damage (21)] in the cortex of hypocaloric induced IUGR pup rats compared to control was observed ($P < 0.0001$, **Figure 6**). We have previously established that oxidative stress during development leads to PV-IR and WFA+ PV cell deficit (22, 23). Indeed the number of PV-IR cell and PV-IR cell intensity in the ACC of IUGR rats were significantly decreased compared to CTL (**Figure 6**, # of PV cell: $P = 0.0044$, and PV-IR cell intensity: $P = 0.047$, not shown).

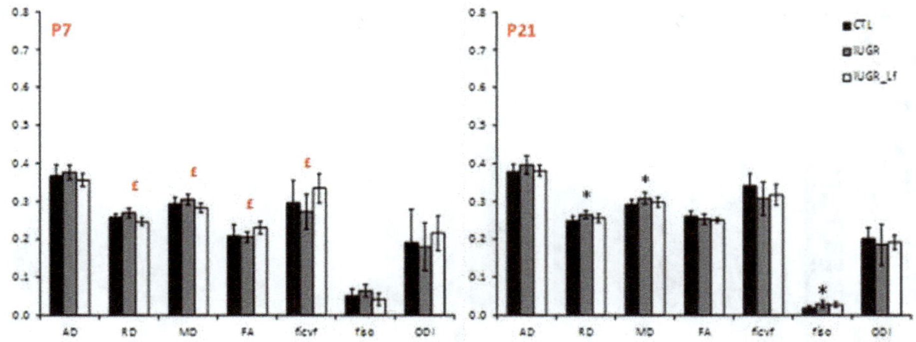

FIGURE 3 | Histogram of diffusivities (Mean, MD; Axial, AD and Radial, RD; $\times 10^{-4}$ $mm^2.s^{-1}$), fractional anisotropy (FA), intra-neurite volume fraction (f_{icvf}), cerebrospinal volume fraction (f_{iso}), and orientation dispersion index (ODI) at P7 and P21 in the cortex. Results are mean ± SD. $P < 0.05$, *CTL vs. IUGR, $CTL vs. IUGR_Lf, £IUGR vs. IUGR_Lf. *Effect of the lesion; £effect of Lf, red positive, black negative; *, £effect of the lesion restored by Lf; *,$effect of lesion but no effect of Lf; *, £,$effect of the lesion partially restored by Lf.

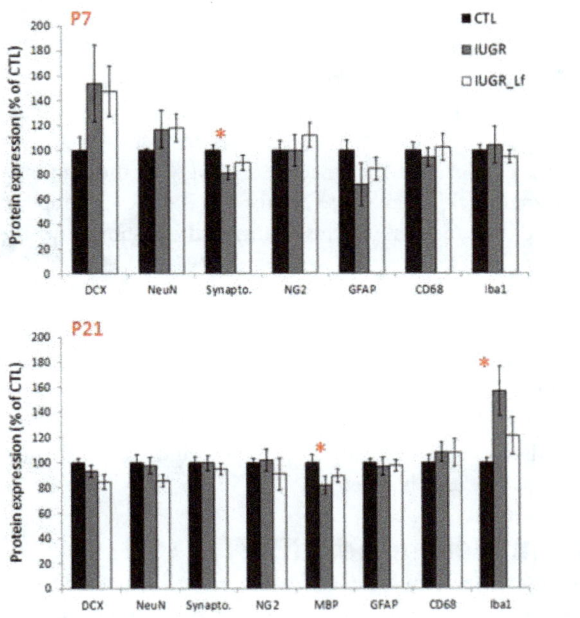

FIGURE 4 | Normalized protein expression to the control group level in CTL, IUGR, and IUGR_Lf pups at P7 (high panel) and P21 (low panel) in the cortex. Results are mean value ± SEM. $N = 5–7$ pups per group (P7) and $N = 9–14$ pups per group (P21). $P < 0.05$ *CTL vs. IUGR. Raw data in **Supplementary Tables 1, 2**.

However, the WFA+ PV cells, which are PV+ cells surrounded by PNN were not strongly affected as the decrease in IUGR rats *vs.* CTL remained at a trend level.

In order to assess the subsequent damages of oxidative stress on PV-IR cells and WFA+ PV (PNNs) during early post-weaning ages, we assessed whether Lf could prevent PV-IR and PNN impairment in ACC of IUGR rats. Indeed, Lf supplementation during development prevented increase of 8-oxo-dG intensity in the ACC of IUGR_Lf rats as compared to IUGR rats ($P < 0.0001$, **Figure 7**). The oxidative stress marker levels, 8-oxo-dG intensity, in ACC of IUGR_Lf rats did not significantly differ from that of in control rats. Lactoferrin also fully restored the number of PV-IR cells in ACC of IUGR_Lf compared to IUGR alone ($P = 0.001$), and compared to CTL rats ($P = 0.65$, NS). Interestingly, the WFA+ PV (PV PNNs) deficit in ACC of IUGR rats was not prevented by Lf ($P = 0.23$, NS).

Striatum

DTI and NODDI derived parameters were measured in the striatum (**Figure 7**). IUGR striatal microstructure integrity presented significant alterations compared to the CTL group. Increase in AD and RD at P7 and P21, as well as decrease in f_{icvf} and increase in f_{iso} at P7 depicted microstructural changes. DTI and NODDI parameter changes were reverted in P7 IUGR_Lf pups and partially at P21.

Structural proteins used as cell markers in the striatum were not differentially expressed between the groups. However, NG2 expression was increased at P7 in IUGR_Lf striatum compared to the IUGR group (**Figure 8**). In striatum, at P7, the apoptotic pathway was potentially affected in IUGR pups with the anti-apoptotic Bcl-2 mRNA expression statistically downregulated and data showed a tendency ($P = 0.053$) to be reversed in IUGR_Lf when compared to IUGR pups. At P21 (**Figure 8**, lower panel), alteration in synaptic plasticity in the IUGR group was depicted by a statistical decrease in βCaMKII expression compared to the CTL group. This altered expression was reverted in the IUGR_Lf group. Fractin quantification was not statistically different among the groups. Growth factor IGF2 was found to be statistically increased in IUGR at P21 with no statistical difference in IUGR_Lf.

External Capsule

DTI and NODDI derived parameters in external capsule white matter tract are shown in **Figure 9**. At P7, RD was significantly increased in IUGR pups and reversed, along with a decrease in AD and MD, in IUGR_Lf when compared to IUGR. In the P7 IUGR_Lf group, f_{icvf} and f_{iso} were also significantly different from the IUGR group and there was no statistical difference between IUGR_Lf and CTL pups.

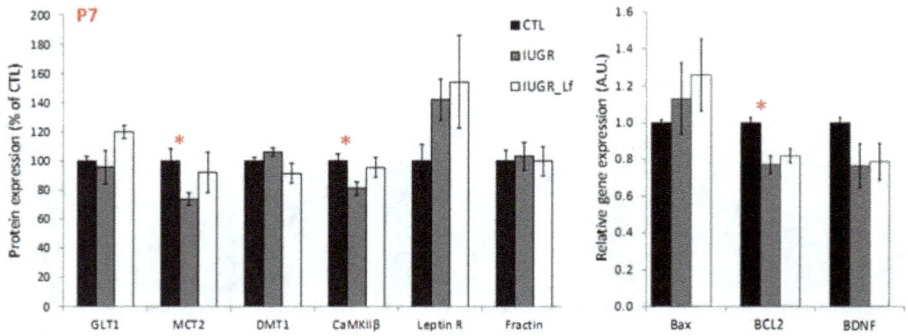

FIGURE 5 | Cortical protein (normalized to the control group level) involved in global brain mechanisms such as metabolism, growth and apoptosis for CTL, IUGR, and IUGR_Lf pups at P7. Quantification was done either after immunoblotting or RT-qPCR. Selection of metabolic transporter and receptor expressions (GLT1, MCT2, DMT1, CaMKIIβ, and Leptin R) and proteic feature of apoptosis (Fractin). Expression of pro- and anti-apoptotic mRNA (Bax and BCL2) and growth factor BDNF mRNA expression (BDNF). Results are mean values ± SEM of $N = 6–7$ pups per group. $P < 0.05$ *CTL vs. IUGR. Raw data in **Supplementary Table 3**.

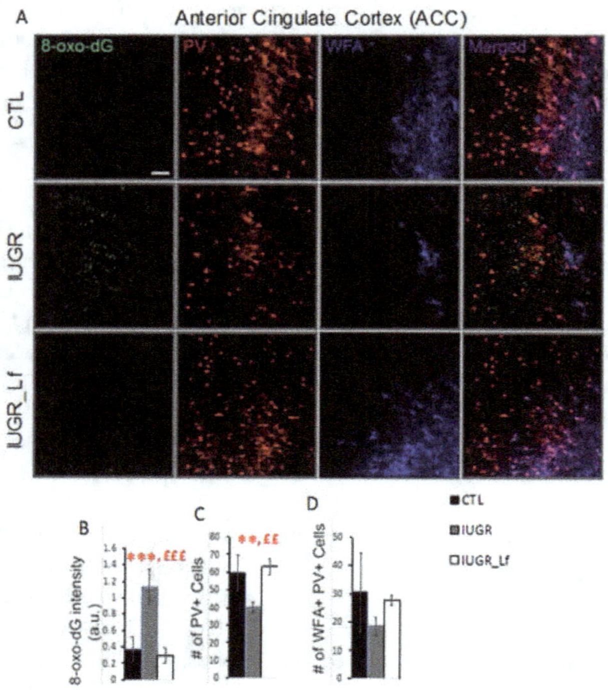

FIGURE 6 | Interneurons assessment in the cortex at P21. **(A)** Micrographs showing labeling for 8-oxo-dG (labels mitochondrial DNA oxidation), PV, and WFA (labels PNN) in ACC of CTL, IUGR, and IUGR_Lf. **(B)** Lactoferrin prevents increase in 8-oxo-dG labeling. **(C)** Quantification reveals that Lactoferrin restores PV immunoreactive cell deficits in hypocaloric induced IUGR rats. **(D)** There is a tendency for lactoferrin to prevent decrease of PNN (WFA + PV) in hypocaloric induced IUGR rats. Bars in all graphs represent SD. For each group $n = 4$ (for each animal 3–4 brain sections). *CTL vs. IUGR, £IUGR vs. IUGR_Lf, number of * or £: 3 $P < 0.001$; 2 $P < 0.01$; Scale bar: 50 μm.

Behavioral Tests

Cognitive and motor functions were assessed by a battery of behavioral tests performed between P31 to P41. These tests target behavioral aspects that could be impaired in IUGR children, such as motor activity, attention, memory and anxiety. Rats were frequently observed and monitored; pups from IUGR groups did not exhibit any abnormalities in motion, activity or basic behavior compared to the controls.

Elevated Plus Maze (EPM)

The elevated plus maze assesses the motor activity as well as the anxiety level. The global activity between the groups was not different and showed the three groups staying more in the closed arms than in the open ones (**Figure 10**). Ratio of time spent in the open to time spent in the closed arms did not show any difference among groups.

Open Field Test (OFT)

This test assesses the exploratory drive, as well as the global activity. Rats usually avoid open spaces and rather prefer exploring the area close to the wall (thigmotaxis). This trend was visible within the three groups (**Figure 10**). However, no differences were observed.

Beam Walking Test (BWT)

Locomotor activity and coordination were assessed by BWT. The number of paw slips was converted into digits and counted as number of mistakes. No statistical differences were found between the groups (**Figure 10**).

Novel Object Recognition (NOR)

The NOR test was used to assess long-term memory. Rats were confronted to two objects in the 2 sessions of testing: two familiar objects (*objects A and A′*) and a new one (*object B*). The data did not detect preferences for the new objects nor differences within groups (**Figure 10**).

Morris Water Maze (MWM)

In the day of the test (Probe Trial) when the platform was removed, the time to find the platform zone was measured (**Figure 10**). CTL pups performed significantly better, crossing the platform region faster than IUGR and IUGR_Lf groups. The ability to learn did not vary between the groups during the training phase.

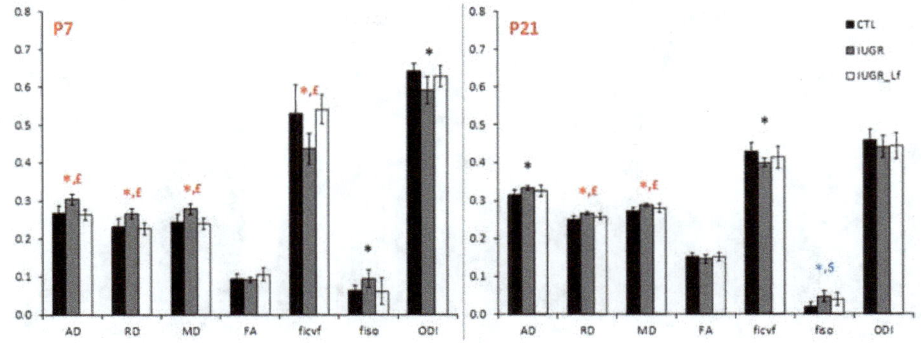

FIGURE 7 | Histogram of diffusivities (Mean, MD; Axial, AD and Radial, RD; $\times 10^{-4}$ $mm^2.s^{-1}$), fractional anisotropy (FA), intra-neurite volume fraction (f_{icvf}), cerebrospinal volume fraction (f_{iso}), and orientation dispersion index (ODI) at P7 and P21 in the striatum. $P < 0.05$, *CTL vs. IUGR, $CTL vs. IUGR_Lf, £IUGR vs. IUGR_Lf. *Effect of the lesion; £effect of Lf, red positive, black negative; *, £effect of the lesion restored by Lf; *,$effect of lesion but no effect of Lf; *, £,$effect of the lesion partially restored by Lf.

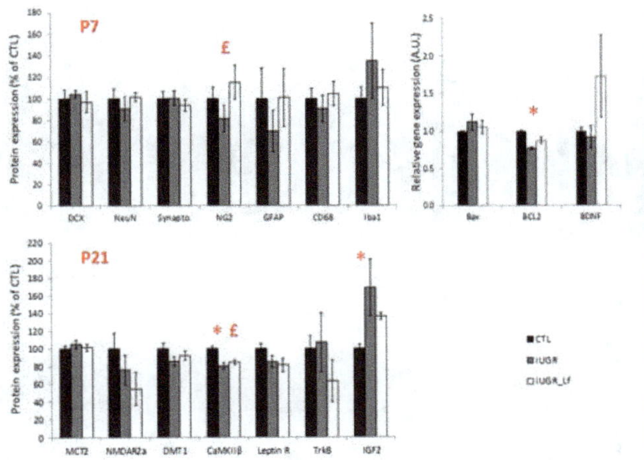

FIGURE 8 | Striatal protein (normalized to the control group level) for CTL, IUGR, and IUGR_Lf pups at P7 (high panel) and P21 (low panel). Structural protein expression at P7 (DCX, NeuN, Synapto., NG2, GFAP, CD68, and Iba1). Expression of striatal pro- and anti-apoptotic mRNA at P7 (Bax and BCL2). Selection of metabolic transporter and receptor expressions in the striatum at P21 (MCT2, NMDar2a, DMT1, CaMKIIβ, and Leptin R). Growth factor molecule and receptor mRNA expression in the striatum at P21 (TrKB and IGF2). Results are mean values ± SEM of $N = 3$ to 14 pups per group. $P < 0.05$ *CTL vs. IUGR, £IUGR vs. IUGR_Lf. Raw data in **Supplementary Tables 4, 5**.

DISCUSSION

In the present study, we explored the potential neuroprotective action of maternal bovine lactoferrin (Lf) supplementation on a 50% CR-induced IUGR model. As IUGR is thought to induce a delay in neurodevelopment, we addressed special focus on brain microstructural integrity, cell markers as well as metabolic proteins and gene expressions, which are important in cerebral development and injury. Further investigations were pursued for behavioral deficits. Analyses were performed at P7, P21 and from P31 to P41. P7 corresponds to the near term equivalent age for humans. P21 corresponds to the peak of myelination and cortical maturation providing already good information about the consequences of IUGR and potential Lf neuroprotection. Behavioral tests were performed at a time period where myelination is nearly completed (P31 to 41, preadolescent human equivalent) and as such potential mental disabilities can be observed in children at this time point. Indeed, these tests target behavioral aspects that could be impaired in IUGR children, such as motor activity, attention, memory and anxiety.

IUGR Model

Despite any effect of Lf supplementation on the weight of the dams, evidences validated our CR-induced IUGR model as it reduced maternal weight gain during gestation and had long-lasting effect during lactation period. While control dams gained 50% of their initial body weight by the end of gestation, restricted animals gained only 17%. This reduced maternal weight gain was also observed in a previous study using a stress induced model (maternal dexamethasone infusion) during the third week of gestation (12) and by others (24). Low birth weight in IUGR newborns is considered as a major indicator of prenatal insults. Pups were weighted at P1, and as both restricted diets were isocaloric, it was not expected that nutritional supplementation with Lf would improve low body weight in P1 IUGR pups indicating that offspring birthweight is highly dependent on the maternal food caloric intake during gestation. However, while IUGR pups receiving Lf through lactation caught up control body weight at P7, IUGR catch-up was only observed at P21. This gives rise to a potentially improved early metabolism in IUGR pups receiving Lf. In a placental insufficiency model, pups with moderate IUGR had a catch-up growth at P7, whereas catch-up growth in severe IUGR pups was not reported (25).

Cortical Impairment and Effects of Lactoferrin

We reported a decrease in cortical synaptophysin expression at P7 in whole cortical homogenate tissue, resulting from caloric restriction. As IUGR neurodevelopment is thought to be delayed due to reduced nutrients during a critical

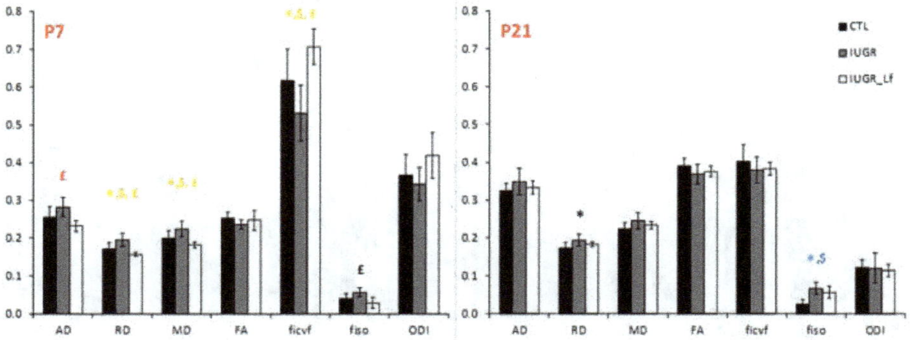

FIGURE 9 | Histogram of diffusivities (Mean, MD; Axial, AD and Radial, RD; $\times 10^{-4}$ mm^2.s^{-1}), fractional anisotropy (FA), intra-neurite volume fraction (f_{icvf}), cerebrospinal volume fraction (f_{iso}), and orientation dispersion index (ODI) at P7 and P21 in the external capsule. $P < 0.05$, *CTL vs. IUGR, $CTL vs. IUGR_Lf, £IUGR vs. IUGR_Lf. *Effect of the lesion; £effect of Lf, red positive, black negative; *, £effect of the lesion restored by Lf; *,$effect of lesion but no effect of Lf; *, £,$: effect of the lesion partially restored by Lf.

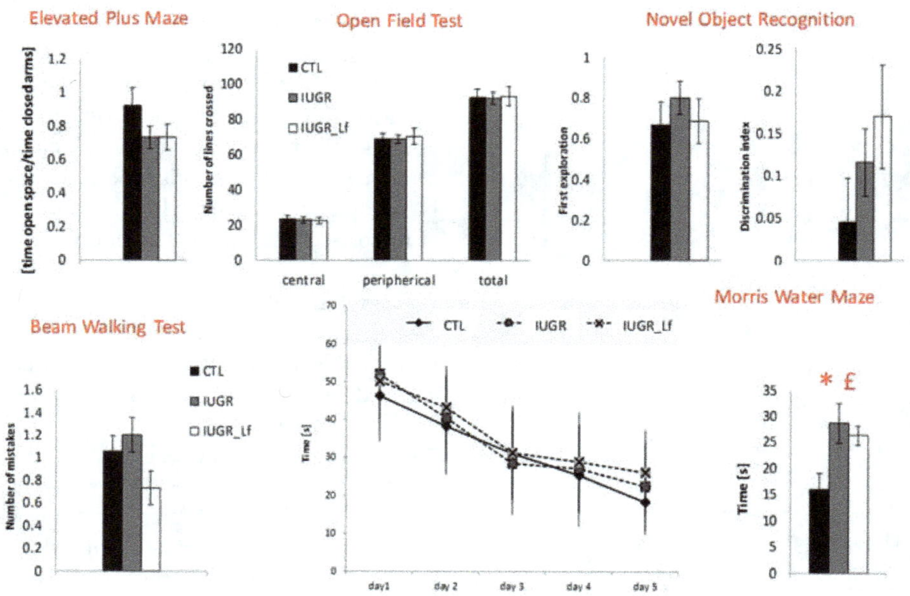

FIGURE 10 | Behavioral test results for CTL, IUGR, and IUGR_Lf pups. Elevated plus maze: ratio measuring the time spent in open space divided by the time spent in closed arm in the elevated plus maze. The center of the apparatus was considered as open space. Open field test: exploratory drive analysis by number of lines crossed in the central and peripherical zone, and in total in the open filed test. Novel object recognition: preferences between familiar and new object in novel object recognition. First object explored (familiar object = 0 and new object = 1) and Discrimination index showing preference for the new object. Beam walking test: number of paw slips during the beam walking test. Morris water maze: time to find the platform zone in the Morris water maze with learning curve displaying the time to find the platform through the five-day training (Day values are the mean of four trials) and time to find the platform zone the day of the test. All results are mean values ± SEM, $N = 16$–26 pups per group. $P < 0.05$ *CTL vs. IUGR, £IUGR vs. IUGR_Lf.

phase of cerebral development (26–28), the present result suggest that IUGR leads to transient delay in synaptogenesis in the cortex in P7 restricted rats. Similarly in sheep (29), impaired fetal environment was induced by an intra-amniotic lipopolysaccharide pro-inflammatory environment and cerebral synaptophysin expression was reported to be decreased in motor, somatosensory and entorhinal cortices causing reduction in density of presynaptical boutons.

A decrease in beta Ca2+/calmodulin-dependent protein kinase II (βCaMKII) expression in the cortex further supports this interpretation. βCaMKII is activated by calcium and is an important kinase targeting substrate responsible for long-term potentiation (30). *In vitro* overexpression induced an increase in the number of neurite extensions and in formation of new synapses (31). Therefore, it is related to morphology and quantity of synapses (32) by modifying the cytoskeletal structure. Along with our previous results on synaptophysin expression, decrease in βCaMKII emphasizes a potentially altered number/size of synapses and supports a transient delay in synaptic formation and possibly function.

Myelin basic protein (MBP) is one of the main components of myelin sheath structure and primordial for its formation and compaction and for axonal. In the current study, MBP expression was reduced in the cortex in IUGR pups at P21. Uterine artery ligation IUGR induced models have been widely used to approach white matter damage linked to perinatal impairments such as prematurity or fetal growth restriction observing a similar reduction in MBP density in the corpus callosum and the cingulum, sign of myelination defect (24).

Moreover, cortical expression of Iba-1, a microglial protein, was increased at P21. As it is expressed in both quiescent and amoeboid form and even though it is upregulated by activation (33), we quantified CD68 expression in order to identify properly activated microglial. However, CD68 analysis failed to identify microglial activation induced by IUGR. In a placental insufficiency rat model, inflammatory microgliosis was reported to impair white matter development (24). Indeed, using another marker (OX42) for immunohistochemistry, a higher density of microglia was observed in IUGR rats. Taken together, myelin integrity alteration concomitant with increased microglia density are in accordance with others work (14). Even though, our current results showed comparatively less microstructural alterations, it may further demonstrate the neuroinflammatory basis for cerebral impaired development in IUGR condition.

Despite an absence of significant differences, a tendency in the up-regulation of βCaMKII, synaptogenesis and MBP levels was observed in the Lf supplemented group providing evidence for a beneficial effect on cortical development. Indeed, DTI and NODDI derived parameters demonstrated a potential conservation of the microstructure in the cortex at P7 in IUGR_Lf rats compared to IUGR even though at P21 remaining impairments detected by diffusion MRI appeared moderates in the IUGR group. Altogether these results suggest that Lactoferrin reduces the delayed and impaired cortical development following caloric restriction.

We have demonstrated that redox dysregulation and oxidative stress (genetic or environmental origin) during development, in several animals models relevant to schizophrenia and autism, at microcircuit levels, leads to excitatory-inhibitory imbalance through impairment of the PV inhibitory network and their PNN (23, 34, 35). Similar redox dysregulation processes during development, at macrocircuit levels, could underlie impaired oligodendrocytes and delayed cortical myelination (34, 36). Parvalbumin immunoreactive (PV-IR) cell, oligodendrocyte and myelination impairment have been reported in schizophrenia (37). Abnormal control of redox system could therefore affect neuronal synchronization important for cognitive processing, and also disturb myelination leading to subsequent white matter injuries. N-acetyl-cysteine (NAC) is an antioxidant demonstrated to prevent oxidative stress during development and as such, to protect PVI and PNN. Clinically, several positive effects of NAC have been observed including an improvement of negative symptoms, a decrease of antipsychotics side effects, and an improvement of mismatch negativity and local neural synchronization in chronic schizophrenic psychosis. Recently, Conus et al. (38) observed on early psychosis patients that NAC add-on therapy for 6 months led to significant improvements in neuro-cognition and a reduced positive symptoms in patients presenting high oxidative status.

In the present study, lactoferrin prevents oxidative stress thus restoring PV-IR cell deficits in ACC of hypocaloric induced IUGR rat pups. Lactoferrin could have prevented oxidative stress and restored PV-IR impairment through anti-inflammatory and antioxidant properties in the same way as NAC does, even without improving MBP expression (myelination). Although beyond the scope of the present study, it may prove vital for the future studies to look into additional functional consequences of hypocaloric induced IUGR, such as mismatch negativity (sensory gating), and fast spiking neuronal synchronization (important for cognitive and social processing), and the effect of lactoferrin supplementation. This would certainly shed additional light on the contribution of a developmental undernutrition in psychiatric disease such as schizophrenia and potential prevention.

Impaired Microstructure in Striatum and Restoration With Lf

MR Imaging of the striatum of IUGR pups showed promising improvement of the neurodevelopment with Lf. The striatum is a vulnerable gray matter area in developing brain (11), which was proposed to be especially affected in case of periventricular leukomalacia and may be related to mild motor deficits (39) but also potentially to psychiatric disorders such as schizophrenia (40). In the present study, at P7, microstructural organization was altered or delayed, as depicted by reduction of the neurite density (f_{icvf}) and dispersion of the fibers (ODI) were reduced whereas isotropic volume fraction (f_{iso}) was increased. No changes in cell markers used in the current study were identified, suggesting alterations of arborization/maturation rather than in neuronal or glial reduced populations. No difference in MBP expression was observed, however, the low level of MBP immunostaining of brain sections at early time-point did not allow a structural assessment in the axonal fascicles. Nonetheless, these parameters were normalized with Lf, promoting a better integrity of the striatum in the first week after birth. Similar neuroprotective effect of Lf was observed at longer term (P21) in the striatum following lipopolysaccharide injection in the rat pup (11). MCT 2 expression in the striatum was decreased as observed in the cortex. Similar to the cortex, striatal mRNA expression of Bcl-2 was also downregulated and normalized with the Lf supplementation. As Bax expression was not affected by IUGR, reduction in anti-apoptotic protein presumed an increased apoptotic rate in IUGR condition (Bax/Bcl-2) (41). However, no increase in fractin expression was visible. Interestingly, βCaMKII protein expression was reduced in IUGR and restored with Lf at P21. Lactoferrin administration also improved striatal expression of βCaMKII. DTI/NODDI and βCaMKII findings suggest reduced arborization as consequence of IUGR reversed by Lf.

External Capsule, IUGR Impact on White Matter Tracts, and Repair With Lf

In external capsule, increased water diffusivity was observed perpendicularly to the main diffusion direction at P7. This abnormal RD was associated with increased f_{iso} and reduced neurite density emphasizing clearly for a defective myelin organization. RD in the external capsule and corpus callosum were also increased in P21 moderate—but not in mild—IUGR pups after placental insufficiency (42). As it was correlated with poor oligodendrocyte density and an abnormal percentage of unmyelinated axons, RD modification was suggested to result readily from this myelin injury. All these studies related impaired neurodevelopment with alteration in the external capsule around 3 weeks of age. By this time, oligodendrocyte and astrocyte proliferations and maturations stage is likely to be finished. However, in our case, the microstructural alterations of external capsule were observed in P7 pups transiently as almost no difference was measured at P21. Positive effect of Lf at 7 days point was obvious. Our model further argues for a potential delay in myelination process rather than a long-lasting injury.

Neuroprotection with Lf was assessed in the inflammatory (11) and hypoxic-ischemic (10) models, as well as in the present CR model. While partial normalization was observed in the case of brain inflammation, diffusivities were fully normalized in the hypoxic-ischemic injured brain, such as the RD in the present study. Supplementation with Lf appeared to improve impaired white matter formation.

Limitation of IUGR Impact and Neuroprotection by Lf

The present study further illustrates the complexity of the IUGR condition, which depends on the timing, the severity, the heterogeneity of risk factors and pathways potentially impaired that are mimicked by various animal models. Maternal stress, placental insufficiency and undernutrition mimicking-models were all reported to interfere with fetal trajectory growth but altered pathways are very likely to differ depending on the risk factor (43). Our present model, moderate undernutrition, using a 50% caloric restriction during gestation, is likely to induce a mild and transient impairment to the neurodevelopment despite the IUGR phenotype. We believe that part of the non-significant changes seen in the model and the partial Lf neuroprotection are due to the mild IUGR model used. It is important to notice that mild IUGR has been also reported in humans with moderate but depicted developmental impairments (44). It is important to notice that this model mimics one type of environmental risk which is necessary but not sufficient by itself alone to reproduce fully the clinical phenotypes. One may need the combination with genetic risks as well. As such, the mildness of the model is evident and may be responsible for absence of behavioral impairments. Furthermore, behavior evaluation was made at childhood age before adulthood where psychiatric symptoms generally occur following IUGR including social problems, poor cognitive performances, anxiety, and schizophrenia (45). Notice that, due to the variability of the caloric restriction model and according to the high number of different techniques used in this study, number of pups in each group was not large enough to assess possible gender differences but it is point to consider in further experiments.

CONCLUSION

In this study, we show that IUGR induced by moderate undernutrition demonstrated mild cerebral impairments. Cortical synaptogenesis and myelination were potentially delayed. Striatal microstructure showed alterations. The white matter integrity assessed in the external capsule presented abnormal development. Lf supplementation showed beneficial restoration in the cortex, in the striatum microstructure and in the white matter organization of the external capsule. Further Lf showed reduced oxidative stress in ACA interneurons. This model does not fully represent the clinical situation as IUGR newborns often cumulate adverse conditions in addition to IUGR, such as hypoxia-ischemia or infection/inflammation. Nevertheless, oral Lf supplementation showed partial neuroprotection in this CR IUGR model. This is also neuroprotective against hypoxia-ischemia and inflammation in the developing brain, and thus represents a very promising tool to reduce developmental diseases in IUGR and preterm infants.

AUTHOR CONTRIBUTIONS

All authors participated to the design of the study. ES performed behavioral analysis. AT performed IUGR model. CL and J-HC performed immunostaining, protein and gene expression analysis. YvdL performed MRI experiments and analyzed the data. YvdL and CL wrote the manuscript. ES, J-HC, AT, KD, and SS revised the manuscript.

FUNDING

ES received a Swiss Excellence Scholarship for Foreign Scholars to perform the study in SVZ laboratory. This study was supported by the Swiss National Fund N° 33CM30-124101/140334 and the Fondation pour Recherches Médicales, Geneva, the Center for Biomedical Imaging (CIBM) of the UNIL, UNIGE, HUG, CHUV, and EPFL, and the Leenaards and Jeantet Foundations.

REFERENCES

1. Batalle D, Eixarch E, Figueras F, Munoz-Moreno E, Bargallo N, Illa M, et al. Altered small-world topology of structural brain networks in infants with intrauterine growth restriction and its association with later neurodevelopmental outcome. *Neuroimage* (2012) 60:1352–66. doi: 10.1016/j.neuroimage.2012.01.059

2. Ramenghi LA, Martinelli A, De Carli A, Brusati V, Mandia L, Fumagalli M, et al. Cerebral maturation in IUGR and appropriate for gestational age preterm babies. *Reprod Sci.* (2011) 18:469–75. doi: 10.1177/1933719110388847
3. Tolsa CB, Zimine S, Warfield SK, Freschi M, Sancho Rossignol A, Lazeyras F, et al. Early alteration of structural and functional brain development in premature infants born with intrauterine growth restriction. *Pediatr Res.* (2004) 56:132–8. doi: 10.1203/01.PDR.0000128983.54614.7E
4. Sandomirsky BP, Galchenko SE, Galchenko KS. Antioxidative properties of lactoferrin from bovine colostrum before and after its lyophilization. *Cryo Lett.* (2003) 24:275–80.
5. Satue-Gracia MT, Frankel EN, Rangavajhyala N, German JB. Lactoferrin in infant formulas: effect on oxidation. *J Agric Food Chem.* (2000) 48:4984–90. doi: 10.1021/jf0002490
6. Ronayne de Ferrer PA, Baroni A, Sambucetti ME, Lopez NE, Ceriani Cernadas JM. Lactoferrin levels in term and preterm milk. *J Am Coll Nutr.* (2000) 19:370–3. doi: 10.1080/07315724.2000.10718933
7. Huang RQ, Ke WL, Qu YH, Zhu JH, Pei YY, Jiang C. Characterization of lactoferrin receptor in brain endothelial capillary cells and mouse brain. *J Biomed Sci.* (2007) 14:121–8. doi: 10.1007/s11373-006-9121-7
8. Haversen L, Ohlsson BG, Hahn-Zoric M, Hanson LA, Mattsby-Baltzer I. Lactoferrin down-regulates the LPS-induced cytokine production in monocytic cells via NF-kappa B. *Cell Immunol.* (2002) 220:83–95. doi: 10.1016/S0008-8749(03)00006-6
9. Manzoni P, Rinaldi M, Cattani S, Pugni L, Romeo MG, Messner H, et al. Bovine lactoferrin supplementation for prevention of late-onset sepsis in very low-birth-weight neonates: a randomized trial. *JAMA* (2009) 302:1421–8. doi: 10.1001/jama.2009.1403
10. van de Looij Y, Ginet V, Chatagner A, Toulotte A, Somm E, Huppi PS, et al. Lactoferrin during lactation protects the immature hypoxic-ischemic rat brain. *Ann Clin Transl Neurol.* (2014) 1:955–67. doi: 10.1002/acn3.138
11. Ginet V, van de Looij Y, Petrenko V, Toulotte A, Kiss J, Huppi PS, et al. Lactoferrin during lactation reduces lipopolysaccharide-induced brain injury. *Biofactors* (2016) 42:323–36. doi: 10.1002/biof.1278
12. Somm E, Larvaron P, van de Looij Y, Toulotte A, Chatagner A, Faure M, et al. Protective effects of maternal nutritional supplementation with lactoferrin on growth and brain metabolism. *Pediatr Res.* (2014) 75:51–61. doi: 10.1038/pr.2013.199
13. Zhang H, Schneider T, Wheeler-Kingshott CA, Alexander DC. NODDI: practical *in vivo* neurite orientation dispersion and density imaging of the human brain. *Neuroimage* (2012) 61:1000–16. doi: 10.1016/j.neuroimage.2012.03.072
14. Rideau Batista Novais A, Pham H, Van de Looij Y, Bernal M, Mairesse J, Zana-Taieb E, et al. Transcriptomic regulations in oligodendroglial and microglial cells related to brain damage following fetal growth restriction. *Glia* (2016) 64:2306–20. doi: 10.1002/glia.23079
15. Berretta S, Pantazopoulos H, Markota M, Brown C, Batzianouli ET. Losing the sugar coating: potential impact of perineuronal net abnormalities on interneurons in schizophrenia. *Schizophr Res.* (2015) 167:18–27. doi: 10.1016/j.schres.2014.12.040
16. Wang D, Fawcett J. The perineuronal net and the control of CNS plasticity. *Cell Tissue Res.* (2012) 349:147–60. doi: 10.1007/s00441-012-1375-y
17. Sanches EF, Van de Looij Y, Toulotte A, da Silva AR, Romero J, Sizonenko SV. Brain metabolism alterations induced by pregnancy swimming decreases neurological impairments following neonatal hypoxia-ischemia in very immature rats. *Front Neurol.* (2018) 9:480. doi: 10.3389/fneur.2018.00480
18. Walf AA, Frye CA. The use of the elevated plus maze as an assay of anxiety-related behavior in rodents. *Nat Protoc.* (2007) 2:322–8. doi: 10.1038/nprot.2007.44
19. Rojas A, Ganesh T, Manji Z, O'Neill T, Dingledine R. Inhibition of the prostaglandin E2 receptor EP2 prevents status epilepticus-induced deficits in the novel object recognition task in rats. *Neuropharmacology* (2016) 110(Pt A):419–30. doi: 10.1016/j.neuropharm.2016.07.028
20. Jones DK, Basser PJ. "Squashing peanuts and smashing pumpkins": how noise distorts diffusion-weighted MR data. *Magn Reson Med.* (2004) 52:979–93. doi: 10.1002/mrm.20283
21. Kasai H. Analysis of a form of oxidative DNA damage, 8-hydroxy-2'-deoxyguanosine, as a marker of cellular oxidative stress during carcinogenesis. *Mutat Res.* (1997) 387:147–63. doi: 10.1016/S1383-5742(97)00035-5
22. Cabungcal JH, Steullet P, Morishita H, Kraftsik R, Cuenod M, Hensch TK, et al. Perineuronal nets protect fast-spiking interneurons against oxidative stress. *Proc Natl Acad Sci USA.* (2013) 110:9130–5. doi: 10.1073/pnas.1300454110
23. Cabungcal JH, Steullet P, Kraftsik R, Cuenod M, Do KQ. Early-life insults impair parvalbumin interneurons via oxidative stress: reversal by N-acetylcysteine. *Biol Psychiatry* (2013) 73:574–82. doi: 10.1016/j.biopsych.2012.09.020
24. Olivier P, Baud O, Bouslama M, Evrard P, Gressens P, Verney C. Moderate growth restriction: deleterious and protective effects on white matter damage. *Neurobiol Dis.* (2007) 26:253–63. doi: 10.1016/j.nbd.2007.01.001
25. Olivier P, Baud O, Evrard P, Gressens P, Verney C. Prenatal ischemia and white matter damage in rats. *J Neuropathol Exp Neurol.* (2005) 64:998–1006. doi: 10.1097/01.jnen.0000187052.81889.57
26. Baschat AA. Neurodevelopment after fetal growth restriction. *Fetal Diagn Ther.* (2014) 36:136–42. doi: 10.1159/000353631
27. Morgane PJ, Austin-LaFrance R, Bronzino J, Tonkiss J, Diaz-Cintra S, Cintra L, et al. Prenatal malnutrition and development of the brain. *Neurosci Biobehav Rev.* (1993) 17:91–128. doi: 10.1016/S0149-7634(05)80234-9
28. Rice D, Barone SJr. Critical periods of vulnerability for the developing nervous system: evidence from humans and animal models. *Environ Health Perspect.* (2000) 108 (Suppl. 3):511–33. doi: 10.1289/ehp.00108s3511
29. Strackx E, Jellema RK, Rieke R, Gussenhoven R, Vles JS, Kramer BW, et al. Intra-amniotic LPS induced region-specific changes in presynaptic bouton densities in the ovine fetal brain. *BioMed Res Int.* (2015) 2015:276029. doi: 10.1155/2015/276029
30. Lisman J, Yasuda R, Raghavachari S. Mechanisms of CaMKII action in long-term potentiation. *Nat Rev Neurosci.* (2012) 13:169–82. doi: 10.1038/nrn3192
31. Fink CC, Bayer KU, Myers JW, Ferrell JEJr, Schulman H, Meyer T. Selective regulation of neurite extension and synapse formation by the beta but not the alpha isoform of CaMKII. *Neuron* (2003) 39:283–97. doi: 10.1016/S0896-6273(03)00428-8
32. Okamoto K, Narayanan R, Lee SH, Murata K, Hayashi Y. The role of CaMKII as an F-actin-bundling protein crucial for maintenance of dendritic spine structure. *Proc Natl Acad Sci USA.* (2007) 104:6418–23. doi: 10.1073/pnas.0701656104
33. Ito D, Tanaka K, Suzuki S, Dembo T, Fukuuchi Y. Enhanced expression of Iba1, ionized calcium-binding adapter molecule 1, after transient focal cerebral ischemia in rat brain. *Stroke* (2001) 32:1208–15. doi: 10.1161/01.STR.32.5.1208
34. Do KQ, Cabungcal JH, Frank A, Steullet P, Cuenod M. Redox dysregulation, neurodevelopment, and schizophrenia. *Curr Opin Neurobiol.* (2009) 19:220–30. doi: 10.1016/j.conb.2009.05.001
35. Steullet P, Cabungcal JH, Coyle J, Didriksen M, Gill K, Grace AA, et al. Oxidative stress-driven parvalbumin interneuron impairment as a common mechanism in models of schizophrenia. *Mol Psychiatry* (2017) 22:936–43. doi: 10.1038/mp.2017.47
36. Monin A, Baumann PS, Griffa A, Xin L, Mekle R, Fournier M, et al. Glutathione deficit impairs myelin maturation: relevance for white matter integrity in schizophrenia patients. *Mol Psychiatry* (2015) 20:827–38. doi: 10.1038/mp.2014.88
37. Lewis DA, Levitt P. Schizophrenia as a disorder of neurodevelopment. *Ann Rev Neurosci.* (2002) 25:409–32. doi: 10.1146/annurev.neuro.25.112701.142754
38. Conus P, Seidman LJ, Fournier M, Xin L, Cleusix M, Baumann PS, et al. N-acetylcysteine in a double-blind randomized placebo-controlled trial: toward biomarker-guided treatment in early psychosis. *Schizophr Bull.* (2018) 44:317–27. doi: 10.1093/schbul/sbx093
39. Pierson CR, Folkerth RD, Billiards SS, Trachtenberg FL, Drinkwater ME, Volpe JJ, et al. Gray matter injury associated with periventricular leukomalacia in the premature infant. *Acta Neuropathol.* (2007) 114:619–31. doi: 10.1007/s00401-007-0295-5
40. Nosarti C, Reichenberg A, Murray RM, Cnattingius S, Lambe MP, Yin L, et al. Preterm birth and psychiatric disorders in young adult life. *Arch Gen Psychiatry* (2012) 69:E1–8. doi: 10.1001/archgenpsychiatry.2011.1374
41. Yang E, Korsmeyer SJ. Molecular thanatopsis: a discourse on the BCL2 family and cell death. *Blood* (1996) 88:386–401.

42. Ruff CA, Faulkner SD, Rumajogee P, Beldick S, Foltz W, Corrigan J, et al. The extent of intrauterine growth restriction determines the severity of cerebral injury and neurobehavioural deficits in rodents. *PLoS ONE* (2017) 12:e0184653. doi: 10.1371/journal.pone.0184653
43. Winterhager E, Gellhaus A. Transplacental nutrient transport mechanisms of intrauterine growth restriction in rodent models and humans. *Front Physiol.* (2017) 8:951. doi: 10.3389/fphys.2017.00951
44. Nardozza LM, Caetano AC, Zamarian AC, Mazzola JB, Silva CP, Marcal VM, et al. Fetal growth restriction: current knowledge. *Arch Gynecol Obstet.* (2017) 295:1061–77. doi: 10.1007/s00404-017-4341-9
45. Calkins K, Devaskar SU. Fetal origins of adult disease. *Curr Probl Pediatr Adolesc Health Care* (2011) 41:158–76. doi: 10.1016/j.cppeds.2011.01.001

12

Neonatal Morbidities of Fetal Growth Restriction: Pathophysiology and Impact

Atul Malhotra[1,2,3†], Beth J. Allison[2,4†], Margie Castillo-Melendez[2,4], Graham Jenkin[2,4], Graeme R. Polglase[2,4] and Suzanne L. Miller[2,4]*

[1] Monash Newborn, Monash Children's Hospital, Melbourne, VIC, Australia, [2] The Ritchie Centre, Hudson Institute of Medical Research, Melbourne, VIC, Australia, [3] Department of Paediatrics, Monash University, Melbourne, VIC, Australia, [4] Department of Obstetrics and Gynaecology, Monash University, Melbourne, VIC, Australia

***Correspondence:**
Atul Malhotra
atul.malhotra@monash.edu

† These authors have contributed equally to this work*

Being born small lays the foundation for short-term and long-term implications for life. Intrauterine or fetal growth restriction describes the pregnancy complication of pathological reduced fetal growth, leading to significant perinatal mortality and morbidity, and subsequent long-term deficits. Placental insufficiency is the principal cause of FGR, which in turn underlies a chronic undersupply of oxygen and nutrients to the fetus. The neonatal morbidities associated with FGR depend on the timing of onset of placental dysfunction and growth restriction, its severity, and the gestation at birth of the infant. In this review, we explore the pathophysiological mechanisms involved in the development of major neonatal morbidities in FGR, and their impact on the health of the infant. Fetal cardiovascular adaptation and altered organ development during gestation are principal contributors to postnatal consequences of FGR. Clinical presentation, diagnostic tools and management strategies of neonatal morbidities are presented. We also present information on the current status of targeted therapies. A better understanding of neonatal morbidities associated with FGR will enable early neonatal detection, monitoring and management of potential adverse outcomes in the newborn period and beyond.

Keywords: IUGR, FGR, bronchopulmonary dysplasia, cardiac, brain injury, necrotizing enterocolitis

OVERVIEW AND DESCRIPTION

Fetal growth restriction (FGR) describes the fetus that does not grow to its expected biological potential *in utero*, and is a relatively common complication of pregnancy. True FGR, as compared to constitutional smallness, is a pathological condition wherein the placental fails to deliver an adequate supply of oxygen and nutrients to the developing fetus, termed placental insufficiency. As a consequence, fetal growth becomes stunted. It is only in the last several years that consensus definitions for pathological FGR have been developed (1), but it remains that many cases of FGR *in utero* remain undetected, and therefore the neonatal description of small for gestational age (SGA) continues to be a useful and necessary proxy for FGR (2). Traditionally, an estimated fetal weight or abdominal circumference of less than the 10th centile for the population at a given gestational age was considered highly suggestive of FGR. However this broad description of SGA includes the many infants (~20%) that are born small, but are otherwise healthy (2). Accordingly, consensus definitions for FGR now incorporate Doppler indices of placental function/ dysfunction during pregnancy (1), to provide a more robust assessment of pathological fetal growth restriction.

Clear and well-defined guidelines for description of FGR subsequent to placental insufficiency are important for two broad reasons, (i) early identification of FGR flags infants who are at significantly elevated risk for neonatal complications, and (ii) early identification of infants with FGR who would benefit from intervention(s) to improve outcomes. The etiology of many adverse consequences of FGR arise *in utero* from fetal hypoxia and nutrient deprivation secondary to placental dysfunction, with fetal hemodynamic adaptations *in utero* laying the foundation for altered organ structure and function in the neonatal period and beyond.

ETIOLOGY AND UTEROPLACENTAL FACTORS

The basic determinants of fetal growth are the individual's genetic makeup, nutrient availability from the mother, and environmental factors, coupled with the capacity of the placenta to adequately transfer nutrients and oxygen to the fetus, and endocrine modulation of these interactions (3, 4). Reduced fetal growth, and subsequent pathological FGR, can be caused by maternal factors (e.g., under nutrition, hypertension, preeclampsia), fetal (chromosomal abnormalities, multiple fetuses) or placental factors (5), however in the majority of cases, FGR results from placental dysfunction (6). Here, the term *placental insufficiency* is broadly used to describe reduced transfer of oxygen and nutrients to the fetus, with adverse effects on fetal development. Antecedents of placental insufficiency can include maternal malnutrition and hypertension, but in up to 60% of cases the placental insufficiency is idiopathic, wherein there is a physiological deficiency in the remodeling of uterine and placental spiral arteries resulting in restricted uteroplacental perfusion (7).

Abnormalities in placental function provide a primary clinical indicator that transfer of oxygen and nutrients is suboptimal, and fetal growth may be adversely affected. In the fetus, placental insufficiency is characterized by preferential blood flow redistribution to the vital organs (brain, myocardium, and adrenal glands), while other organs, including the gastrointestinal tract, skin, and others may be deprived of sufficient blood flow. This fetal redistribution of blood flow occurs as a direct result of hypoxia, and can be detected as altered umbilical, uterine and/or middle cerebral artery Doppler flows (8). Large population studies of small but otherwise healthy infants at birth (Apgar $\geq$ 7 at 5 min of life) demonstrates that severely growth restricted infants at the third birth weight centile are indeed chronically hypoxic; umbilical vein median pO_2 13 mmHg (FGR) versus 26 mmHg (normally grown infants), and median SaO_2 16 vs. 55% respectively (9, 10).

In addition to the fundamental roles of oxygen and glucose for development, fetal growth is dependent on a number of key anabolic hormones—placental, pancreatic, thyroid, adrenal and pituitary hormones—any disruption in these can also lead to FGR (11, 12). The insulin-like growth factors -I and -II (IGF-I and IGF-II) are both proposed to play central roles in normal fetal growth, stimulating fetal cell proliferation, differentiation, protein and glycogen synthesis, where these actions are mediated via their receptors and the IGF-binding proteins (IGFBPs). The two IGFs are detected in the fetal circulation in early gestation, and in particular it is noted that decreased serum IGF-1 is correlated with reduced fetal growth (3, 13). IGF-1 also has a central role in brain growth, white matter development and brain connectivity (14). Pregnancy-associated plasma protein-A (PAPP-A), secreted by the placental decidua, cleaves IGFBP-4, which in turn is a potent inhibitor of IGF bioactivity. Accordingly, low levels of PAPP-A in early pregnancy are linked with an increased risk for FGR, although the predictive value of this biomarker still remains poor (15). A recent study has investigated whether administration of IGF-1 into the amniotic fluid can improve postnatal growth and metabolism in a sheep model of FGR, and results from this study look promising (16) (see Interventions for Improved Outcomes section). Glucocorticoid hormones play a central role in the development and maturation of fetal organs, while growth hormone, which is the major hormonal regulator of postnatal growth, has no demonstrable effect on fetal growth *per se* (17). Exogenous glucocorticoids are administered to pregnant women at imminent risk of preterm birth to mature the fetal lungs, and preterm birth is a common complication of FGR. Preclinical and clinical evidence demonstrates that antenatal steroids may exacerbate growth restriction (particularly repeat doses) (18) and that the FGR fetus differentially responds to antenatal steroids compared to appropriately-grown fetuses, likely mediated via altered placental response to steroids (19). Antenatal glucocorticoids may not significantly improve neonatal outcomes in FGR preterm infants (20), and indeed, may have adverse effects on brain development (21, 22). Further research is clearly needed in this area.

The fetus mounts a critical hemodynamic response to hypoxia, aimed at ensuring the most important fetal organs maximize their oxygen supply. This adaptive response redistributes blood flow away from peripheral vascular beds which is preferentially shunted toward essential organs, termed *brain sparing* (23). This results in preferential supply of blood flow to favor the brain, heart, and adrenals, at the expense of the gut, kidney, hematologic organs, and peripheral vascular beds. When fetal hypoxia is chronic in nature, as occurs with placental insufficiency, the persistent fetal hemodynamic shift has significant consequences for the fetus and neonate. Characteristically, prolonged fetal hypoxia reduces fetal weight overall, but also does so in an asymmetric manner, with relatively spared head size and a thin and/or shorter body length. While hemodynamic redistribution may be an attempt to protect vital organs from hypoxic injury, an adverse impact on fetal organ development and vascular remodeling is increasingly being recognized (23, 24). For example, the shunting of blood flow away from the kidneys is now recognized as contributing to suboptimal renal development with reduced nephron endowment (25). Further, sustained vasoconstriction of peripheral vascular beds alters local arterial wall properties including endothelial vasodilator dysfunction and sympathetic hyperinnervation, and consequently contributes to cardiac remodeling (26). The short and long-term consequences of sustained redistribution of cardiac output are profound, for both spared and non-spared organs, and these will be discussed in more detail below.

The overall incidence of FGR depends on the diagnostic criteria used, and the population being examined. It is estimated that between 3 and 9% of pregnancies in the developed world, and up to 25% of pregnancies in low-middle income countries are affected by FGR (27, 28). Factors that influence FGR rates in communities include maternal nutrition, maternal and paternal smoking rates, alcohol and drug addiction, socio-economic status, maternal activity, stress during pregnancy and genetic make-up (29). The incidence of FGR is significantly higher in low- and middle- income countries, compared to high-income countries, and this is notably contributed by a large number of FGR infants born in the Asian continent, which accounts for approximately 75% of all affected infants in the world, followed by Africa and South America (30).

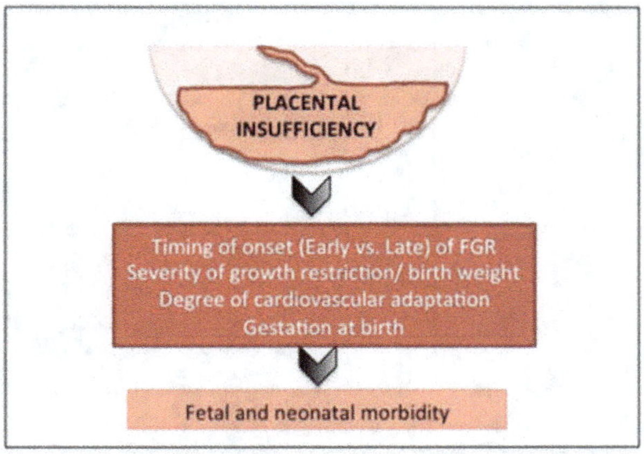

FIGURE 1 | Factors that affect outcomes in FGR.

CLASSIFICATION TYPES OF FGR

FGR can be classified as early- or late-onset, reflecting the gestational age when growth restriction is diagnosed. Early onset FGR (<32 weeks gestation) is the more severe phenotype, associated with significant disruption to placental perfusion leading to chronic fetal hypoxia, and with subsequent fetal cardiovascular adaptation *in utero* (31). Fetuses with early-onset placental insufficiency are more likely to be born preterm, to deteriorate over weeks, and have a high risk of morbidity or mortality. Late onset FGR (≥32 weeks gestation) is the more common presentation of growth restriction (up to 80% of FGR cases), and is generally linked with a milder placental deficit, together with a lesser degree of fetal hemodynamic adaptation. Although placental dysfunction is mild, this group has a high risk of deteriorating rapidly, such that they have an elevated risk of stillbirth (31). This broad distinction between early- and late-onset FGR demonstrates that the timing when placental function becomes rate limiting for the fetus is a principal factor affecting outcome.

Advances in obstetric monitoring mean that it is increasingly likely that placental insufficiency and fetal growth restriction are detected during pregnancy. However, a significant proportion (up to 50%) of FGR fetuses remain undiagnosed, and are first recognized only very late in pregnancy or at birth (32–34). Furthermore, debate continues around the utility of third trimester ultrasound for the detection of late-onset FGR (35), with a recent study reporting that undiagnosed FGR does not lead to increased incidence of morbidity in neonates (36). These data likely reflect that it is predominantly the early-onset FGR infants with severe placental insufficiency, and worse neonatal outcomes, who are more straightforward to detect during pregnancy. Currently, no effective antenatal therapy exists for FGR, hence, delivery of the fetus remains the only viable option for a severely affected pregnancy; this often occurs preterm, introducing further risk of morbidity and mortality (37, 38). Together these data are indicative that the timing of the onset of placental insufficiency (early vs. late), gestation at birth, and severity of compromise/birth weight are the most predictive factors for neonatal outcomes (39) (**Figure 1**).

PERINATAL MORBIDITIES

A typical FGR infant at term age and an appropriately grown infant at term are shown in **Figure 2**. Key pathophysiological mechanisms driving fetal growth restriction and the resulting *in-utero* and postnatal consequences are highlighted in **Figure 3**. Placental pathology and FGR are strongly associated with fetal demise *in utero*, and stillbirth (40–42). FGR is the greatest risk factor for stillbirth; overall it is shown that up to 50% of infants who are stillborn were small for gestational age or growth restricted (43). The detection, early diagnosis, surveillance and delivery of the severely growth restricted fetus are paramount to decrease stillbirth, but it remains that 40% of severe FGR infants (<3rd centile for birth weight) remain undetected *in utero* (44).

After birth, FGR infants are more likely to spend a significantly longer time in NICU compared to gestation age-matched infants (45). Accordingly, financial costs associated with the care of FGR infants are high, given that many of them will remain in NICU for prolonged periods (46, 47). FGR infants demonstrate elevated rates of intolerance to feeds/ milk, feeding difficulties and necrotizing enterocolitis (NEC). NEC is predominantly seen in infants who are born preterm, but late preterm infants are more likely to develop NEC if they were growth restricted (48). It is likely that *in utero* chronic fetal hypoxia and subsequent cardiovascular redistribution of blood flow away from the gastrointestinal tract contribute to immature gut development (49). FGR newborns, especially with abnormal flows in the umbilical artery prior to birth, are shown to have more feed intolerance when compared to their well-grown preterm counterparts (50). Superior mesenteric artery blood flows have been used as a marker for splanchnic perfusion in neonates and decreased flows correlate with feed intolerance (51). Application of near infra-red spectroscopy in the neonatal period as an assessment tool for monitoring gut perfusion can detect changes in splanchnic oxygen delivery, which may be reduced in FGR

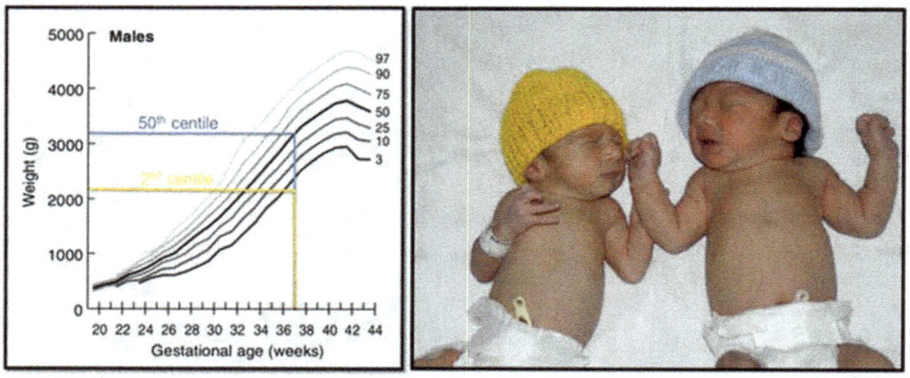

Monash Children's Hospital

HUDSON

FIGURE 2 | Example of a FGR (2nd centile weight for age, yellow), and an appropriately grown (50th centile weight for age, blue) infant born at 37 weeks gestation.

infants and may predict feeding intolerance and development of NEC (52). Studies have shown that preterm FGR infants do not tolerate enteral feeds in the first few days of life (53) but conversely there is evidence that delaying enteral feeds in preterm FGR infants does not confer any protection against feed intolerance or NEC (54). In fact, it may delay establishment of feeds and increase length of stay in the neonatal unit (55).

Malnutrition and low birth weight puts FGR infants at an increased risk of a number of transient neonatal morbidities including hypothermia, altered glucose metabolism (hypoglycemia, hyperglycemia), hypocalcemia, polycythemia, jaundice and sepsis (5). Increased risk of infection is also common, potentially related to depressed immunological state and competence (56). FGR infants born preterm also have an increased risk of retinopathy of prematurity (57). FGR is linked to altered nephrogenesis, due to suboptimal tubular development caused by intrauterine hypoxia (58), and in turn, urinary Cystatin-C excretion is increased in FGR infants compared to appropriately-grown infants which is seen to reflect reduced renal volume (59). It is therefore suggested that increased secretion of Cystatin-C signifies nephron loss as a result of the negative impact of FGR on kidney development. Factors involved in nephron loss may include intrauterine hypoxia, decreased antioxidant capacity, and altered levels of growth factors.

SPECIFIC NEONATAL MORBIDITIES (TABLE 1)

Cardiovascular Morbidity

Clinical Features

In addition to chronic hypoxia, placental insufficiency imposes other important stressors for the developing fetus, such as oxidative stress, inflammation and increased hemodynamic stress. This leads to elevated cardiac afterload due to high placental vascular resistance, which in turn directly and indirectly impacts on the developing cardiovascular system. It is now accepted that the fetal adaptations to these combined stressors sets the fetus, and future offspring, on a path of predetermined increased risk of cardiovascular disease (60, 61). It is also now apparent that subclinical or subtle evidence of cardiovascular dysfunction is present in fetal and/or early neonatal life, well before the onset of significant cardiovascular or metabolic disease in adulthood, supporting the notion of perinatal programming (60).

Advances in Doppler ultrasonography of the placental and fetal circulations provide a window of opportunity to observe and quantify fetal cardiovascular function, and early dysfunction. In early-onset FGR, severe placental insufficiency is characterized by high vascular resistance within placental vascular beds, resulting in absent or reversed diastolic umbilical artery flow, as well as high pulsatility index in the ductus venosus and increased dilation of cerebral vessels evident of fetal brain sparing (31). In late-onset FGR, umbilical artery flow may be normal, representing a milder placental insufficiency. Despite this, brain sparing is still evident, with increased cerebral to placental blood flow driven primarily by vasodilation within the middle cerebral artery in response to hypoxia (62). In both early- and late-onset FGR, increasing vasodilation within cerebral vascular beds is indicative of a worsening fetal state (63). Increased myocardial performance index, an index incorporating both diastolic and systolic function to assess global cardiac function/dysfunction, is evident from 24 weeks gestation in early onset-FGR fetuses (64). An increase in myocardial performance index is not indicative of improved performance, but rather demonstrates an increased time of systolic relaxation evident in early-onset FGR. Increased myocardial dysfunction is also present in late-onset FGR from >35 weeks gestation. In this population, late-onset placental insufficiency and FGR results in fetuses with larger, more globular hearts and early indices of functional deficits with impaired relaxation (65). This study is the first to show that late-onset placental insufficiency and FGR induces cardiac dysfunction that is detectable in the third trimester of pregnancy (~35 weeks gestation), indicating the presence of cardiac programming prior to birth. It has also been shown that

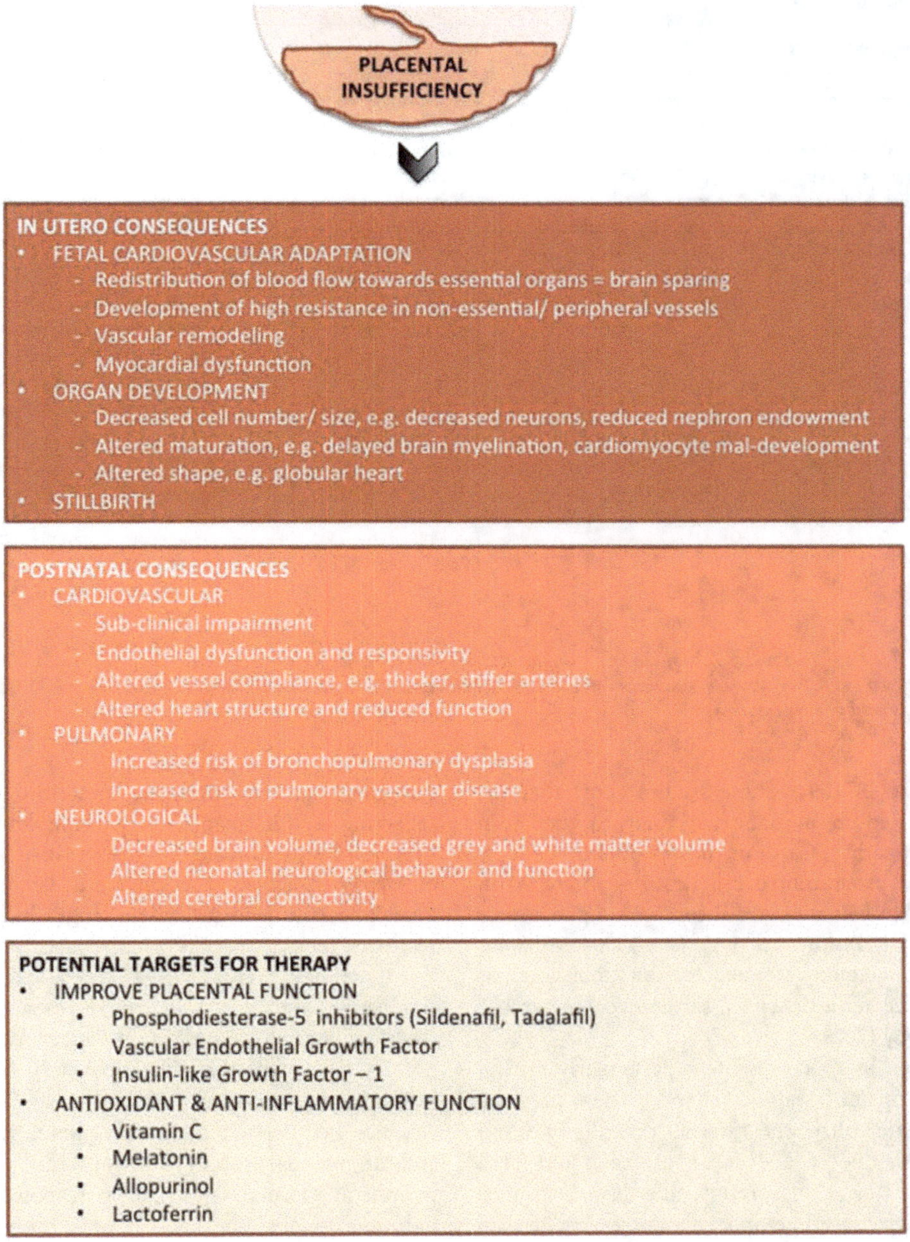

FIGURE 3 | *In-utero* and postnatal consequences of FGR and potential targeted therapies.

cardiac dysfunction and markers of cardiac injury such as BNP and H-FABP become increasingly worse as the severity of fetal compromise progresses (66).

Pathophysiology

In the presence of very high placental resistance associated with a sub-optimal pregnancy, the fetal heart contracts against an increased afterload, thereby increasing the work required to contract with each beat, resulting in increased heart wall stress and hypertrophy (65). Over a sustained period, hypertrophy increases wall thickness altering ventricular compliance. Increased afterload is evidenced by the presence of increased serum B-natriuretic peptide in infants born growth restricted (67).

Where placental insufficiency is present, the fetal heart must also adapt to a reduced supply of glucose, with the fetal heart producing ATP from glycolysis and oxidation of lactate. Despite this, cardiac glucose consumption is not altered in growth restriction due to increase in insulin receptor GLUT4 in the heart, which increases insulin transport to maintain glucose consumption (68). Thus, glucose availability is not considered a primary limiting factor for fetal cardiac function. More in-depth analysis of the effects of suboptimal oxygen and glucose supply to the developing heart can be examined

TABLE 1 | Neonatal morbidities in fetal growth restriction.

	Cardiovascular morbidity	Respiratory morbidity	Neurological morbidity	Others
Neonatal period	Early hypotension Persistent fetal circulation/PPHN Structural heart changes Vessel wall rigidity Cardiac function issues Late systemic hypertension Secondary pulmonary hypertension	Increased need for respiratory/ventilator support Meconium aspiration syndrome Pulmonary hemorrhage Bronchopulmonary dysplasia	Perinatal asphyxia Microcephaly Cranial ultrasound abnormalities (IVH, PVL) White matter and gray matter changes on MRI Functional and DTI MRI changes General movement assessment abnormalities EEG abnormalities	Poor transition Hypoglycemia Hypocalcemia Hypothermia Sepsis Jaundice Polycythemia Prolonged NICU stay Feed intolerance Delay in establishment of feeds Necrotizing enterocolitis Renal tubular injury Retinopathy of prematurity
Long term impact	Hypertension Ischemic heart disease Stroke Atherosclerosis	Chronic respiratory insufficiency Reactive airway disease	Neurodevelopmental issues Behavioral problems Learning difficulties Cerebral palsy Dementia Mental health issues	Failure to thrive Obesity Immune dysfunction Osteoporosis Metabolic syndrome Renal issues Hormonal issues Cancer Shortened life span

PPHN, persistent pulmonary hypertension; IVH, intraventricular hemorrhage; PVL, periventricular leukomalacia; MRI, magnetic resonance imaging; DTI, diffusion tensor imaging; EEG, electroencephalography; NICU, neonatal intensive care unit.

in animal studies of FGR (69). These studies show that the fetal heart is remodeled in a manner similar to that seen in dilated cardiomyopathy. Cardiomyocyte development is adversely affected and programmed cell death is increased in growth restricted fetal guinea pigs and sheep, with a persistence of the mononucleated, primitive cell type (70, 71). Permanent alterations in heart morphology are detected into adulthood, as evidenced by persistence in the deficits in cardiomyocyte number and cardiac hypertrophy (70).

The transition to ex utero represents a particularly critical period where the heart must rapidly adapt to new pressure and flow demands. After birth, the external pressures around the heart are reduced, due to alleviation of the liquid-filled lungs and amniotic fluid. Concurrently, the low resistance placental circulation is removed, temporarily decreasing cardiac output and increasing afterload, and thus heart rate, end-diastolic pressure and stroke volume must all be increased to maintain adequate cardiac output. In response to these altered pressure demands throughout the transition to ex-utero life, the myocardium undergoes rapid changes in cardiac muscle protein expression (72). One critical change precipitated by such pressure changes at birth is a shift in the fibrous component of sarcomeres toward smaller isoforms, which increase the passive tension within with postnatal heart (72). It is postulated that the growth-restricted fetus undergoes these changes *in utero*, due to the presence of increased afterload secondary to high placental resistance, and resulting in altered cardiac compliance (73). In human infants and in experimental animal models of FGR, the heart is shown to have shorter sarcomeres, which likely contributes to decreased contractile strength (73, 74). Further, changes in the large sarcomere protein titin are described in the FGR heart, reflecting a shift from a large compliant isoform toward a small and stiff isoform (73). As titin is a major determinant of sarcomere length, this change in isoform is consistent with overall reduction in sarcomere length in the hearts of growth-restricted fetuses, and has consequences for cardiac development and function.

Changes in the hearts of growth-restricted fetuses are directly coupled with changes in the wider cardiovascular system, notably the vasculature. It is now well described that vascular responses to placental insufficiency and chronic hypoxia are vascular bed-dependent. In peripheral vascular beds, human and animal data show that sustained vasoconstriction and peripheral vascular resistance in response to chronic hypoxia induces arterial stiffness and elevated central pulse pressure (75–77). Growth restriction induced via chronic hypoxia increases peripheral vascular tone via numerous methods, including endothelial dysfunction (76), increased sympathetic nervous system activation (69) and oxidative stress (78). Oxidative stress, induced via increased reactive oxygen species generation, quenches nitric oxide (NO), thereby reducing its bioavailability and increasing peripheral vascular tone. We have previously described an increase in plasma urate levels arising from chronic fetal hypoxia (78) suggesting activation of a potent oxidative enzyme, xanthine oxidase. Importantly, it is this altered vascular tone in fetal life that sets up developmental programming for future hypertension, as evidenced in both FGR animals (79) and human cohorts (61). Central vessels, such as the aorta and carotid arteries, have increased wall thickness (80) and increased stiffness (81) in FGR humans and animals. The vascular changes described above persist into adulthood, however, they are more pronounced in peripheral vascular beds compared to central vascular bed (82).

Vascular compensation is observed in FGR offspring, wherein remodeling of the arterial wall, collagen and elastin content contribute to altered vascular mechanics (83). Rodent and guinea pig studies show that interruption of fetal growth in mid gestation coincides with a crucial period of elastin production within vasculature, attenuating elastin deposition and subsequently content, such that elastin is reduced and collagen increased (84, 85). This remodeling greatly impacts on vascular mechanics, as collagen is 100-times stiffer than elastin and, as a consequence, vascular stiffness is significantly increased (85). These changes in vessel biomechanics are most notably in the lower body arteries of growth-restricted offspring (83). Following low protein diet restriction, the aorta from adolescent rodents are not only stiffer, they also have increased fibrotic tendency, despite being normotensive (67). However, a more profound effect on vascular extracellular matrix remodeling is seen with placental dysfunction-induced growth restriction, compared to other factors such as diet (high fat) or fetal sex. These data are suggestive that vascular remodeling occurs primarily in response to changes in pressure and flow caused by chronic hypoxia and adaptive hemodynamic redistribution, rather than metabolic or hormone alterations.

Impact

The evidence presented above all indicates that exposure to placental insufficiency and chronic hypoxia significantly alters *fetal* development of the cardiovascular system. Unsurprisingly, the fetal cardiovascular alterations subsequent to placental insufficiency persist into clearly detectable structural and functional changes in the early postnatal period. After birth, tissue Doppler imaging (TDI) has allowed detection of persistent sub-clinical changes in movement and timing of the myocardium throughout the cardiac cycle, in particular during myocardial relaxation (86). In the first days of life, infants who were growth restricted show altered cardiac structure detectable on ultrasound with decreased sphericity index (a more globular shape), together with increased interventricular septum and left ventricle wall thickness (77). Further, load-dependent diastolic function is impaired (77, 87) this often represents impaired cardiac relaxation resulting in the transition from contraction to relaxation occurring prior to aortic valve opening, a situation which is common in hearts exposed to chronically high afterload. Frequently, FGR does not alter overall cardiac output, however components of cardiac output are altered with decreased stroke volume and increased heart rate often presenting in the FGR newborn (86). With increasing severity of FGR there is increased biomarkers of myocardiac cell damage, such as heart fatty acid binding protein (H-FABP), and incremental worsening of both systolic and diastolic dysfunction and in particular heart relaxation is altered (66). These alterations are indicative of hemodynamic compromise and are linked to worsening outcomes including fetal demise (88). Early signs of alteration in blood pressure in association with FGR remains contentious—we have documented increased blood pressure in the early postnatal period (80), whilst others show no change in blood pressure (82); these differences may reflect the difference between clinical and pre-clinical studies or the severity of the growth restriction induced.

In turn, *in utero* cardiac and vascular remodeling in FGR neonates programs for cardiovascular disease into adulthood. Indeed, the consequences of growth restriction on adult cardiovascular function are now well studied, and are central to the Developmental Origins of Health and Disease (DOHAD) hypothesis. These findings are apparent from both human epidemiological and experimental paradigms in growth-restricted offspring (76, 85) and adults (60). Long-term evidence of the link between low birth weight and developmental programming is available in the infants born in famine conditions in Europe in the 1900s wherein SGA is linked with significantly higher blood pressure in later life (89), and with increased risk of ischemic heart disease and cerebrovascular disease (90). Precursors of long-term suboptimal outcomes such as stroke and hypertension (91) have been proposed to be evident in growth restriction offspring as pre-atherosclerotic vascular damage in both newborns (92) and 18 month old FGR offspring (93).

Despite excellent evidence of the link between FGR and adult cardiovascular disease, there is some difficulty in dissociating the potentially separate effects of placental insufficiency/FGR and preterm birth. Growth restricted fetuses are often born preterm, particularly early-onset severe FGR infants, and preterm birth is also associated with adverse effects on the developing cardiovascular system (94). A recent study by Cohen et al. (87) followed both preterm and preterm FGR infants to 6 months of age to determine cardiac morphology. They found that changes in cardiac structure and function associated with preterm birth alone were sub-clinical, and normalized in childhood, while only thickened ventricular walls persisted into 6 months of age in FGR infants (87). This study goes some way to delineate the separate effects of prematurity and growth restriction and suggests a possible persistence of structural changes in FGR over and above the effects of prematurity.

Respiratory Morbidity

Clinical Features

There is heterogeneity in descriptions of pulmonary complications associated with FGR, which probably reflect the heterogeneity in growth restriction itself. There is however good evidence that chronic hypoxia associated with FGR interrupts normal pulmonary development, and increases susceptibility to both short- and long-term respiratory compromise. Preterm FGR newborns are 45% more likely to have bronchopulmonary dysplasia (BPD) or die from respiratory complications after birth as compared to well-grown infants (45). Further, even FGR infants born at term have worse respiratory outcomes than appropriately grown infants (95). FGR infants spend a significantly increased time in NICU and on mechanical ventilation compared to age-matched control infants, and rates of respiratory distress syndrome (70) and BPD are increased with FGR (45, 96, 97). Indeed, large multicenter trials for early-onset FGR describe that BPD is the most common morbidity for this population. The risk of BPD is greater when FGR and preterm birth are co-morbidities. Growth restriction is also associated with pulmonary hypertension of the newborn (96). FGR is associated with impaired lung function in children (98) that can persist to adulthood (99).

Pathophysiology

Human FGR cohort studies and preclinical animal studies describe that FGR can result in altered lung development; in some cases these are subtle structural and/or biochemical changes, wherein the timing and severity of compromise modulates effect. In animal studies, an early onset placental or hypoxic compromise mediates a more pronounced adverse outcome. Chronic hypoxia in fetal sheep resulting in FGR induces an adaptive response within the developing lung, where genes regulating hypoxic signaling, lung liquid reabsorption and surfactant maturation are increased (100). A 2-week exposure to hypoxia alone in rats disrupts alveolarization, reducing alveolar number via reduced septation (101). In fetal sheep we have induced late-onset placental insufficiency and FGR to examine lung morphology in preterm and term-born lambs. Lambs born naturally at term have simplified lung architecture with decreased secondary crest abundance and increased elastin deposition (102). Lambs that are delivered preterm and exposed to 2 h of mechanical ventilation do not demonstrate a difference in lung structure between FGR and appropriately-grown lambs, with no difference in the ratio of lung tissue to airspace or septal crest density, however the early tissue injury marker cyr61 is significantly increased in FGR lambs (103). Further, we observed that both FGR and appropriately grown lambs had similar ventilation requirements in the first hours of life. These findings extend previous results in FGR animal experiments from our group (104) and others (105, 106), which find no overt difference in pulmonary structure of FGR offspring. When we compare results between our preterm and term lamb cohorts, it is evident that the timing and duration of placental insufficiency is a critical determinant of lung dysfunction. We have recently examined the effects of early-onset placental insufficiency on lung structure and function, finding that lung cellular morphological changes are present (unpublished results). Accordingly, we propose that altered lung structural development is dependent on the timing of compromise, rather than the severity of growth restriction. Further, in early-onset FGR, the severity of fetal hypoxia has an inverse relationship with pulmonary surfactant production leading to decreased surfactant, a relationship not maintained in late-onset FGR (107). It is well accepted that without adequate surfactant, the newborn is at increased risk of pulmonary complications after birth, particularly when the infant is born preterm.

As discussed above, chronic hypoxia results in the fetal adaptive response of redistribution of cardiac output. MRI studies have confirmed that in late gestation of human fetuses, growth restriction is associated with an increased superior vena cava flow and, consequently, decreased pulmonary artery flow (108). This hemodynamic response is contributed by increased pulmonary vascular resistance (97). Increased pulmonary vascular resistance also reduces venous return to the left heart (109) and enhances right ventricular afterload. Combined ventricular output is thus maintained (108). Postnatally, FGR does not alter pulmonary blood flow during the transition to ex utero life, but left ventricular output is lower (110). Thus it is apparent that the hemodynamic adaptation to chronic hypoxia also has important implications for pulmonary vascular development, and accordingly, lung structure and function in FGR offspring.

A handful of studies have also examined fetal breathing movements in the developing fetus, and undertaken comparison in FGR versus appropriately grown fetuses. Fetal breathing movements are an important component of normal lung development, as they provide a stretch stimulus for growth throughout gestation (111). In FGR sheep, fetal breathing movements are significantly reduced in late gestation, although it is noted that not all experimental models of placental insufficiency show such changes (69). The cessation of fetal breathing movements in response to placental insufficiency is thought to occur by way of physiological response to reduce metabolic rate and thus conservation of oxygen, and is associated with disrupted alveolarization (112).

Deficits in pulmonary development subsequent to placental compromise are not confined to lung alveolar morphology. There is a growing understanding of the link between poor alveolar development and poor lung vascular development (113–115), called the *Vascular Hypothesis*. Growth restriction, induced via hyperthermia in pregnant sheep, impairs both lung alveolar and vascular development in the developing fetus (116). In complimentary experiments, lung alveolar cells isolated from the same growth-restricted fetuses demonstrate reduced cell growth, migration and branching, which are key components of normal lung development (116). These findings are confirmed *in vivo* in which growth-restricted offspring demonstrate diminished pulmonary vascular function and density, together with decreased pulmonary alveolarization (116, 117). Abnormal pulmonary vascular development in growth restricted fetuses is likely to be a key mechanism increasing the risk of BPD, pulmonary hypertension and life-long reduction in respiratory capacity, such as seen in chronic obstructive disease (116).

Impact

BPD is a chronic lung disease characterized by arrested airway and parenchymal development and resulting in long-term respiratory complications, with a high susceptibility in preterm and growth restricted infants. BPD is a multifactorial condition, however it is primarily thought to result from chronic ventilation-induced injury in preterm infants, contributed by lung exposure to excess oxygen and inflammation. FGR is an independent risk factor for BPD in human infants (118–120). Being born subsequent to placental insufficiency and growth restricted is associated with a 3.6-fold higher risk of developing BPD than age-matched control infants (120), despite FGR infants having similar RDS rates as appropriately-grown counterparts. Lio et al. (121) have also recently shown that FGR infants with placental dysfunction have a 6-fold increased risk of developing BPD compared to low birth weight/ SGA infants. Further, they noted that birth weight *per se* and not ventilation duration, or other neonatal morbidities, contributed to the presence of BPD.

Maternal vascular unit deficiency, a marker for pre-eclampsia, is a common placental pathology associated with FGR, and it has also been shown that maternal vascular unit dysfunction doubles the risk of BPD in preterm human infants (118). Thus, human and animal data strongly support that the foundations of postnatal lung deficits and BPD are laid down *in utero* in FGR infants with placental insufficiency, and that vascular pathology is likely to be a contributing factor.

Neonatal pulmonary hypertension is highly associated with decreasing gestational age and low birth weight, and is a common complication of BPD (96). Pulmonary hypertension is characterized by hypoxemia of the newborn and right-to left shunting through the ductus arteriosus, due to maintenance of high pressures within the pulmonary circulation. Accordingly, neonatal pulmonary hypertension occurs via a failure of structural cardiovascular remodeling after birth, and is likely developmentally programmed *in utero* (122). In post mortem tissue analysis it is shown that newborns with pulmonary hypertension displayed reduced pulmonary vascular surface area with increased muscularization of distal pulmonary vasculature (123). These data suggest a strong association with FGR induced by vascular remodeling in chronically hypoxic fetuses, resulting in impaired control of vascular tone within the pulmonary circulation after birth. Altered pulmonary vascular composition has been more closely examined in growth restricted rats, demonstrating increased pulmonary vasoconstriction caused by local endothelial dysfunction and excessive collagen and reduced elastin in the pulmonary vasculature (124). Animal models of FGR also provide strong evidence that the hallmarks of pulmonary hypertension are already present in the growth-restricted fetus and offspring soon after birth. Our group and others have shown vascular changes, including decreased vascular density and dysfunction in fetal sheep (116) and in 2-h-old lambs (110). Thus, even prior to birth, FGR is associated with pulmonary hypertension.

The long-term effects of low birth weight have been examined in adult offspring conceived during the 1940s Dutch famine, who show an increased risk of obstructive airway disease (89). Further analysis of this cohort determined that neither serum immunoglobulin E concentration nor mean lung volumes were different (125). The authors speculate that bronchial reactivity must be the cause of the airway disease following growth restriction.

Neurological Morbidity

Clinical Features

FGR is strongly linked to suboptimal brain development, and long-term neurological dysfunctions in motor ability, cognition and learning, and behavior. We have recently reviewed the consequences of placental insufficiency and FGR on the developing brain (28), and describe that the age of onset and severity of FGR, together with gestational age at birth, play important modulatory roles in altered brain structure and function. The first indication of structural anomalies of the FGR brain can be derived from magnetic resonance imaging (MRI) during fetal development. MRI of the fetal brain during development demonstrates reduced brain volume, and altered cortical folding and brain morphology in FGR fetuses (126, 127). Arthurs et al. (128) showed lower diffusion weighted imaging values in parts of the brain in severe FGR fetuses as compared to normal age-matched controls, which were suggestive of an abnormal maturational profile. Postnatally, at term-equivalent age, MRI detects reduced intracranial volume, particularly contributed by decreased cortical gray matter volume in FGR infants (129), and altered developmental profile of white matter myelination (130), the hippocampus (131) and the basal ganglia (132) of growth-restricted infants, compared to appropriately grown infants. Functional MRI is also an upcoming tool to study whole brain functional networks in newborn infants for the assessment of altered organization and prediction of long-term neurodevelopment (133). Diffusion tensor imaging (DTI) and connectivity-based analysis of the FGR brain in the neonatal period is also being increasingly investigated (134).

MRI has the ability to detect even relatively small volume, structural, and organizational differences within the brain of FGR and appropriately-grown infants (135) but MRI capability and expertise in analysis is not readily available at all birth centers. In contrast, neonatal cranial US is widely used, but shows less sensitivity for detection of these subtle, but important neurological changes associated with neuropathology in FGR infants (136). Cranial ultrasound is frequently used as an assessment tool in premature infants, and term infants with severe FGR, to identify significant neuropathology in the neonatal period. There remains uncertainty as to whether cranial ultrasound can adequately detect neuropathology associated with FGR when compared to age-matched appropriately grown preterm infants (135, 136). Certainly in older preterm and term FGR infants, the benefit of routine cranial ultrasound screening in the neonatal period is questionable (137). We did not find evidence of altered cerebral ventricular volume using ultrasound imaging in FGR infants <10th centile, however we did observe a correlation between increasing ventricular volume and a decrease in functional motor scores (138). Cruz-Martinez et al. (139) have suggested that FGR infants with signs of middle cerebral artery and other Doppler abnormalities (indicative of significant brain sparing) are more likely to have neuropathology that can be detected on neonatal cranial ultrasound. This is interesting, as it further supports that the term *brain sparing* is a misnomer, and while it represents an appropriate survival response in the fetus, it is actually associated with worsening fetal condition and greater brain injury (28).

FGR infants frequently have a reduced head circumference compared to age-matched appropriately-grown infants, which is likely due to reduced brain volume (129), and reduced brain volume persists to 12 months of age (140). Cerebellar and hippocampal volumes may also be reduced (130). Brain myelination and connectivity have been shown to be adversely affected in FGR infants in the first 12 months of life, representative of white matter injury (141). Diffusion MRI of the human brain shows that the overall neuronal network complexity and connectivity of the FGR brain is reduced, with reduced global and local axonal circuits (142). Long-range cortical-basal ganglia (thalamocortical) connections are decreased in children born preterm with FGR, compared to children born preterm but appropriately-grown (142), indicating that brain connectivity is significantly worse in children who were FGR compared to children who were preterm but well-grown. Deficits in brain connectivity correlate with neurobehavioral impairments including hyperactivity and poor cognition at school in children who were born FGR (143).

Neonatal functional assessment may detect early problems with neurological processing and behavior in infants who were born growth restricted. Tolsa et al. (129) showed that FGR newborns had specific alterations of brain structure as studied by volumetric MRI at preterm and term age, with reduced cortical gray matter volume correlating with deficits in attention and responsivity at term-equivalent age. General movement assessments (Prechtl movements) provide an early motor analysis, wherein abnormalities are predictive for cerebral palsy, and general movements may be adversely affected in some FGR infants (144). Similarly, electroencephalography performed early in the neonatal period has been shown to be affected and may correlate with adverse neurodevelopment in studies of FGR infants (145, 146). There is however limited data on early detection of functional deficits in growth-restricted infants, reflecting challenges in detecting delayed neurodevelopment in the neonatal period.

Pathophysiology

It is now well established that the traditional brain sparing physiology does not necessarily mean normal cerebral development *in utero* (28). In fact, fetuses with the most severe brain sparing are at the highest risk of adverse neurodevelopment in childhood. Prenatal loss of vasoreactivity in FGR has been suggested as a mechanism for poor outcomes, in which fetuses who do not adjust their cerebral circulatory control in response to hypoxic challenge may be more at risk of impaired cerebrovascular regulation (147). There are also reports of preferential perfusion and cerebral redistribution of brain blood flow in FGR fetuses, leading to some brain regions being at higher risk of injury (148). This is supported by work in fetal sheep to demonstrate that FGR is associated with regional cerebral blood flow redistribution, with the most notable differences between FGR and appropriately grown fetuses seen in the cerebral cortex and periventricular white matter (21).

Cerebral blood flow frequently continues to be abnormal for the first few days after birth in FGR human infants, but whether this puts infants at an increased risk of acute brain injury is not known. It has been reported the cerebral blood flow remains elevated after birth in FGR infants (149), even when the neonate is no longer exposed to a hypoxic environment and is no longer in need of a compensatory change in cardiac output. Postnatally, elevated cerebral blood flow might potentiate hyperoxia and oxidative stress within the fragile brain, which could also contribute to further neurological damage.

Animal models of chronic hypoxia and growth restriction have helped us to understand the development of neuropathology associated with placental insufficiency and FGR (28, 150–152). Adverse effects on brain gray matter development, white matter, and cerebellum have been described both in sheep, rabbit and rat models of FGR (153–155). In fetal sheep, we showed that early-onset placental dysfunction is associated with more widespread and severe white matter brain injury and neuroinflammation compared with late-onset, however both early- and late-onset FGR demonstrate complex patterns of gray and white matter neuropathology (154). Animal studies also show that the severity of brain injury, and the resultant neurodevelopment deficits, depends on the extent and severity of brain involvement in FGR (156). Hypomyelination and delayed myelination due to oligodendrocyte maturational deficits have been identified as possible mechanisms causing the white matter injury seen in FGR infants (157). Deficits in neuronal connectivity have also been described in animal models (158). Our group, and others, has observed that deficits in various components of the neurovascular unit play a significant role in the brain injury seen in animal models of FGR (159). Prematurity is a confounder in human FGR, but studies in FGR animals allow the separation of growth restriction and preterm birth. The individual contributions of preterm birth and/or neonatal ventilation of the FGR newborn on the progression of brain injury are now being examined (160, 161). These studies have determined that preterm birth and ventilation synergistically predispose the vulnerable FGR brain to neuropathology.

Impact

FGR infants are at increased risk of adverse neurodevelopmental outcomes in childhood. Neurological morbidities related to motor deficits, including cerebral palsy, behavioral issues, and cognitive impairment is significantly increased in young children and adolescents who were diagnosed as growth restricted at birth (28, 162–164). The risk of cerebral palsy is 30-fold greater in FGR infants, compared to those that are well grown (165), and increases with worsening growth restriction. Overall, >40% of children who have cerebral palsy had a low birth weight; that is, they were growth restricted, born preterm, or both (166). This is important, as FGR and preterm birth are frequent co-morbidities. In addition to motor deficits, preterm FGR infants followed-up at 1, 2, and 3 years of age showed deficits in cognition and behavioral outcomes compared to preterm age-matched appropriately-grown infants (167). Further, a longitudinal study observing FGR offspring with evidence of brain sparing from birth to middle school age (9–10 years old) found a complex set of neurodevelopmental deficits, such as a significant reduction in IQ, compared to age-matched appropriately-grown children (168). Multiple follow-up studies of FGR infants into school age describe diminished gross and fine motor skills, cognition, memory, and academic ability, as well as neuropsychological dysfunctions encompassing poor attention, hyperactivity and altered mood (143, 169–171). FGR infants born preterm and those with fetal circulatory redistribution are at the greatest risk for the worst outcomes (172). These adverse outcomes can continue into adolescence and young adulthood (173). It is apparent that determining the neurodevelopmental consequences of FGR is complicated by the severity of FGR, early- or late-onset, and the gestational age at delivery (28). However, in both early- and late-onset FGR, the presence of cardiovascular redistribution and brain-sparing is associated with abnormal neurodevelopmental outcomes (28).

Interventions for Improved Outcomes

Management of pregnancies complicated by FGR represents a balance between antenatal compromise, often with worsening chronic hypoxia that contributes to subpotimal organ development, and the risks associated with preterm delivery and postnatal intensive care, which may also contribute to morbidities. In high-income countries, about half of fetuses with moderate- to severe-growth restriction are detected antenatally and are therefore amenable to treatment during pregnancy, but it remains that nearly 40% of infants born at the 3rd centile for weight are not detected *in utero* (44). With this in mind, both antenatal and postnatal therapies must be considered. Currently, no specific treatment is available for FGR. Potential treatments should target maldevelopment of multiple organs, various injurious pathways, cell types, and structural deficits that manifest over different developmental stages. Here we will provide an overview of the current state of understanding for a handful of treatments for FGR (**Figure 3**).

Antenatal

Antenatal treatments are principally aimed at improving placental function and thereby increasing fetal growth *in utero*. To date, the best studied of these has been sildenafil citrate. Sildenafil is a potent phosphodiesterase type 5 (PDE5) inhibitor that is an effective smooth muscle relaxant where the PDE5 enzyme is present in an organ or tissue, as is the case for the human placenta (174). The effects of sildenafil on smooth muscle are mediated via an enhanced and prolonged nitric oxide release leading to vasodilatation. Both *in vitro* and *in vivo* studies demonstrate that sildenafil vasodilates human myometrium vessels from normal (175, 176) and growth restricted placenta. Most experimental studies to date support that sildenafil increases fetal weight in compromised rat, sheep and human pregnancies (177). In contrast, we have shown that antenatal sildenafil administration to pregnant sheep with placental insufficiency decreases fetal weight and worsens fetal hypoxia (178). Although initial preclinical evidence for the multinational STRIDER trial suggested improved outcomes for FGR infants, this trial has now been aborted due to unexpected baby deaths (179), leading to a call for increased preclinical studies underpinning clinical trials (180), and improved understanding of the effects of sildenafil on the fetus given that it crosses the placenta (181). The longer acting tadalafil remains an active clinical experimental treatment of interest as an antenatal therapy for FGR and, given that tadalafil does not cross placenta (174), it may be more favorable as a targeted placental treatment.

The EVERREST Project is also investigating a targeted approach to improve placental function in pregnancies complicated by FGR using gene therapy to inject vascular endothelial growth factor (VEGF) into uterine arteries (182). VEGF is known for its role in inducing angiogenesis and in the EVERREST Project it is hypothesized that application of adenovirus VEGF in, or near placental arteries will induce a local and acute increase in VEGF expression, and subsequent angiogenesis of the placental vasculature. Preclinical studies have shown promise with improved blood flow (183) and fetal weight gain (184) in animal models of growth restriction, resulting from the improved vascularization of the placenta. The clinical trial is ongoing.

A recent large animal (sheep) study examined intra-amniotic administration of the growth-promoting protein insulin-like growth factor-1 (IGF-1) (16). This work showed that increasing the bioavailability of IGF-1 in pregnancies complicated by placental insufficiency and FGR improved birth weight in female lambs, but not males, and modified postnatal catch-up growth in both females and males. Intrauterine IGF-1 also mediated expression of key somatotrophic and metabolic genes, indicative that antenatal treatment could be utilized to positively affect postnatal growth and wellbeing.

A number of antenatal treatments have been explored preclinically that aim to restore fetal oxidative tone via maternal antioxidant administration, using agents such as allopurinol, melatonin and vitamin C (75, 79, 185). Antioxidant treatment has principally targeted improved cardiovascular and neurological outcomes in growth-restricted offspring. To date, melatonin has been the most widely studied, given melatonin's established safety profile, ease of administration, and strong antioxidant benefits. In sheep, we have shown that maternal melatonin administration to ewes carrying a growth restricted fetus results in a significant improvement in vascular function and reduced arterial stiffness, two vital pathologies evident in FGR offspring, which predispose to cardiovascular disease (75). Melatonin administration also resulted in improved cardiac function in the right ventricle. Further, this study showed that maternal melatonin improved fetal oxygenation and increased birth weight (75), however other ovine studies show either no improvement in birth weight (186) or exacerbation of growth restriction with melatonin (187). In cultured human umbilical vein endothelial cells (HUVECs), melatonin improves vascular endothelial integrity, likely via combined anti-oxidant and anti-inflammatory mechanisms (188). Exposure to antenatal melatonin does not reverse alveolar simplification in FGR newborn lambs (102), but does improve pulmonary vascular structure and function (189), and pulmonary tone may be maintained long term via alteration to receptor populations (190). As our understanding of perturbations to lung growth in FGR offspring continues to be explored, so too does the opportunity for targeting novel pathways. For example, recent work has shown that NPY is down regulated in FGR, where NPY is a sympathetic neurotransmitter that is critical for normal lung growth (191).

The effects of maternal melatonin administration on brain development have also been examined. Antenatal melatonin crosses the placental and the blood brain barrier, and melatonin is a strong antioxidant and also demonstrates anti-inflammatory benefits in the developing brain (186, 192–194). In pregnancies complicated by placental insufficiency and FGR, maternal melatonin improves white matter brain development via increased myelination and decreased axonopathy in the fetal brain, and subsequently, neurobehavior of FGR+MLT lambs is significantly improved after birth (186). Melatonin has also been shown to have beneficial effects on cerebral vasculature by preventing FGR-related apoptosis and disruption of blood brain barrier instability via improved vascular interactions with astrocytes and pericytes (195). Antenatal melatonin has been examined in pilot studies to treat FGR (186) and preeclampsia (188) with results supporting that melatonin is an effective anti-oxidant that is safe for the mother and baby, and may extend pregnancy (196).

Emerging evidence supports that the glycoprotein lactoferrin shows potential as an antenatal treatment for pregnancies complicated by FGR, particularly for the developing brain (197). Lactoferrin is a glycoprotein that demonstrates strong antioxidant, anti-inflammatory and anti-microbial effects—important factors that could mediate neuroprotective benefits. In rats, lactoferrin supplementation during pregnancy shows positive benefits for dexamethasone-induced fetal growth restriction (197). Maternal lactoferrin significantly increased birth weight of control rat pups, and FGR offspring exposed to lactoferrin showed a normalized weight at postnatal day 21. Lactoferrin supplementation also improved brain hippocampal structure and stimulated brain derived neurotrophic factor (BDNF) (197), important observations in light of the neuropathology associated with human FGR. Nutritional supplementation (glucose, amino acids and electrolytes) into the amniotic sac of FGR rabbits has also recently been explored, with some promising results suggesting that survival rate for FGR offspring was improved with treatment, although birth weight and cardiac function deficits were not improved (198).

Postnatal

As mentioned above, nearly 40% of human infants with severe FGR are not detected antenatally (44), and therefore not amenable to antenatal treatments. In light of this we must continue to investigate therapies to improve multi-organ dysfunctions in growth restricted infants. We have highlighted in this paper that deficits in cardiovascular, pulmonary and cerebral development are already present at birth in FGR infants, principally caused by chronic hypoxia *in utero*. Therefore any potential postnatal therapy would aim to be reparative and to prevent progression of ongoing multi-organ damage.

Lactoferrin shows great potential as a postnatal therapy, in addition to positive effects antenatally. Lactoferrin is highly abundant in human colostrum and milk, and it reaches the brain after oral administration (197, 199). In this regard, breastfed infants show higher total anti-oxidant capacity and a lower oxidative stress index compared to non-breastfed infants. Importantly, randomized controlled trials with nutritional lactoferrin supplementation in premature neonates demonstrate a promising reduction in late onset sepsis and necrotizing enterocolitis (200). Lactoferrin supplementation during lactation is protective for neonatal rats exposed to either hypoxia-ischemia or lipopolysaccharide-induced systemic inflammation (201, 202). Analysis of the neonatal rat brain using a combination of advanced MRI analysis and histology demonstrates that gray and white matter microstructure is normalized with lactoferrin supplementation, myelination is protected and measures of axonal integrity and brain organization are restored in rats with lactoferrin supplementation (201). Early environment enrichment or postnatal stimulation has also been shown to have some benefits in brain connectivity in a rabbit model of FGR (203). While there are no current published studies on stem cell therapy for FGR related brain injury, our lab and others are working on testing their applications in FGR and other pregnancy complications (204). The application of postnatal therapies to improve multi-organ deficits associated with FGR should remain a foremost preclinical research area.

CONCLUSIONS

Understanding the pathophysiological mechanisms that underlie neonatal morbidities that are particularly associated with FGR provide the fundamental basis for improving short- and long-term outcomes in growth restricted offspring. It is clear that placental compromise and chronic fetal hypoxia program the fetus for suboptimal growth and development, with fetal cardiovascular dysfunctions and altered organ development already apparent in the FGR fetus during pregnancy. The timing of the onset of placental insufficiency, the severity of growth restriction, the degree of cardiovascular adaptation, and gestational age at birth are all critical factors that modify outcome for FGR infants. In the neonatal period, FGR infants demonstrate early evidence of cardiac, vascular, pulmonary, neurological and other deficits, which can lead to long durations in neonatal intensive care, and long-term health problems. Improved antenatal detection, and both antenatal and postnatal therapies that target the key pathophysiological mechanisms underlying altered multi organ structure and function must be considered critical research areas.

AUTHOR CONTRIBUTIONS

AM and BA critically researched literature, co-wrote the first draft of the manuscript and approved the final version. MC-M, GJ, GP, and SM reviewed the manuscript, contributed to various sections and approved the final version.

ACKNOWLEDGMENTS

The authors wish to thank their funding supports: National Health and Medical Research Council (NH&MRC) project grant, Cerebral Palsy Alliance grant, Royal Australasian College of Physicians Foundation Fellowship (AM); NH&MRC Research Fellowships (GP and SM), National Heart Foundation of Australia (GP), Australian Research Council Future Fellowship (SM) and the Victorian Government's Operational Infrastructure Support Program.

REFERENCES

1. Gordijn SJ, Beune IM, Thilaganathan B, Papageorghiou A, Baschat AA, Baker PN, et al. Consensus definition of fetal growth restriction: a Delphi procedure. *Ultrasound Obstetr Gynecol.* (2016) 48:333–9. doi: 10.1002/uog.15884
2. McCowan LM, Figueras F, Anderson NH. Evidence-based national guidelines for the management of suspected fetal growth restriction: comparison, consensus, and controversy. *Am J Obstetr Gynecol.* (2018) 218:S855–68. doi: 10.1016/j.ajog.2017.12.004
3. Owens JA. Endocrine and substrate control of fetal growth: placental and maternal influences and insulin-like growth factors. *Reprod Fertil Dev.* (1991) 3:501–17. doi: 10.1071/RD9910501
4. Vorherr H. Factors influencing fetal growth. *Am J Obstetr Gynecol.* (1982) 142:577–88. doi: 10.1016/0002-9378(82)90765-7
5. Sharma D, Shastri S, Sharma P. Intrauterine growth restriction: antenatal and postnatal aspects. clinical medicine insights. *Pediatrics* (2016) 10:67–83. doi: 10.4137/CMPed.S40070
6. Burton GJ, Jauniaux E. Pathophysiology of placental-derived fetal growth restriction. *Am J Obstetr Gynecol.* (2018) 218:S745–61. doi: 10.1016/j.ajog.2017.11.577
7. Ghidini A. Idiopathic fetal growth restriction: a pathophysiologic approach. *Obstetr Gynecol Survey* (1996) 51:376–82. doi: 10.1097/00006254-199606000-00023
8. Figueras F, Gratacos E. An integrated approach to fetal growth restriction. *Best Pract Res Clin Obstet Gynaecol.* (2017) 38:48–58. doi: 10.1016/j.bpobgyn.2016.10.006
9. Helwig JT, Parer JT, Kilpatrick SJ, Laros RK Jr. Umbilical cord blood acid-base state: what is normal? *Am J Obstetr Gynecol.* (1996) 174:1807–12. discussion: 1812–4.
10. Arikan GM, Scholz HS, Petru E, Haeusler MC, Haas J, Weiss PA. Cord blood oxygen saturation in vigorous infants at birth: what is normal? *BJOG* (2000) 107:987–94. doi: 10.1111/j.1471-0528.2000.tb10401.x
11. Fowden AL, Forhead AJ. Endocrine mechanisms of intrauterine programming. *Reproduction* (2004) 127:515–26. doi: 10.1530/rep.1.00033
12. Murphy VE, Smith R, Giles WB, Clifton VL. Endocrine regulation of human fetal growth: the role of the mother, placenta, and fetus. *Endocrine Rev.* (2006) 27:141–69. doi: 10.1210/er.2005-0011
13. Agrogiannis GD, Sifakis S, Patsouris ES, Konstantinidou AE. Insulin-like growth factors in embryonic and fetal growth and skeletal development (Review). *Mol Med Reports* (2014) 10:579–84. doi: 10.3892/mmr.2014.2258
14. Netchine I, Azzi S, Le Bouc Y, Savage MO. IGF1 molecular anomalies demonstrate its critical role in fetal, postnatal growth and brain development. *Best Pract ResClin Endocrinol Metab.* (2011) 25:181–90. doi: 10.1016/j.beem.2010.08.005
15. Morris RK, Bilagi A, Devani P, Kilby MD. Association of serum PAPP-A levels in first trimester with small for gestational age and adverse pregnancy outcomes: systematic review and meta-analysis. *Prenatal Diagnosis* (2017) 37:253–65. doi: 10.1002/pd.5001
16. Spiroski AM, Oliver MH, Jaquiery AL, Prickett CR, Espiner EA, Harding JE, et al. Postnatal effects of intrauterine treatment of the growth-restricted ovine fetus with intra-amniotic insulin-like growth factor-1. *J Physiol* (2017) 596:5925–45. doi: 10.1113/JP274999
17. Waters MJ, Kaye PL. The role of growth hormone in fetal development. *Growth Horm IGF Res.* (2002) 12:137–46. doi: 10.1016/S1096-6374(02)00018-7
18. Romejko-Wolniewicz E, Teliga-Czajkowska J, Czajkowski K. Antenatal steroids: can we optimize the dose? *Curr Opin Obstetr Gynecol.* (2014) 26:77–82. doi: 10.1097/GCO.0000000000000047
19. Wallace EM, Baker LS. Effect of antenatal betamethasone administration on placental vascular resistance. *Lancet* (1999) 353:1404–7. doi: 10.1016/S0140-6736(98)08229-4
20. Kim WJ, Han YS, Ko HS, Park IY, Shin JC, Wie JH. Antenatal corticosteroids and outcomes of preterm small-for-gestational-age neonates in a single medical center. *Obstetr Gynecol Sci.* (2018) 61:7–13. doi: 10.5468/ogs.2018.61.1.7
21. Miller SL, Supramaniam VG, Jenkin G, Walker DW, Wallace EM. Cardiovascular responses to maternal betamethasone administration in the intrauterine growth-restricted ovine fetus. *Am J Obstetr Gynecol.* (2009) 201:613.e1-8. doi: 10.1016/j.ajog.2009.07.028
22. Miller SL, Chai M, Loose J, Castillo-Melendez M, Walker DW, Jenkin G, et al. The effects of maternal betamethasone administration on the intrauterine growth-restricted fetus. *Endocrinology* (2007) 148:1288–95. doi: 10.1210/en.2006-1058
23. Giussani DA. The fetal brain sparing response to hypoxia: physiological mechanisms. *J Physiol.* (2016) 594:1215–30. doi: 10.1113/JP271099
24. Morrison JL. Sheep models of intrauterine growth restriction: fetal adaptations and consequences. *Clin Exp Pharmacol Physiol.* (2008) 35:730–43. doi: 10.1111/j.1440-1681.2008.04975.x
25. Schreuder MF, Nauta J. Prenatal programming of nephron number and blood pressure. *Kidney Int.* (2007) 72:265–8. doi: 10.1038/sj.ki.5002307
26. Miller SL, Wallace EM. Effect of antenatal steroids on haemodynamics in the normally grown and growth restricted fetus. *Curr Pediatr Rev.* (2013) 9:67–74. doi: 10.2174/1573396311309010014
27. Suhag A, Berghella V. Intrauterine Growth Restriction (IUGR): Etiology and Diagnosis. *Curr Obstetr Gynecol Rep.* (2013) 2:102–11. doi: 10.1007/s13669-013-0041-z
28. Miller SL, Huppi PS, Mallard C. The consequences of fetal growth restriction on brain structure and neurodevelopmental outcome. *J Physiol.* (2016) 594:807–23. doi: 10.1113/JP271402
29. Romo A, Carceller R, Tobajas J. Intrauterine growth retardation (IUGR): epidemiology and etiology. *Pediatr Endocrinol Rev.* (2009) 6(Suppl. 3):332–6.
30. de Onis M, Blossner M, Villar J. Levels and patterns of intrauterine growth retardation in developing countries. *Eur J Clin Nutr.* (1998) 52(Suppl. 1):S5–15.
31. Baschat AA. Planning management and delivery of the growth-restricted fetus. *Best Pract Res Clin Obstetr Gynaecol.* (2018) 49:53–65. doi: 10.1016/j.bpobgyn.2018.02.009
32. Lappen JR, Myers SA. The systematic error in the estimation of fetal weight and the underestimation of fetal growth restriction. *Am J Obstetr Gynecol.* (2017) 216:477–83. doi: 10.1016/j.ajog.2017.02.013
33. Ernst SA, Brand T, Reeske A, Spallek J, Petersen K, Zeeb H. Care-related and maternal risk factors associated with the antenatal nondetection of intrauterine growth restriction: a case-control study from Bremen, Germany. *BioMed Res Int.* (2017) 2017:1746146. doi: 10.1155/2017/1746146
34. Chauhan SP, Beydoun H, Chang E, Sandlin AT, Dahlke JD, Igwe E, et al. Prenatal detection of fetal growth restriction in newborns classified as small for gestational age: correlates and risk of neonatal morbidity. *Am J Perinatol.* (2014) 31:187–94. doi: 10.1055/s-0033-1343771
35. Callec R, Lamy C, Perdriolle-Galet E, Patte C, Heude B, Morel O. Impact on obstetric outcome of third-trimester screening for small-for-gestational-age fetuses. *Ultrasound Obstetr Gynecol.* (2015) 46:216–20. doi: 10.1002/uog.14755
36. Larkin JC, Chauhan SP, Simhan HN. Small for gestational age: the differential mortality when detected versus undetected antenatally. *Am J Perinatol.* (2017) 34:409–14. doi: 10.1055/s-0036-1592132
37. Zeitlin J, Ancel PY, Saurel-Cubizolles MJ, Papiernik E. The relationship between intrauterine growth restriction and preterm delivery: an empirical approach using data from a European case-control study. *BJOG* (2000) 107:750–8. doi: 10.1111/j.1471-0528.2000.tb13336.x
38. Parker SE, Werler MM. Epidemiology of ischemic placental disease: a focus on preterm gestations. *Semin Perinatol.* (2014) 38:133–8. doi: 10.1053/j.semperi.2014.03.004
39. Monier I, Ancel PY, Ego A, Jarreau PH, Lebeaux C, Kaminski M, et al. Fetal and neonatal outcomes of preterm infants born before 32 weeks of gestation according to antenatal vs postnatal assessments of restricted growth. *Am J Obstetr Gynecol.* (2017) 216:516.e1–e10. doi: 10.1016/j.ajog.2017.02.001
40. Ananth CV, Friedman AM. Ischemic placental disease and risks of perinatal mortality and morbidity and neurodevelopmental outcomes. *Semin Perinatol.* (2014) 38:151–8. doi: 10.1053/j.semperi.2014.03.007
41. Bukowski R, Hansen NI, Willinger M, Reddy UM, Parker CB, Pinar H, et al. Fetal growth and risk of stillbirth: a population-based case-control study. *PLoS Med.* (2014) 11:e1001633. doi: 10.1371/journal.pmed.1001633
42. Malacova E, Regan A, Nassar N, Raynes-Greenow C, Leonard H, Srinivasjois R, et al. Risk of stillbirth, preterm delivery, and fetal growth restriction

following exposure in a previous birth: systematic review and meta-analysis. *BJOG* (2018) 125:183–92. doi: 10.1111/1471-0528.14906

43. Gardosi J, Kady SM, McGeown P, Francis A, Tonks A. Classification of stillbirth by relevant condition at death (ReCoDe): population based cohort study. *BMJ* (2005) 331:1113–7. doi: 10.1136/bmj.38629.587639.7C
44. Victorian Perinatal Services Performance Indicators, 2012-2013. Available online at: www.health.vic.gov.au/CCOPMM
45. Sasi A, Abraham V, Davies-Tuck M, Polglase GR, Jenkin G, Miller SL, et al. Impact of intrauterine growth restriction on preterm lung disease. *Acta Paediatr.* (2015) 104:e552-6. doi: 10.1111/apa.13220
46. Marzouk A, Filipovic-Pierucci A, Baud O, Tsatsaris V, Ego A, Charles A, et al. Prenatal and post-natal cost of small for gestational age infants: a national study. *BMC Health Serv Res.* (2017) 17:221. doi: 10.1186/s12913-017-2155-x
47. Lim G, Tracey J, Boom N, Karmakar S, Wang J, Berthelot JM, et al. CIHI survey: hospital costs for preterm and small-for-gestational age babies in Canada. *Healthcare Q.* (2009) 12:20–4. doi: 10.12927/hcq.2013.21121
48. Gephart SM, Hanson CK. Preventing necrotizing enterocolitis with standardized feeding protocols: not only possible, but imperative. *Adv Neonatal Care* (2013) 13:48–54. doi: 10.1097/ANC.0b013e31827ece0a
49. Bozzetti V, Tagliabue PE. Enteral feeding of intrauterine growth restriction preterm infants: theoretical risks and practical implications. *La Pediatria Medica e Chirurgica* (2017) 39:160. doi: 10.4081/pmc.2017.160
50. Ahamed MF, Dar P, Vega M, Kim M, Gao Q, Havranek T. Early feeding tolerance in small for gestational age infants with normal versus abnormal antenatal Doppler characteristics. *J Neonatal-Perinatal Med.* (2017) 10:43–48. doi: 10.3233/NPM-1682
51. Bozzetti V, Paterlini G, De Lorenzo P, Gazzolo D, Valsecchi MG, Tagliabue PE. Impact of continuous vs bolus feeding on splanchnic perfusion in very low birth weight infants: a randomized trial. *J Pediatr.* (2016) 176:86–92.e2. doi: 10.1016/j.jpeds.2016.05.031
52. Fortune PM, Wagstaff M, Petros AJ. Cerebro-splanchnic oxygenation ratio (CSOR) using near infrared spectroscopy may be able to predict splanchnic ischaemia in neonates. *Intensive Care Med.* (2001) 27:1401–7. doi: 10.1007/s001340100994
53. Kempley S, Gupta N, Linsell L, Dorling J, McCormick K, Mannix P, et al. Feeding infants below 29 weeks' gestation with abnormal antenatal Doppler: analysis from a randomised trial. *Arch Dis Childhood.* (2014) 99:F6–F11. doi: 10.1136/archdischild-2013-304393
54. Leaf A, Dorling J, Kempley S, McCormick K, Mannix P, Linsell L, et al. Early or delayed enteral feeding for preterm growth-restricted infants: a randomized trial. *Pediatrics* (2012) 129:e1260–8. doi: 10.1542/peds.2011-2379
55. Zecca E, Costa S, Barone G, Giordano L, Zecca C, Maggio L. Proactive enteral nutrition in moderately preterm small for gestational age infants: a randomized clinical trial. *J Pediatr.* (2014) 165:1135–1139.e1. doi: 10.1016/j.jpeds.2014.08.065
56. Longo S, Borghesi A, Tzialla C, Stronati M. IUGR and infections. *Early Hum Dev.* (2014) 90(Suppl. 1):S42–4. doi: 10.1016/S0378-3782(14)70014-3
57. Lee JW, VanderVeen D, Allred EN, Leviton A, Dammann O. Prethreshold retinopathy in premature infants with intrauterine growth restriction. *Acta Paediatr* (2015) 104:27–31. doi: 10.1111/apa.12799
58. Aisa MC, Cappuccini B, Barbati A, Orlacchio A, Baglioni M, Di Renzo GC. Biochemical parameters of renal impairment/injury and surrogate markers of nephron number in intrauterine growth-restricted and preterm neonates at 30-40 days of postnatal corrected age. *Pediatr Nephrol.* (2016) 31:2277–87. doi: 10.1007/s00467-016-3484-4
59. Barbati A, Cappuccini B, Aisa MC, Grasselli C, Zamarra M, Bini V, et al. Increased urinary cystatin-C levels correlate with reduced renal volumes in neonates with intrauterine growth restriction. *Neonatology* (2016) 109:154–60. doi: 10.1159/000441273
60. Menendez-Castro C, Rascher W, Hartner A. Intrauterine growth restriction - impact on cardiovascular diseases later in life. *Mol Cell Pediatr.* (2018) 5:4. doi: 10.1186/s40348-018-0082-5
61. Barker DJ, Bull AR, Osmond C, Simmonds SJ. Fetal and placental size and risk of hypertension in adult life. *BMJ* (1990) 301:259–62. doi: 10.1136/bmj.301.6746.259
62. Oros D, Figueras F, Cruz-Martinez R, Meler E, Munmany M, Gratacos E. Longitudinal changes in uterine, umbilical and fetal cerebral Doppler indices in late-onset small-for-gestational age fetuses. *Ultrasound Obstetr Gynecol.* (2011) 37:191–5. doi: 10.1002/uog.7738
63. Ghosh GS, Gudmundsson S. Uterine and umbilical artery Doppler are comparable in predicting perinatal outcome of growth-restricted fetuses. *BJOG* (2009) 116:424–30. doi: 10.1111/j.1471-0528.2008.02057.x
64. Hassan WA, Brockelsby J, Alberry M, Fanelli T, Wladimiroff J, Lees CC. Cardiac function in early onset small for gestational age and growth restricted fetuses. *Eur J Obstet Gynecol Reprod Biol.* (2013) 171:262–5. doi: 10.1016/j.ejogrb.2013.09.020
65. Perez-Cruz M, Cruz-Lemini M, Fernandez MT, Parra JA, Bartrons J, Gomez-Roig MD, et al. Fetal cardiac function in late-onset intrauterine growth restriction vs small-for-gestational age, as defined by estimated fetal weight, cerebroplacental ratio and uterine artery Doppler. *Ultrasound Obstet Gynecol.* (2015) 46:465–71. doi: 10.1002/uog.14930
66. Crispi F, Hernandez-Andrade E, Pelsers MM, Plasencia W, Benavides-Serralde JA, Eixarch E, et al. Cardiac dysfunction and cell damage across clinical stages of severity in growth-restricted fetuses. *Am J Obstetr Gynecol.* (2008) 199:254.e1–8. doi: 10.1016/j.ajog.2008.06.056
67. Menendez-Castro C, Fahlbusch F, Cordasic N, Amann K, Munzel K, Plank C, et al. Early and late postnatal myocardial and vascular changes in a protein restriction rat model of intrauterine growth restriction. *PLoS ONE* (2011) 6:e20369. doi: 10.1371/journal.pone.0020369
68. Barry JS, Rozance PJ, Brown LD, Anthony RV, Thornburg KL, Hay WW Jr. Increased fetal myocardial sensitivity to insulin-stimulated glucose metabolism during ovine fetal growth restriction. *Exp Biol Med (Maywood)* (2016) 241:839–47. doi: 10.1177/1535370216632621
69. Poudel R, McMillen IC, Dunn SL, Zhang S, Morrison JL. Impact of chronic hypoxemia on blood flow to the brain, heart, and adrenal gland in the late-gestation IUGR sheep fetus. *Am J Physiol Regul Integr Comp Physiol.* (2015) 308:R151–62. doi: 10.1152/ajpregu.00036.2014
70. Masoumy EP, Sawyer AA, Sharma S, Patel JA, Gordon MK, Regnault RH, et al. The lifelong impact of fetal growth restriction on cardiac development. *Pediatr Res.* (2018) 84:537–44. doi: 10.1038/s41390-018-0069-x
71. Bubb KJ, Cock ML, Black MJ, Dodic M, Boon WM, Parkington HC, et al. Intrauterine growth restriction delays cardiomyocyte maturation and alters coronary artery function in the fetal sheep. *J Physiol.* (2007) 578:871–81. doi: 10.1113/jphysiol.2006.121160
72. Opitz CA, Linke WA. Plasticity of cardiac titin/connectin in heart development. *J Muscle Res Cell Motil.* (2005) 26:333–42. doi: 10.1007/s10974-005-9040-7
73. Torre I, Gonzalez-Tendero A, Garcia-Canadilla P, Crispi F, Garcia-Garcia F, Bijnens B, et al. Permanent cardiac sarcomere changes in a rabbit model of intrauterine growth restriction. *PLoS ONE* (2014) 9:e113067. doi: 10.1371/journal.pone.0113067
74. Iruretagoyena JI, Gonzalez-Tendero A, Garcia-Canadilla P, Amat-Roldan I, Torre I, Nadal A, et al. Cardiac dysfunction is associated with altered sarcomere ultrastructure in intrauterine growth restriction. *Am J Obstet Gynecol.* (2014) 210:550.e1–7. doi: 10.1016/j.ajog.2014.01.023
75. Tare M, Parkington HC, Wallace EM, Sutherland AE, Lim R, Yawno T, et al. Maternal melatonin administration mitigates coronary stiffness and endothelial dysfunction, and improves heart resilience to insult in growth restricted lambs. *J Physiol.* (2014) 592:2695–709. doi: 10.1113/jphysiol.2014.270934
76. Brain KL, Allison BJ, Niu Y, Cross CM, Itani N, Kane AD, et al. Induction of controlled hypoxic pregnancy in large mammalian species. *Physiol Rep.* (2015) 3:e12614. doi: 10.14814/phy2.12614
77. Sehgal A, Allison BJ, Gwini SM, Miller SL, Polglase GR. Cardiac morphology and function in preterm growth restricted infants: relevance for clinical sequelae. *J Pediatr.* (2017) 188:128–134.e2. doi: 10.1016/j.jpeds.2017.05.076
78. Allison BJ, Brain KL, Niu Y, Kane AD, Herrera EA, Thakor AS, et al. Fetal *in vivo* continuous cardiovascular function during chronic hypoxia. *J Physiol.* (2016) 594:1247–64. doi: 10.1113/JP271091
79. Allison BJ, Kaandorp JJ, Kane AD, Camm EJ, Lusby C, Cross CM, et al. Divergence of mechanistic pathways mediating cardiovascular aging and developmental programming of cardiovascular disease. *FASEB J.* (2016) 30:1968–75. doi: 10.1096/fj.201500057

80. Sehgal A, Allison BJ, Gwini SM, Menahem S, Miller SL, Polglase GR. Vascular aging and cardiac maladaptation in growth-restricted preterm infants. *J Perinatol.* (2017) 38:92–7. doi: 10.1038/jp.2017.135
81. Dodson RB, Rozance PJ, Petrash CC, Hunter KS, Ferguson VL. Thoracic and abdominal aortas stiffen through unique extracellular matrix changes in intrauterine growth restricted fetal sheep. *Am J Physiol Heart Circ Physiol.* (2014) 306:H429–37. doi: 10.1152/ajpheart.00472.2013
82. Kuo AH, Li C, Huber HF, Clarke GD, Nathanielsz PW. Intrauterine growth restriction results in persistent vascular mismatch in adulthood. *J Physiol.* (2017) 596:5777–90. doi: 10.1113/JP275139
83. Canas D, Herrera EA, Garcia-Herrera C, Celentano D, Krause BJ. Fetal growth restriction induces heterogeneous effects on vascular biomechanical and functional properties in guinea pigs (Cavia porcellus). *Front Physiol.* (2017) 8:144. doi: 10.3389/fphys.2017.00144
84. Martyn CN, Greenwald SE. Impaired synthesis of elastin in walls of aorta and large conduit arteries during early development as an initiating event in pathogenesis of systemic hypertension. *Lancet* (1997) 350:953–5. doi: 10.1016/S0140-6736(96)10508-0
85. Dodson RB, Miller TA, Powers K, Yang Y, Yu B, Albertine KH, et al. Intrauterine growth restriction influences vascular remodeling and stiffening in the weanling rat more than sex or diet. *Am J Physiol Heart Circ Physiol.* (2017) 312:H250–64. doi: 10.1152/ajpheart.00610.2016
86. Fouzas S, Karatza AA, Davlouros PA, Chrysis D, Alexopoulos D, Mantagos S, et al. Neonatal cardiac dysfunction in intrauterine growth restriction. *Pediatr Res.* (2014) 75:651–7. doi: 10.1038/pr.2014.22
87. Cohen E, Whatley C, Wong FY, Wallace EM, Mockler JC, Odoi A, et al. Effects of foetal growth restriction and preterm birth on cardiac morphology and function during infancy. *Acta Paediatr.* (2017) 107:450–5. doi: 10.1111/apa.14144
88. Verburg BO, Jaddoe VW, Wladimiroff JW, Hofman A, Witteman JC, Steegers EA. Fetal hemodynamic adaptive changes related to intrauterine growth: the Generation R Study. *Circulation* (2008) 117:649–59. doi: 10.1161/CIRCULATIONAHA.107.709717
89. Roseboom T, de Rooij S, Painter R. The Dutch famine and its long-term consequences for adult health. *Early Hum Dev.* (2006) 82:485–91. doi: 10.1016/j.earlhumdev.2006.07.001
90. Leon DA, Lithell HO, Vagero D, Koupilova I, Mohsen R, Berglund L, et al. Reduced fetal growth rate and increased risk of death from ischaemic heart disease: cohort study of 15 000 Swedish men and women born 1915-29. *BMJ* (1998) 317:241–5. doi: 10.1136/bmj.317.7153.241
91. Fukuoka H. DOHaD (Developmental Origins of Health and Disease) and Birth Cohort Research. *J Nutr Sci Vitaminol.* (2015) 61(Suppl.):S2–4. doi: 10.3177/jnsv.61.S2
92. Skilton MR, Evans N, Griffiths KA, Harmer JA, Celermajer DS. Aortic wall thickness in newborns with intrauterine growth restriction. *Lancet* (2005) 365:1484–6. doi: 10.1016/S0140-6736(05)66419-7
93. Zanardo V, Fanelli T, Weiner G, Fanos V, Zaninotto M, Visentin S, et al. Intrauterine growth restriction is associated with persistent aortic wall thickening and glomerular proteinuria during infancy. *Kidney Int.* (2011) 80:119–23. doi: 10.1038/ki.2011.99
94. Singhal A, Kattenhorn M, Cole TJ, Deanfield J, Lucas A. Preterm birth, vascular function, and risk factors for atherosclerosis. *Lancet* (2001) 358:1159–60. doi: 10.1016/S0140-6736(01)06276-6
95. Kotecha SJ, Watkins WJ, Heron J, Henderson J, Dunstan FD, Kotecha S. Spirometric lung function in school-age children: effect of intrauterine growth retardation and catch-up growth. *Am J Respirat Crit Care Med.* (2010) 181:969–74. doi: 10.1164/rccm.200906-0897OC
96. Check J, Gotteiner N, Liu X, Su E, Porta N, Steinhorn R, et al. Fetal growth restriction and pulmonary hypertension in premature infants with bronchopulmonary dysplasia. *J Perinatol.* (2013) 33:553–7. doi: 10.1038/jp.2012.164
97. Sehgal A, Gwini SM, Menahem S, Allison BJ, Miller SL, Polglase GR. Preterm growth restriction and bronchopulmonary dysplasia: the vascular hypothesis and related physiology. *J Physiol.* (2018). doi: 10.1113/JP276040. [Epub ahead of print].
98. Ronkainen E, Dunder T, Kaukola T, Marttila R, Hallman M. Intrauterine growth restriction predicts lower lung function at school age in children born very preterm. *Arch Dis Childhood* (2016) 101:F412–7. doi: 10.1136/archdischild-2015-308922
99. Barker DJ, Godfrey KM, Fall C, Osmond C, Winter PD, Shaheen SO. Relation of birth weight and childhood respiratory infection to adult lung function and death from chronic obstructive airways disease. *BMJ* (1991) 303:671–5. doi: 10.1136/bmj.303.6804.671
100. McGillick EV, Orgeig S, Allison BJ, Brain KL, Niu Y, Itani N, et al. Maternal chronic hypoxia increases expression of genes regulating lung liquid movement and surfactant maturation in male fetuses in late gestation. *J Physiol.* (2017) 595:4329–50. doi: 10.1113/JP273842
101. Ambalavanan N, Nicola T, Hagood J, Bulger A, Serra R, Murphy-Ullrich J, et al. Transforming growth factor-beta signaling mediates hypoxia-induced pulmonary arterial remodeling and inhibition of alveolar development in newborn mouse lung. *Am J Physiol.* (2008) 295:L86–95. doi: 10.1152/ajplung.00534.2007
102. Polglase GR, Barbuto J, Allison BJ, Yawno T, Sutherland AE, Malhotra A, et al. Effects of antenatal melatonin therapy on lung structure in growth-restricted newborn lambs. *J Appl Physiol.* (2017) 123:1195–203. doi: 10.1152/japplphysiol.00783.2016
103. Allison BJ, Hooper SB, Coia E, Zahra VA, Jenkin G, Malhotra A, et al. Ventilation-induced lung injury is not exacerbated by growth restriction in preterm lambs. *Am J Physiol.* (2016) 310:L213–23. doi: 10.1152/ajplung.00328.2015
104. Sutherland AE, Crossley KJ, Allison BJ, Jenkin G, Wallace EM, Miller SL. The effects of intrauterine growth restriction and antenatal glucocorticoids on ovine fetal lung development. *Pediatr Res.* (2012) 71:689–96. doi: 10.1038/pr.2012.19
105. Maritz GS, Cock ML, Louey S, Joyce BJ, Albuquerque CA, Harding R. Effects of fetal growth restriction on lung development before and after birth: a morphometric analysis. *Pediatr Pulmonol.* (2001) 32:201–10. doi: 10.1002/ppul.1109
106. Gortner L, Hilgendorff A, Bahner T, Ebsen M, Reiss I, Rudloff S. Hypoxia-induced intrauterine growth retardation: effects on pulmonary development and surfactant protein transcription. *Biol Neonate* (2005) 88:129–35. doi: 10.1159/000085895
107. Orgeig S, Crittenden TA, Marchant C, McMillen IC, Morrison JL. Intrauterine growth restriction delays surfactant protein maturation in the sheep fetus. *Am J Physiol.* (2010) 298:L575–83. doi: 10.1152/ajplung.00226.2009
108. Zhu MY, Milligan N, Keating S, Windrim R, Keunen J, Thakur V, et al. The hemodynamics of late-onset intrauterine growth restriction by MRI. *Am J Obstetr Gynecol.* (2016) 214:367.e1–367.e17. doi: 10.1016/j.ajog.2015.10.004
109. Kiserud T, Ebbing C, Kessler J, Rasmussen S. Fetal cardiac output, distribution to the placenta and impact of placental compromise. *Ultrasound Obstetr Gynecol.* (2006) 28:126–36. doi: 10.1002/uog.2832
110. Polglase GR, Allison BJ, Coia E, Li A, Jenkin G, Malhotra A, et al. Altered cardiovascular function at birth in growth-restricted preterm lambs. *Pediatr Res.* (2016) 80:538–46. doi: 10.1038/pr.2016.104
111. Hooper SB, Harding R. Fetal lung liquid: a major determinant of the growth and functional development of the fetal lung. *Clin Exp Pharmacol Physiol.* (1995) 22:235–47. doi: 10.1111/j.1440-1681.1995.tb01988.x
112. Harding R. Fetal pulmonary development: the role of respiratory movements. *Equine Vet J Suppl.* (1997) 32–9. doi: 10.1111/j.2042-3306.1997.tb05076.x
113. Filby CE, Hooper SB, Wallace MJ. Partial pulmonary embolization disrupts alveolarization in fetal sheep. *Respir Res.* (2010) 11:42. doi: 10.1186/1465-9921-11-42
114. Thebaud B, Abman SH. Bronchopulmonary dysplasia: where have all the vessels gone? Roles of angiogenic growth factors in chronic lung disease. *Am J Respir Crit Care Med.* (2007) 175:978–85. doi: 10.1164/rccm.200611-1660PP
115. Galambos C, Ng YS, Ali A, Noguchi A, Lovejoy S, D'Amore PA, et al. Defective pulmonary development in the absence of heparin-binding vascular endothelial growth factor isoforms. *Am J Respir Cell Mol Biol.* (2002) 27:194–203. doi: 10.1165/ajrcmb.27.2.4703
116. Rozance PJ, Seedorf GJ, Brown A, Roe G, O'Meara MC, Gien J, et al. Intrauterine growth restriction decreases pulmonary alveolar and vessel growth and causes pulmonary artery endothelial cell

dysfunction *in vitro* in fetal sheep. *Am J Physiol.* (2011) 301:L860–71. doi: 10.1152/ajplung.00197.2011
117. Karadag A, Sakurai R, Wang Y, Guo P, Desai M, Ross MG, et al. Effect of maternal food restriction on fetal rat lung lipid differentiation program. *Pediatr Pulmonol.* (2009) 44:635–44. doi: 10.1002/ppul.21030
118. Mestan KK, Check J, Minturn L, Yallapragada S, Farrow KN, Liu X, et al. Placental pathologic changes of maternal vascular underperfusion in bronchopulmonary dysplasia and pulmonary hypertension. *Placenta* (2014) 35:570–4. doi: 10.1016/j.placenta.2014.05.003
119. Eriksson L, Haglund B, Odlind V, Altman M, Ewald U, Kieler H. Perinatal conditions related to growth restriction and inflammation are associated with an increased risk of bronchopulmonary dysplasia. *Acta Paediatr.* (2015) 104:259–63. doi: 10.1111/apa.12888
120. Gagliardi L, Rusconi F, Da Frè M, Mello G, Carnielli V, Di Lallo D, et al. Pregnancy disorders leading to very preterm birth influence neonatal outcomes: results of the population-based ACTION cohort study. *Pediatr Res.* (2013) 73:794–801. doi: 10.1038/pr.2013.52
121. Lio A, Rosati P, Pastorino R, Cota F, Tana M, Tirone C, et al. Fetal Doppler velocimetry and bronchopulmonary dysplasia risk among growth-restricted preterm infants: an observational study. *BMJ Open* (2017) 7:e015232. doi: 10.1136/bmjopen-2016-015232
122. Papamatheakis DG, Chundu M, Blood AB, Wilson SM. Prenatal programming of pulmonary hypertension induced by chronic hypoxia or ductal ligation in sheep. *Pulmonary Circ.* (2013) 3:757–80. doi: 10.1086/674767
123. Berkelhamer SK, Mestan KK, Steinhorn RH. Pulmonary hypertension in bronchopulmonary dysplasia. *Semin Perinatol.* (2013) 37:124–31. doi: 10.1053/j.semperi.2013.01.009
124. Joss-Moore LA, Wang Y, Yu X, Campbell MS, Callaway CW, McKnight RA, et al. IUGR decreases elastin mRNA expression in the developing rat lung and alters elastin content and lung compliance in the mature rat lung. *Physiol Genom.* (2011) 43:499–505. doi: 10.1152/physiolgenomics.00183.2010
125. Lopuhaä CE, Roseboom TJ, Osmond C, Barker DJ, Ravelli AC, Bleker OP, et al. Atopy, lung function, and obstructive airways disease after prenatal exposure to famine. *Thorax* (2000) 55:555–61. doi: 10.1136/thorax.55.7.555
126. Egana-Ugrinovic G, Sanz-Cortes M, Figueras F, Bargallo N, Gratacos E. Differences in cortical development assessed by fetal MRI in late-onset intrauterine growth restriction. *Am J Obstetr Gynecol.* (2013) 209:126.e1-8. doi: 10.1016/j.ajog.2013.04.008
127. Huppi PS. Cortical development in the fetus and the newborn: advanced MR techniques. *Top Magn Reson. Imaging* (2011) 22:33–8. doi: 10.1097/RMR.0b013e3182416f78
128. Arthurs OJ, Rega A, Guimiot F, Belarbi N, Rosenblatt J, Biran V, et al. Diffusion-weighted magnetic resonance imaging of the fetal brain in intrauterine growth restriction. *Ultrasound Obstetr Gynecol.* (2017) 50:79–87. doi: 10.1002/uog.17318
129. Tolsa CB, Zimine S, Warfield SK, Freschi M, Sancho Rossignol A, Lazeyras F, et al. Early alteration of structural and functional brain development in premature infants born with intrauterine growth restriction. *Pediatr. Res.* (2004) 56:132–8. doi: 10.1203/01.PDR.0000128983.54614.7E
130. Ramenghi LA, Martinelli A, De Carli A, Brusati V, Mandia L, Fumagalli M, et al. Cerebral maturation in IUGR and appropriate for gestational age preterm babies. *Reprod Sci.* (2011) 18:469–75. doi: 10.1177/1933719110388847
131. Lodygensky GA, Seghier ML, Warfield SK, Tolsa CB, Sizonenko S, Lazeyras F, et al. Intrauterine growth restriction affects the preterm infant's hippocampus. *Pediatr Res.* (2008) 63:438–43. doi: 10.1203/PDR.0b013e318165c005
132. Bruno CJ, Bengani S, Gomes WA, Brewer M, Vega M, Xie X, et al. MRI differences associated with intrauterine growth restriction in preterm infants. *Neonatology* (2017) 111:317–23. doi: 10.1159/000453576
133. Batalle D, Munoz-Moreno E, Tornador C, Bargallo N, Deco G, Eixarch E, et al. Altered resting-state whole-brain functional networks of neonates with intrauterine growth restriction. *Cortex* (2016) 77:119–31. doi: 10.1016/j.cortex.2016.01.012
134. van de Looij Y, Dean JM, Gunn AJ, Huppi PS, Sizonenko SV. Advanced magnetic resonance spectroscopy and imaging techniques applied to brain development and animal models of perinatal injury. *Int J Dev Neurosci.* (2015) 45:29–38. doi: 10.1016/j.ijdevneu.2015.03.009
135. Malhotra A, Ditchfield M, Fahey MC, Castillo-Melendez M, Allison BJ, Polglase GR, et al. Detection and assessment of brain injury in the growth-restricted fetus and neonate. *Pediatr Res.* (2017) 82:184–93. doi: 10.1038/pr.2017.37
136. Malhotra A, Yahya Z, Sasi A, Jenkin G, Ditchfield M, Polglase GR, et al. Does fetal growth restriction lead to increased brain injury as detected by neonatal cranial ultrasound in premature infants? *J Paediatr Child Health* (2015) 51:1103–8. doi: 10.1111/jpc.12910
137. Krishnamurthy MB, Popiel A, Malhotra A. Screening investigations in small-for-gestational-age near-term and term infants. *Eur J Pediatr.* (2017) 176:1707–12. doi: 10.1007/s00431-017-3031-8
138. McLean G, Hough C, Sehgal A, Ditchfield M, Polglase GR, Miller SL. Three-dimensional ultrasound cranial imaging and early neurodevelopment in preterm growth-restricted infants. *J Paediatr Child Health* (2018) 54:420–5. doi: 10.1111/jpc.13808
139. Cruz-Martinez R, Tenorio V, Padilla N, Crispi F, Figueras F, Gratacos E. Risk of ultrasound-detected neonatal brain abnormalities in intrauterine growth-restricted fetuses born between 28 and 34 weeks' gestation: relationship with gestational age at birth and fetal Doppler parameters. *Ultrasound Obstetr Gynecol.* (2015) 46:452–9. doi: 10.1002/uog.14920
140. Padilla N, Falcon C, Sanz-Cortes M, Figueras F, Bargallo N, Crispi F, et al. Differential effects of intrauterine growth restriction on brain structure and development in preterm infants: a magnetic resonance imaging study. *Brain Res.* (2011) 1382:98–108. doi: 10.1016/j.brainres.2011.01.032
141. Padilla N, Junque C, Figueras F, Sanz-Cortes M, Bargallo N, Arranz A, et al. Differential vulnerability of gray matter and white matter to intrauterine growth restriction in preterm infants at 12 months corrected age. *Brain Res.* (2014) 1545:1–11. doi: 10.1016/j.brainres.2013.12.007
142. Batalle D, Eixarch E, Figueras F, Munoz-Moreno E, Bargallo N, Illa M, et al. Altered small-world topology of structural brain networks in infants with intrauterine growth restriction and its association with later neurodevelopmental outcome. *Neuroimage* (2012) 60:1352–66. doi: 10.1016/j.neuroimage.2012.01.059
143. Fischi-Gomez E, Vasung L, Meskaldji DE, Lazeyras F, Borradori-Tolsa C, Hagmann P, et al. Structural brain connectivity in school-age preterm infants provides evidence for impaired networks relevant for higher order cognitive skills and social cognition. *Cereb Cortex* (2015) 25:2793–805. doi: 10.1093/cercor/bhu073
144. Tanis JC, Schmitz DM, Boelen MR, Casarella L, van den Berg PP, Bilardo CM, et al. Relationship between general movements in neonates who were growth restricted *in utero* and prenatal Doppler flow patterns. *Ultrasound Obstetr Gynecol.* (2016) 48:772–8. doi: 10.1002/uog.15903
145. Yerushalmy-Feler A, Marom R, Peylan T, Korn A, Haham A, Mandel D, et al. Electroencephalographic characteristics in preterm infants born with intrauterine growth restriction. *J Pediatr.* (2014) 164:756–761.e1. doi: 10.1016/j.jpeds.2013.12.030
146. Cohen E, Wong FY, Wallace EM, Mockler JC, Odoi A, Hollis S, et al. EEG power spectrum maturation in preterm fetal growth restricted infants. *Brain Res.* (2018) 1678:180–6. doi: 10.1016/j.brainres.2017.10.010
147. Arduini D, Rizzo G, Romanini C, Mancuso S. Fetal haemodynamic response to acute maternal hyperoxygenation as predictor of fetal distress in intrauterine growth retardation. *BMJ* (1989) 298:1561–2. doi: 10.1136/bmj.298.6687.1561
148. Hernandez-Andrade E, Figueroa-Diesel H, Jansson T, Rangel-Nava H, Gratacos E. Changes in regional fetal cerebral blood flow perfusion in relation to hemodynamic deterioration in severely growth-restricted fetuses. *Ultrasound Obstetr Gynecol.* (2008) 32:71–6. doi: 10.1002/uog.5377
149. Ishii H, Takami T, Fujioka T, Mizukaki N, Kondo A, Sunohara D, et al. Comparison of changes in cerebral and systemic perfusion between appropriate- and small-for-gestational-age infants during the first three days after birth. *Brain Dev.* (2014) 36:380–7. doi: 10.1016/j.braindev.2013.06.006
150. Hunter DS, Hazel SJ, Kind KL, Owens JA, Pitcher JB, Gatford KL. Programming the brain: common outcomes and gaps in knowledge from animal studies of IUGR. *Physiol Behav.* (2016) 164:233–48. doi: 10.1016/j.physbeh.2016.06.005

151. Basilious A, Yager J, Fehlings MG. Neurological outcomes of animal models of uterine artery ligation and relevance to human intrauterine growth restriction: a systematic review. *Dev Med Child Neurol.* (2015) 57:420–30. doi: 10.1111/dmcn.12599
152. Swanson AM, David AL. Animal models of fetal growth restriction: considerations for translational medicine. *Placenta* (2015) 36:623–30. doi: 10.1016/j.placenta.2015.03.003
153. McDougall ARA, Wiradjaja V, Azhan A, Li A, Hale N, Wlodek ME, et al. Intrauterine growth restriction alters the postnatal development of the rat cerebellum. *Dev Neurosci.* (2017) 39:215–27. doi: 10.1159/000470902
154. Alves de Alencar Rocha AK, Allison BJ, Yawno T, Polglase GR, Sutherland AE, Malhotra A, et al. Early- versus late-onset fetal growth restriction differentially affects the development of the fetal sheep brain. *Dev Neurosci.* (2017) 39:141–55. doi: 10.1159/000456542
155. Eixarch E, Batalle D, Illa M, Munoz-Moreno E, Arbat-Plana A, Amat-Roldan I, et al. Neonatal neurobehavior and diffusion MRI changes in brain reorganization due to intrauterine growth restriction in a rabbit model. *PLoS ONE* (2012) 7:e31497. doi: 10.1371/journal.pone.0031497
156. Ruff CA, Faulkner SD, Rumajogee P, Beldick S, Foltz W, Corrigan J, et al. The extent of intrauterine growth restriction determines the severity of cerebral injury and neurobehavioural deficits in rodents. *PLoS ONE* (2017) 12:e0184653. doi: 10.1371/journal.pone.0184653
157. Tolcos M, Petratos S, Hirst JJ, Wong F, Spencer SJ, Azhan A, et al. Blocked, delayed, or obstructed: what causes poor white matter development in intrauterine growth restricted infants? *Prog Neurobiol.* (2017) 154:62–77. doi: 10.1016/j.pneurobio.2017.03.009
158. Bisignano M, Rees S. The effects of intrauterine growth retardation on synaptogenesis and mitochondrial formation in the cerebral and cerebellar cortices of fetal sheep. *Int J Dev Neurosci.* (1988) 6:453–60. doi: 10.1016/0736-5748(88)90051-2
159. Castillo-Melendez M, Yawno T, Allison BJ, Jenkin G, Wallace EM, Miller SL. Cerebrovascular adaptations to chronic hypoxia in the growth restricted lamb. *Int J Dev Neurosci.* (2015) 45:55–65. doi: 10.1016/j.ijdevneu.2015.01.004
160. Allison BJ, Hooper SB, Coia E, Jenkin G, Malhotra A, Zahra V, et al. Does growth restriction increase the vulnerability to acute ventilation-induced brain injury in newborn lambs? Implications for future health and disease. *J Dev Orig Health Dis.* (2017) 8:556–65. doi: 10.1017/S204017441700037X
161. Malhotra A, Castillo-Melendez M, Allison BJ, Sutherland AE, Nitsos I, Pham Y, et al. Neuropathology as a consequence of neonatal ventilation in premature growth restricted lambs. *Am J Physiol Regul Integr Comp Physiol.* (2018) 315:R1183–1194. doi: 10.1152/ajpregu.00171.2018
162. Blair EM, Nelson KB. Fetal growth restriction and risk of cerebral palsy in singletons born after at least 35 weeks' gestation. *Am J Obstetr Gynecol.* (2015) 212:520.e1-7. doi: 10.1016/j.ajog.2014.10.1103
163. Morsing E, Asard M, Ley D, Stjernqvist K, Marsal K. Cognitive function after intrauterine growth restriction and very preterm birth. *Pediatrics* (2011) 127:e874–82. doi: 10.1542/peds.2010-1821
164. Baschat AA. Neurodevelopment after fetal growth restriction. *Fetal Diagn Ther.* (2014) 36:136–42. doi: 10.1159/000353631
165. MacLennan AH, Thompson SC, Gecz J. Cerebral palsy: causes, pathways, and the role of genetic variants. *Am J Obstet Gynecol.* (2015) 213:779–88. doi: 10.1016/j.ajog.2015.05.034
166. Report of the Australian Cerebral Palsy Register, Birth Years 1993-2006 (February 2013).
167. Sung IK, Vohr B, Oh W. Growth and neurodevelopmental outcome of very low birth weight infants with intrauterine growth retardation: comparison with control subjects matched by birth weight and gestational age. *J Pediatr.* (1993) 123:618–24. doi: 10.1016/S0022-3476(05)80965-5
168. Leitner Y, Fattal-Valevski A, Geva R, Eshel R, Toledano-Alhadef H, Rotstein M, et al. Neurodevelopmental outcome of children with intrauterine growth retardation: a longitudinal, 10-year prospective study. *J Child Neurol.* (2007) 22:580–7. doi: 10.1177/0883073807302605
169. Low JA, Handley-Derry MH, Burke SO, Peters RD, Pater EA, Killen HL, et al. Association of intrauterine fetal growth retardation and learning deficits at age 9 to 11 years. *Am J Obstet Gynecol.* (1992) 167:1499–505. doi: 10.1016/0002-9378(92)91727-R
170. Geva R, Eshel R, Leitner Y, Fattal-Valevski A, Harel S. Memory functions of children born with asymmetric intrauterine growth restriction. *Brain Res.* (2006) 1117:186–94. doi: 10.1016/j.brainres.2006.08.004
171. Geva R, Eshel R, Leitner Y, Valevski AF, Harel S. Neuropsychological outcome of children with intrauterine growth restriction: a 9-year prospective study. *Pediatrics* (2006) 118:91–100. doi: 10.1542/peds.2005-2343
172. Murray E, Fernandes M, Fazel M, Kennedy SH, Villar J, Stein A. Differential effect of intrauterine growth restriction on childhood neurodevelopment: a systematic review. *BJOG* (2015) 122:1062–72. doi: 10.1111/1471-0528.13435
173. Larroque B, Bertrais S, Czernichow P, Leger J. School difficulties in 20-year-olds who were born small for gestational age at term in a regional cohort study. *Pediatrics* (2001) 108:111–5. doi: 10.1542/peds.108.1.111
174. Walton RB, Reed LC, Estrada SM, Schmiedecke SS, Villazana-Kretzer DL, Napolitano PG, et al. Evaluation of sildenafil and tadalafil for reversing constriction of fetal arteries in a human placenta perfusion model. *Hypertension* (2018) 72:167–76. doi: 10.1161/HYPERTENSIONAHA.117.10738
175. Khan RN, Hamoud H, Warren A, Wong LF, Arulkumaran S. Relaxant action of sildenafil citrate (Viagra) on human myometrium of pregnancy. *Am J Obstetr Gynecol.* (2004) 191:315–21. doi: 10.1016/j.ajog.2003.11.005
176. Wareing M, Myers JE, O'Hara M, Baker PN. Sildenafil citrate (Viagra) enhances vasodilatation in fetal growth restriction. *J Clin Endocrinol Metab.* (2005) 90:2550–5. doi: 10.1210/jc.2004-1831
177. Paauw ND, Terstappen F, Ganzevoort W, Joles JA, Gremmels H, Lely AT, et al. Sildenafil During pregnancy: a preclinical meta-analysis on fetal growth and maternal blood pressure. *Hypertension* (2017) 70:998–1006. doi: 10.1161/HYPERTENSIONAHA.117.09690
178. Miller SL, Loose JM, Jenkin G, Wallace EM. The effects of sildenafil citrate (Viagra) on uterine blood flow and well being in the intrauterine growth-restricted fetus. *Am J Obstetr Gynecol.* (2009) 200:102.e1-7. doi: 10.1016/j.ajog.2008.08.029
179. Hawkes N. Trial of Viagra for fetal growth restriction is halted after baby deaths. *BMJ* (2018) 362:k3247. doi: 10.1136/bmj.k3247
180. Smith GCS. The STRIDER trial: one step forward, one step back. *Lancet* (2018) 2:80–1. doi: 10.1016/S2352-4642(17)30176-1
181. Pellicer B, Herraiz S, Cauli O, Rodrigo R, Asensi M, Cortijo J, et al. Haemodynamic effects of long-term administration of sildenafil in normotensive pregnant and non-pregnant rats. *BJOG* (2011) 118:615–23. doi: 10.1111/j.1471-0528.2010.02839.x
182. Spencer R, Ambler G, Brodszki J, Diemert A, Figueras F, Gratacos E, et al. EVERREST prospective study: a 6-year prospective study to define the clinical and biological characteristics of pregnancies affected by severe early onset fetal growth restriction. *BMC Preg Childbirth* (2017) 17:43. doi: 10.1186/s12884-017-1226-7
183. David AL, Torondel B, Zachary I, Wigley V, Abi-Nader K, Mehta V, et al. Local delivery of VEGF adenovirus to the uterine artery increases vasorelaxation and uterine blood flow in the pregnant sheep. *Gene Ther.* (2008) 15:1344–50. doi: 10.1038/gt.2008.102
184. Carr DJ, Wallace JM, Aitken RP, Milne JS, Martin JF, Zachary IC, et al. Peri- and postnatal effects of prenatal adenoviral VEGF gene therapy in growth-restricted sheep. *Biol Reproduct.* (2016) 94:142. doi: 10.1095/biolreprod.115.133744
185. Kane AD, Herrera EA, Camm EJ, Giussani DA. Vitamin C prevents intrauterine programming of *in vivo* cardiovascular dysfunction in the rat. *Circul J.* (2013) 77:2604–11. doi: 10.1253/circj.CJ-13-0311
186. Miller SL, Yawno T, Alers NO, Castillo-Melendez M, Supramaniam VG, VanZyl N, et al. Antenatal antioxidant treatment with melatonin to decrease newborn neurodevelopmental deficits and brain injury caused by fetal growth restriction. *J Pineal Res.* (2014) 56:283–94. doi: 10.1111/jpi.12121
187. Gonzalez-Candia A, Veliz M, Araya C, Quezada S, Ebensperger G, Seron-Ferre M, et al. Potential adverse effects of antenatal melatonin as a treatment for intrauterine growth restriction: findings in pregnant sheep. *Am J Obstetr Gynecol.* (2016) 215:245.e1-7. doi: 10.1016/j.ajog.2016.02.040
188. Hobson SR, Gurusinghe S, Lim R, Alers NO, Miller SL, Kingdom JC, et al. Melatonin improves endothelial function *in vitro* and prolongs pregnancy

in women with early-onset preeclampsia. *J Pineal Res.* (2018) 65:e12508. doi: 10.1111/jpi.12508
189. Astorga CR, Gonzalez-Candia A, Candia AA, Figueroa EG, Canas D, Ebensperger G, et al. Melatonin decreases pulmonary vascular remodeling and oxygen sensitivity in pulmonary hypertensive newborn lambs. *Front Physiol.* (2018) 9:185. doi: 10.3389/fphys.2018.00185
190. Torres F, Gonzalez-Candia A, Montt C, Ebensperger G, Chubretovic M, Seron-Ferre M, et al. Melatonin reduces oxidative stress and improves vascular function in pulmonary hypertensive newborn sheep. *J Pineal Res.* (2015) 58:362–73. doi: 10.1111/jpi.12222
191. Thangaratnarajah C, Dinger K, Vohlen C, Klaudt C, Nawabi J, Lopez Garcia E, et al. Novel role of NPY in neuroimmune interaction and lung growth after intrauterine growth restriction. *Am J Physiol.* (2017) 313:L491–l506. doi: 10.1152/ajplung.00432.2016
192. Welin AK, Svedin P, Lapatto R, Sultan B, Hagberg H, Gressens P, et al. Melatonin reduces inflammation and cell death in white matter in the mid-gestation fetal sheep following umbilical cord occlusion. *Pediatr Res.* (2007) 61:153–8. doi: 10.1203/01.pdr.0000252546.20451.1a
193. Yawno T, Mahen M, Li J, Fahey MC, Jenkin G, Miller SL. The beneficial effects of melatonin administration following hypoxia-ischemia in preterm fetal sheep. *Front Cell Neurosci.* (2017) 11:296. doi: 10.3389/fncel.2017.00296
194. Miller SL, Yan EB, Castillo-Melendez M, Jenkin G, Walker DW. Melatonin provides neuroprotection in the late-gestation fetal sheep brain in response to umbilical cord occlusion. *Dev Neurosci.* (2005) 27:200–10. doi: 10.1159/000085993
195. Castillo-Melendez M, Yawno T, Sutherland A, Jenkin G, Wallace EM, Miller SL. Effects of antenatal melatonin treatment on the cerebral vasculature in an ovine model of fetal growth restriction. *Dev Neurosci.* (2017) 39:323–37. doi: 10.1159/000471797
196. Hobson SR, Lim R, Gardiner EE, Alers NO, Wallace EM. Phase I pilot clinical trial of antenatal maternally administered melatonin to decrease the level of oxidative stress in human pregnancies affected by pre-eclampsia (PAMPR): study protocol. *BMJ Open* (2013) 3:e003788. doi: 10.1136/bmjopen-2013-003788
197. Somm E, Larvaron P, van de Looij Y, Toulotte A, Chatagner A, Faure M, et al. Protective effects of maternal nutritional supplementation with lactoferrin on growth and brain metabolism. *Pediatr Res.* (2014) 75:51–61. doi: 10.1038/pr.2013.199
198. Gumus HG, Illa M, Pla L, Zamora M, Crispi F, Gratacos E. Nutritional intra-amniotic therapy increases survival in a rabbit model of fetal growth restriction. *PLoS ONE* (2018) 13:e0193240. doi: 10.1371/journal.pone.0193240
199. Jahan M, Kracht S, Ho Y, Haque Z, Bhattachatyya BN, Wynn PC, et al. Dietary lactoferrin supplementation to gilts during gestation and lactation improves pig production and immunity. *PLoS ONE* (2017) 12:e0185817. doi: 10.1371/journal.pone.0185817
200. Manzoni P, Rinaldi M, Cattani S, Pugni L, Romeo MG, Messner H, et al. Bovine lactoferrin supplementation for prevention of late-onset sepsis in very low-birth-weight neonates: a randomized trial. *JAMA* (2009) 302:1421–8. doi: 10.1001/jama.2009.1403
201. van de Looij Y, Ginet V, Chatagner A, Toulotte A, Somm E, Huppi PS, et al. Lactoferrin during lactation protects the immature hypoxic-ischemic rat brain. *Ann Clin Transl Neurol.* (2014) 1:955–67. doi: 10.1002/acn3.138
202. Ginet V, van de Looij Y, Petrenko V, Toulotte A, Kiss J, Huppi PS, et al. Lactoferrin during lactation reduces lipopolysaccharide-induced brain injury. *BioFactors* (2016) 42:323–36. doi: 10.1002/biof.1278
203. Illa M, Brito V, Pla L, Eixarch E, Arbat-Plana A, Batalle D, et al. Early environmental enrichment enhances abnormal brain connectivity in a rabbit model of intrauterine growth restriction. *Fetal Diagn Ther.* (2017) 44:184–93. doi: 10.1159/000481171
204. James JL, Srinivasan S, Alexander M, Chamley LW. Can we fix it? Evaluating the potential of placental stem cells for the treatment of pregnancy disorders. *Placenta* (2014) 35:77–84. doi: 10.1016/j.placenta.2013.12.010

13

Postnatal Catch-Up Growth after Suspected Fetal Growth Restriction at Term

Linda van Wyk[1,2], Kim E. Boers[3], Aleid G. van Wassenaer-Leemhuis[4], Joris A. M. van der Post[4], Henk A. Bremer[5], Friso M. C. Delemarre[6], Sanne J. Gordijn[2], Kitty W. M. Bloemenkamp[1], Frans J. M. E. Roumen[7], Martina Porath[8], Jan M. M. van Lith[1], Ben W. J. Mol[9], Saskia le Cessie[10] and Sicco A. Scherjon[2] for the DIGITAT study group*

[1] Departments of Obstetrics, Leiden University Medical Centre, Leiden, Netherlands, [2] Department of Obstetrics, University Medical Centre Groningen, Groningen, Netherlands, [3] Haaglanden Medical Centre, The Hague, Netherlands, [4] Academic Medical Centre, Amsterdam, Netherlands, [5] Reinier de Graaf Hospital, Delft, Netherlands, [6] Elkerliek Hospital, Helmond, Netherlands, [7] Atrium Medical Centre, Heerlen, Netherlands, [8] Maxima Medical Centre, Veldhoven, Netherlands, [9] Department of Obstetrics, Monash University Medical Centre, Clayton, VIC, Australia, [10] Department of Clinical Epidimiology, Leiden University Medical Centre, Leiden, Netherlands

***Correspondence:**
Linda van Wyk
vwyklinda@gmail.com

Objective: The aim of this study was to study growth patterns of children born after suspected fetal growth restriction (FGR) at term and to compare the effect of induction of labor (IoL) and expectant management (EM), also in relation to neurodevelopmental and behavioral outcome at age 2.

Methods: We performed a 2 years' follow-up of growth of children included in the Disproportionate Intrauterine Growth Restriction Trial at Term (DIGITAT) study, a Randomized Controlled Trial (RCT) comparing IoL with EM in pregnancies with suspected FGR at term. We collected data on child growth until the age of 2 years. Standard deviation scores (SDSs) for height and weight were calculated at different ages. We assessed the effects of IoL compared with EM and the effects of a birth weight below or above the 3rd or 10th centile on catch-up growth. Target height SDSs were calculated using the height of both parents.

Results: We found a significant increase in SDS in the first 2 years. Children born after EM showed more catch-up growth in the first month [height: mean difference −0.7 (95% CI: 0.2; 1.3)] and weight [mean difference −0.5 (95% CI: 0.3; 0.7)]. Children born with a birth weight below the 3rd and 10th centiles showed more catch-up growth after 1 year [mean difference −0.8 SDS (95% CI: −1.1; −0.5)] and after 2 years [mean difference −0.7 SDS (95% CI: −1.2; −0.2)] as compared to children with a birth weight above the 3rd and 10th centiles. SDS at birth had the strongest effect on adverse neurodevelopmental outcome at 2 years of age.

Conclusion: After FGR at term, postnatal catch-up growth is generally present and associated with the degree of FGR. Obstetric management in FGR influences postnatal growth. Longer-term follow-up is therefore needed and should be directed at growth and physical health.

Clinical Trial Registration: www.ClinicalTrials.gov, identifier SRCTN10363217.

Keywords: intrauterine growth restriction, fetal growth restriction, catch-up growth, Disproportionate Intrauterine Growth Restriction Trial at Term, follow-up

INTRODUCTION

Catch-up growth is considered to be a process of compensatory accelerated growth after a period of poor growth intrauterine. Many studies have shown that growth-restricted children show catch-up growth in the first years after birth (1–6). Catch-up growth is recognized when a child shows accelerated growth, which is visualized as an upward crossing of its centiles in length or weight growth.

Long-term consequences of fetal growth restriction (FGR) and catch-up growth have been studied extensively in the last two decades. It is now generally accepted that low birth weight as a consequence of growth restriction is a risk factor for cardiovascular disease later in life (7–9). It however remains debatable whether this is caused by the catch-up growth itself or the underlying pathophysiology of FGR, by the (extent of) postnatal catch-up growth, or perhaps by a combination. Studies have shown that FGR intrauterine growth restriction itself is associated with an alteration of genetic programming, independent of Body Mass Index (BMI), related to metabolic and cardiovascular diseases (10). On the contrary, others have shown that it is the postnatal catch-up growth and accelerated weight gain that lead to the increased risk (11).

Wit et al. suggest that catch-up growth can be either *complete* or *incomplete* (12). Catch-up growth is considered to be complete in case a mean final height is reached close to the mean target height based on the height of both parents (12). In case of incomplete catch-up growth, the target height range will not be reached and is associated with increased neurodevelopmental problems when compared to children with complete catch-up growth (13–15).

In the Disproportionate Intrauterine Growth Restriction Trial at Term (DIGITAT) trial (16)—a multicenter randomized controlled trial—the effects of induction of labor (IoL) vs. expectant management (EM) in pregnancies suspected of intrauterine growth restriction at term were compared. Suspected intrauterine growth restriction was defined as fetal abdominal circumference below the 10th percentile, estimated fetal weight below the 10th percentile, flattening of the growth curve in the third trimester (as judged by a clinician), or the presence of all three factors.

Data were also collected of women who refused randomization but gave permission for follow-up. Pregnant women with a singleton fetus in the cephalic position, beyond 36 weeks of gestation, and suspected FGR were counseled for trial participation. Primary fetal and maternal outcomes were comparable. Gestational age at birth was lower in the induction group (mean difference –iff (95% CI: –I%fe to –o%fe as was birth weight (mean difference 130 g, 95% CI: –I%f to –o%f $P < 0.001$) when compared to the expectant monitoring group. Despite this difference in (absolute) weight in favor of the children in the group with expectant monitoring, more babies in the expectant group were severely growth restricted, with a birth weight below the third percentile (31 vs. 13%; difference –if%, 95% CI: –I%fe to –o%fer $P < 0.001$) (16).

At 2 years of age, a neurodevelopmental and behavioral follow-up study was performed and showed that children with low birth weights, especially if the birth weight was below the 3rd centile, had a greater risk [adjusted OR 3.6 (95% CI: 1.5–8.8)] for abnormal scores on the Ages and Stages Questionnaire (ASQ). The prevalence of these abnormalities was directly related to the severity of growth restriction (17).

The objective of the present study was to (1) analyze whether obstetric management (IoL vs. EM) policy influences catch-up growth, (2) assess whether children born in the DIGITAT trial (participants and nonparticipants) exhibit catch-up growth until age 2, and (3) assess long-term behavioral and neurodevelopmental outcomes in relation to catch-up growth.

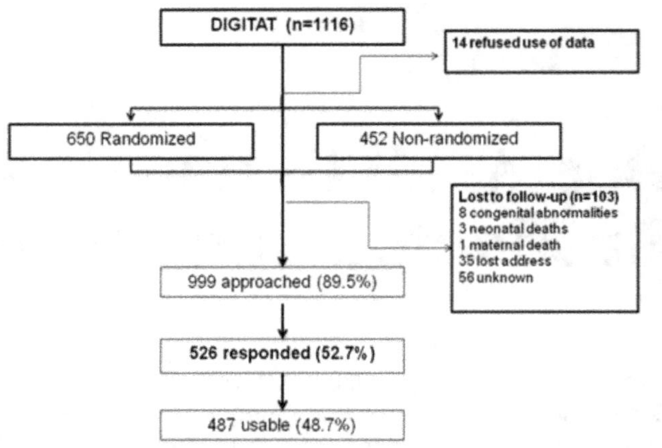

FIGURE 1 | Flowchart of trial participants.

METHODS

Participants

The study population consisted of children born to mothers who participated in the DIGITAT trial (16). During the study period, 1,116 women were eligible for the trial, of whom 14 refused participation, 452 women refused randomization but gave permission for use of their medical data and for follow-up, and 650 women were randomized to either induction of labor (IoL) or an expectant management (EM) (**Figure 1**). Both the randomized and nonrandomized women are included in this study.

Baseline Characteristics

Baseline characteristics of the mothers and children were collected at study inclusion and at birth and have been described elsewhere (16).

Abbreviations: ASQ, Ages and Stages Questionairre; CBCL, Child Behavior Checklist; CI, confidence interval; DIGITAT, Disproportionate Intrauterine Growth Restriction Trial at Term; IQR, interquartile range; FGR, fetal growth restriction; SD, standard deviation; SDS, standard deviation score.

Procedure

We collected growth data until the age of 2 of children born to mothers of the DIGITAT trial. General health, height, weight, and developmental milestones of children in the Netherlands are assessed regularly and free of charge in a national program at the Child Health Center's periodically. Parents were asked to participate in a postal inquiry and to send us the recorded growth data (height and weight) of their child until the age of 2 years and to report the height of the father. Maternal height was already recorded at baseline. Standard deviation scores (SDSs) or *Z* scores were calculated for height, weight, and weight for height at different ages based on, respectively, calculated target height- and population-based growth curves (18). Head circumference was not recorded.

Neurodevelopmental and behavioral outcomes of these children were also assessed at 2 years of age using two standardized parental questionnaires: the Ages and Stages Questionnaire (ASQ) (19) and the Child Behavior Checklist (CBCL) (20). The mean scores of both questionnaires were compared between groups,

TABLE 1 | Baseline characteristics.

Characteristic	Respondent (*n* = 526)	Non-respondent (*n* = 473)	Difference in % or mean (95% CI)
Maternal age (years)	29.7 (26.3; 33.8)	27.7 (23.3; 31.9)	2.2 (1.5; 2.8)**
Maternal Body Mass Index at study entry†	21.8 (19.7; 24.6)	21.8 (19.5; 24.8)	0.04 (−0.6; 0.7)
Maternal smoking in pregnancy§	134 (25.5)	201 (44.7)	−17.1 (−23.2; −11.1)**
Caucasian‡	448 (91.1)	354 (73.9)	17.2 (12.5; 21.8)**
EDUCATION			
Lower professional	200 (69.9)	243 (81.8)	−11.9 (−18.8;−5.0)**
Higher professional	86 (30.1)	54 (18.2)	11.9 (5.0; 18.8)**
Gestational age at birth	272.3 (265.6; 280.4)	272.5 (264.6; 280.8)	−0.02 (−1.2; 1.2)
Male sex	186 (38.9)	198 (38.4)	−0.4 (−5.673, 6.454)
Birth weight (grams)	2,505 (2,215; 2,771)	2,505 (2,281; 2,769)	30.0 (−77.4; 19.2)
Birth weight <10th centile	382 (72.7)	336 (71.1)	1.5 (−4.0; 7.2)
Birth weight <3rd centile	121 (25.4)	129 (25.2)	0.2 (−5.2; 5.7)
Composite adverse neonatal outcome	30 (5.7)	24 (5.1)	0.6 (−2.2; 3.4)

$^{**}p < 0.001$. CI, confidence interval.
Table shows median [IQR: 25th to 75th percentile) or number (%)].
Data were compared using the Student's t-test, chi-square, or Fisher's exact test.
†n = 457 for respondents; n = 394 for non-respondents.
§n = 485 for respondents; n = 449 for non-respondents.
‡n = 492 for respondents; n = 479 for non-respondents.

TABLE 2 | Baseline characteristics of randomized participants (induction vs. expectant monitoring).

Characteristic	Induction (*n* = 158)	Expectant monitoring (*n* = 134)	Difference in % or mean (95% CI)
Maternal age (years)	28.03 (25.13; 32.07)	28.19 (24.69; 31.51)	−0.14 (−1.28; 0.99)
Maternal BMI at study entry†	22.1 (19.9; 25.8)	22.3 (20.2; 25.3)	−0.05 (−1.26; 1.15)
Maternal smoking in pregnancy§	34 (36.8)	43 (35.0)	0.02 (−0.1; 0.13)
Caucasian‡	12 (7.9)	13 (10.2)	−0.02 (−0.09; 0.05)
Education (higher professional)	16 (16.2%)	19 (22.9)	−0.07 (−0.18; 0.05)
Gestational age at birth	266.4 (261.5; 271.2)	277.5 (269.8; 283.6)	−9.91 (−11.85; −7.97)*
Male sex	57 (36.5)	53 (39.6)	− 3.1 (−8.0; 1.4)
Birth weight (grams)	2,435 (2,174; 2,660)	2,600 (2,230; 2,850)	−134 (−221; −46)*
Birth weight <10th centile	21 (13.3)	37 (27.8)	−14.5 (−24; −5.0)*
Birth weight <3rd centile	103 (65.2)	102 (76.7)	−11.5 (−22.0; −1.0)*
Composite adverse neonatal outcome&	7 (4.9)	7 (6.0)	−1.1 (−7; 4)

$^{*}p < 0.05$.
Table shows median [(IQR: 25th to 75th percentile) or number (%)].
Data were compared using the Student t-test, chi-square, or Fisher exact test.
†n = 141 for induction; n = 122 for expectant management.
§n = 144 for induction; n = 123 for expectant management.
‡n = 151 for induction; n = 127 for expectant management.
&n = 143 for induction; n = 116 for expectant management.

TABLE 3 | Age, height, weight, and standard deviation score (SDS) for height, weight, weight for height, height SDS below target height, and difference between SDS in height and weight from birth.

Age (months)	Height (cm) (n)	Weight(g) (n)	SDS height	SDS weight	SDS weight for height (n)	SDS height-target height (n)	Difference in SDS height from birth (n)	95% CI	Difference in SDS weight from birth (n)	95% CI
Birth	46.4 ± 2.7 (236)	2,493 ± 397 (526)	−1.6 ± 1.3	−2.0 ± 0.86	NA	−1.4 ± 1.4	NA		NA	
1	50.7 ± 2.4 (370)	3,411 ± 476 (392)	−1.7 ± 1.1	−1.8 ± 1.0	−0.5 ± 1.1	−1.5 ± 1.2	0.2 (n = 161)	−0.4; 0.03	0.2 (n = 388)	0.1; 0.3;
3	57.7 ± 2.7 (419)	5,074 ± 685 (433)	−1.2 ± 1.1	−1.1 ± 1.0	−0.2 ± 1.2	−0.9 ± 1.1	0.4 (n = 188)	0.2; 0.6	0.9 (n = 429)	0.8; 1.0
6	64.7 ± 2.8 (439)	6,790 ± 825 (451)	−1.0 ± 1.1	−1.0 ± 1.1	−0.3 ± 1.1	−0.7 ± 1.2	0.6 (n = 202)	0.5; 0.8	1.1 (n = 446)	1.0; 1.2
9	69.9 ± 2.8 (355)	8,037 ± 937 (360)	−0.9 ± 1.1	−0.9 ± 1.1	−0.4 ± 1.0	−0.5 ± 1.0	0.8 (n = 159)	0.6; 0.9	1.1 (n = 356)	1.0; 1.2
12	72.8 ± 3.0 (296)	8,669 ± 1,103(301)	−0.8 ± 1.1	−1.0 ± 1.1	−0.5 ± 1.1	−0.5± 1.1	0.7 (n = 148)	0.5; 0.9	1.0 (n = 299)	0.9; 1.2
18	80.1 ± 3.3 (190)	10,101 ± 1,103 (192)	−0.9 ± 1.1	−1.1 ± −0.96	−0.8 ± 0.9	−0.5 ± 1.0	0.7 (n = 87)	0.4; 1.0	1.0 (n = 191)	0.8; 1.1
24	85.3 ± 4.2 (98)	11,362 ± 1,513 (100)	−0.9 ± 1.3	−1.0 ± 1.2	−0.7 ± 1.1	−0.6 ± 1.2	0.6 (n = 43)	0.2; 1.0	0.9 (n = 99)	0.7; 1.2

Table shows mean (n) and standard deviation or 95% CI.

and the numbers of children with abnormal scores were also compared.

We found no commonly used or accepted definition of catch-up growth, and different studies use different definitions. We defined "complete catch-up growth" of height if the measured height SDS minus the target SDS was above −1.6. For weight and for weight for height, an SDS above −2 was used as an indication of complete catch-up growth (21).

Statistical Analysis

SDSs at birth were calculated using birth weight and height centiles, corrected for gestational age, using the formula of Niklasson (22). "Growth Analyser" v. 3.5 was used to calculate SDSs for height and weight at different ages using Dutch population-based curves (18). The formula of van Dommelen et al. (23) was used to calculate target height SDSs. This formula includes the height of both parents.

Continuous variables were presented as means with standard deviations (SDs), or medians with interquartile ranges (IQRs). Differences between groups were presented as differences in means or percentages with 95% confidence intervals (CIs). Continuous variables were compared using the Student's *t*-test or the nonparametric Mann–Whitney *U* test. The chi-square test and the Fisher's exact test were used for categorical variables.

We assessed whether catch-up growth was influenced by the following factors: IoL compared with EM (only for children included in the randomized study), the effects of birth weight below the 3rd or 10th centile, adverse neonatal outcome at birth (defined as 5-min Apgar score of <7, umbilical artery pH of <7.05, or admission to neonatal intensive care), birth weight centile, maternal smoking, breastfeeding, and gestational age at birth. Parents of the children included in the trial completed two questionnaires, the Ages and Stages Questionnaire (ASQ) and Child Behavior Checklist (CBCL), for presence of neurodevelopmental and behavioral problems, respectively.

The target height SD score was compared to the actual SD score using a paired *t*-test. Changes in SDS scores between different time points were calculated and compared between subgroups using non-paired *t*-tests. Repeated SDS measurements were analyzed using a linear mixed model, which accounts for missing values during follow-up with random person and age effects and fixed group effects. Since the relation between age and SDS scores was expected to be nonlinear, we used quadratic spline functions with knots on 1, 3, 6, 9, 12, and 18 months to model this relation. The results of these analyses are presented graphically.

We performed a logistic regression analysis to study the effect of gestational age and birth weight SDS. In a second analysis, we studied the additional effect of catch-up growth on the outcome. Multiple imputation was used to handle missing observations.

Analyses were carried out in Statistical Package for the Social Sciences (SPSS) 20. The repeated-measures analyses were carried out in R, version 3.02.

RESULTS

Baseline characteristics of respondents (completion of questionnaires) and non-respondents are shown in **Table 1**.

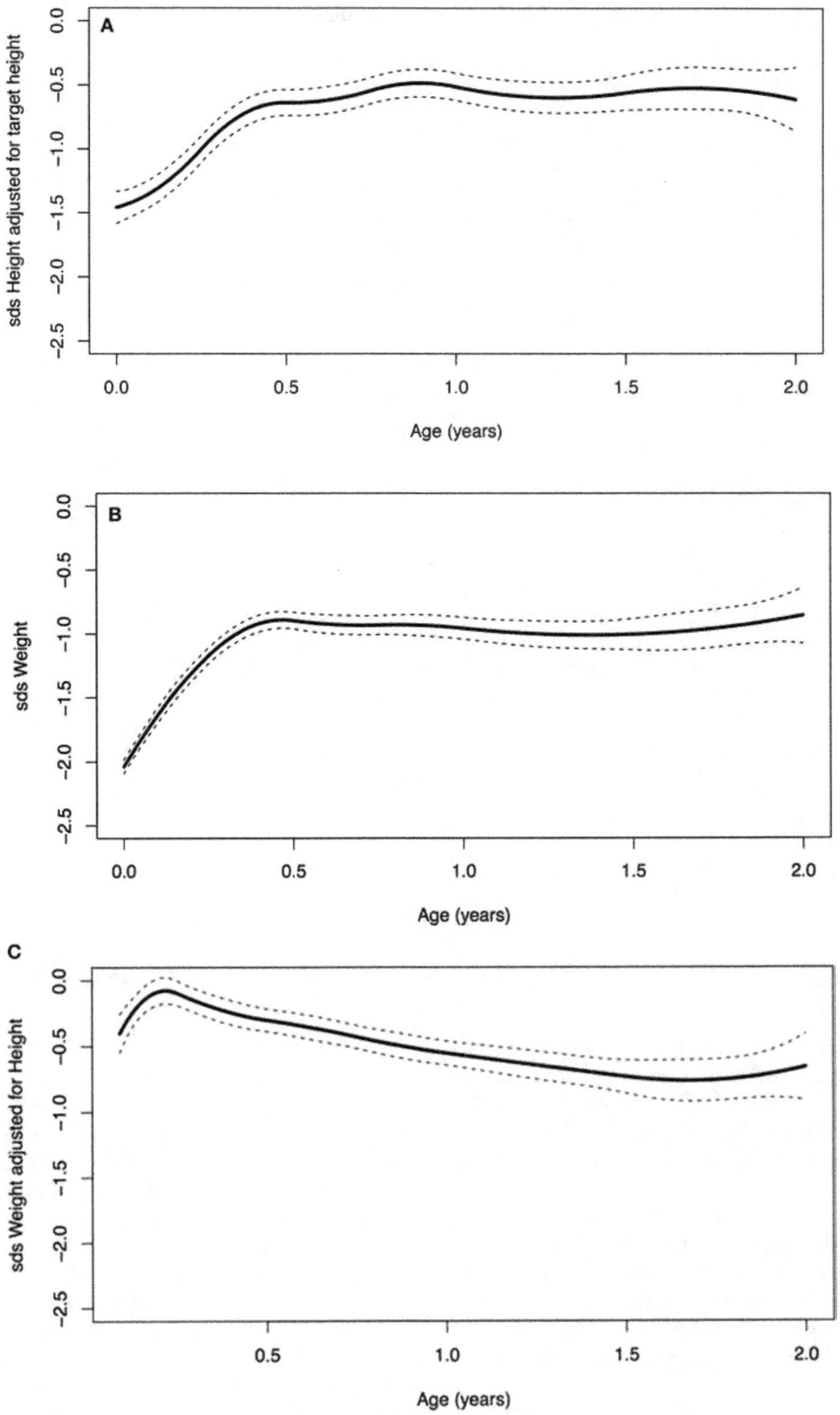

FIGURE 2 | (A) Age vs. standard deviation score (SDS) height adjusted for target height, **(B)** SDS weight, and **(C)** SDS weight for height.

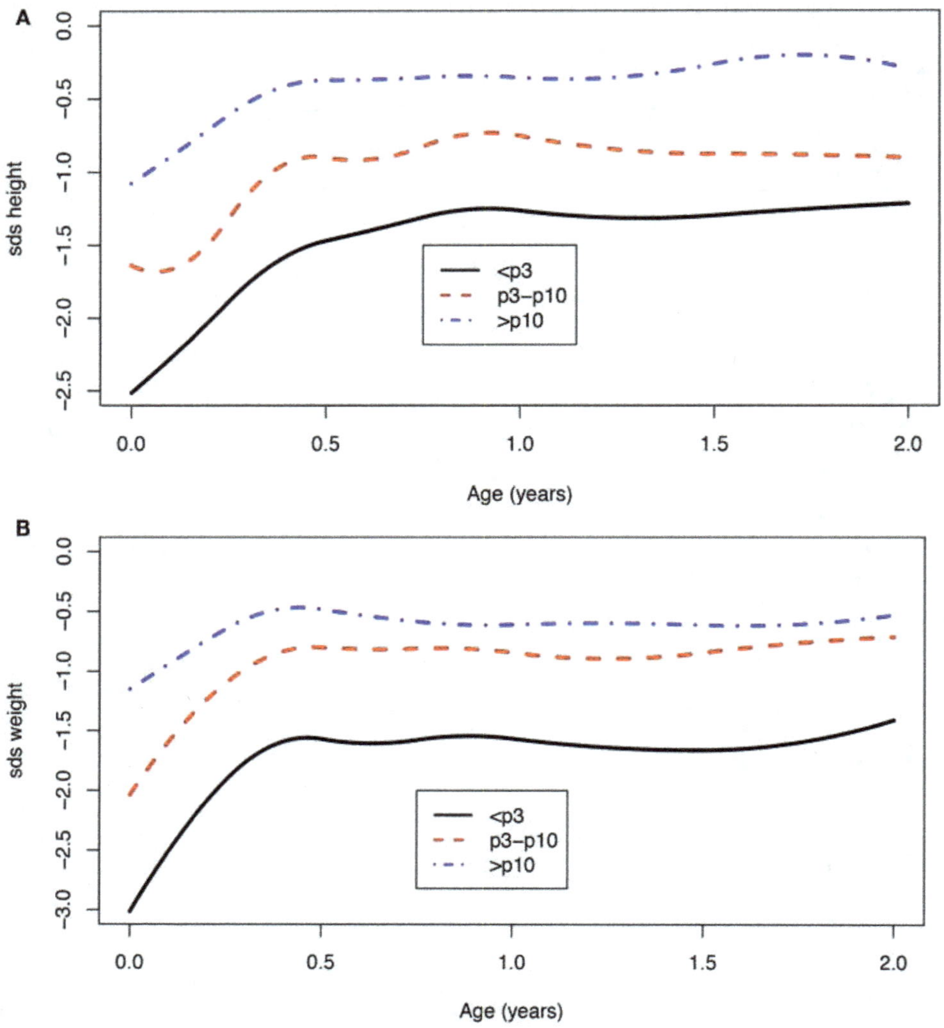

FIGURE 3 | (A,B) Age vs. SDS height and SDS weight for a birth weight below the 3rd, between 3rd and 10th, and above the 10th centile.

Respondents were slightly older, smoked less, higher educated, and more often Caucasian than non-responders. Baseline characteristics of the IoL group vs. EM are shown in **Table 2**. Babies born after EM were more severely growth restricted (birth with below the 3rd centile) than babies born after a policy of IoL (65.2 vs. 75.7%, $p < 0.05$).

The response rate was 53% ($n = 526$) (**Figure 1**). Of these patients, 292 were in the "randomized" group. For 487 children, at least 1 measurement of weight was available; for 458 children, 5 or more weight measurements were available; and for 71 children, 10 weight measurements were available. At 2 years of age, height measurement of 98 children and weight measurement of 100 children were available.

A significant increase in SDS in the first 2 years of life was seen (**Table 3**). At birth, the average SDS was −1.6 for height and −2.0 for weight in the entire group. At 2 years of age, the average SDS was −0.9 [mean increase from birth 0.7 (95% CI: 0.2; 1.0)] for height and −1.0 [mean increase from birth 1.0 (95% CI: 0.7; 1.2)] for weight (**Table 3** and **Figure 2**).

Children with a birth weight below the 10th centile ($<p10$) were born with a mean SDS of −1.8 for height ($n = 171$) and −2.4 for weight ($n = 382$), and at 2 years of age, the SDS was −1.1 for height ($n = 67$) and −1.2 for weight ($n = 69$). For children who were born with a birth weight that equals or was above the 10th centile ($>p10$), the mean SDS at birth was −1.1 for height ($n = 63$) and −1.2 for weight ($n = 141$), and at 2 years of age, −0.4 for height ($n = 30$) and −0.6 for weight ($n = 30$). Children born with a birth weight $<p10$ showed significantly more catch-up growth in weight at age 1 [mean difference −0.8 SDS (95% CI: −1.1; −0.5)] as well as at age 2 [mean difference −0.7 SDS (95% CI: −1.2; −0.2)] when compared to children born with a birth weight $>p10$ (**Figure 3**). The same effect was seen for children with a birth weight below the third centile (**Figure 3**). These children remain lower in SDS height and weight compared to the children born with a birth weight above the 3rd and 10th centiles.

Girls had lower weight SDS at birth [mean difference 0.3 SDS (95% CI: 0.1; 0.4)] and show more catch-up growth in weight

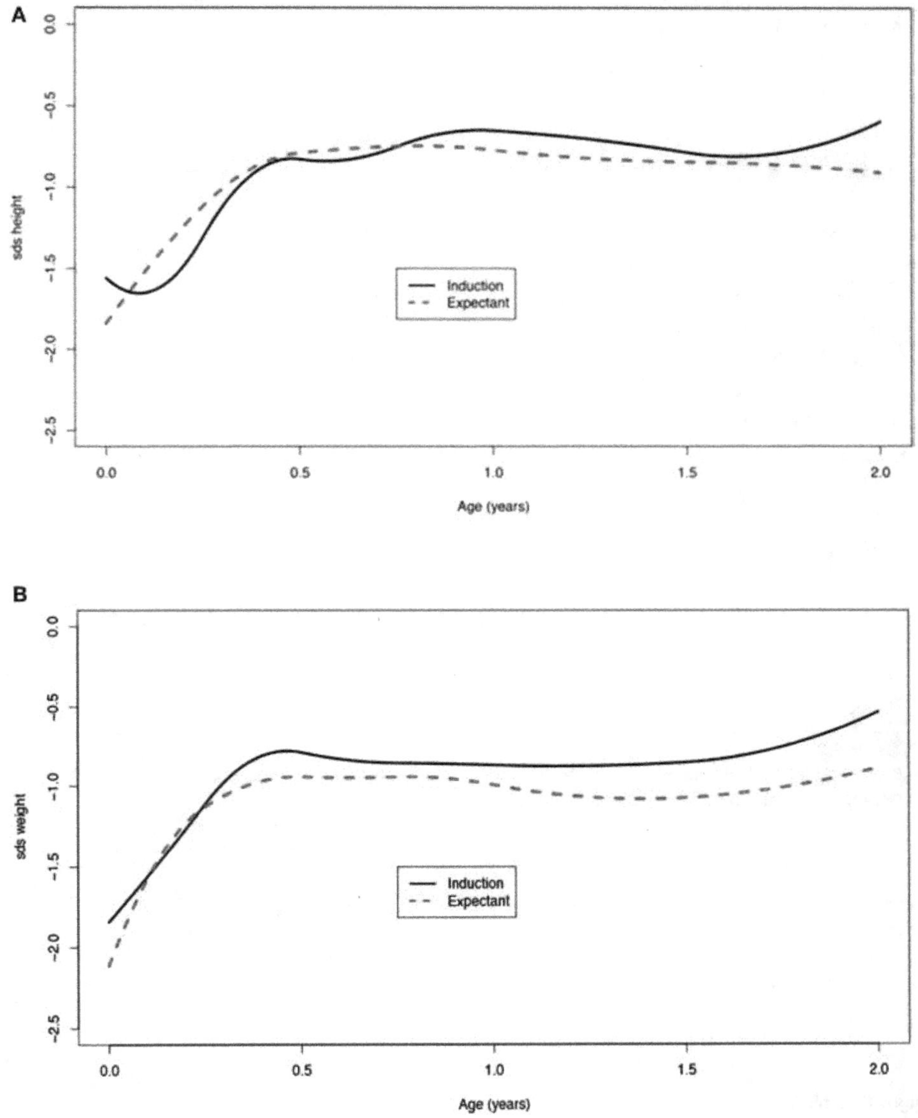

FIGURE 4 | (A,B) Age vs. SDS height and weight for induction of labor vs. expectant management.

particularly in the first month compared to boys (results in **Supplementary Material**).

Children born after obstetric policy of EM compared to children born after IoL showed significantly more catch-up growth in height [mean difference 0.7 (95% CI: 0.2; 1.3)] and weight [mean difference 0.5 (95% CI: 0.3; 0.7)] during the first month after birth. Thereafter, the growth patterns of the two groups were similar (**Figure 4**, **Table 4**).

Children with adverse neonatal outcome had lower SDS birth weight. We did not observe significantly more catch-up growth in this group, but numbers were low (**Supplementary Material**). Smoking during pregnancy resulted in 0.3 SDS (95% CI: −0.5; −0.1) lower birth weight in comparison to nonsmoking; a significant difference was seen in catch-up growth in the first 6 months after birth between children from smoking vs. nonsmoking mothers: after 6 months, the SDS scores were very similar in both groups (**Supplementary Material**). We did not see any effect of breastfeeding (**Supplementary Material**).

Complete catch-up growth in height was seen in 86% ($n = 311$) of children, and 84% ($n = 335$) complete catch-up in weight after 1 year. The mean target height SDS for the entire group was −0.3 SDS; the mean observed SD height score at 2 years of age was −0.9 SD, which is still significantly lower than the expected target height SD ($p = 0.000$).

When looking at neurodevelopmental and behavioral outcome problems at 2 years of age found by the ASQ and CBCL, we found that children with an abnormal score on the ASQ and were 6 and 12 months of age showed more catch-up in weight and were more below their target height when compared to the children with a normal ASQ (**Table 5**). We found no difference in catch-up height or weight in children with an adverse outcome for the CBCL (**Supplementary Material**). In a multivariate

TABLE 4 | Mean SDS height corrected for target height (TH), SDS weight, and catch-up growth (SDS weight–SDS birth) (± standard deviation) at different ages compared between children randomized for induction or expectant monitoring.

		Induction			Expectant management			Mean difference (95% CI)	*p*-value
		N	**Mean**	**SD**	***N***	**Mean**	**SD**		
SDS height-TH (SD)	1 month	97	−1.6	1.2	83	−1.2	1.1	−0.4 (−0.8;−0.1)	0.014
	6 months	112	−0.7	1.1	103	−0.5	1.2	−0.2 (−0.5; 0.1)	0.251
	9 months	92	−0.4	1.0	84	−0.3	0.9	−0.1 (−0.4; 0.2)	0.413
	12 months	78	−0.4	0.8	62	−0.4	1.3	0.1 (−0.3; 0.4)	0.759
	18 months	48	−0.5	0.8	51	−0.5	1.1	0.0 (−0.4; 0.4)	0.917
SDS birth weight	Birth	148	−1.8	0.7	121	−2.1	0.9	0.3 (0.1;0.5)	0.005
	1 month	115	−1.9	1.0	97	−1.7	1.0	−0.2 (−0.4; 0.1)	0.233
	3 months	125	−1.0	0.9	104	−1.1	0.9	0.1 (−0.2; 0.3)	0.633
	6 months	129	−0.9	1.0	112	−1.0	1.1	0.1 (−0.2; 0.4)	0.424
	9 months	105	−0.8	1.0	92	−0.9	1.0	0.1 (−0.2; 0.4)	0.600
	12 months	92	−0.9	0.9	66	−1.1	1.3	0.2 (−0.2; 0.5)	0.333
	18 months	57	−1.0	0.8	53	−1.0	0.9	0.0 (−0.3; 0.4)	0.879
Catch-up growth	1 month	115	0.1	0.9	97	−0.4	0.8	0.5 (0.3; 0.7)	0.000
SDS weight–SDS birth	3 months	125	−0.8	1.0	104	−1.0	0.9	0.2 (0.0; 0.5)	0.069
	6 months	129	−1.0	1.1	112	−1.1	1.1	0.2 (−0.1; 0.5)	0.205
	9 months	105	−1.0	1.2	92	−1.2	1.1	0.2 (−0.2; 0.5)	0.322
	12 months	92	−0.9	1.2	66	−1.0	1.1	0.1 (−0.3; 0.4)	0.667
	18 months	57	−0.9	0.8	53	−1.1	1.1	0.3 (−0.1; 0.6)	0.163

TABLE 5 | Mean SDS height corrected for target height (TH), SDS birth weight and catch up growth (SDS weight-SDS birth) (± standard deviation) at different ages compared between neurodevelopmental outcomes at age 2.

	Abnormal ASQ			
	Yes	**No**	**Difference in mean (95% CI)**	***p*-value**
SDS height-TH (SD)				
6 months ($n = 376$)	−1.1 (1.1)	−0.6 (1.1)	−0.5 (−0.8; 0.2)	0.002
12 months ($n = 268$)	−1.1 (1.1)	−0.4 (1.0)	−0.7 (−1.0; −0.3)	0.002
18 months ($n = 355$)	−0.9 (1.2)	−0.5 (0.9)	−0.4 (−0.9; 0.2)	0.1
SDS Birth weight	−2.7 (0.8)	−1.9 (0.8)	−0.8 (−1.0; −0.6)	<0.001
Catch-up growth SDS weight-SDS birth				
6 months ($n = 443$)	1.3 (0.9)	1.0 (1.0)	0.3 (0.04; 0.6)	0.03
12 months ($n = 355$)	1.3 (0.9)	1.0 (1.1)	0.3 (0.005; 0.7)	0.047
18 months ($n = 188$)	1.2 (1.3)	0.9 (1.0)	0.3 (−0.2; 0.7)	0.3

logistic model, birth weight SDS had a strong association with an abnormal outcome of ASQ [a decrease of 1 birth weight SDS yielded a 2.6 (95% CI: 1.8; 3.5) times higher odds on an abnormal ASQ score]. Also, a moderate effect of gestational age [a 1-week longer gestational age increased the odds on an abnormal ASQ score by 1.21 (95% CI: 0.98; 1.50)] was found. Adding growth variables during the first month did not significantly improve the model and did not remarkably change these odds ratios.

DISCUSSION

Children born after EM of labor in FGR were more severely growth restricted at birth than children born after IoL (16), and these children exhibited more catch-up growth during the first month after birth. Also, growth-restricted children with a birth weight below the 10th centile showed more catch-up growth than those born with birth weights above the 10th centile. Catch-up growth occurs fastest in the first months after birth.

The fact that children born with a birth weight below the 10th centile showed significantly more catch-up growth than children born with a birth weight above the 10th centile indicates that more of these children were truly growth restricted and therefore might be at greater risk of developing metabolic syndrome in later life (7–9, 24). Children born after an EM also showed more catch-up growth during the first month after birth than children born after IoL. The difference in gestational age at birth between these children is on average 10 days. One could argue that keeping a fetus in an undernourished intrauterine environment for 10 days longer leads to more serious growth restriction and, in turn, also to more catch-up growth. It is therefore likely that the antenatal decision either to actively end the undernourished status by inducing labor or to "wait and see"—an EM—influences long-term outcome and puts these children at a greater risk for metabolic and cardiovascular problems in later life. The long-term effects in relation to catch-up growth (i.e., during the first month, first years, etc.). remain unclear, and therefore, the long-term effects of catch-up growth during the first month after birth are undefined.

In children with neurodevelopmental problems at 2 years of age, more catch-up was seen in weight and height when compared to children with a normal neurodevelopmental outcome. This effect, however, disappears when correcting for weight SDS and gestational age at birth. We previously found that birth weight centile is the most important factor of influence on neurodevelopmental outcome at age 2, reflecting the dose effect of the severity of FGR (placental insufficiency) (17).

At 2 years of age, the majority of children of the DIGITAT cohort have height higher than 1.6 SD below their target height range and weight above −2 SDS, indicating that catch-up growth is, for the greatest part, complete (12). However, height and height SDS corrected for mid-parental height (target height SDS) and weight SDS are still significantly lower than expected in these children based on the norm population.

Our study is the first study to compare the effects of IoL with EM on postnatal catch-up growth in FGR. Previous studies have shown that children born after FGR exhibit catch-up growth in height and weight (1–3, 5, 6, 9, 12), but none of these studies studied catch-up growth in relation to obstetric policies to growth at 2 years of age. Another unique aspect of our study is that we included children based on suspected FGR and not based on actual birth weight, making comparisons with children with a birth weight above the 10th possible.

A weakness of our study is a possible response bias as data were obtained through postal inquiries and data were completed by the parents. We do, however, believe our measurements are reliable, as the children were measured by child health care professionals during routine scheduled child health care visits and parents were asked to provide us with those measurements. Respondents (mothers of the children) were slightly older, smoked less, higher educated, and more frequently Caucasian. Whereas, the percentage of growth-restricted children was comparable between non-respondents and respondents, there might have been more healthy life and feeding styles in respondent families; we do not know, however, to which direction our results would shift if the total sample would have been available. Unfortunately, our response rate was only around 50%, and the number of measurements at the age of 2 years is much lower. Within the group of respondents, we do not expect the group of children of whom we have measurements at age 2 to differ from the group of children without measurements at age 2. We suspect that missing values at 2 years are due to logistical reasons: the questionnaires were sent out around the age of 2 years (22–26 months of age) when a considerable group of parents had not yet been to the child health clinic for the scheduled 2-year visit and therefore did not have the measurements. We, therefore, do not expect a bias in our results, but it does influence our sample sizes.

The timing of IoL remains difficult however, as IoL before 38 weeks' gestation increases risks of complications due to late prematurity (25, 26). There are no known applicable biophysical markers that reflect maturation of fetuses; the best timing of induction depends, for the greatest part, on clinical assessment. We hypothesize that IoL in suspected FGR is optimal around 38 weeks (25), minimizing negative effects of being born late premature and hopefully preventing the risks from FGR and catch-up growth.

CONCLUSION

The majority of children born after FGR at term exhibit catch-up growth after birth and show complete catch-up growth after 2 years. After an EM policy, more children are severely growth restricted and show more catch-up growth during the first month after birth. A lower birth weight percentile was found as the most important factor influencing adverse neurodevelopmental outcome at age 2.

AUTHOR CONTRIBUTIONS

LW, SC, and KBo performed the analyses, drafted the initial manuscript, and approved the final manuscript as submitted. SS conceptualized and designed the study, interpreted the data, and critically reviewed the manuscript. JP, AW-L, HB, SG, FD, MP, KBl, FR, JL, and BM critically reviewed the manuscript. All authors have seen and approved the final manuscript.

REFERENCES

1. Albertsson-Wikland K, Karlberg J. Postnatal growth of children born small for gestational age. *Acta Paediatr Suppl.* (1997) 423:193–5. doi: 10.1111/j.1651-2227.1997.tb18413.x
2. Hokken-Koelega AC, De Ridder MA, Lemmen RJ, Den Hartog H, De Muinck Keizer-Schrama SM, Drop SL. Children born small for gestational age: do they catch up? *Pediatr Res.* (1995) 38:267–71. doi: 10.1203/00006450-199508000-00022
3. Karlberg J, Albertsson-Wikland K. Growth in full-term small-for-gestational-age infants: from birth to final height. *Pediatr Res.* (1995) 38:733–9. doi: 10.1203/00006450-199511000-00017
4. Karlberg JP, Albertsson-Wikland K, Kwan EY, Lam BC, Low LC. The timing of early postnatal catch-up growth in normal, full-term infants born short for gestational age. *Horm Res.* (1997) 48(Suppl. 1):17–24. doi: 10.1159/000191279

5. Albertsson-Wikland K, Karlberg J. Natural growth in children born SGA with and without catch up growth. *Horm Res.* (2003) 59(Suppl. 1):129. doi: 10.1159/000067839
6. Beukers F, Cranendonk A, de Vries JI, Wolf H, Lafeber HN, Vriesendrop HC, et al. Catch-up growth in children born growth restricted to mothers with hypertensive disorders of pregnancy. *Arch Dis Child.* (2013) 98:30–5. doi: 10.1136/archdischild-2012-302510
7. de Boo HA, Harding JE. The developmental origins of adult disease (barker) hypothesis. *Aust N Z J Obstet Gynaecol.* (2006) 46:4–14. doi: 10.1111/j.1479-828X.2006.00506.x
8. Barker DJ. The origins of the developmental origins theory. *J Intern Med.* (2007) 261:412–7. doi: 10.1111/j.1365-2796.2007.01809.x
9. Claris O, Beltrand J, Levy-Marchal C. Consequences of intrauterine growth and early neonatal catch-up growth. *Semin Perinatol.* (2010) 34:207–10. doi: 10.1053/j.semperi.2010.02.005
10. Crume TL, Scherzinger A, Stamm E, McDuffie R, Bischoff KJ, Hamman RF, et al. The long-term impact of intrauterine growth restriction in a diverse U.S. cohort of children: the EPOCH study. *Obesity.* (2014) 22:608–15. doi: 10.1002/oby.20565
11. Neitzke U, Harder T, Schellong K, Melchior K, Ziska T, Rodekamp E, et al. Intrauterine growth restriction in a rodent model and developmental programming of the metabolic syndrome: a critical appraisal of the experimental evidence. *Placenta.* (2008) 29:246–54. doi: 10.1016/j.placenta.2007.11.014
12. Wit JM, Boersma B. Catch-up growth: definition, mechanisms, and models. *J Pediatr Endocrinol Metab.* (2002) 15(Suppl. 5):1229–41.
13. Gibson AT, Carney S, Cavazzoni E, Wales JK. Neonatal and post-natal growth. *Horm Res.* (2000) 53(Suppl. 1):42–9. doi: 10.1159/0000 53204
14. Ross G, Krauss AN, Auld PA. Growth achievement in low-birth-weight premature infants: relationship to neurobehavioral outcome at one year. *J Pediatr.* (1983) 103:105–8. doi: 10.1016/S0022-3476(83) 80791-4
15. Leitner Y, Fattal-Valevski A, Geva R, Bassan H, Posner E, Kutai M, et al. Six-year follow-up of children with intrauterine growth retardation: long-term, prospective study. *J Child Neurol.* (2000) 15:781–6. doi: 10.1177/088307380001501202
16. Boers KE, Vijgen SM, Bijlenga D, van der Post JA, Bekedam DJ, Kwee A, et al. Induction versus expectant monitoring for intrauterine growth restriction at term: randomised equivalence trial (DIGITAT). *BMJ.* (2010) 341:c7087. doi: 10.1136/bmj.c7087
17. van Wyk L, Boers KE, van der Post JA, van Pampus MG, van Wassenaer AG, van Baar AL, et al. Effects on (neuro)developmental and behavioral outcome at 2 years of age of induced labor compared with expectant management in intrauterine growth-restricted infants: long-term outcomes of the DIGITAT trial. *Am J Obstet Gynecol.* (2012) 206:406.e1–e7. doi: 10.1016/j.ajog.2011.10.054
18. Dutch Growth Foundation (2008). *Growth Analyser (Version 3.5.204).*
19. Squires J, Twombly E, Bricke D, Potter L. *ASQ-3 User's Guide.* 3rd ed. Paul H Brookes, Plaats van oublicatie (2009).
20. Achenbach TM, Rescorla LA. *ASEBA Pre-school Forms and Profiles.* Burlington, NJ: University of Vermont, Research Center for Children, Youth and Families (2000).
21. Ford GW, Doyle LW, Davis NM, Callanan C. Very low birth weight and growth into adolescence. *Arch Pediatr Adolesc Med.* (2000) 154:778–84. doi: 10.1001/archpedi.154.8.778
22. Niklasson A, Ericson A, Fryer JG, Karlberg J, Lawrence C, Karlberg P. An update of the Swedish reference standards for weight, length and head circumference at birth for given gestational age (1977-1981). *Acta Paediatr Scand.* (1991) 80:756–62. doi: 10.1111/j.1651-2227.1991.tb11945.x
23. van Dommelen P, Schonbeck Y, van Buuren S. A simple calculation of the target height. *Arch Dis Child.* (2012) 97:182–2. doi: 10.1136/archdischild-2011-301095
24. Gluckman PD, Hanson MA, Cooper C, Thornburg KL. Effect of in utero and early-life conditions on adult health and disease. *N Engl J Med.* (2008) 359:61–73. doi: 10.1056/NEJMra0708473
25. Boers KE, van Wyk L, van der Post JA, Kwee A, van Pampus MG, Spaanderdam ME, et al. Neonatal morbidity after induction vs expectant monitoring in intrauterine growth restriction at term: a subanalysis of the DIGITAT RCT. *Am J Obstet Gynecol.* (2012) 206:344.e1–e7. doi: 10.1016/j.ajog.2012.01.015
26. Teune MJ, Bakhuizen S, Gyamfi Bannerman C, Opmeer BC, van Kaam AH, van Wassenaer AG, et al. A systematic review of severe morbidity in infants born late preterm. *Am J Obstet Gynecol.* (2011) 205:374.e1–9. doi: 10.1016/j.ajog.2011.07.015

14

Mechanisms Underpinning Adaptations in Placental Calcium Transport in Normal Mice and those with Fetal Growth Restriction

Christina E. Hayward[1,2], Kirsty R. McIntyre[1,2], Colin P. Sibley[1,2], Susan L. Greenwood[1,2] and Mark R. Dilworth[1,2]*

[1] Maternal and Fetal Health Research Centre, Division of Developmental Biology and Medicine, Faculty of Biology, Medicine and Health, School of Medical Sciences, University of Manchester, Manchester, United Kingdom, [2] Manchester Academic Health Science Centre, St. Mary's Hospital, Manchester University NHS Foundation Trust, Manchester, United Kingdom

*Correspondence:
Mark R. Dilworth
m.r.dilworth@manchester.ac.uk

Fetal delivery of calcium, via the placenta, is crucial for appropriate skeletal mineralization. We have previously demonstrated that maternofetal calcium transport, per gram placenta, is increased in the placental specific insulin-like growth factor 2 knockout mouse (P0) model of fetal growth restriction (FGR) compared to wild type littermates (WTL). This effect was mirrored in wild-type (WT) mice comparing lightest vs. heaviest (LvH) placentas in a litter. In both models increased placental calcium transport was associated with normalization of fetal calcium content. Despite this adaptation being observed in small normal (WT), and small dysfunctional (P0) placentas, mechanisms underpinning these changes remain unknown. Parathyroid hormone-related protein (PTHrP), elevated in cord blood in FGR and known to stimulate plasma membrane calcium ATPase, might be important. We hypothesized that PTHrP expression would be increased in LvH WT placentas, and in P0 vs. WTL. We used calcium pathway-focused PCR arrays to assess whether mechanisms underpinning these adaptations in LvH WT placentas, and in P0 vs. WTL, were similar. PTHrP protein expression was not different between LvH WT placentas at E18.5 but trended toward increased expression (139%; $P = 0.06$) in P0 vs. WTL. PCR arrays demonstrated that four genes were differentially expressed in LvH WT placentas including increased expression of the calcium-binding protein calmodulin 1 (1.6-fold; $P < 0.05$). Twenty-four genes were differentially expressed in placentas of P0 vs. WTL; significant reductions were observed in expression of S100 calcium binding protein G (2-fold; $P < 0.01$), parathyroid hormone 1 receptor (1.7-fold; $P < 0.01$) and PTHrP (2-fold; $P < 0.05$), whilst serum/glucocorticoid-regulated kinase 1 (SGK1), a regulator of nutrient transporters, was increased (1.4 fold; $P < 0.05$). Tartrate resistant acid phosphatase 5 (TRAP5 encoded by Acp5) was reduced in placentas of both LvH WT and P0 vs. WTL (1.6- and 1.7-fold, respectively; $P < 0.05$). Signaling events underpinning adaptations in calcium transport are distinct between LvH placentas of WT mice and those in P0 vs. WTL. Calcium binding proteins appear important in functional adaptations in the former whilst PTHrP and SGK1 are also implicated in the latter. These data facilitate understanding of mechanisms underpinning placental calcium transport adaptation in normal and growth restricted fetuses.

Keywords: placenta, calcium, adaptation, FGR, IUGR, mouse

INTRODUCTION

Placental dysfunction, associated with reduced rates of nutrient uptake (1–3), is a major cause of fetal growth restriction (FGR), the failure of a fetus to reach its growth potential (4). FGR is a significant risk factor for stillbirth (5, 6). Additionally, FGR infants demonstrate increased incidence of childhood diseases such as cerebral palsy, and adulthood diseases including heart disease, stroke, diabetes and osteoporosis (7–11). The current lack of therapies for FGR (12) emphasizes the need for better understanding of how fetal development is normally achieved and how it is dysregulated in FGR.

Placental transfer of calcium increases over gestation to match fetal demand and ensure appropriate fetal skeletal mineralization (13). Poor fetal provision of calcium *in utero* has been linked with an increased risk of developing osteoporosis later in life (14). Maternofetal transfer of calcium across the placenta involves calcium moving from maternal blood into the syncytiotrophoblast (transporting epithelium of the placenta) down an electrochemical gradient through calcium permeable cation channels (e.g., TRPV6, transient receptor potential vanilloid type 6) on the maternal-facing microvillous membrane (MVM) (15–17). Once in the trophoblast cytosol calcium is buffered to avoid overly increasing the intracellular concentration, and shuttled to the fetal-facing basal membrane (BM) by calcium binding proteins such as calbindin-D_{9K} (16). Calcium is actively transported across the BM by plasma membrane calcium ATPases (PMCA) into the fetal compartment. The actions of PMCA help to maintain calcium concentrations in the fetus above those found in maternal blood. Unlike the activity of other nutrient, and especially amino acid, transport systems that are reduced in placentas of growth restricted fetuses (1–3), the activity of PMCA is increased in human FGR (18) as is the maternofetal transfer of calcium in a rodent model of FGR, the placental-specific insulin-like growth factor *2* (P0) knockout mouse (19).

Optimal fetal growth depends on adequate nutrient delivery and placental supply can be adapted to meet the metabolic needs of the developing fetus. In pregnancies with normal outcomes, adaptation of placental transport in relation to placental size appears important in both women and mice (20–22). Our previous studies of wild-type (WT) mouse litters demonstrated that maternofetal calcium transfer across the lightest placentas is adaptively up-regulated, compared to the heaviest placentas, so that all fetuses, whether with relatively lighter or heavier placentas, accrue an appropriate level of calcium relative to their size near term (22). We suggested that this increased maternofetal transfer of calcium (per gram placenta), which coincides with increased placental calbindin-D_{9K} expression at embryonic day (E)18.5, is an example of a placental adaptation that promotes fetal calcium acquisition despite a relatively small placental size. We also found a normalization of fetal calcium accretion by E18.5, following a reduction at E16.5, which may be indicative of a fetus signaling to its placenta, by as yet unknown mechanisms, to increase maternofetal transfer of calcium. The gestational timing of this adaptation in WT mice was similar to that which we previously observed in the P0 knockout mouse (19), and points to a role for fetal nutrient demand in driving this adaptation via altered expression of placental calcium binding proteins. These data showed that placental adaptations are an important feature of both normal and compromised fetal growth and help to ensure appropriate calcium acquisition relative to the size of the fetus.

Nothing is yet known regarding the underlying mechanisms that affect adaptation of placental calcium transport and in particular the fetal and/or placental signals that may be important in this process. Therefore, in this study we investigated mechanisms underlying the adaptive up-regulation of maternofetal calcium transfer. Initially, parathyroid hormone-related protein (PTHrP) was investigated as a candidate fetal signal. PTHrP is produced in a number of tissues including, but not limited to, the placenta, fetal membranes and fetal brain, liver, bone and parathyroid glands (23). In these tissues, there are multiple secretory mature peptides which have a range of different biological functions that can be elicited through endocrine, paracrine, autocrine and intracrine mechanisms [reviewed by (24)]. In women, the concentration of PTHrP in maternal serum, and PTHrP expression in amnion and choriodecidua, are both increased in late gestation in parallel with the rapid increase in fetal growth and calcium accretion (25–27). Previous studies in rodents have demonstrated the importance of PTHrP and its receptor, the PTH/PTHrP receptor, in fetal development. Deletion of these genes in mice results in neonatal death, due to skeletal dysplasia (28) or death *in utero* mid gestation due to growth restriction (29). In a spontaneously hypertensive rat model, inappropriate levels of PTHrP in the placenta, fetal plasma and amniotic fluid were associated with compromised fetal growth (30, 31). Enhancing endogenous levels of PTHrP, by the addition of a PTH/PTHrP receptor antagonist, improves fetal growth in this rat model (31). In PTHrP knockout mice, maternofetal calcium transfer and fetal calcium accretion are increased despite fetal hypocalcaemia and lack of a maternal fetal calcium gradient (32–34). In human pregnancies complicated by FGR, PTHrP expression in fetal membranes and placenta is increased in cases of preterm FGR (35), and concentrations are elevated in cord blood (18). PTHrP also stimulates PMCA activity in BM vesicles isolated from human placenta (36). Thus, we hypothesized that PTHrP is a candidate signal stimulating an increase in calcium transfer and would be elevated in: (1) placental tissue and tissues from fetuses of the lightest vs. heaviest (LvH) placentas in WT mice; and (2) in placentas of P0 fetuses compared to their WT littermates (WTL). Using calcium pathway-focused PCR arrays we also tested the hypothesis that placental mechanisms underpinning the adaptive increase in calcium transfer in WT mice and in P0 mice would be similar.

MATERIALS AND METHODS

Animals

Experiments were performed in accordance with the UK Animals (Scientific Procedures) Act of 1986 under the authority of a UK Home office project license (PPLs 40/3385 and P9755892D) and were authorized by the Animal Welfare and Ethical Review Board of the University of Manchester. The methods stated in this study adhere to the ARRIVE guidelines (37) and comply with the animal ethical principles under which the journal operates.

Wild-type C57Bl/6J (Envigo, UK) females (10–16 weeks old) and males (12–26 weeks old) were mated and discovery of a copulation plug was used to define embryonic day (E)0.5 (term = E19.5). Mice were provided with nesting material and communally housed (with the exception of stud males that were individually housed) in individually ventilated cages under a constant 12 h light/dark cycle at 21–23°C with free access to food (Beekay Rat and Mouse diet, Bantin and Kingman) and water (Hydropac, Denver, US). Pregnant female mice were euthanized (cervical dislocation appropriate under ASPA schedule 1) and a laparotomy and hysterotomy performed. All fetuses were rapidly killed by cervical dislocation.

On E18.5 ($N = 20$ litters), pregnant WT females were euthanized and fetuses and placentas were rapidly harvested, blotted and wet weights measured. The lightest ($n = 20$) and heaviest ($n = 20$) placentas were identified in each litter. All placentas and fetuses were snap frozen and stored at −80°C. In 9/20 litters, brains ($n = 18$; 9 from the lightest placental group, 9 from the heaviest) and livers ($n = 18$; 9 from lightest, 9 from heaviest) from fetuses corresponding to the lightest and heaviest placentas were immediately dissected, snap frozen and stored at −80°C. Fetal weight histograms were constructed and a non-linear regression performed (Gaussian distribution) from which individualized fetal weight centiles were calculated as described previously (38).

Placental specific insulin-like growth factor 2 (*Igf2*) (P0) knockout mice ($N = 10$ litters), which had deletion of the U2 exon of the *Igf2* gene, were generated as previously described (39) and were a kind gift from Dr Miguel Constância and Professor Wolf Reik. C57BL/6J female mice (8–14 weeks old) and males heterozygous for the P0 deletion (10–32 weeks old) were mated and produced mixed litters of WTL fetuses and growth restricted fetuses [P0; reported birthweight 78% compared to WTL at E19 equivalent to E18.5 in the current study (40)]. Embryonic day was defined as above. At E18.5, placentas and fetuses (40 WTL; 38 P0 from 10 litters) were weighed, snap frozen and stored at −80°C. Fetal tail tips were collected from all fetuses and stored at −20°C for genotype determination.

The aim of the study, comparing lightest vs. heaviest placentas or those from WTL vs. P0 mice within a single litter, meant that randomization or blinding of the samples was not possible.

Genotyping of P0 Knockout Mice

Genotype (WTL or P0) was determined for all fetuses from P0 mice according to a previously published genotyping protocol (19, 41). In brief, genomic DNA was extracted from fetal tail tips using a DNeasy kit (Qiagen, Manchester, UK). *Igf2* $P0^{+/-}$ mutants were identified with a specific primer pair to amplify a 740 bp fragment across the 5 kb deletion (P0 dF 5′-TCCTGTACCTCCTAACTACCAC−3′ and P0 dR 5′-GAGCCAGAAGCAAACT−3′) and a primer to amplify a 495 bp fragment from the WT allele (5′-CAATCTGCTCCTGCCTG−3′). PCR conditions were as follows: 4 min denaturation at 94°C; 35 cycles of 1 min at 94°C, 1 min at 56°C, 1 min at 72°C; and 10 min final extension at 72°C. Samples were loaded with bromophenol blue and run on a 1.5% agarose gel. Bands were visualized using an InGenius transilluminator (Sygene Bio, Cambridge, UK).

Protein Expression

The lightest and heaviest placentas from WT mice ($N = 7$ litters) and placentas of P0 and WTL ($N = 8$ litters, 1 paired P0 and WTL placenta per litter selected at random) were homogenized and processed as described previously (19). Briefly, whole homogenates were separated, by means of centrifugation, into cytosolic fractions. Due to the small amount of starting tissue, whole homogenates of fetal tissues (brains and livers; $N = 9$ litters) were used for protein expression studies.

SDS-PAGE was performed followed by electrotransfer to Immobilon-FL PVDF membranes (Millipore UK Ltd., Watford, UK). Primary antibodies included: rabbit polyclonal antibodies for serum/glucocorticoid-regulated kinase 1 (SGK1; 1 μg/ml; ab43606; Abcam, Cambridge, UK) and calmodulin (CaM; 2 μg/ml; sc-5537; Santa Cruz Biotechnology c/o Insight Biotechnology Ltd, Wembley, UK); rabbit monoclonal antibody for tartrate-resistant acid phosphatase (TRAP; 0.9 μg/ml; ab191406; Abcam); and goat polyclonal antibody for PTHrP (1 μg/ml; N-19, sc-9680; Santa Cruz Biotechnology). β-actin (0.5 μg/ml; ab8227; Abcam) or β-tubulin (0.9 μg/ml; ab6046; Abcam) was used as a loading control; when used no difference was observed in β-actin or β-tubulin expression between groups. Negative controls were by omission of primary antibody. Immunoreactive species were detected with fluorescent-conjugated secondary antibodies (Li-COR Biosciences, Cambridge, UK) and membranes imaged using an Odyssey Sa Infrared Imaging System (Li-COR). Signal density was measured using Image Studio Lite (Li-COR). All signals were in the linear range of detection. Protein expression was compared separately between the lightest and heaviest placentas, fetal tissues from lightest and heaviest placentas, and WT and P0 samples.

RT² Profiler PCR Arrays

RNA was extracted from whole placentas ($N = 7$ litters: $n = 7$ lightest, $n = 7$ heaviest; $N = 6$–7 litters: $n = 6$–7 WTL, $n = 6$–7 P0, 1 paired P0 and WTL placenta per litter selected at random) using an RNeasy Mini Kit (74104; Qiagen, Manchester, UK), RNase-Free DNase set (79254; Qiagen) and measured by a Thermo Scientific NanoDrop 2000C spectrophotometer (A_{260}/A_{280} range 2.06–2.12). Any contaminating genomic DNA was removed and cDNA was synthesized from 0.5 μg RNA per sample using the RT² first strand kit (330401; Qiagen; genomic DNA elimination mix for 5 min at 42°C, on ice for 1 min; reverse transcription mix for 42°C for 15 min followed by 5 min at 95°C). Expression of 168 related genes, 5 reference genes and quality controls was measured in each placenta using RT² Profiler PCR arrays (PAMM-066Z mouse cAMP/calcium signaling pathway finder and PAMM-170Z mouse osteoporosis array; 96-well format; Qiagen) with RT² SYBR® Green ROX™ qPCR mastermix (330523; Qiagen) on a Stratagene MX3005P®, according to the manufacturer's instructions (10 min at 95°C, 40 cycles of 15 s at 95°C followed by 1 min at 60°C; dissociation curve 1 min at 95°C, 30 s at 55°C, 30 s at 95°C). Data were analyzed using SA Bioscience PCR Array Data Analysis 3.5 Web Portal (http://dataanalysis.sabiosciences.com/pcr/arrayanalysis.php).

Data and Statistical Analysis

Data are presented as the lightest placenta as a percentage of the heaviest in a litter (dotted line = 100%), placentas of P0 fetuses as a percentage of WTL (dotted line = 100%), or median and [range] where the experimental N = number of litters, n = number of placentas or fetuses. The solid line on graphs represents the median value. For P0 and WTL fetal and placental weights, average fetal weights for each genotype per litter were calculated and data are shown as a mean of these average weights. Data were analyzed by Wilcoxon matched-pairs signed-rank test or Mann Whitney test. $P < 0.05$ was considered statistically significant.

PCR array data were analyzed using SA Bioscience PCR Array Data Analysis 3.5 Web Portal (http://pcrdataanalysis.sabiosciences.com/pcr/arrayanalysis.php). Fold change [2∧(- Delta Delta Ct)] is the normalized gene expression [2∧(- Delta Ct)] in the test sample (lightest placenta or placenta of P0 fetus) divided by the normalized gene expression [2∧(- Delta Ct)] in the control sample (heaviest placenta or placenta of WTL fetus). Fold-change values >1 indicate an up-regulation in expression, and fold-change values <1 demonstrate a down-regulation (**Supplementary Tables 1, 2**). Fold regulation values are shown in **Tables 2, 3**.

RESULTS

Fetal and Placental Weights

As expected, lightest placentas from WT mice demonstrated significantly reduced placental weight vs. heaviest placentas at E18.5 ($P < 0.0001$, **Table 1**). Fetal weight was significantly reduced ($P < 0.01$) and fetal weight: placental weight (F:P) ratio increased ($P < 0.0001$), in fetuses from lightest vs. heaviest WT placentas (**Table 1**). Mean fetal weight centiles were lower in the lightest compared to the heaviest placenta group (39th vs. 56th centile; $P < 0.05$) but were not considered growth restricted (normal range 10th–90th centile). Consistent with previous studies (19, 40, 41), placentas from P0 fetuses compared to WTL fetuses were lighter, fetal weight was lower and F:P ratio higher at E18.5 (all $P < 0.0001$, **Table 1**).

PTHrP Protein Expression

There were no significant differences in PTHrP protein expression between the lightest and heaviest placentas of WT mice, or within brains and livers of those fetuses from the lightest and heaviest placentas (**Figures 1A–C,E**). There was a trend toward increased PTHrP protein expression in placental tissue of P0 vs. WTL fetuses (139%; $P = 0.06$; **Figures 1D–E**). The PTHrP antibody used for these studies was discontinued during the timecourse of the project and so we were unable to assess PTHrP expression in fetal brains and livers of fetuses in P0 vs. WTL mice. Attempts to use different antibodies targeted to PTHrP failed to show reproducible amplification of signal.

TABLE 1 | Placental weight, fetal weight and fetal weight:placental weight (F:P) ratio in the lightest and heaviest placental groups of wild-type (WT) mice and in P0 and wild-type littermates (WTL) at embryonic day (E) 18.5.

	Lightest	Heaviest	Lightest/ Heaviest (%)	*P*-value
Placental weight (g)	0.068 (0.052–0.080)	0.087 (0.076–0.100)	78.0 (64.0–89.0)	<0.0001
Fetal weight (g)	1.151 (0.924–1.289)	1.191 (1.018–1.441)	94.5 (79.0–108.0)	0.01
F:P ratio	16.8 (12.8–24.0)	14.2 (11.4–16.8)	119.5 (92.0–166.0)	<0.0001
	P0	**WTL**	**P0/WTL (%)**	***P*-value**
Placental weight (g)	0.065 (0.048–0.100)	0.096 (0.050–0.113)	64.0 (58.3–83.1)	<0.0001
Fetal weight (g)	0.977 (0.735–1.218)	1.179 (0.854–1.386)	80.9 (68.1–85.6)	<0.0001
F:P ratio	14.5 (10.91–18.4)	12.6 (10.0–17.1)	110.6 (100.5–146.4)	<0.0001

Data are median (range) or presented as the lightest placenta as a percentage of the heaviest in a litter (lightest/heaviest (%) column) in WT mice or as the litter average of P0 fetuses as a percentage of the litter average of their WT littermates (P0/WTL (%) column). Data are analyzed by Wilcoxon matched-pairs signed rank test (lightest vs. heaviest; P0 vs. WTL). $P < 0.05$ was considered statistically significant.

TABLE 2 | Results of the cAMP/Ca^{2+} signaling pathway finder and osteoporosis RT^2 profiler PCR arrays in the lightest compared to the heaviest placentas from WT mice.

Gene	Product	Fold regulation	*P*-value
Calm1	Calmodulin 1	+1.6	0.04*
Alpl	Alkaline Phosphatase	+1.2	0.04*
Acp5	Acid Phosphatase 5 Tartrate Resistant	−1.6	0.04*
Hspa5	Heat Shock 70 kDa Protein 5	−1.8	0.01*

*Fold regulation is the normalized gene expression in the lightest placentas divided by the normalized gene expression in the heaviest placentas. Fold regulation values +1 indicate an up-regulation in expression, whilst fold regulation values −1 demonstrate a down-regulation. *$P < 0.05$.*

RT^2 Profiler PCR Arrays

PCR arrays demonstrated significant changes in the expression of four genes (**Table 2**); an increase in calmodulin 1 (*Calm1*; $P < 0.05$) and alkaline phosphatase (*Alpl*; $P < 0.05$) expression, and a decreased expression of tartrate resistant acid phosphatase 5 (*Acp5*; $P < 0.05$) and heat shock protein 5 (*Hspa5*; $P < 0.05$) in the lightest vs. heaviest WT placentas ($N = 6$). Placental protein expression of calmodulin (CaM; 107%; **Figure 2A**) and tartrate resistant acid phosphatase 5 (TRAP; 89%; **Figure 2B**) measured by Western blot was not different between lightest and heaviest placenta groups.

Twenty-four genes were differentially expressed in placentas from P0 vs. WTL fetuses in the same litter as shown in **Table 3**. Of note, significantly reduced expression was observed in the genes encoding calbindin-D_{9K}, S100 calcium binding protein G (*S100g*; −1.9-fold, $P < 0.01$), PTHrP (*Pthlh*; −2-fold, $P <$

TABLE 3 | Results of the cAMP/Ca^{2+} signaling pathway finder and osteoporosis RT^2 profiler PCR arrays between placentas from P0 compared to wild-type littermate (WTL) fetuses.

Gene	Product	Fold regulation	*P*-value
Ar	Androgen Receptor	+1.7	0.04*
Esr1	Estrogen Receptor	+1.5	0.02*
Sgk1	Serum/Glucocorticoid-Regulated Kinase 1	+1.4	0.03*
Eno2	Enolase 2, γ Neuronal	+1.4	0.03*
Tnfrsf11b	Tumor Necrosis Factor Receptor Superfamily, 11b	+1.4	0.001**
Tgfb3	Transforming Growth Factor, β3	−1.2	0.04*
Rb1	Retinoblastoma 1	−1.3	0.02*
Pck2	Phosphoenolpyruvate Carboxykinase 2 (Mitochondrial)	−1.3	0.04*
Junb	Jun-B Oncogene	−1.3	0.04*
Fosb	FBJ Osteosarcoma Oncogene B	−1.4	0.02*
Crem	cAMP Responsive Element Modulator	−1.4	0.03*
Per1	Period Homolog 1 (Drosophila)	−1.4	0.04*
Nos2	Nitric Oxide Synthase 2, Inducible	−1.4	0.006**
Brca1	Breast Cancer 1	−1.5	0.01*
Acp5	Acid Phosphatase 5, Tartrate Resistant	−1.7	0.02*
Cyp17a1	Cytochrome P450 Family 17, a1	−1.7	0.03*
Ltbp2	Latent Transforming Growth Factor β Binding Protein 2	−1.8	0.03*
Gem	GTP Binding Protein (over-expressed in skeletal muscle)	−1.8	0.04*
S100g	S100 Calcium Binding Protein G	−1.9	0.004**
Dkk1	Dickkopf Homolog 1	−1.9	0.005**
Wnt10b	Wingless Related MMTV Integration Site 10b	−1.9	0.04*
Car2	Carbonic Anhydrase 2	−2.0	0.009**
Pthrp	Parathyroid Hormone-Related Protein	−2.0	0.02*
Ncam1	Neural Cell Adhesion Molecule 1	−2.0	0.002**

Fold regulation is the normalized gene expression in placentas of P0 fetuses divided by the normalized gene expression in placentas of WTL fetuses. Fold regulation values +1 indicate an up-regulation in expression, whilst fold regulation values −1 demonstrate a down-regulation. $^*P < 0.05$; $^{**}P < 0.01$.

0.05) and parathyroid hormone 1 receptor (*Pth1r*; −1.7-fold, $P < 0.01$). Expression of serum/glucocorticoid-regulated kinase 1 (*Sgk1*; 1.4-fold, $P < 0.05$), a kinase involved in the regulation of a range of membrane transporters, ion channels and transcription factors as well as cell survival (42–46) was increased. There was no difference in serum/glucocorticoid-regulated kinase 1 (SGK1; 88%; **Figure 3**) protein expression between placentas of P0 and WT mice.

There was only one similar change in gene expression between the two study groups; tartrate resistant acid phosphatase 5 (*Acp5*, −1.6-and −1.7-fold, respectively) was reduced to the same extent in the lightest placentas of WT mice and placentas of P0 fetuses (**Tables 2, 3**). Whilst TRAP protein expression was no different between lightest and heaviest WT placentas, gene expression of TRAP was increased in placentas of P0 compared to WT littermates (TRAP; 144%; **Figure 2C**).

DISCUSSION

We have previously observed similar adaptive increases in maternofetal calcium transport in small placentas from WT mice, and in small pathological placentas of the P0 knockout mouse model of FGR, with accompanying changes in calbindin-D_{9K} expression (19, 22). Here we demonstrate that the underlying mechanisms of these adaptations in the two models appear to be distinct. Contrary to our hypothesis, expression of PTHrP was not different between lightest compared with heaviest (LvH) WT placentas, but there was a trend toward increased expression in P0 vs. WTL placentas; PTHrP has been shown to influence placental calcium transport in most (32, 33, 36), but not all studies (47). As such, any change in PTHrP expression in placentas near term may be important in the increased maternofetal calcium transfer observed in P0 vs. WTL.

As shown by our previous studies, calbindin-D_{9K} is implicated as a mediator of placental adaptation in calcium transfer both in WT mice (22) and in the P0 mouse (19). However, the lack of change in placental calcium transfer in the calbindin-D_{9K} knockout mouse indicates that other candidates, including calbindin-D_{28K}, TRPV5/6 and the sodium-calcium exchanger, might also be involved (48, 49). Thus, we adopted a holistic approach to compare the expression of genes related to calcium transfer and signaling in WT mice and P0 mice. We speculated that these experiments would identify similar calcium-specific pathways altered in the lightest and/or P0 placentas and provide insight into potential regulators of the observed placental adaptation. The number of genes showing altered expression was limited in lightest vs. heaviest WT placentas but mRNA expression of calmodulin-1 was increased in the lightest placentas at E18.5. Whilst this may act as a further indicator of the

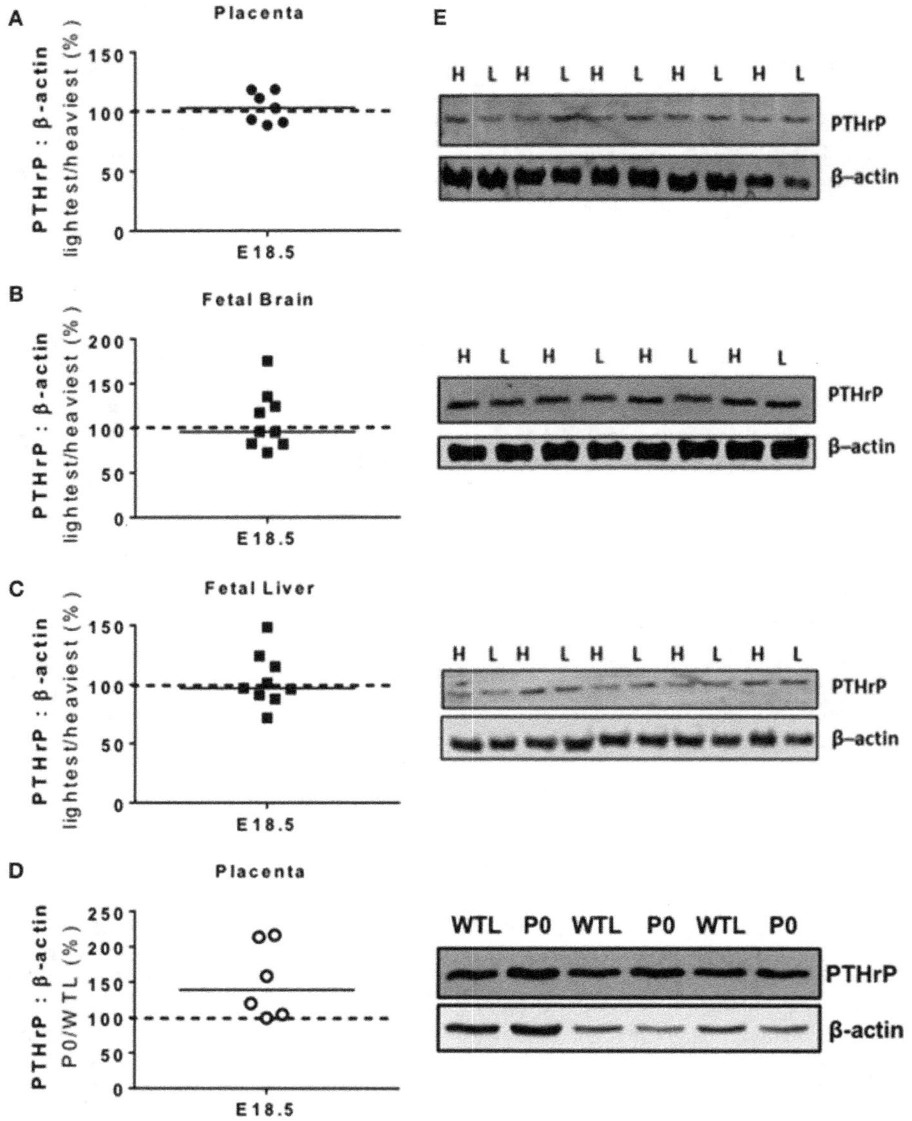

FIGURE 1 | Placental and fetal protein expression of parathyroid hormone-related protein (PTHrP). PTHrP protein expression was not significantly different in paired lightest (L) and heaviest (H) placentas from the same litter **(A)** or in the brains **(B)** and livers **(C)** of the fetuses from these placentas. **(D)** There was a trend for higher PTHrP protein expression in placentas of paired placental-specific insulin-like growth factor 2 knockout (P0) and wild-type (WTL) fetuses ($P = 0.06$) from the same litter. **(E)** Representative Western blots of PTHrP (26 kDa) with the corresponding loading control (β-actin; 42 kDa). Black line = median; dotted line 100% = H or WTL placenta.

importance of calcium binding proteins in the previously observed adaptation, this altered expression was not mirrored at the protein level; the importance of the change in gene expression therefore requires further elucidation.

In contrast to the lightest and heaviest placentas in WT mice, multiple genes were differentially expressed in placentas of P0 vs. WT littermates. This is perhaps unsurprising given that P0 mice represent a model of fetal growth restriction whereas lightest vs. heaviest placentas represent extremes of placental weight in a "normal" WT population. Despite the increased maternofetal calcium transport at E18.5, expression of placental calcium-related genes was generally reduced in P0 vs. WTL. Significant reductions were observed in the expression of *S100g* (encoding calbindin-D_{9K}), *Pth1r* and *Pthrp*, whilst *Sgk1*, a regulator of epithelial ion transport and cell survival, was up-regulated. SGK1 is a downstream effector of the PI3K/AKT signaling pathway, and in support of the observations here, this pathway is dysregulated in the placentas of P0 knockout mice in late gestation (50). The trend for reduced gene expression near to term could be the result of timing in gestation, i.e., gene expression increased earlier in gestation to promote changes in placental nutrient transport might be downregulated nearer to term having already resulted in increased transcription of the target protein, as previously observed for calbindin-D_{9K} in

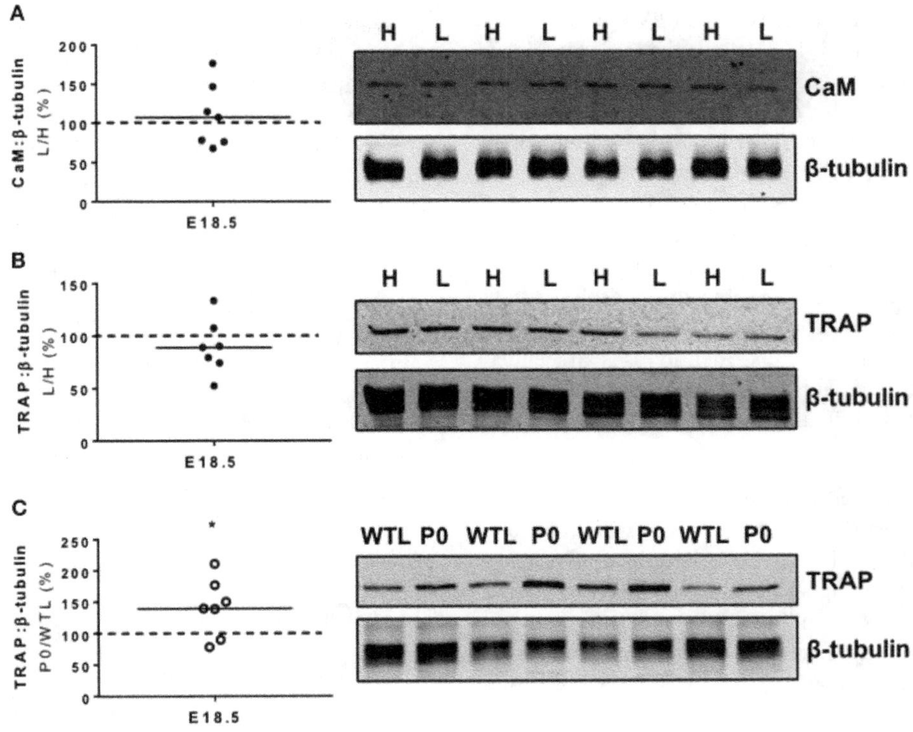

FIGURE 2 | Placental protein expression of calmodulin (CaM) and tartrate resistant acid phosphatase 5 (TRAP). **(A)** CaM and **(B)** TRAP protein expression was not significantly different in paired lightest (L) and heaviest (H) WT placentas from the same litter. **(C)** TRAP protein expression was increased in placentas of placental-specific insulin-like growth factor 2 knockout (P0) compared to wild-type littermates (WTL) from the same litter (*$P < 0.05$; Wilcoxon signed rank test). Black line = median; dotted line 100% = heaviest WT placenta **(A,B)** or WTL placenta **(C)**. Detected band sizes from representative western blots were as follows; CaM (17 KDa), TRAP (42 kDa) and ß-tubulin loading control (50 kDa).

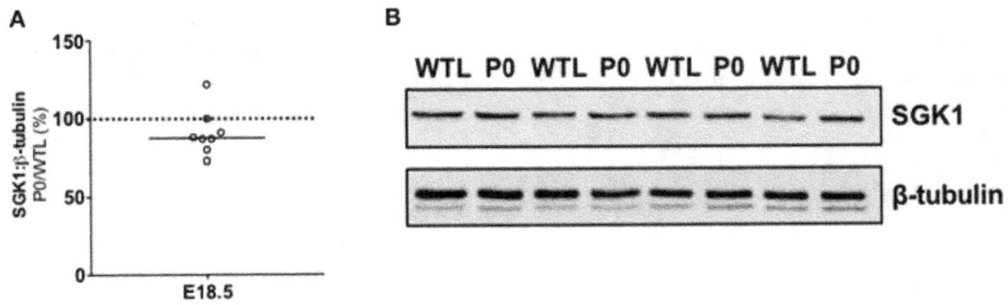

FIGURE 3 | Placental protein expression of serum/glucocorticoid-regulated kinase 1 (SGK1). **(A)** SGK1 protein expression was not significantly different in paired placentas of placental-specific insulin-like growth factor 2 knockout (P0) and wild-type (WTL) fetuses from the same litter. **(B)** Representative Western blots of SGK1 (49 kDa) with the corresponding loading control (β-tubulin; 50 kDa). Black line = median; dotted line 100% = WTL placenta.

lightest vs. heaviest WT placentas (22). The choice of E18.5 for these studies reflected the timepoint at which the adaptation (increased placental calcium transport) was previously observed (19, 22) but analyses earlier in gestation would offer further insight into the timing of these changes. With regards to the trend for reduced gene expression near term in P0 vs. WTL, altered gene expression may not be the driving force in these placentas; instead post-translational processing of binding proteins and/or receptors (e.g., TRPV6) may underlie the adaptive changes in calcium transfer. Mechanisms will need to be explored further in future experiments. Whilst the discrepancy in *S100g* gene and calbindin-D_{9K} protein expression at E18.5 will need elucidating, calbindin-D_{9K} does appear to be important in the previously reported changes in placental calcium transport in mouse models of FGR (19, 22).

Increased *Sgk1* expression in P0 vs. WT warrants further investigation to assess whether SGK1, and its activated phosphorylated isoform, play an important role in these adaptive responses by the placenta. SGK1 influences intracellular calcium by up-regulating store operated calcium entry (SOCE), increasing calcium release-activated calcium channel (CRAC) current, and increasing the activity of TRPV5 and 6 (46). Expression and activation of SGK1 is enhanced by higher levels of cytosolic calcium thus SGK1 has been suggested as an amplifier of calcium entry; influx of extracellular calcium through SOCE combined with activation of calcium/calmodulin protein kinase signaling up-regulates levels and activity of SGK1 (42–44). Activation of SGK1 also occurs through other mechanisms, including through the phosphatidylinositol-3-kinase pathway that when stimulated by growth factors activates the mechanistic target of rapamycin complex 2 triggering the phosphorylation of 3-phosphoinositide-dependent kinase PDK1 and subsequent phosphorylation of SGK1 (45, 51). Identifying extracellular regulators stimulating SGK1 intracellular activity may provide potential candidate signals initiating placental adaptations.

Placental *Acp5* gene expression was lower in the lightest compared to the heaviest placentas and in P0 fetuses compared to their WTLs. In contrast, TRAP5 protein expression (encoded by *Acp5*) was not different between the lightest and heaviest placentas, and significantly higher in placentas of P0 compared to WTLs. Previous studies in animal models indicate *Acp5* has an essential role in modeling, remodeling and mineralization of developing bone and cartilage (52), as well as participating in iron transfer from mother to fetus (53). Hansson et al. (54) demonstrated increased placental *Acp5* gene expression in pre-eclampsia compared to normal pregnancy and suggested that this increase might be a compensatory mechanism for poor placentation to prevent fetal malnutrition (54). The elevated expression of TRAP5 protein in placentas of P0 vs. WTL fetuses, which may be as a result of increased gene expression earlier in gestation leading to increased protein translation, supports a regulatory role for TRAP5 in this mouse model of FGR; the added complexity of the opposing direction of change in gene and protein expression, suggest post-translational modification is very important.

For all of the studies described herein, there was an unequal distribution of fetal sex when considering the placental samples analyzed. For the studies comparing lightest vs. heaviest placentas in WT mice, there was a bias toward females having the lightest placentas and males having the heaviest placentas. Whilst we have previously reported that adaptive changes in maternofetal calcium transport do not appear to be influenced by fetal sex (22), future studies investigating the mechanisms underpinning these adaptations should also consider sex-dependent effects. Likewise, fetal sex should be taken into account when assessing mechanisms underpinning placental adaptations in P0 vs. WTL mice.

In summary this study has shown differences in the mechanisms underlying adaptations in placental calcium transport in normal pregnancy vs. that affected by growth restriction. Our data suggest that calcium binding proteins in normal mouse pregnancy, and PTHrP and *Acp5*/TRAP in FGR (P0) pregnancy, are candidate adaptation regulatory proteins worthy of further investigation.

AUTHOR CONTRIBUTIONS

KM performed research. SG and CS contributed to the conception and design of the work. CH and MD contributed to the conception and design of the work and performed research. All authors were involved in drafting the paper.

ACKNOWLEDGEMENTS

We would like to thank the staff of the Biological Services Facility at the University of Manchester for their assistance with this project. Infrastructure support was provided by the National Institute for Health Research Manchester Biomedical Research Centre and Tommy's the Baby Charity.

REFERENCES

1. Glazier JD, Cetin I, Perugino G, Ronzoni S, Grey AM, Mahendran D, et al. Association between the activity of the system A amino acid transporter in the microvillous plasma membrane of the human placenta and severity of fetal compromise in intrauterine growth restriction. *Pediatr Res.* (1997) 42:514–9. doi: 10.1203/00006450-199710000-00016
2. Jansson T, Scholtbach V, Powell TL. Placental transport of leucine and lysine is reduced in intrauterine growth restriction. *Pediatr Res.* (1998) 44:532–7. doi: 10.1203/00006450-199810000-00011
3. Shibata E, Hubel CA, Powers RW, von Versen-Hoeynck F, Gammill H, Rajakumar A, et al. Placental system A amino acid transport is reduced in pregnancies with small for gestational age (SGA) infants but not in preeclampsia with SGA infants. *Placenta* (2008) 29:879–82. doi: 10.1016/j.placenta.2008.07.001
4. Brodsky D, Christou H. Current concepts in intrauterine growth restriction. *J Intensive Care Med.* (2004) 19:307–19. doi: 10.1177/08850666042 69663
5. Flenady V, Koopmans L, Middleton P, Frøen JF, Smith GC, Gibbons K, et al. Major risk factors for stillbirth in high-income countries: a systematic review and meta-analysis. *Lancet* (2011) 377:1331–40. doi: 10.1016/S0140-6736(10)62233-7
6. Gardosi J, Kady SM, McGeown P, Francis A, Tonks A. Classification of stillbirth by relevant condition at death (ReCoDe): population based cohort study. *Br Med J.* (2005) 331:1113–7. doi: 10.1136/bmj.38629.587639.7C
7. Barker DJ. Fetal nutrition and cardiovascular disease in later life. *Br Med Bull.* (1997) 53:96–108. doi: 10.1093/oxfordjournals.bmb.a011609
8. Barker DJ, Bull AR, Osmond C, Simmonds SJ. Fetal and placental size and risk of hypertension in adult life. *Br Med J.* (1990) 301:259–62. doi: 10.1136/bmj.301.6746.259
9. Javaid MK, Cooper C. Prenatal and childhood influences on osteoporosis. *Best Pr Res Clin Endocrinol Metab.* (2002) 16:349–67. doi: 10.1053/beem.2002.0199
10. McIntire DD, Bloom SL, Casey BM, Leveno KJ. Birth weight in relation to morbidity and mortality among newborn infants. *N Engl J Med.* (1999) 340:1234–8. doi: 10.1056/NEJM199904223401603
11. Osmond C, Kajantie E, Forsen TJ, Eriksson JG, Barker DJ. Infant growth and stroke in adult life: the Helsinki birth cohort study. *Stroke* (2007) 38:264–70. doi: 10.1161/01.STR.0000254471.72186.03
12. Fisk NM, Atun R. Market failure and the poverty of new drugs in maternal health. *PLoS Med.* (2008) 5:e22. doi: 10.1371/journal.pmed.0050022

13. Strid H, Powell TL. ATP-dependent Ca2+ transport is up-regulated during third trimester in human syncytiotrophoblast basal membranes. *Pediatr Res.* (2000) 48:58–63. doi: 10.1203/00006450-200007000-00012
14. Tobias JH, Cooper C. PTH/PTHrP activity and the programming of skeletal development *in utero*. *J Bone Miner Res.* (2004) 19:177–82. doi: 10.1359/JBMR.0301235
15. Bernucci L, Henríquez M, Díaz P, Riquelme G. Diverse calcium channel types are present in the human *placental* syncytiotrophoblast basal membrane. *Placenta* (2006) 27:1082–95. doi: 10.1016/j.placenta.2005.12.007
16. Haché S, Takser L, LeBellego F, Weiler H, Leduc L, Forest JC, et al. Alteration of calcium homeostasis in primary preeclamptic syncytiotrophoblasts: effect on calcium exchange in placenta. *J Cell Mol Med.* (2011) 15:654–67. doi: 10.1111/j.1582-4934.2010.01039.x
17. Yang H, Kim TH, An BS, Choi KC, Lee HH, Kim JM, et al. Differential expression of calcium transport channels in placenta primary cells and tissues derived from preeclamptic placenta. *Mol Cell Endocrinol.* (2013) 367:21–30. doi: 10.1016/j.mce.2012.12.012
18. Strid H, Bucht E, Jansson T, Wennergren M, Powell TL. ATP dependent Ca2+transport across basal membrane of human syncytiotrophoblast in pregnancies complicated by intrauterine growth restriction or diabetes. *Placenta* (2003) 24:445–52. doi: 10.1053/plac.2002.0941
19. Dilworth MR, Kusinski LC, Cowley E, Ward BS, Husain SM, Constancia M, et al. Placental-specific Igf2 knockout mice exhibit hypocalcemia and adaptive changes in placental calcium transport. *Proc Natl Acad Sci USA.* (2010) 107:3894–9. doi: 10.1073/pnas.0911710107
20. Coan PM, Angiolini E, Sandovici I, Burton GJ, Constância M, Fowden AL, et al. Adaptations in placental nutrient transfer capacity to meet fetal growth demands depend on placental size in mice. *J Physiol.* (2008) 586:4567–76. doi: 10.1113/jphysiol.2008.156133
21. Godfrey KM, Matthews N, Glazier J, Jackson A, Wilman C, Sibley CP. Neutral amino acid uptake by the microvillous plasma membrane of the human placenta is inversely related to fetal size at birth in normal pregnancy. *J Clin Endocrinol Metab.* (1998) 83:3320–6.
22. Hayward CE, Renshall LJ, Sibley CP, Greenwood SL, Dilworth MR. Adaptations in maternofetal calcium transport in relation to placental size and fetal sex in mice. *Front Physiol.* (2017) 8:1050. doi: 10.3389/fphys.2017.01050
23. Simmonds CS, Kovacs CS. Role of parathyroid hormone (PTH) and PTH-related protein (PTHrP) in regulating mineral homeostasis during fetal development. *Crit Rev Eukaryot Gene Expr.* (2010) 20:235–73. doi: 10.1615/CritRevEukarGeneExpr.v20.i3.40
24. Philbrick WM, Wysolmerski JJ, Galbraith S, Holt E, Orloff JJ, Yang KH, et al. Defining the roles of parathyroid hormone-related protein in normal physiology. *Physiol Rev.* (1996) 76:127–73. doi: 10.1152/physrev.1996.76.1.127
25. Ardawi MSM, Nasrat HA, BA'Aqueel HS. Calcium-regulating hormones and parathyroid hormone-related peptide in normal human pregnancy and postpartum: a longitudinal study. *Eur. J. Endocrinol.* (1997) 137:402–9.
26. Curtis NE, Ho PW, King RG, Farrugia W, Moses EK, Gillespie MT, et al. The expression of parathyroid hormone-related protein mRNA and immunoreactive protein in human amnion and choriodecidua is increased at term compared with preterm gestation. *J Endocrinol.* (1997) 154:103–12. doi: 10.1677/joe.0.1540103
27. Moniz C, Burton PB, Malik AN, Dixit M, Banga JP, Nicolaides K, et al. Parathyroid hormone-related peptide in normal human fetal development. *J Mol Endocrinol.* (1990) 5:259–66. doi: 10.1677/jme.0.0050259
28. Karaplis AC, Luz A, Glowacki J, Bronson RT, Tybulewicz VL, Kronenberg HM, et al. Lethal skeletal dysplasia from targeted disruption of the parathyroid hormone-related peptide gene. *Genes Dev.* (1994) 8:277–89. doi: 10.1101/gad.8.3.277
29. Lanske B, Karaplis AC, Lee K, Luz A, Vortkamp A, Pirro A, et al. PTH/PTHrP receptor in early development and Indian hedgehog-regulated bone growth. *Science* (1996) 273:663–6. doi: 10.1126/science.273.5275.663
30. Wlodek ME, Westcott KT, Ho PW, Serruto A, Di Nicolantonio R, Farrugia W, et al. Reduced fetal, placental, and amniotic fluid PTHrP in the growth-restricted spontaneously hypertensive rat. *Am J Physiol Regul Integr Comp Physiol.* (2000) 279:R31–8. doi: 10.1152/ajpregu.2000.279.1.R31
31. Wlodek ME, Di Nicolantonio R, Westcott KT, Farrugia W, Ho PWM, Moseley JM. PTH/PTHrP receptor and mid-molecule PTHrP regulation of intrauterine PTHrP: PTH/PTHrp receptor antagonism increases SHR fetal weight. *Placenta* (2004) 25:53–61. doi: 10.1016/j.placenta.2003.08.001
32. Bond H, Dilworth MR, Baker B, Cowley E, Requena Jimenez A, Boyd RD, et al. Increased maternofetal calcium flux in parathyroid hormone-related protein-null mice. *J Physiol.* (2008) 586:2015–25. doi: 10.1113/jphysiol.2007.149104
33. Kovacs CS, Lanske B, Hunzelman JL, Guo J, Karaplis AC, Kronenberg HM. Parathyroid hormone-related peptide (PTHrP) regulates fetal-placental calcium transport through a receptor distinct from the PTH/PTHrP receptor. *Proc Natl Acad Sci USA.* (1996) 93:15233–8. doi: 10.1073/pnas.93.26.15233
34. Kovacs CS, Manley NR, Moseley JM, Martin TJ, Kronenberg HM. Fetal parathyroids are not required to maintain placental calcium transport. *J Clin Invest.* (2001) 107:1007–15. doi: 10.1172/JCI11321
35. Curtis NE, King RG, Moseley JM, Ho PWM, Rice GE, Wlodek ME. Preterm fetal growth restriction is associated with increased parathyroid hormone-related protein expression in the fetal membranes. *Am J Obstet Gynecol.* (2000) 183:700–5. doi: 10.1067/mob.2000.106593
36. Strid H, Care A, Jansson T, Powell T. Parathyroid hormone-related peptide (38-94) amide stimulates ATP-dependent calcium transport in the basal plasma membrane of the human syncytiotrophoblast. *J Endocrinol.* (2002) 175:517–24. doi: 10.1677/joe.0.1750517
37. Kilkenny C, Browne WJ, Cuthill IC, Emerson M, Altman DG. Improving bioscience research reporting: the ARRIVE guidelines for reporting animal research. *PLoS Biol.* (2010) 8:e1000412. doi: 10.1371/journal.pbio.1000412
38. Dilworth MR, Kusinski LC, Baker BC, Renshall LJ, Greenwood SL, Sibley CP, et al. Defining fetal growth restriction in mice: a standardized and clinically relevant approach. *Placenta* (2011) 32:914–6. doi: 10.1016/j.placenta.2011.08.007
39. Constancia M, Dean W, Lopes S, Moore T, Kelsey G, Reik W. Deletion of a silencer element in Igf2 results in loss of imprinting independent of H19. *Nat Genet.* (2000) 26:203–6. doi: 10.1038/79930
40. Constância M, Hemberger M, Hughes J, Dean W, Ferguson-Smith A, Fundele R, et al. Placental-specific IGF-II is a major modulator of placental and fetal growth. *Nature* (2002) 417:945–8. doi: 10.1038/nature00819
41. Constância M, Angiolini E, Sandovici I, Smith P, Smith R, Kelsey G, et al. Adaptation of nutrient supply to fetal demand in the mouse involves interaction between the Igf2 gene and placental transporter systems. *Proc Natl Acad Sci USA.* (2005) 102:19219–24. doi: 10.1073/pnas.0504468103
42. Brickley DR, Agyeman AS, Kopp RF, Hall BA, Harbeck MC, Belova L, et al. Serum- and glucocorticoid-induced protein kinase 1 (SGK1) is regulated by store-operated Ca2+entry and mediates cytoprotection against necrotic cell death. *J Biol Chem.* (2013) 288:32708–19. doi: 10.1074/jbc.M113.507210
43. Eylenstein A, Gehring E-MM, Heise N, Shumilina E, Schmidt S, Szteyn K, et al. Stimulation of Ca2+-channel Orai1/STIM1 by serum- and glucocorticoid-inducible kinase 1 (SGK1). *FASEB J.* (2011) 25:2012–21. doi: 10.1096/fj.10-178210
44. Imai S, Okayama N, Shimizu M, Itoh M. Increased intracellular calcium activates serum and glucocorticoid-inducible kinase 1 (SGK1) through a calmodulin-calcium calmodulin dependent kinase kinase pathway in Chinese hamster ovary cells. *Life Sci.* (2003) 72:2199–209. doi: 10.1016/S0024-3205(03)00092-4
45. Lang F, Artunc F, Vallon V. The physiological impact of the serum and glucocorticoid-inducible kinase SGK1. *Curr Opin Nephrol Hypertens.* (2009) 18:439–48. doi: 10.1097/MNH.0b013e32832f125e
46. Sopjani M, Kunert A, Czarkowski K, Klaus F, Laufer J, Föller M, et al. Regulation of the Ca2+ channel TRPV6 by the Kinases SGK1, PKB/Akt, and PIKfyve. *J Membr Biol.* (2010) 233:35–41. doi: 10.1007/s00232-009-9222-0
47. Shaw AJ, Mughal MZ, Maresh MJA, Sibley CP. Effects of two synthetic parathyroid hormone-related protein fragments on maternofetal transfer of calcium and magnesium and release of cyclic AMP by the in-situ perfused rat placenta. *J Endocrinol.* (1991) 129:399–404. doi: 10.1677/joe.0.1290399
48. Koo TH, Yang H, An BS, Choi KC, Hyun SH, Jeung EB. Calcium transport genes are differently regulated in maternal and fetal placenta in the knockout

mice of calbindin-D(9k) and -D(28k). *Mol Reprod Dev.* (2012) 79:346–55. doi: 10.1002/mrd.22033
49. Lee GS, Lee KY, Choi KC, Ryu YH, Paik SG, Oh GT, et al. Phenotype of a calbindin-D9k gene knockout is compensated for by the induction of other calcium transporter genes in a mouse model. *J Bone Min Res* (2007) 22:1968–78. doi: 10.1359/jbmr.070801
50. Sferruzzi-Perri AN, Vaughan OR, Coan PM, Suciu MC, Darbyshire R, Constancia M, et al. Placental-specific Igf2 deficiency alters developmental adaptations to undernutrition in mice. *Endocrinology* (2011) 152:3202–12. doi: 10.1210/en.2011-0240
51. García-Martínez JM, Alessi DR. mTOR complex 2 (mTORC2) controls hydrophobic motif phosphorylation and activation of serum- and glucocorticoid-induced protein kinase 1 (SGK1). *Biochem J.* (2008) 416:375–85. doi: 10.1042/BJ20081668
52. Hayman ARR, Jones SJJ, Boyde A, Foster D, Colledge WHH, Carlton MBB, et al. Mice lacking tartrate-resistant acid phosphatase (Acp 5) have disrupted endochondral ossification and mild osteopetrosis. *Development* (1996) 122:3151–62.
53. Buhi WC, Ducsay CA, Bartol FF, Bazer FW, Roberts RM. A function of the allantoic sac in the metabolism of uteroferrin and maternal iron by the fetal pig. *Placenta* (1983) 4 Spec No:45 5–69.
54. Hansson SR, Chen Y, Brodszki J, Chen M, Hernandez-Andrade E, Inman JM, et al. Gene expression profiling of human placentas from preeclamptic and normotensive pregnancies. *Mol Hum Reprod.* (2006) 12:169–79. doi: 10.1093/molehr/gal011

15

Impact of Intrauterine Growth Restriction on Cognitive and Motor Development at 2 Years of Age

Julia Hartkopf[1,2,3], Franziska Schleger[1,2,3], Jana Keune[4], Cornelia Wiechers[5], Jan Pauluschke-Froehlich[6], Magdalene Weiss[3,6], Annette Conzelmann[7], Sara Brucker[6], Hubert Preissl[1,2,3,8] and Isabelle Kiefer-Schmidt[3,6]*

[1] *Institute for Diabetes Research and Metabolic Diseases of the Helmholtz Center Munich at the University of Tuebingen, Tuebingen, Germany,* [2] *German Center for Diabetes Research (DZD e.V.), Tuebingen, Germany,* [3] *fMEG Center, University of Tuebingen, Tuebingen, Germany,* [4] *Department of Neurology, Klinikum Bayreuth GmbH, Bayreuth, Germany,* [5] *Department of Neonatology, University of Tuebingen, Tuebingen, Germany,* [6] *Department of Women's Health, University of Tuebingen, Tuebingen, Germany,* [7] *Department of Child and Adolescent Psychiatry, Psychosomatics and Psychotherapy, University of Tuebingen, Tuebingen, Germany,* [8] *Department of Internal Medicine, Division of Endocrinology, Diabetology, Angiology, Nephrology and Clinical Chemistry, University of Tuebingen, Tuebingen, Germany*

***Correspondence:**
Julia Hartkopf
Julia.hartkopf@med.uni-tuebingen.de

Intrauterine growth restriction (IUGR), which is already known to be a risk factor for pathological intrauterine development, perinatal mortality, and morbidity, is now also assumed to cause both physical and cognitive alterations in later child development. In the current study, effects of IUGR on infantile brain function were investigated during the fetal period and in a follow-up developmental assessment during early childhood. During the fetal period, visual and auditory event-related responses (VER and AER) were recorded using fetal magnetoencephalography (fMEG). VER latencies were analyzed in 73 fetuses (14 IUGR fetuses) while AER latencies were analyzed in 66 fetuses (11 IUGR fetuses). Bayley Scales of Infant Development, Second Edition (BSID-II) were used to assess the developmental status of the infants at the age of 24 months. The Mental Development Index (MDI) was available from 66 children (8 IUGR fetuses) and the Psychomotor Development Index (PDI) from 63 children (7 IUGR fetuses). Latencies to visual stimulation were more delayed in IUGR than in small for gestational age (SGA) or appropriate for gestational age (AGA) fetuses, albeit not to any significant extent (p = 0.282). The MDI in former IUGR infants was significantly lower (p = 0.044) than in former SGA and AGA infants. However, IUGR had no impact on PDI (p = 0.213). These findings support the hypothesis that IUGR may constitute a risk factor for neurodevelopmental delay. Further investigation of the possible underlying mechanisms, as well as continued long-term developmental research, is therefore necessary.

Keywords: intrauterine growth restriction, child development, fetal magnetoencephalography, visual event-related responses (VER), auditory event-related responses (AER)

Abbreviations: AER, auditory event-related responses; AGA, appropriate for gestational age; BSID-II, Bayley Scales of Infant Development, Second Edition; BSID-III, Bayley Scales of Infant and Toddler Development, Third Edition; fMEG, fetal magnetoencephalography; fT, femto Tesla; GA, gestational age; Hz, Hertz; ISI, inter-stimulus interval; IUGR, intrauterine growth restriction; MDI, Mental Development Index; ms, millisecond; PDI, Psychomotor Development Index; SGA, small for gestational age; VER, visual event-related responses.

INTRODUCTION

Over the last few decades, it has become evident that events during early development in humans - even during the prenatal phase - can have long-term effects on health and disease. This concept is commonly known as Developmental Origins of Health and Disease (Barker, 2007; Wadhwa et al., 2009).

One trademark of anomalous prenatal development is intrauterine growth restriction (IUGR). Intrauterine growth restriction is characterized by a pathological restriction of fetal weight, as is presumed to be the case when a fetus is "small for gestational age" (SGA), i.e., when its estimated fetal weight and birth weight are below the 10th percentile for gestational age (GA). The literature and practice often does not distinguish clearly between IUGR and SGA. Consistent criteria are therefore required to establish general valid guidelines in diagnosis and treatment (Barker et al., 2013; Unterscheider et al., 2014; Levine et al., 2015). SGA, which is a more general term for those fetuses and infants whose estimated and actual birth weights are below the 10th percentile, is not necessarily connected with a pathological finding. The term also includes cases of below-average weight caused by genetic preconditions. By contrast, IUGR is associated with pathological intrauterine changes that cause restricted fetal growth. It is also linked to a higher risk of perinatal mortality and morbidity and requires appropriate medical support (Craigo, 1994; Bamberg and Kalache, 2004). It is important to distinguish between pathologically growth-restricted fetuses and constitutionally small fetuses. Placental insufficiency, the most frequently observed pathological cause for restricted fetal growth, should be diagnosed by the umbilical artery Doppler velocity (Figueras and Gardosi, 2011). Placental insufficiency is associated with metabolic and hormonal influences on the fetuses and manifests itself by reduced fetal growth and weight gain during pregnancy. These processes can lead to specific alterations in later physical and cognitive development known as "fetal programming" (Godfrey and Barker, 2001; Martin-Gronert and Ozanne, 2012). Since this influence begins during pregnancy, an early investigational approach is advisable.

Recent follow-up studies with former IUGR infants often used only reduced body size or abnormal Doppler for diagnosis of IUGR. A review by Murray et al. (2015) showed that only a small number of studies on the neurodevelopmental outcome in children with IUGR born at 35 weeks of gestation or later used both abnormal Doppler and small size as diagnostic criteria. The authors reported that IUGR is associated with an increased risk for neurodevelopmental delay. Children with fetal circulatory redistribution (i.e., a pathological Doppler) were reported to be more severely affected.

Neurodevelopmental impairments in IUGR infants are reflected by morphological and structural brain alterations and impaired brain function even in utero (D'Hooghe and Odendaal, 1991; Vindla et al., 1997; Nijhuis et al., 2000; Tolsa et al., 2004; Dubois et al., 2008; Lodygensky et al., 2008). In earlier trials, changes in body movements and heart rate were the two main indicators for stimulus processing for investigating the influence of IUGR on functional brain development in utero. Following acoustic or vibroacoustic stimulation, heart rate responses in IUGR fetuses were delayed and their body movement patterns lower than in controls (Gagnon et al., 1988, 1989; Kisilevsky et al., 2014).

Fetal magnetoencephalography (fMEG) is a non-invasive method for measuring fetal brain activity. From the GA of 28 weeks onward, fetal auditory event-related brain responses (AER) and visual event-related brain responses (VER) can be recorded and a decrease of latency can be assumed to be a marker of the maturation and integrity of functional fetal brain development (Schleussner et al., 2001; Eswaran et al., 2002; Schleussner and Schneider, 2004; Holst et al., 2005; Kiefer et al., 2008). Against this background, by demonstrating that IUGR fetuses have slower VER than their appropriate for gestational age (AGA) control counterparts, we recently ascertained that VER latency is associated with fetal outcome (Morin et al., 2015). A follow-up study to determine the impact of VER latencies on early childhood development, i.e., from birth to 24 months of age, is currently under way.

In the present study, we aimed to determine whether fetal outcome affects early childhood development. This entailed a developmental assessment using BSID-II that was performed at the age of 24 months in former IUGR, SGA, and AGA children. Furthermore, we investigated whether VER and AER latencies, as assessed by fMEG, differed between the fetal outcome groups.

MATERIALS AND METHODS

Participants

One hundred and seven women with singleton pregnancies were recruited by the Department of Obstetrics and Gynecology at the University Hospital, Tuebingen. They gave written informed consent of their and their infant's participation prior to the study, which was approved by the local Ethical Committee of the Medical Faculty of the University of Tuebingen (No. 476/2008MPG1). The study was performed in accordance with the relevant guidelines and regulations.

Fifteen of the infants had birth weights below the 10th percentile, and an increased umbilical artery pulsatility index above the 90th percentile for the respective GA was observed during pregnancy. These 15 fetuses were classified as IUGR due to an insufficient placental blood supply. Although 32 of the infants were born with weights below the 10th percentile, they had a normal umbilical artery Doppler during pregnancy and no placental insufficiency was found. These 32 fetuses were classified as constitutionally SGA. Sixty healthy children with an AGA birth weight were included as controls.

fMEG Measurement

To investigate potential differences in brain development already during pregnancy, all participants underwent an fMEG measurement with visual and auditory stimulation to record event-related brain responses of the fetuses from 28 weeks of GA. The fMEG measurement was performed with a magnetoencephalographic system for fetal and neonatal studies (SARA II: SQUID Array for Reproductive Assessment,

VSM MedTech Ltd., Port Coquitlam, BC, Canada). During the measurement, the woman placed her abdomen in an ergonomically shaped array containing 156 primary and 29 reference sensors. Visual stimuli were presented during 10 min of the measurement and consisted of light flashes delivered by fiber optic wire to an LED-light pad that was placed on the maternal abdomen near the location of a fetal eye, as determined via ultrasound. The light flashes had a wavelength of 625 nm and an intensity of 8000 lux; stimulus duration was 500 ms and the ISI was set at random between 1.5 and 2.5 s (Morin et al., 2015).

Auditory stimulation consisted of an oddball-paradigm with pure tones and was presented for a further 10 min of the measurement. Stimulus duration was 500 ms and the ISI was randomly selected between 1900 and 2100 ms. Standard tones, presented with a frequency of 500 Hz, were interspersed with deviant tones presented at 750 Hz to avoid habituation to the standard tone. Stimuli were delivered into a balloon via an air-filled tube placed on the maternal abdomen. The sequence of visual and auditory stimulation was randomized over subjects. Fetal data were recorded with a sampling rate of 610.352 Hz (Muenssinger et al., 2013).

fMEG Data Analysis

Recorded fetal auditory and visual datasets were filtered offline with a high-pass filter of 0.5 Hz and were transformed by a first-order gradiometer to eliminate any external interference. Maternal and fetal heart signals were attenuated by signal space projection (McCubbin et al., 2006). The data was cut into segments ranging from 200 ms before to 1000 ms after the stimulus. A 10 Hz low-pass filter was applied and the average of the segments was calculated. VER and AER were analyzed by visual examination and defined as a peak in a time window of 80–500 ms after the stimulus, with a minimal amplitude of 4 fT in at least four sensors around the fetal head coil. The latency between stimulus onset and peak was documented for further statistical analysis.

Developmental Test

Two years after fMEG measurement, all families were invited to participate in an assessment of their child's development with BSID-II. Of a total of 107 participants, 66 returned for the follow-up assessment. The 41 participants who discontinued were distributed as follows: IUGR group: 7 of 15 children (46.7%), SGA group: 14 of 32 children (43.8%) and AGA group: 20 of 40 children (50%). The most common reasons for non-participation are summarized in **Figure 1**.

The BSID-II was developed for the measurement of the current developmental state of infants and children between 1 and 42 months of age (Nellis and Gridley, 1994). An experienced and trained psychologist, who was unaware of the medical history of the infant, conducted the test with the child in the presence of a parent. The BSID-II is divided into two scales: the MDI and PDI. The cognitive and psychomotor development of a child can therefore be assessed separately. MDI and PDI both have a mean of 100 and a standard deviation (SD) of 15.

Statistics

Data was described as mean ± SD. A preliminary assumption check revealed that data was normally distributed, as assessed by Shapiro–Wilk test ($p > 0.05$), and that there were no univariate or multivariate outliers, as assessed by boxplot and Mahalanobis distance ($p > 0.001$), respectively. MDI, PDI, VER latency, and AER latency were analyzed for differences between fetal outcome groups (IUGR, SGA, and AGA) using one-way ANOVA and Welch's test of unequal variances, respectively. *Post hoc* analyses were performed using the Games-Howell correction method. PASW Statistics 21 (SPSS Inc., Chicago, IL, United States) was used for statistical analysis and the significance level was set to $p < 0.05$.

RESULTS

Auditory event-related responses and VER latencies were measured using fMEG in 107 fetuses. Of these, 15 were IUGR fetuses, 32 were SGA fetuses and 60 were AGA fetuses. **Table 1** shows mean and SD for GA at birth and birth weight. VER latencies could be analyzed in a total of 73 fetuses (14 IUGR, 22 SGA, and 37 AGA) at a mean GA of 34.1 weeks. AER latencies were detectable in a total of 66 fetuses (11 IUGR, 22 SGA, and 33 AGA) at a mean GA of 34.0 weeks.

Mental Development Index and PDI were assessed using BSID-II at a mean (± SD) age of 24.10 (± 0.79) months. MDI was assessed in 66 children (8 IUGR, 18 SGA, and 40 AGA) and was 96 (± 6), 100 (± 16), and 103 (± 13), respectively. PDI was assessed in 63 children (7 IUGR, 16 SGA, and 40 AGA) and was 94 (± 7), 96 (± 11), and 100 (± 10), respectively. Results are presented as box plots in **Figure 2**.

Table 2 shows the results of the univariate one-way ANOVA in a comparison of MDI, PDI, VER latency, and AER latency in the IUGR, SGA, and AGA groups. There were no statistically significant differences between PDI ($p = 0.213$), VER latency ($p = 0.282$), and AER latency ($p = 0.206$). However, the MDI differed significantly between groups ($p = 0.044$) and increased from the IUGR (96 ± 6) to the SGA (100 ± 16) as well as to the AGA group (103 ± 13). Games-Howell *post hoc* analysis (**Table 3**) revealed that the difference between IUGR and AGA was statistically significant ($p = 0.035$).

DISCUSSION

In the current study, we aimed to investigate the impact of IUGR on early child development. At the age of two, children's developmental status was assessed using BSID-II. The MDI was significantly lower in the IUGR than in the AGA group. Although scores for the PDI decreased from AGA to SGA, and IUGR, these differences were not statistically significant. In addition, fetal brain responses to visual and sound stimulation were assessed via fMEG before birth. We observed an increase in VER latencies from AGA over SGA to IUGR fetuses. These latency differences were, however, not statistically significant. Our results suggest that functional brain development maybe

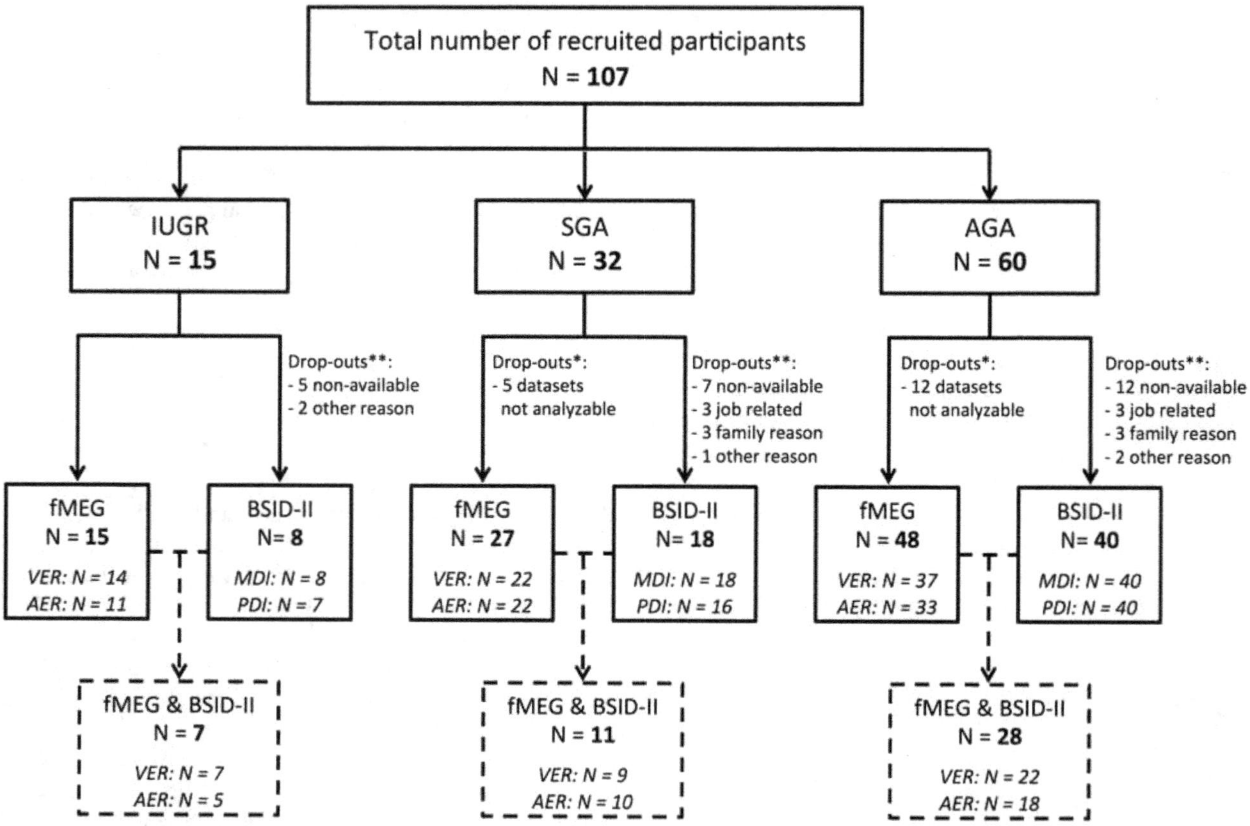

FIGURE 1 | Flow chart showing enrollment and follow-up. All 107 infants were evaluated using fMEG. At the age of 2 years, developmental assessment was performed using BSID-II. *Indicates the number of fMEG data sets that were not analyzable. **Indicates the number of children that were lost to follow-up. At the bottom of the figure, the number of children for whom BSID-II and fMEG was available is shown.

TABLE 1 | Mean weeks (wks) of gestational age (GA) at the time of VER measurement, AER measurement and birth as well as birth weight in grams (g) of IUGR versus SGA versus AGA fetus.

Fetal group		GA at VER (wks)	GA at AER (wks)	GA at birth (wks)	Birth weight (g)
IUGR	Mean	33.6	33.8	35.5	1720
	N	14	11	15	15
	SD	2.7	2,6	2.8	405
SGA	Mean	34.7	34.1	38.6	2446
	N	22	23	32	32
	SD	3.0	3.4	2.1	401
AGA	Mean	33.9	33.9	40.0	3454
	N	37	34	60	60
	SD	3.0	3.1	1,6	412

already altered during gestation and might cause an alteration in the neurological developmental trajectory in later life. However, it must be emphasized that these findings are based on a relatively small group of children.

Intrauterine growth restriction, a pathologic growth restriction of fetuses, is associated with significant neonatal morbidity and mortality (Nardozza et al., 2017). It is also believed to impact morphological and structural brain development (D'Hooghe and Odendaal, 1991; Vindla et al., 1997; Nijhuis et al., 2000; Tolsa et al., 2004; Dubois et al., 2008; Lodygensky et al., 2008). We recently reported that latencies of fetal AER and VER assessed by fMEG are delayed in fetuses with IUGR (Morin et al., 2015). In the present study, however, the differences in VER and AER latencies between IUGR, SGA, and AGA fetuses were not statistically different. A possible explanation for these seemingly contradictory findings may be due to the fact that we had used a case control approach in the previous study to match subjects for GA and fetal behavioral state. Since our primary focus in the present study was on the effect of IUGR on neurodevelopmental changes at 2 years of age, we decided to increase sample size by including not only matched pairs of SGA-AGA and IUGR-AGA subjects but also of all other subjects. For proof of the possible predictive value of fMEG, further studies with larger population sizes and longitudinal assessment of functional brain development are necessary.

In the current study, we used simple tone stimulation only. However, since several cognitive capabilities such as discrimination and habituation are already established in the last trimester of gestation, it would be worthwhile to apply these stimulation paradigms to determine whether they are

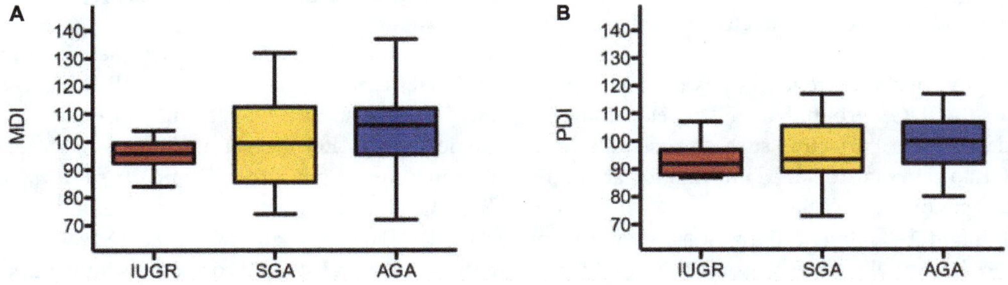

FIGURE 2 | Box plots of MDI **(A)** and PDI **(B)** in IUGR, SGA, and AGA group. Box plots represent median, interquartiles, and ranges.

TABLE 2 | MDI, PDI, VER latency and AER latency in IUGR, SGA, and AGA groups as calculated using one-way ANOVA.

		N	Mean	*SD*	*p*-value
MDI	IUGR	8	96	6	
	SGA	18	100	16	
	AGA	40	103	13	
	Total	66	101	13	0.044*
PDI	IUGR	7	94	7	
	SGA	16	96	11	
	AGA	40	100	10	
	Total	63	98	10	0.213
VER latency	IUGR	14	233	59	
	SGA	22	217	64	
	AGA	37	204	57	
	Total	73	213	60	0.282
AER latency	IUGR	11	204	65	
	SGA	22	220	61	
	AGA	33	188	69	
	Total	66	201	67	0.206

*Welch's t-test was used on account of unequal variances and sample-sizes and *indicates a significant group difference.*

TABLE 3 | Comparisons of the MDI between the IUGR, SGA, and AGA groups.

	IUGR	SGA	AGA
IUGR	–	−4.44 (± 4.33) $p = 0.568$	−7.83 (± 2.91) $p = 0.035$
SGA	4.44 (± 4.33) $p = 0.568$	–	−3.38 (± 4.26) $p = 0.710$
AGA	7.83 (± 2.91) $p = 0.035$	3.38 (± 4.26) $p = 0.710$	–

The differences of mean MDI values (± standard error) are shown and the respective p-values were calculated by Games-Howell post hoc analysis.

more specific for alterations of early fetal brain development (Draganova et al., 2005; Matuz et al., 2012; Muenssinger et al., 2013; Hartkopf et al., 2016). Interestingly, intrauterine auditory stimulation with the maternal voice in growth-restricted fetuses has been proposed as a potential tool to compensate brain alterations that might be responsible for later language impairment (Kisilevsky et al., 2014).

When it came to childhood development, we observed lower cognitive and psychomotor abilities in IUGR than in AGA children, although only the differences in cognitive (mental) scores were of statistical significance. In line with our results, earlier trials showed that former IUGR infants are more liable to achieve lower scores in neurocognitive and/or motor developmental assessment tests than control children without IUGR (for a review, see Murray et al., 2015). The comparability of studies on neurocognitive development of IUGR children, is, however, limited due to the selection criteria for growth restriction. Unlike reduced growth in SGA fetuses, which is usually constitutional, the growth delay in IUGR has a pathological cause. We therefore identified IUGR fetuses by using ultrasound to estimate fetal weight as well as to measure the umbilical artery pulsatility index. The latter is a marker of placental blood supply and a clinical standard to monitor intrauterine malnutrition (Murray et al., 2015). In a follow-up sample of 83 very-low-birth-weight infants, Leppanen et al. used the mental scale of BSID-II to show that only the subgroup with a pathological Doppler was affected by an altered cognitive outcome at the age of 2 years, whereas motor development remained unaffected (Leppanen et al., 2010). This is akin to the present study: PDI of BSID-II did not reveal any differences in psychomotor development between IUGR, SGA, and AGA children at 2 years of age. Several other studies investigating motor outcomes in IUGR children also reported that no differences were observed (Wienerroither et al., 2001; Eixarch et al., 2008; Padilla et al., 2010). Some study results indicate an influence of prematurity and severity of IUGR on motor development (Gazzolo et al., 1995; Padilla et al., 2011).

The MDI of the BSID-II includes measures for different cognitive skills, i.e., active and passive speech development, problem solving, or memory performance. The updated version "Bayley Scales of Infant and Toddler Development, Third Edition" (BSID-III) provides more specific subscores: a cognitive scale, a receptive language and an expressive language scale. To establish specific approaches to support affected infants and their families with early interventions, the assessment should be performed with the updated version in future investigations. However, the German version of the third edition was not available at the time of this study, nor is a behavioral scale, as provided by the original versions of BSID-II and BSID-III, available in the German language to date. Results of studies investigating behavioral changes in former IUGR children indicate that attention, social-interactive skills or mood might also be affected (Roza et al., 2008; Beukers et al., 2017).

The major limitation of the current study is the low sample size, particularly for the IUGR group. Future studies with larger sample sizes should consider co-factors such as onset, duration and severity of IUGR to gain more detailed information about the impact of different types of IUGR (Miller et al., 2016). Moreover, loss to follow-up might be influenced by socioeconomic or demographic factors and might therefore bias our results (see **Figure 1** for drop-out at the different stages).

CONCLUSION

The results of this study support the hypothesis that IUGR might be a risk factor for a delay in neurocognitive development (MDI) in two-year old children. However, the differences were only modest, and not significant with respect to the PDI, and the three study groups did not differ significantly in fetal event-related brain activity. The investigation of underlying physiological processes and their impact on human brain development should be the focus of further research. Moreover, larger trials with a standardized definition of IUGR and well-defined outcome measures are required to identify factors that impact the role of IUGR on child development. These findings would be instrumental in developing specific treatment and support for the affected infants and their families.

AUTHOR CONTRIBUTIONS

JH, HP and IK-S conceived and designed the study. MW, JP-F, SB, and IK-S recruited the participants. JP-F, SB, and IK-S performed fetal ultrasound and Doppler measurements. JH, JK, and MW carried out fMEG measurements. CW conducted the physical examination of neonates. JK and JH performed Bayley testing. JH, AC, FS and HP analyzed the data and were responsible for statistics. JH, FS, HP and IK-S prepared the draft manuscript. All authors made substantial corrections for the final manuscript.

FUNDING

This work was partly supported by the German Research Foundation (DFG BI 195/50 and KI 1306/3-1), the University of Tuebingen (E.05.00303 and E.05.0259.1), Federal Ministry of Education and Research (BMBF) to the German Center for Diabetes Research (DZD e.V.), and the Foundation of Baden-Wuerttemberg. We acknowledge support by the German Research Foundation and Open Access Publishing Fund of University of Tuebingen.

ACKNOWLEDGMENTS

We are very grateful to all the families who participated in our study.

REFERENCES

1. Bamberg, C., and Kalache, K. D. (2004). Prenatal diagnosis of fetal growth restriction. *Semin. Fetal Neonatal. Med.* 9, 387–394. doi: 10.1016/j.siny.2004.03.007
2. Barker, D. J. (2007). The origins of the developmental origins theory. *J. Intern. Med.*261, 412–417. doi: 10.1111/j.1365-2796.2007.01809.x
3. Barker, E. D., McAuliffe, F. M., Alderdice, F., Unterscheider, J., Daly, S., Geary, M. P., et al. (2013). The role of growth trajectories in classifying fetal growth restriction. *Obstet. Gynecol.* 122(2 Pt 1), 248–254. doi: 10.1097/AOG.0b013e31829ca9a7
4. Beukers, F., Aarnoudse-Moens, C. S. H., van Weissenbruch, M. M., Ganzevoort, W., van Goudoever, J. B., and van Wassenaer-Leemhuis,
5. A. G. (2017). Fetal growth restriction with brain sparing: neurocognitive and behavioral outcomes at 12 years of age. *J. Pediatr.* 188:e102. doi: 10.1016/j.jpeds.2017.06.003
6. Craigo, S. D. (1994). The role of ultrasound in the diagnosis and management of intrauterine growth retardation. *Semin. Perinatol.* 18, 292–304.
7. D'Hooghe, T. M., and Odendaal, H. J. (1991). Fewer accelerations and decreased long term variability in the heart rate of small for gestational age fetuses. *Int. J. Gynaecol. Obstet.* 35, 133–138. doi: 10.1016/0020-7292(91)90816-N
8. Draganova, R., Eswaran, H., Murphy, P., Huotilainen, M., Lowery, C., and Preissl, H. (2005). Sound frequency change detection in fetuses and newborns, a magnetoencephalographic study. *Neuroimage* 28, 354–361. doi: 10.1016/j.neuroimage.2005.06.011
9. Dubois, J., Benders, M., Borradori-Tolsa, C., Cachia, A., Lazeyras, F., Ha-Vinh Leuchter, R., et al. (2008). Primary cortical folding in the human newborn: an early marker of later functional development. *Brain* 131(Pt 8), 2028–2041. doi: 10.1093/brain/awn137
10. Eixarch, E., Meler, E., Iraola, A., Illa, M., Crispi, F., Hernandez-Andrade, E., et al. (2008). Neurodevelopmental outcome in 2-year-old infants who were small-for-gestational age term fetuses with cerebral blood flow redistribution. *Ultrasound Obstet. Gynecol.* 32, 894–899. doi: 10.1002/uog.6249
11. Eswaran, H., Wilson, J., Preissl, H., Robinson, S., Vrba, J., Murphy, P., et al. (2002). Magnetoencephalographic recordings of visual evoked brain activity in the human fetus. *Lancet* 360, 779–780. doi: 10.1016/S0140-6736(02)09905-1
12. Figueras, F., and Gardosi, J. (2011). Intrauterine growth restriction: new concepts in antenatal surveillance, diagnosis, and management. *Am. J. Obstet. Gynecol.* 204, 288–300. doi: 10.1016/j.ajog.2010.08.055
13. Gagnon, R., Hunse, C., Carmichael, L., and Patrick, J. (1989). Vibratory acoustic stimulation in 26- to 32-week, small-for-gestational-age fetus. *Am. J. Obstet. Gynecol.* 160, 160–165. doi: 10.1016/0002-9378(89)90111-7
14. Gagnon, R., Hunse, C., Fellows, F., Carmichael, L., and Patrick, J. (1988). Fetal heart rate and activity patterns in growth-retarded fetuses: changes after vibratory acoustic stimulation. *Am. J. Obstet. Gynecol.* 158, 265–271. doi: 10.1016/0002-9378(88)90135-4
15. Gazzolo, D., Visser, G. H., Santi, F., Magliano, C. P., Scopesi, F., Russo, A., et al. (1995). Behavioural development and Doppler velocimetry in relation to perinatal outcome in small for dates fetuses. *Early. Hum. Dev* 43, 185–195. doi: 10.1016/0378-3782(95)01676-7
16. Godfrey, K. M., and Barker, D. J. (2001). Fetal programming and adult health. *Public Health Nutr.* 4, 611–624. doi: 10.1079/PHN2001145
17. Hartkopf, J., Schleger, F., Weiss, M., Hertrich, I., Kiefer-Schmidt, I., Preissl, H., et al. (2016). Neuromagnetic signatures of syllable processing in fetuses and infants provide no evidence for habituation. *Early. Hum. Dev.* 100, 61–66. doi: 10.1016/j.earlhumdev.2016.04.002
18. Holst, M., Eswaran, H., Lowery, C., Murphy, P., Norton, J., and Preissl, H. (2005). Development of auditory evoked fields in human fetuses and newborns: a longitudinal MEG study. *Clin. Neurophysiol.* 116, 1949–1955. doi: 10.1016/j.clinph.2005.04.008
19. Kiefer, I., Siegel, E., Preissl, H., Ware, M., Schauf, B., Lowery, C., et al. (2008). Delayed maturation of auditory-evoked responses in growth-restricted fetuses revealed by magnetoencephalographic recordings. *Am. J. Obstet. Gynecol.* 199, 503.e1–503.e7. doi: 10.1016/j.ajog.2008.04.014
20. Kisilevsky, B. S., Chambers, B., Parker, K. C. H., and Davies, G. A. L. (2014). Auditory processing in growth-restricted fetuses and newborns and

later language development. *Clin. Psychol. Sci.* 2, 495–513. doi: 10.1177/2167702613509371

21. Leppanen, M., Ekholm, E., Palo, P., Maunu, J., Munck, P., Parkkola, R., et al. (2010). Abnormal antenatal Doppler velocimetry and cognitive outcome in very-low- birth-weight infants at 2 years of age. *Ultrasound Obstet Gynecol.* 36, 178–185. doi: 10.1002/uog.7694
22. Levine, T. A., Grunau, R. E., McAuliffe, F. M., Pinnamaneni, R., Foran, A., and Alderdice, F. A. (2015). Early childhood neurodevelopment after intrauterine growth restriction: a systematic review. *Pediatrics* 135, 126–141. doi: 10.1542/peds.2014-1143
23. Lodygensky, G. A., Seghier, M. L., Warfield, S. K., Tolsa, C. B., Sizonenko, S., Lazeyras, F., et al. (2008). Intrauterine growth restriction affects the preterm infant's hippocampus. *Pediatr. Res.* 63, 438–443. doi: 10.1203/PDR.0b013e318165c005
24. Martin-Gronert, M. S., and Ozanne, S. E. (2012). Mechanisms underlying the developmental origins of disease. *Rev. Endocr. Metab. Disord.* 13, 85–92. doi: 10.1007/s11154-012-9210-z
25. Matuz, T., Govindan, R. B., Preissl, H., Siegel, E. R., Muenssinger, J., Murphy, P., et al. (2012). Habituation of visual evoked responses in neonates and fetuses: a MEG study. *Dev. Cogn. Neurosci.* 2, 303–316. doi: 10.1016/j.dcn.2012.03.001
26. McCubbin, J., Robinson, S. E., Cropp, R., Moiseev, A., Vrba, J., Murphy, P., et al. (2006). Optimal reduction of MCG in fetal MEG recordings. *IEEE Trans. Biomed. Eng.* 53, 1720–1724. doi: 10.1109/TBME.2006.876619
27. Miller, S. L., Huppi, P. S., and Mallard, C. (2016). The consequences of fetal growth restriction on brain structure and neurodevelopmental outcome. *J. Physiol.* 594, 807–823. doi: 10.1113/JP271402
28. Morin, E. C., Schleger, F., Preissl, H., Braendle, J., Eswaran, H., Abele, H., et al. (2015). Functional brain development in growth-restricted and constitutionally small fetuses: a fetal magnetoencephalography case-control study. *BJOG* 122, 1184–1190. doi: 10.1111/1471-0528.13347
29. Muenssinger, J., Matuz, T., Schleger, F., Kiefer-Schmidt, I., Goelz, R., Wacker-Gussmann, A., et al. (2013). Auditory habituation in the fetus and neonate: an fMEG study. *Dev. Sci.* 16, 287–295. doi: 10.1111/desc.12025
30. Murray, E., Fernandes, M., Fazel, M., Kennedy, S. H., Villar, J., and Stein, A. (2015). Differential effect of intrauterine growth restriction on childhood neurodevelopment: a systematic review. *BJOG* 122, 1062–1072. doi: 10.1111/1471-0528.13435
31. Nardozza, L. M., Caetano, A. C., Zamarian, A. C., Mazzola, J. B., Silva, C. P., Marcal, V. M., et al. (2017). Fetal growth restriction: current knowledge. *Arch. Gynecol. Obstet.* 295, 1061–1077. doi: 10.1007/s00404-017-4341-9
32. Nellis, L., and Gridley, B. E. (1994). Review of the bayley scales of infant development—second edition. *J. Sch. Psychol.* 32, 201–209. doi: 10.1016/0022- 4405(94)90011-6
33. Nijhuis, I. J., ten Hof, J., Mulder, E. J., Nijhuis, J. G., Narayan, H., Taylor, D. J., et al. (2000). Fetal heart rate in relation to its variation in normal and growth retarded fetuses. *Eur. J. Obstet. Gynecol. Reprod. Biol.* 89, 27–33. doi: 10.1016/S0301-2115(99)00162-1
34. Padilla, N., Falcon, C., Sanz-Cortes, M., Figueras, F., Bargallo, N., Crispi, F., et al. (2011). Differential effects of intrauterine growth restriction on brain structure and development in preterm infants: a magnetic resonance imaging study. *Brain Res.* 1382, 98–108. doi: 10.1016/j.brainres.2011.01.032
35. Padilla, N., Perapoch, J., Carrascosa, A., Acosta-Rojas, R., Botet, F., and Gratacos, E. (2010). Twelve-month neurodevelopmental outcome in preterm infants with and without intrauterine growth restriction. *Acta Paediatr.* 99, 1498–1503. doi: 10.1111/j.1651-2227.2010.01848.x
36. Roza, S. J., Steegers, E. A., Verburg, B. O., Jaddoe, V. W., Moll, H. A., Hofman, A., et al. (2008). What is spared by fetal brain-sparing? Fetal circulatory redistribution and behavioral problems in the general population. *Am. J. Epidemiol.* 168, 1145–1152. doi: 10.1093/aje/kwn233
37. Schleussner, E., and Schneider, U. (2004). Developmental changes of auditory-evoked fields in fetuses. *Exp. Neurol.* 190(Suppl. 1), S59–S64. doi: 10.1016/j.expneurol.2004.04.008
38. Schleussner, E., Schneider, U., Kausch, S., Kahler, C., Haueisen, J., and Seewald, H. J. (2001). Fetal magnetoencephalography: a non-invasive method for the assessment of fetal neuronal maturation. *BJOG* 108, 1291–1294.
39. Tolsa, C. B., Zimine, S., Warfield, S. K., Freschi, M., Sancho Rossignol, A., Lazeyras, F., et al. (2004). Early alteration of structural and functional brain development in premature infants born with intrauterine growth restriction. *Pediatr. Res.* 56, 132–138. doi: 10.1203/01.PDR.0000128983.54614.7E
40. Unterscheider, J., Daly, S., Geary, M. P., Kennelly, M. M., McAuliffe, F. M., O'Donoghue, K., et al. (2014). Definition and management of fetal growth restriction: a survey of contemporary attitudes. *Eur. J. Obstet. Gynecol. Reprod. Biol.* 174, 41–45. doi: 10.1016/j.ejogrb.2013.11.022
41. Vindla, S., James, D. K., Sahota, D. S., and Coppens, M. (1997). Computerised analysis of behaviour in normal and growth-retarded fetuses. *Eur. J. Obstet. Gynecol. Reprod. Biol.* 75, 169–175. doi: 10.1016/S0301-2115(97)00131-0
42. Wadhwa, P. D., Buss, C., Entringer, S., and Swanson, J. M. (2009). Developmental origins of health and disease: brief history of the approach and current focus on epigenetic mechanisms. *Semin. Reprod. Med.* 27, 358–368. doi: 10.1055/s-0029- 1237424
43. Wienerroither, H., Steiner, H., Tomaselli, J., Lobendanz, M., and Thun-Hohenstein, L. (2001). Intrauterine blood flow and long-term intellectual, neurologic, and social development. *Obstet. Gynecol.* 97, 449–453.

16

Failure of Decidualization and Maternal Immune Tolerance Underlies Uterovascular Resistance in Intra Uterine Growth Restriction

Caroline Dunk[1], Melissa Kwan[1], Aleah Hazan[1], Sierra Walker[1], Julie K. Wright[1], Lynda K. Harris[2,3,4], Rebecca Lee Jones[3,4], Sarah Keating[5], John C. P. Kingdom[1,5], Wendy Whittle[5], Cynthia Maxwell[5] and Stephen J. Lye[1,5,6]*

[1] Research Centre for Women's and Infants' Health, Lunenfeld Tanenbaum Research Institute, Mount Sinai Hospital, Sinai Health System, Toronto, ON, Canada, [2] Division of Pharmacy and Optometry, University of Manchester, Manchester, United Kingdom, [3] Faculty of Biology Medicine and Health, Maternal and Fetal Health Research Centre, University of Manchester, Manchester, United Kingdom, [4] Academic Health Science Centre, St Mary's Hospital, Manchester, United Kingdom, [5] Department of Obstetrics and Gynaecology, Faculty of Medicine, University of Toronto, Toronto, ON, Canada, [6] Department of Physiology, Faculty of Medicine, University of Toronto, Toronto, ON, Canada

***Correspondence:**
Caroline Dunk
dunk@lunenfeld.ca

Failure of uterine vascular transformation is associated with pregnancy complications including Intra Uterine Growth Restriction (IUGR). The decidua and its immune cell populations play a key role in the earliest stages of this process. Here we investigate the hypothesis that abnormal decidualization and failure of maternal immune tolerance in the second trimester may underlie the uteroplacental pathology of IUGR. Placental bed biopsies were obtained from women undergoing elective caesarian delivery of a healthy term pregnancy, an IUGR pregnancy or a pregnancy complicated by both IUGR and preeclampsia. Decidual tissues were also collected from second trimester terminations from women with either normal or high uterine artery Doppler pulsatile index (PI). Immunohistochemical image analysis and flow cytometry were used to quantify vascular remodeling, decidual leukocytes and decidual status in cases vs. controls. Biopsies from pregnancies complicated by severe IUGR with a high uterine artery pulsatile index (PI) displayed a lack of: myometrial vascular transformation, interstitial, and endovascular extravillous trophoblast (EVT) invasion, and a lower number of maternal leukocytes. Apoptotic mural EVT were observed in association with mature dendritic cells and T cells in the IUGR samples. Second trimester pregnancies with high uterine artery PI displayed a higher incidence of small for gestational age fetuses; a skewed decidual immunology with higher numbers of; CD8 T cells, mature CD83 dendritic cells and lymphatic vessels that were packed with decidual leukocytes. The decidual stromal cells (DSCs) failed to differentiate into the large secretory DSC in these cases, remaining small and cuboidal and expressing lower levels of the nuclear progesterone receptor isoform B, and DSC markers Insulin Growth Factor Binding protein-1 (IGFBP-1) and CD10 as compared to controls. This study shows that defective progesterone mediated decidualization and a hostile maternal immune response against the invading endovascular EVT contribute to the failure of uterovascular remodeling in IUGR pregnancies.

Keywords: IUGR, uterovascular transformation, decidua, EVT, immunology, T cells, dendritic, progesterone

INTRODUCTION

Healthy pregnancies display uterine spiral arteries where the endothelial layer has been replaced with placentally-derived EVT and the muscular and elastic layers have been replaced with fibrinoid matrix. This results in their transformation from narrow, vasoactive arteries to flaccid, maximally dilated vessels unresponsive to vasomotor stimuli, and is necessary in order to increase maternal blood flow to the intervillous space for optimal fetal growth (1). Failed transformation of the spiral arteries in contrast is postulated as a contributing cause to several disorders of pregnancy including preeclampsia (PE), intrauterine growth restriction (IUGR), spontaneous preterm labor, preterm premature rupture of the membranes, and miscarriage (2–6). These cases are characterized by reduced utero-placental blood flow, documented by the observation of persistent high resistance waveforms using color/pulsed Doppler ultrasound of the proximal uterine spiral arteries (6–8). Such women do not exhibit any 2nd trimester fall in blood pressure (9) and placental bed biopsies (PBBx) from these subjects at delivery show failure of EVT invasion into the myometrial portions of spiral arteries despite adequate decidual interstitial EVT invasion (10–12). Histologic findings in these pathological PBBx represent varying combinations of the following features—collectively termed as decidual vasculopathy—on hematoxylin eosin stained sections; persistent muscularization of the spiral artery segments, a lack of endovascular trophoblast; apoptosis of endovascular EVT; a maternal leukocyte infiltrate, capable of inducing trophoblast apoptosis; atherosis and further narrowing of the vessel lumens or thrombosis in the spiral artery(2, 3, 5, 13–15). To date most studies have focused on the uteroplacental pathology of PE pregnancies while less is known about the uteroplacental pathology of IUGR. It is also unknown if this failure of uterovascular remodeling is primarily due to an EVT defect or in fact to a defect of decidualization. Recently, Brosens et al. have proposed that defective differentiation of the secretory endometrium to the decidua in the earliest stages of pregnancy may be a significant contributor to the development of the Great Obstetrical Conditions (16, 17).

Human decidualization occurs independently of pregnancy and is initiated following ovulation every menstrual cycle. In the mid-late secretory phase, the actions of progesterone, estradiol, and cAMP coordinate to promote the differentiation of the estrogen-primed endometrium into a receptive tissue prepared for blastocyst implantation in the event of fertilization. This process is referred to as decidualization and requires the coordination of a number of key events including; the differentiation of fibroblast-like endometrial stromal cells into large, rounded, secretory decidual stromal cells (DSC), the growth and elongation of the uterine spiral arteries, and the recruitment and specialization of a unique angiogenic decidual immune population (18, 19). The decidual leukocytes rapidly increase in number during the late secretory period to the effect that they comprise up to 40% of all decidual cells in the first trimester of pregnancy (20, 21). They are recruited from the periphery by chemokines secreted by the differentiated DSC, or proliferate within the decidua as it differentiates (22–24). The leukocyte populations include uterine natural killer cells (uNK, 50–70%), macrophage (20%), T-cells (10%), and myeloid dendritic cells (2%) and play a critical role in the development and transformation of the uterine spiral arteries (25–28).

Following fertilization and blastocyst attachment utero vascular remodeling is initiated early in gestation in both decidual and myometrial junctional zone segments of the spiral arteries. These changes occur prior to the presence of trophoblast in the tissue and are associated with disorganization of the perivascular smooth muscle cells (VSMC) layers, and coincide with the presence of large numbers of maternal leukocytes within the decidua (29–31). In decidual vessels undergoing active transformation numerous perivascular uNK and macrophages are found in close association with and infiltrating the disrupted VSMC layers both *in vivo* and *in vitro* (32–34). We have recently shown that these leukocytes secrete matrix metalloproteinases 2,–7,–9,–11,–16, and–19 which they utilize to disrupt ECM of the vascular wall (31, 35, 36). This leads to separation and disorganization of the VSMC layers and ultimately dedifferentiation and death of the VSMC (34, 37, 38).Vessels newly dilated by trophoblast-independent remodeling are further transformed and stabilized through trophoblast-dependent vascular remodeling, through which maximal dilation of the spiral arteries is finally achieved (39). We have suggested that the influx of decidual leukocytes into the vessel wall may also provide a chemokine stimulus to draw endovascular EVT up the vascular lumen to mediate the last stabilization of the transformed artery (19, 40). It has been shown that uNK secrete CCL8, CXCL-10, and CCL5 to promote EVT invasion via CXCR1 and CXCR3 receptors (40). Interestingly numbers of uNK are reduced in the decidua of term IUGR pregnancies (41), suggesting that altered uNK-EVT interactions may contribute to the failure of endovascular invasion associated with uteroplacental pathology.

The importance of leukocytes in the uterine vascular remodeling of the first trimester is well-established, yet new functions mediated by specific leukocyte populations and interactions between different decidual leukocyte populations and EVT are still being discovered (42). However, less is known about the second trimester decidual leukocyte populations although uterovascular transformation continues well into the 2nd trimester (43). In general studies support the development of a Th2 dominant tolerogenic immune environment in the second trimester under the control of rising levels of placental progesterone (44). Mechanisms employed by the various cell populations, including the DSC, act primarily to either reduce dNK cytotoxicity, or prevent activation of T-cell mediate immune responses either directly or indirectly by altering the phenotypes of antigen-presenting cells (macrophage and dendritic cells) (45, 46). We have previously shown that in the second trimester decidua macrophage differentiate to an alternate M2c proangiogenic tissue remodeling phenotype, T cells increase and are dominated by CD4 T helper cells and T-reg, and dendritic cells are maintained in an immature phenotype (27).

In this study we investigated the hypothesis that decidualization would be compromised in the 2nd trimester of pregnancies from women displaying high uterine artery pulsatile index (PI) and that this would be identified by both disturbances in the development, recruitment, and adaptation of the decidual leukocyte populations and decidualization of the DSC. We focused our investigation on 2nd trimester pregnancies carrying small for gestational age (SGA) fetuses in an aim to inform our observations in the 3rd trimester placental bed biopsies from IUGR pregnancies and thus contribute to the understanding of the development of uterovascular pathology in these cases.

METHODS

Tissue Collection

This study was carried out in accordance with the recommendations of Mount Sinai Hospital Research Ethics Board, Sinai Health System. The protocol was approved by the Mount Sinai Hospital Research Ethics Board, Sinai Health System REB# 02-0061A and 12-0007E]. All subjects gave written informed consent in accordance with the Declaration of Helsinki. All research using human tissues was performed in a class II certified laboratory by qualified staff trained in biological and chemical safety protocols, and in accordance with Health Canada guidelines and regulations.

Placental bed biopsies were collected from healthy women undergoing elective caesarian section at term (n = 15) and from women with high uterine artery Doppler pulsatile index (PI > 1.5) undergoing caesarian section and carrying a IUGR fetus <10% expected fetal weight (n = 8). Five women with preeclampsia, a high uterine artery PI (>1.5) and carrying an IUGR fetus were also recruited for comparison. PI is calculated from measurement of (systolic velocity-diastolic velocity)/mean velocity of the uterine or umbilical artery. Biopsies were collected immediately following delivery of the fetus and placenta under direct visualization via the introduction of the punch biopsy forceps through the uterine incision. Three biopsies were collected; two from the placental site and one from the opposing wall of the uterus. Patient demographic data is presented in **Table 1**; placental pathology is presented in **Table 2**.

Decidual tissue was obtained from healthy women undergoing elective termination for medical reasons between 14 and 19 weeks of gestation at the Second Trimester Interruption of Pregnancy (STIPS) clinic. Second trimester tissues were obtained via dilation and evacuation 24 h after insertion of a cervical laminaria. Uterine artery Doppler assessment was performed prior to the termination procedure. Of the second trimester cases collected, 6 had normal uterine artery Doppler and 6 had elevated uterine artery Doppler (PI > 1.6). Fetal size was also measured by ultrasound (**Table 3**). The increase in the PI cut-off in this group is to account for the higher uterine artery PI normally observed at this gestational age (47).

Immunohistochemistry and Image Analysis

Serial 5 μm sections of each biopsy were immunostained using an avidin-biotin peroxidase technique as previously described (32). Antigen retrieval was performed by either heat mediated 10 mM sodium citrate (pH 6) solution or 1 mM EDTA (pH9) as determined by optimization studies and is indicated in **Table 4**.

TABLE 1 | Patient demographics of the placental bed biopsy study.

Diagnosis	Control (n = 15)	IUGR (n = 8)	IUGR and PE (n = 5)
No. of primigravid	2	1	0
Race (% white)	60%	50%	20%*
Umbilical artery Doppler	Normal, 15	AEDV, 3 REDV, 3 Increased PI, 2	AEDV, 4 Increased PI, 1
Uterine artery Doppler	Normal, 15	Increased PI, 7 Abnormal, 5 Not recorded, 1	Increased PI, 5 Abnormal, 1
No. of vessels examined	Decidual (44) Myometrial (56)	Decidual (21) Myometrial (19)	Decidual (12) Myometrial (13)
Maternal age, (year)	36 (4.3)	37.4 (4.7)	31.6 (5.1)
Systolic BP,(mm Hg)	104.07 (31.05)	120.0 (10.43)	148.80 (35.46)*
Diastolic BP, (mm Hg)	68.71 (11.86)	78.38 (8.42)	91.60 (11.08)*
Gestational age, week	>37, 15	<34, 6* >37, 2	< 34, 4* >37, 1
Birth weight, kg	3.3 (0.52)	1.30 (0.43)*	1.17 (0.36)*
Birth weight percentile	>50%, 15	5th–10th, 6 <5th, 2	5th–10th, 1 <5th, 4
Proteinuria	Abnormal 1, Not recorded, 14	Abnormal, 1 Not recorded, 8	Abnormal, 4 Not recorded, 1

*A/REDV, Absent/reduced endovascular doppler velocity. BP, blood pressure *P < 0.05 compared to healthy term controls.*

TABLE 2 | Placental histopathology in cases and controls.

Placental pathology	Normal (n = 15)	IUGR (n = 8)
Small placenta <25%	0	5
Distal villous hypoplasia	0	2
Fetal thrombotic vasculopathy	1	3
Advanced villous maturity	0	3
Decidual vasculopathy	0	2
Multifocal infarction	0	3
>1 significant lesion	0	2
Villitis of unknown etiology	0	2
Umbilical cord abnormalities	1	4

Blocking was performed for 1 h using Dako Protein Serum-Free Blocking Solution (Dako). Slides were then incubated with primary antibodies to identify EVT (CK7 and HLAG), myometrial and VSMC (Smooth muscle actin), endothelial cells (CD31), and decidual leukocytes (CD45) diluted in PBS or negative IgG controls (specific to the species in which primary antibodies were raised) and incubated overnight at 4°C. Further leukocyte subsets were investigated using antibodies against: CD56 (uNK), CD68 (macrophage), CD3, CD4, and CD8 (T Cells) and CD209 and CD83 (immature and mature dendritic cells). Antibodies are detailed in **Table 4**. Following incubation with species appropriate secondary biotinylated antibodies slides were washed with PBS, developed using the Liquid DAB+ (3,3-diaminobenzidine) Chromogen System (Dako), and counterstained with diluted Gill's No. 1 Hematoxylin

TABLE 3 | Patient demographics of the 2nd trimester decidua study.

Diagnosis	Control ($n = 6$)	High Ut A PI ($n = 6$)
Gestational age, week	14–19	17–19
Uterine artery Doppler	Normal, 6	Increased PI, 6 Abnormal, 5
No. of vessels examined	Decidual (22)	Decidual (34)
Maternal age, y	33 (2.3)	35.4 (3.1)
Systolic BP, mm Hg	119.23 (12.9)	120.0 (5.52)
Diastolic BP, mm Hg	76.71 (7.83)	80.12 (5.47)
Small for gestational age	0	4
FETAL ABNORMALITIES:		
Chromosomal	2	2
Genetic	2	1
Hydrops	1	0
Limb abnormalities	1	1
No heart beat	1	1
Severe IUGR	0	1

(Sigma-Aldrich, Oakville, ON). True PBBx were confirmed by the presence of myometrium, decidua, one or more uterine spiral arteries, and positive staining for HLA-G or CK7 (indicating trophoblast presence). For negative controls, the specific primary antibody was replaced by normal mouse or rabbit IgG at the same antibody concentration used to stain test samples. No staining of the negative controls was observed. Terminal deoxynucleotidyl transferase dUTP nick end labeling (TUNEL) staining was performed using the in situ cell death detection kit-POD and according to the manufacturer's instructions (R and D systems, Oakville, Canada).

Analysis of Structural Alterations in the Placental Bed

Structural alternations in the placental bed biopsies were scored based on previous publications (14, 48). Sections were scored by 2 observers (C.D. and S.K.) blinded to the sections identity and showed good agreement between observers. Decidual and myometrial vessels were considered separately. Disruption of the vessel wall was graded into 3 groups (preserved, disorganized (disorganization and some loss of the media) and absent/grossly disorganized (little or no media remains). Interstitial EVT (inEVT) found > 50 μm from the vessel wall were graded as absent (0), low density (1) or high density (2). Intramural EVT (mEVT) and endovascular EVT (enEVT) were scored as present or absent if within the vessel media, or where it once was, or lumen, respectively.

Image Analysis and Quantification

Quantification of leukocyte subtypes and decidual markers in the PBBx samples controls ($n = 15$ basalis, $n = 15$ paretalis) and IUGR ($n = 8$) and IUGR with maternal PE ($n = 5$) or second trimester human decidual samples from pregnancies with high uterine artery PI ($n = 6$) or normal uterine artery PI ($n = 6$) was performed using an Olympus BX61 microscope equipped with an Olympus DP72 camera, and the newCAST software (Visopharm). Firstly 2 separate masks were established covering the decidual and myometrial areas of the PBBx section. Counts were performed using a standard protocol that assigned random counting frames covering 5% of each total masked tissue area. Brown, positively-staining cells and blue, negatively-staining cells (haematoxylin-stained) were counted at 10X magnification. A positively stained ratio was generated by dividing the total numbers of brown, positively-staining cells by the total number of cells counted in the tissue area).

Isolation of Decidual Leukocytes

Decidual tissue was processed as described in Kwan et al. (27). Briefly, decidua was washed and minced finely and flushed with HBSS$^{+/+}$ 2 to 3 times to ensure maximal release of leukocytes. Decidual cells were collected via filtration through 100 and 70 μm sieves and centrifugation (700 g for 10 min at 4°C). Isolated cells were suspended in RPMI-1640 + 10% FBS and fibroblasts eliminated through differential attachment to tissue culture plates (37°C for 20 min). Following incubation, remaining cells were passed through a 40 μm filter and incubated in erythrocyte lysis buffer EL (Qiagen, Toronto, ON, Canada) for 20 min at 4°C. The final cell suspension was incubated in serum-free protein block (Dako, Burlington, ON, Canada) for 1 h on ice and diluted to a final concentration of 10^6cells/mL.

Cell Labeling and FACS Analysis Gating Strategy

Isolated cells were incubated with fluorochrome-conjugated mouse monoclonal antibodies in 200 μl staining volume for 45 min at 4°C in the dark. Cells were washed in PBS and re-suspended in 200 μl stabilizing-fixative permeabilization buffer (BD Biosciences, Mississauga, ON, Canada) to prevent dissociation of tandem dyes and analyzed using a FACSAria flow cytometer (BD Biosciences, Mississauga, ON, Canada) and FlowJo software (Tree Star, Ashland, OR, USA). Cell debris and aggregates were excluded by gating on forward vs. side scatter, then by height vs. width of forward and side scatter plots prior to population discrimination. Non-leukocyte events were excluded from analysis using threshold gates set on CD45 fluorescence. Positive leukocyte subpopulations were identified upon comparison of fully-stained samples to fluorescence minus one (FMO) and isotype controls. Dendritic cell populations were assessed in more detail within the high side scatter gate within the CD45 positive leukocyte population. Antibodies used are listed in **Table 4**.

Statistical Analysis

Outliers were identified using Grubb's test and excluded from subsequent analysis. Prism 5 (GraphPad, La Jolla, CA, USA) was used to perform ANOVA or unpaired Student's *t*-tests assessing changes in means ± standard deviation of the mean (SD) of patient demographics compared to control term pregnancies and leukocyte populations between second trimester normal and high uterine artery PI cases. Data was tested for normality prior to ANOVA analysis Leukocyte populations were quantified as a percentage of total CD45$^+$ leukocytes except where specified; $p < 0.05$ or greater was considered statistically significant.

TABLE 4 | Flow cytometry and immunohistochemistry antibody information.

Antibody	Clone	Company (cat no)	Dilution/Ag Retrieval	Specificity
CD45 APC-Cy7	2D1	BD 557833	1:33	Common Leukocyte Antigen
CD3 FITC	HIT3a	BD 555339	1:25	T Lymphocytes
CD56 PE-Cy7	B159	BD 557747	1:33	Uterine Natural Killer Cells (NCAM)
CD68 PE	Y1-82A	BD 555743	1:6.6	Mac-1 Integrin (Activation Marker)
CD209 PerCP-Cy5.5	DCN-46	BD 558263	1:10	Immature Dendritic Cells (DC)
CD205 PE	MG38	BD 558069	1:25	Intermediate/Antigen Uptake Receptor DC
CD83 APC	HB15e	BD 551073	1:5	Mature Antigen Presentation DC
CK-7	OV-TL 12/30	Dako M7018	1:200 1 mM EDTA pH9. Heat	Epithelial Cells
HLA-G	4H84	Exbio 11-499-C	1:300 10 mM Na Citrate pH6. Heat	Extravillous Trophoblast
SMA	1A4	Dako M0851	1:100 10 mM Na Citrate pH6. Heat	Smooth Muscle Cells
CD31	JC70A	Dako M0823	1:50 10 mM Na Citrate pH6. Heat	Endothelial Cells
CD45	2B11+PD7/26	Dako M0701	1:100 10 mM Na Citrate pH6. Heat	Common Leukocyte Antigen
CD56/NCAM	123C3	Dako M7204	1:50 1 mM EDTA pH9. Heat	Uterine Natural Killer Cells
CD68	PG-M1	Dako M0876	1:200 10 mM Na Citrate pH6. Heat	Macrophage
CD3	F7.2.38	Dako M7254	1:50 1 mM EDTA pH9.Heat	T cells
CD4	EPR6855	Abcam Ab133616	1:200 10 mM Na Citrate pH6. Heat	T helper cells
CD8	EP1150Y	Abcam Ab93278	1:200 10 mM Na Citrate pH6. Heat	Cytotoxic T cells
CD209	120612	R and D systems MAB1621	1:200 1 mM EDTA pH9. Heat	Immature DC
CD83	HB15e	E Bioscience 14-0839-82	1:50 10 mM Na Citrate pH6. Heat	Mature Antigen Presentation DC
D240/podoplanin	730-01	Covance SIG-3730	1:50 1 mM EDTA pH9. Heat	Lymphatic endothelium
IGFBP-1	H-120	SC Biotech sc-13097	1:200 10 mM Na Citrate pH6 Heat	IGF binding protein 1
CD10	97C5	SC Biotech sc-19993	1:50 1 mM EDTA pH9. Heat	Common acute lymphocytic leukemia antigen
Mouse IgG	DAK-501	Dako X0931	1:300	Mouse Fc
Rabbit IgG	Rabbit Ig fraction	Dako X0903	1:300	Rabbit Fc

RESULTS

Failure of Uterine Vascular Transformation Is Associated With Apoptotic EVT and Altered Maternal Immune Status in IUGR Placental Bed Biopsies

In comparison to healthy term pregnancies in the control group (Normal, $n = 15$) the idiopathic IUGR patient group had; significantly higher uterine artery pulsatile indices (PI), absent (AEDV) or reversed (REDV) umbilical end-diastolic velocity in their umbilical artery, babies born at <10th %tile of weight for gestational age, and placental pathology indicative of IUGR ($n = 8$). A further 5 cases of severe IUGR were collected from women with preeclampsia defined according to the ACOG criteria, showing elevated maternal blood pressure, proteinuria and indicators of end organ damage (**Tables 1, 2**).

Uterine spiral arteries in the myometrial decidual junction of PBBx from healthy term pregnancies displayed significant disorganization and complete disruption of their vascular smooth muscle (VSMC) media and loss of the endothelium, associated with the presence of both enEVT and inEVT (**Figure 1**, Patient 1). Full transformation was associated with

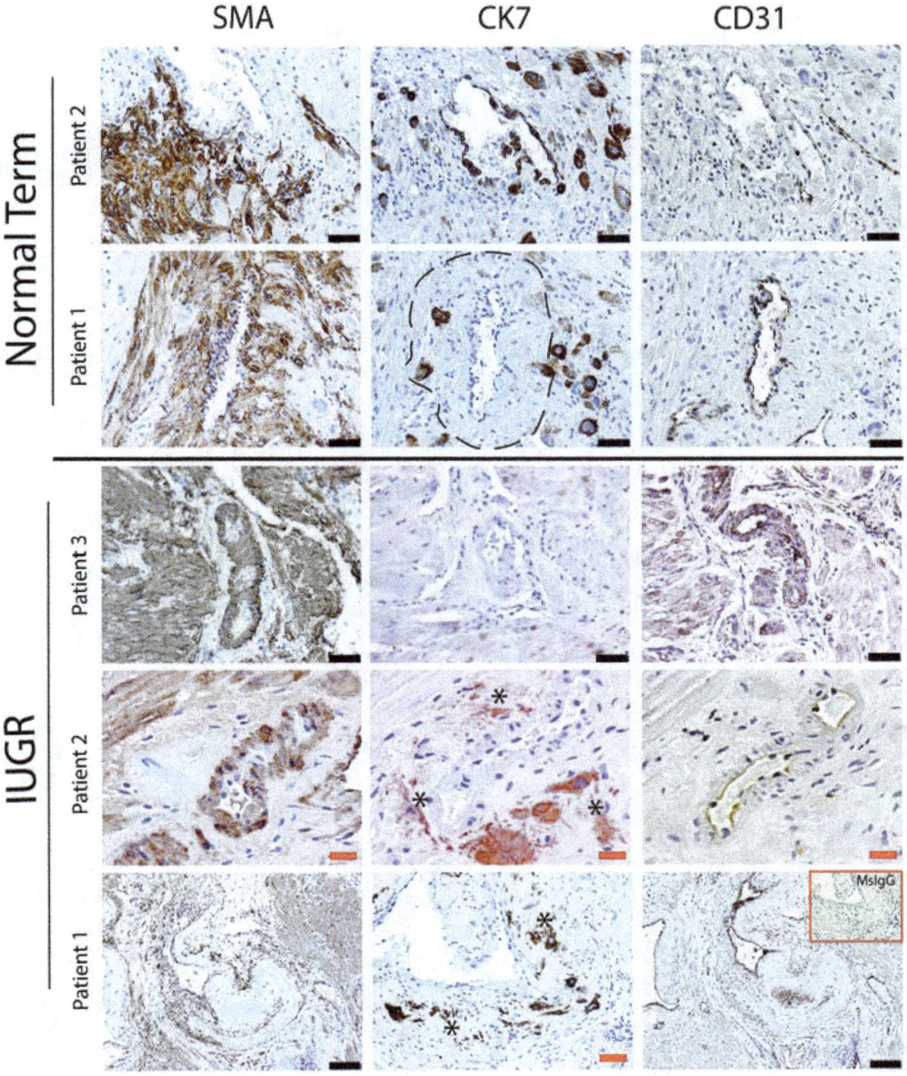

FIGURE 1 | Failed uterovascular transformation in IUGR is associated with persistance of vascular media and failure of interstitial and endovascular invasion. Immunohistochemical staining was performed to determine the degree of uterine artery transformation in PBBx biopsies using antibodies against smooth muscle actin (SMA, Column 1) cytokeratin 7 (CK7, Column 2) and PECAM (CD31, Column 3). Representative serial sections of control (n = 2/15) and IUGR PBBx (n = 3/8) uterine spiral arteries at the decidual myometrial junction are shown. Asterisks denote the presence of fragmented likely apopototic mural EVT in the IUGR cases. Fibrin deposition in the fully transformed artery is shown in patient 1 Normal marked by the hatched line. Negative control mouse IgG1 is shown in the inset lower right. Scale bars: black = 50 μM, 100x magnification; red = 20 μM, 200x.magnification.

mEVT and fibrin deposition in the arterial media (marked area, Patient 2). In contrast, and as expected, PBBx from IUGR pregnancies showed a higher number of preserved uterine arteries with thick organized vascular smooth muscle media and intact endothelium (**Figure 1**, Patients 1–3). Quantitation of all myometrial vessels across the patient subgroups showed that showed that the IUGR biopsies had significantly higher numbers of preserved arteries and a significantly lower number of destroyed vessels compared to controls ($p < 0.05$, **Figure 2**). This was associated with a lack of both inEVT and enEVT invasion into the myometrium (**Supplemental Figure 1A** and **Tables 5, 6**). Placental bed biopsies from IUGR and preeclamptic pregnancies showed a similar lack of enEVT invasion but surprisingly inEVT was unaffected and vascular transformation was not as compromised (**Figure 2, Tables 5–7**, and **Supplemental Figure 1A**). Scoring of decidual vessels and trophoblast invasion showed a small increase in preserved vessels and a low number of interstitial EVT in the IUGR samples as compared to healthy controls (**Table 5** and **Supplemental Figure 1B**).

Interestingly numbers of uterine arteries with an absence of mEVT were equal between controls and pure IUGR samples (**Table 7**). However, in the IUGR cases these mural EVT often displayed signs of fragmentation, nuclear condensation, blebbing, and loss of cytokeratin immunoreactivity, indicative of apoptosis (**Figure 1**, IUGR patient 2 and 3, asterisks). TUNEL

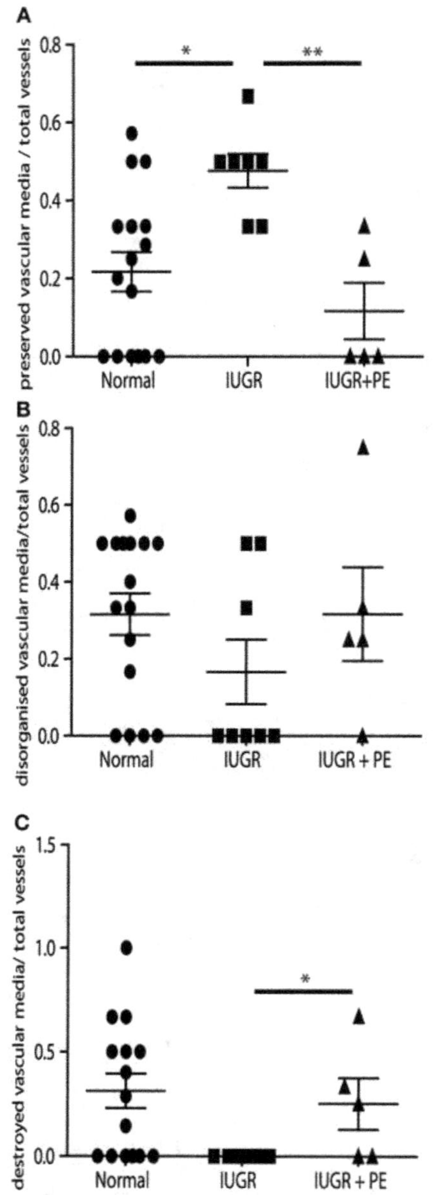

FIGURE 2 | IUGR PBBx display high numbers of preserved uterine spiral arteries. Graphs show quantitation of the degree of remodeling of all myometrial vessels control (circle), IUGR (square) and IUGR with preeclampsia (triangle) groups. Preserved vessels were scored when intact multi layered vascular smooth muscle media was present **(A)**. Disorganized vessels were scored when the vascular media was separated and smooth muscle cells were migrating away from the outer layers of the media **(B)**. Destroyed vessels were scored when all media had been lost and replaced with fibrin **(C)**. $^*p < 0.05$, $^{**}p < 0.01$.

staining confirmed that these mural EVT were indeed apoptotic (arrows) showing positive staining of condensed nuclei in the IUGR cases, however the inEVT in the decidua were unaffected. Controls did not show any TUNEL reactivity in any of the EVT subtypes (**Figure 3**).

Further investigation of the maternal leukocyte populations in the PBBx was initially undertaken by immunostaining and image

TABLE 5 | Interstitial EVT are reduced in the IUGR myometrium and decidua.

Interstitial EVT	Myometrium			Decidua	
% of vessels	Absent	Low	High	Low	High
Normal	0.00	57.14	42.86	54.55	40.91
IUGR	**89.47**	10.53	0.00	**66.67**	33.33
IUGR and PE	0.00	30.77	69.23	33.33	**66.67**

Data is presented as a percentage of all vessels in each PBBx section. Bold text indicates a significant difference from non-bold text, assessed by unpaired T-test with Welch's correction, P < 0.05.

TABLE 6 | Endovascular EVT are absent in IUGR and IUGR and PE myometrium.

Endovascular EVT	Myometrium		Decidua	
% of vessels	Present	Absent	Present	Absent
Normal	32.14	67.86	61.36	38.64
IUGR	15.79	**84.21**	57.14	42.86
IUGR and PE	7.69	**92.31**	50.00	50.00

Data is presented as a percentage of all vessels in each PBBx section. Bold text indicates a significant difference from non-bold text, assessed by unpaired T-test with Welch's correction, P < 0.05.

TABLE 7 | Intramural EVT are reduced in the IUGR decidua and myometrium.

Intramural EVT	Myometrium		Decidua	
% of vessels	Present	Absent	Present	Absent
Normal	37.50	**62.50**	**75.00**	25.00
IUGR	31.58	**68.42**	52.38	47.62
IUGR and PE	15.38	**84.62**	**83.33**	16.67

Data is presented as a percentage of all vessels in each PBBx section. Bold text indicates a significant difference from non-bold text, assessed by unpaired T-test with Welch's correction, P < 0.05.

analysis to count the numbers of $CD45^+$ leukocytes present in the decidua vs. the myometrium (**Figure 4A**). Predominantly leukocytes were found in the decidua, while the few leukocytes observed in the myometrium were usually associated with the vascular plexus of the uterine vasculature (**Figure 4B**). When we compared the biopsies from the placental site (decidua basalis) with the non-placental site (decidua paretalis in the control samples we found there was no difference in the number of CD45+ leukocytes (data not shown). In contrast the numbers of CD45+ leukocytes were shown to be significantly lower in the IUGR decidua basalis as compared to control ($p < 0.001$) (**Figure 4C**). There was no significant difference between IUGR and IUGR complicated by preeclampsia. However, decidua from severe early onset preeclampsia with a normal weight baby (for gestational age) showed a significantly higher number of leukocytes in comparison to all other groups ($p < 0.0001$). In serial sections $CD45^+$ leukocytes were more commonly observed in dense clusters in the IUGR placental bed biopsies, and in close association with the apoptotic mural EVT (**Figure 4D**). Identification of the immune cell subtypes in these clusters showed the presence of immunoreactive CD68$^+$ macrophage, CD3$^+$ T cells and both immature CD209$^+$ and mature CD83$^+$ dendritic cells (arrows) (**Figure 4D**, IUGR Patient 1 and 2 matches to **Figure 1**). In control placental bed biopsies leukocytes were not found in association with mural EVT in the fibrin matrix of transformed vessels and mature CD83 dendritic cells were very infrequent (**Supplemental Figure 2**).

Failed Decidualization and Immune Dysregulation in the 2nd Trimester Is Associated With High Uterine Artery PI and Growth Retardation

To gain insight into the origin of the failed vascular transformation and potential immune dysregulation observed in the third trimester IUGR samples we collected decidua from women undergoing 2nd trimester termination for medical reasons. Prior to the surgical procedure uterine artery Doppler analysis was performed. Patients were grouped by uterine artery Doppler indices specific to the 2nd trimester into normal ($n = 6$), and high uterine artery PI (>1.6) with early end-diastolic notches ($n = 6$) which has been shown to be associated with an increased incidence of preeclampsia at this time point in gestation (49). Fetal abnormalities were chromosomal (T21, T18), genetic (Turners syndrome, Amniotic band syndrome, or 48XY deletion) or no fetal heartbeat. Interestingly when patient data was collated 4 of the 6 high uterine artery PI group had small for gestational age (SGA) fetuses (fetal size was assessed crown to rump length by ultrasound and was noted as expected size of 2 weeks earlier than actual gestational age). In this study we have designated this group as high uterine artery PI and small for gestational age (SGA). We do however acknowledge that we cannot exclude an effect of the fetal abnormality on the fetal size due to the small size of the patient groups; only one pregnancy was terminated at 18-weeks for pure severe IUGR. The control group had normal uterine artery indices and all fetuses were of the expected size for gestational age. Equal numbers and types of fetal abnormality were found in each group (**Table 3**).

Uterovascular remodeling and 2nd trimester decidual leukocyte populations were assessed by immunolocalization, image analysis and multi-color flow cytometry studies. In the 2nd trimester control group interstitial trophoblast staining positively for both CK7 and the EVT marker HLA-G were observed in the walls of Stage III actively remodeling decidual arterioles that had disrupted VSMC and lost their endothelial cells (**Figure 5**, top panel 18 weeks normal). Fully transformed Stage IV vessels were also observed lined with enEVT. As we have previously shown in the first trimester (34), this active vascular transformation was associated with the presence of uNK and macrophage within the vessel wall (lower panel 18 weeks normal). Significant numbers of CD3$^+$ T cells were also observed in association with the vessels.

In contrast the decidua from the high uterine artery PI SGA group was characterized by the presence of InEVT in association with the vasculature, but no enEVT were observed (**Figure 5**, lower 2 panels). In 2 SGA cases abnormal smooth muscle actin staining was seen in the DSCs and arterioles maintained their VSMC wall and intact endothelium. Most importantly, we consistently observed an increased number of small lymphatic vessels leukocytes marked by both CD31 and D240/podoplanin expression (black arrow, SGA and red arrow, IUGR). Moreover, abnormal D240/podoplanin expression lining the DSCs was also observed in the high uterine artery and SGA cases These micro-lymphatics between the DSC are densely packed with CD56$^+$ uNK, CD68$^+$ macrophage and CD3$^+$ T cells (**Figure 5**, 18 weeks SGA and high magnification 18 weeks IUGR). Indeed, the majority of the decidual leukocytes appear to be restricted within the lymphatic vasculature in the high PI SGA cases and were not distributed in the decidual stroma, or associated with transforming vessels, as they are in normal pregnancies. In the IUGR case trophoblast were also observed within the lymphatic vasculature (CK, arrow).

Further investigation of the decidual leukocyte subsets by flow cytometry showed that numbers of total CD45$^+$ leukocytes, CD56$^+$ uNK, and CD68$^+$ macrophage were not different between normal and high uterine artery PI SGA groups and conformed to expected ratios in the second trimester when gated within either total live cells or the CD45$^+$ leukocyte population (CD56$^+$ uNK at 50–60% and CD68$^+$ macrophage at 10–20%, **Figure 6A**). In contrast, numbers of CD3$^+$ T cells were doubled in the high uterine artery with SGA fetuses' groups as compared to the controls (13.57 vs. 7.23%, $p < 0.01$, **Figure 6B**) when gated within the CD45$^+$ population. This significant increase was not seen in the total cell comparison, probably due to an increase in numbers of small DSCs in the high uterine artery PI SGA group (observed in the image analysis of DSCs described below). The T cell subpopulations were further investigated by immunostaining serial sections of decidua with anti-CD4 and antiCD8 antibodies and quantifying T cell number using image analysis. In comparison to controls the high uterine artery PI SGA group had significantly higher numbers of cytotoxic CD8$^+$ T cells ($p < 0.001$, **Figure 6C**) and a significantly decreased CD4/CD8 ratio (1.61 ± 0.39 vs. 1.212 ± 0.35, $p = 0.0028$). Both CD4$^+$ and CD8$^+$ T cells were found in increased density in the SGA cases surrounding untransformed uterine spiral arteries (arrows, **Figure 6D**). In the controls CD4$^+$ T cells were associated with the transforming vessels but CD8$^+$ T cells were very small and infrequent **Figure 6D**, arrows).

The maturation status of decidual dendritic populations was assessed in more detail in the high granular CD45$^+$ gate by flow cytometry using CD209/DC-SIGN (immature), CD205 (intermediate), and CD83 (mature antigen presenting) antibodies. A representative comparison of 18 weeks normal and high Uterine artery PI SGA cases is shown in **Figure 7A**. As can be seen, and as we have previously shown (27), dendritic cells in the normal 2nd trimester decidua are maintained in an immature state only expressing CD209 and CD205. In contrast the high uterine artery PI IUGR case shows the appearance of a significant CD205$^+$ CD83$^+$ population that is absent in the control (45.96 vs. 3.58%). Quantification within the CD45 gate across all cases in the respective groups showed that the increase in numbers of CD83$^+$ mature dendritic cells was common to the high Uterine artery PI SGA group (**Figure 7B**, $p < 0.001$).

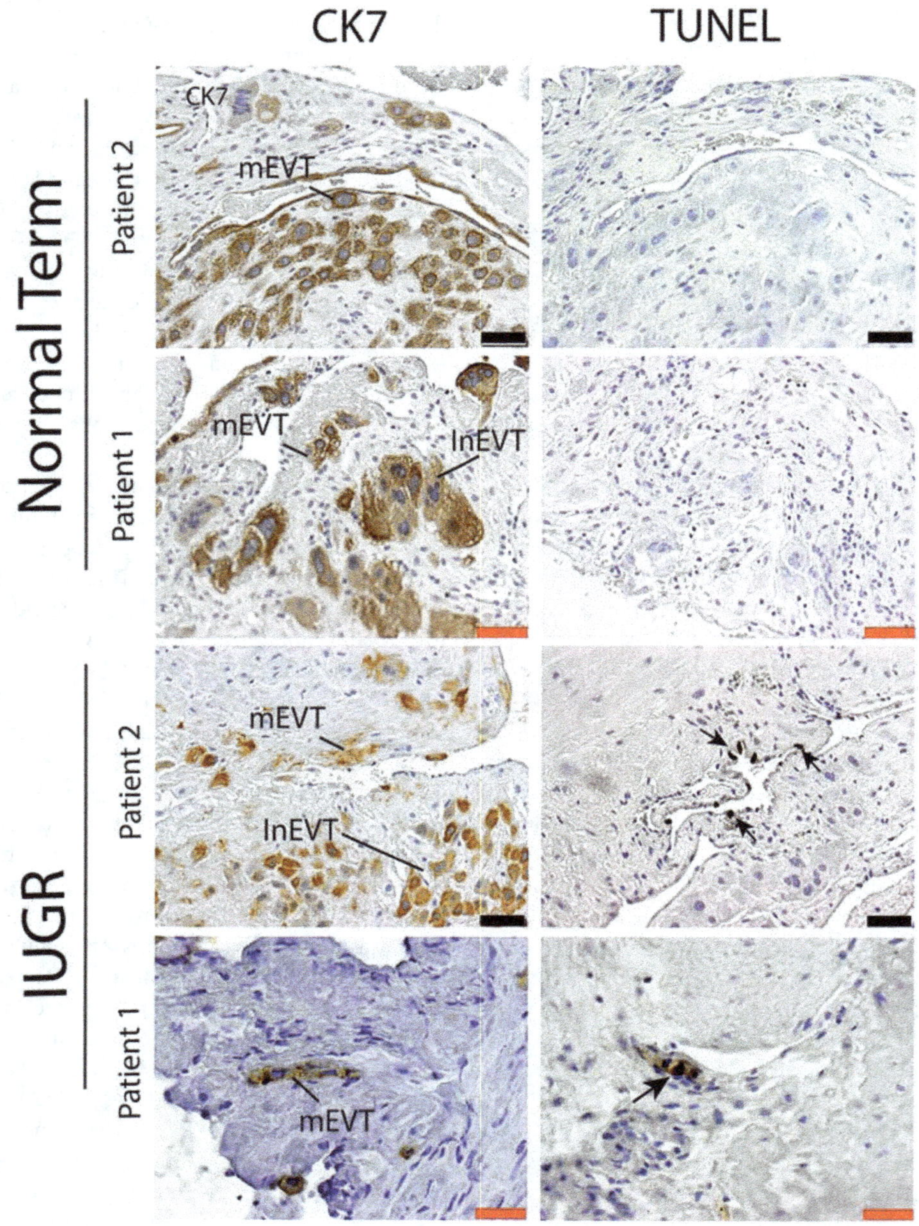

FIGURE 3 | Failed uterovascular transformation in IUGR is associated with the presence of apoptotic mural EVT. Immunohistochemical staining for cytokeratin 7 (CK7, Column 1) and Terminal deoxynucleotidyl transferase dUTP nick end labeling (TUNEL, Column 2) was perfomed to confirm that the fragmented mural EVT that we observed in the IUGR cases were apoptotic. Representative serial sections of control ($n = 2/15$) and IUGR PBBx ($n = 2/8$) uterine spiral arteries at the decidual myometrial junction are shown. Arrows indicate the TUNEL positively nuclei of the mural EVT (mEVT) showing cytokeratin loss in the matching serial sections in the IUGR samples. No TUNEL staining was seen in the interstitial EVT (inEVT) of the IUGR cases or any of the EVT populations of the control term samples. Scale bars: black = 50 μM, 100x magnification; red = 20 μM, 200x.magnification.

These CD83^{+} dendritic cells were observed in leukocyte clusters in association with unremodeled vessels and in lymphatic vessels in the high uterine artery PI SGA cases (**Figure 7C**, SGA, arrows).

Correlation of the above results supported our hypothesis that the initial failure of early decidualization may underlie the resulting uteroplacental pathology of severe IUGR. To investigate this final step in our hypothesis we investigated DSC differentiation status using 3 markers. Progesterone is known to play a key role in the decidualization of DSCs by binding to its nuclear receptor PR-B (50). IGFBP-1 is expressed by DSC as they differentiate to their secretory phenotype (51) and CD10 is expressed by mature DSC (52). To investigate if lower levels of these DSC markers correlated with the above changes in the high uterine artery PI decidua, we performed immunostaining and image analysis to count the numbers of PR-B positive nuclei in the DSC or quantify the intensity of staining in the IGFBP-1 and CD10 slides. DSC size was also quantified by ellipsoid area measurements of 3 random fields

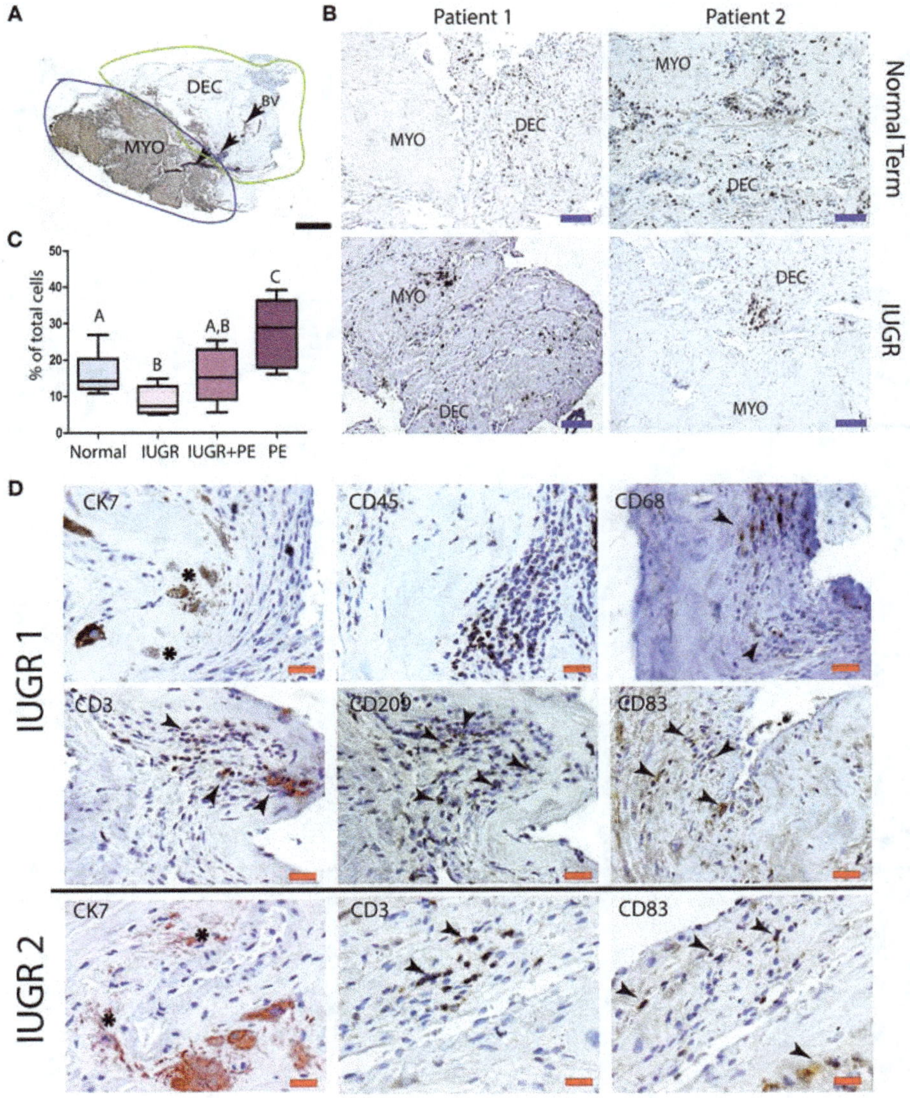

FIGURE 4 | Low decidual leukocyte number and increased mature dendritic cells in association with apoptotic EVT in IUGR. Visiopharm Newcast image analysis system was used to define decidual and myometrial regions based on smooth muscle actin staining of the myometrium **(A)**. Representative stained decidual and myometrial sections from normal term PBBx upper panel and IUGR PBBx lower panel **(B)**. Numbers of brown stained CD45+ leukocytes and blue hematoxylin stained decidual stromal cells or myometrial muscle cells were counted in corresponding serial sections across 5% of the respective region using Visiopharm Newcast image analysis system and random meander sampling **(C)**: Normal $n = 15$, IUGR $n = 8$, IUGR and PE $n = 5$, PE $n = 8$) ($^{A,B}p < 0.01$, $^{A-C}p < 0.0001$, $^{B,C}p < 0.001$). Representative serial sections of IUGR PBBx show that the apoptotic mural EVT (CK7, asterisks) that were observed in these biopsies were associated with leukocyte clusters (CD45) containing CD68+ macrophage and elevated number of CD3 T cells and CD83+ mature dendritic cells (**D**, arrows). Scale bars: black = 500 μM, 20x magnification, blue = 250 μM, 40x magnification, red = 20 μM, 200x.magnification.

of each decidual section (**Figure 8A**). Control 2nd trimester decidua was characterized by large plump pale DSC with large pale nuclei, known to be indicative of a highly active cell. In contrast, the decidual cells of the decidua were physically much smaller, stained more intensely with hematoxylin and displayed small dark staining nuclei. Area measurements showed that control DSC were much larger than decidual cells from the high uterine artery PI SGA cases (930.8 ± 116.6 vs. 670.7 ± 175.9, $p < 0.05$). In the 2 SGA cases showing the decidua also displayed elongated rectangular cells arranged in bands separated by ECM that also expressed abnormal focal points of SMA (**Figure 8D**). Many gaps were also observed between the decidual cells in the high uterine artery PI decidua corresponding to the elevated number of lymphatic vessels reported above (**Figure 8D,** arrow). In the markers of decidualization analysis more DSC expressed strong nuclear PR-B staining in the control normal samples (38.84 ± 2.57% vs. 23.56 ± 6.66%, $p < 0.0001$) (**Figure 8C**). Interestingly IGFBP-1 was restricted to areas surrounding the uterine spiral arteries in 14 and 15 weeks samples and increased to the majority of control DSC at 17–19 weeks of

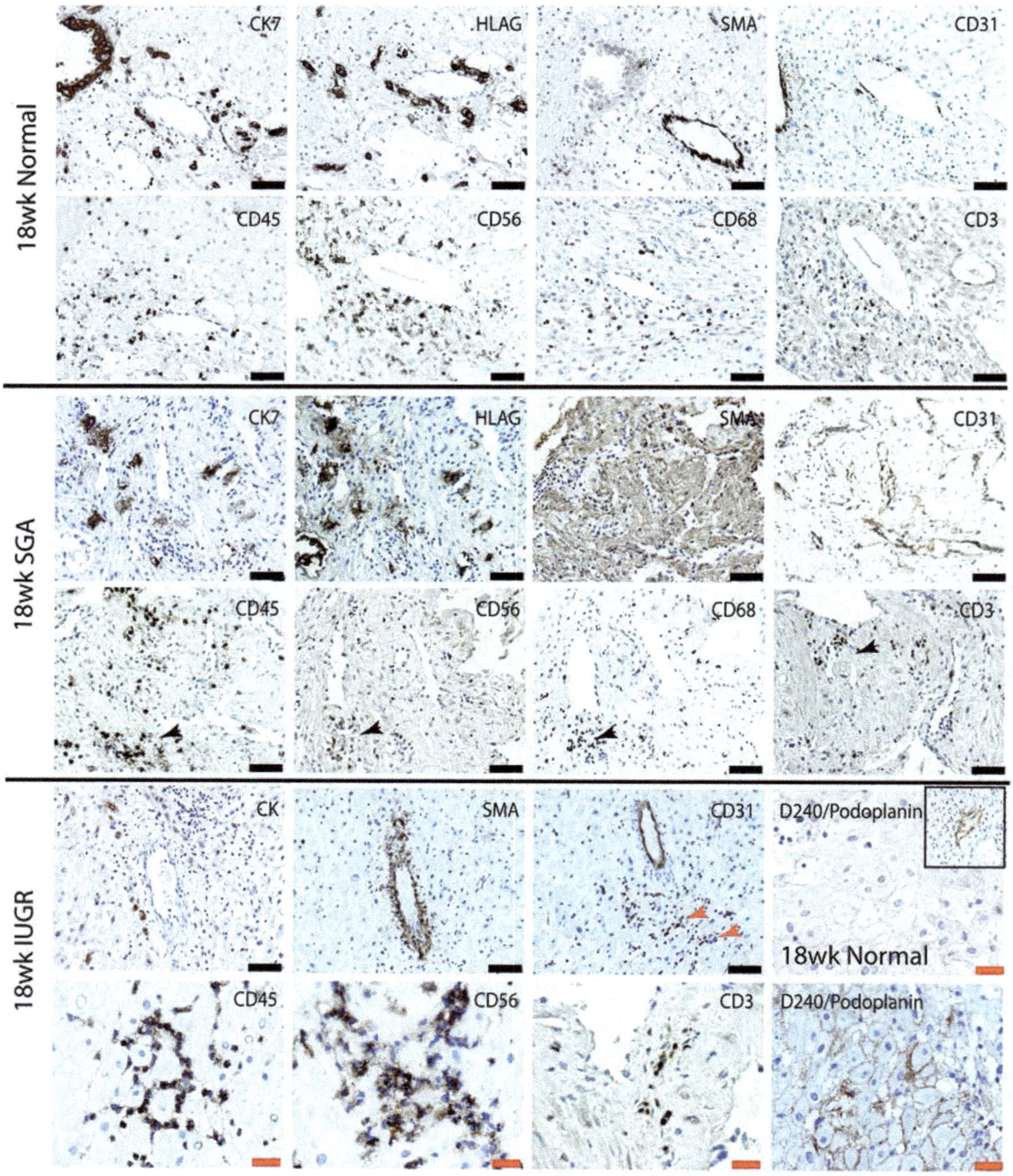

FIGURE 5 | Lymphatic vessel density is increased, and leukocytes are abnormally distributed in the high uterine artery PI SGA decidua. Representative serial sections from normal 18 week trimester decidua (top panel), an 18 week high uterine artery PI SGA case (middle panel) and a 18 week high uterine artery case of IUGR (lower panel) stained with antibodies against CK7 (trophoblast) HLAG (EVT), SMA (VSMC), CD31 (endothelial), CD45 (leukocytes) CD56 (uNK) CD68 (macrophage and CD3 (T cells). Lymphatic vessels were identified by staining with D240/podoplanin (lower right 2 images control and IUGR). In the SGA high numbers of small CD31 vessels full of leukocytes were seen (black arrows) In the IUGR decidua this was more pronounced (red arrow), abnormal D240 podoplanin lymphatic endothelial expression was found surrounding the DSC (lower right panel) creating micro-lymphatic vessels that were packed with uNK (CD56) and T cells (CD3). In controls the DSC were negative and only the larger lymphatic vessels stained positive (inset). Scale bars: black = 50 μM, 100x magnification, red= 20μM, 200x magnification.

gestation (**Figure 8C**). CD10 was similarly expressed throughout the cytoplasm of control DSC (**Figure 8D**). In contrast both IGFBP-1 and CD10 levels were significantly reduced, sporadic, or undetectable in the high uterine artery PI SGA decidua (**Figures 8C,D**).

DISCUSSION

In summary this paper has shown that PBBx from idiopathic IUGR pregnancies with abnormal uterine artery PI (>1.5) demonstrate a higher number of intact uterine spiral arteries,

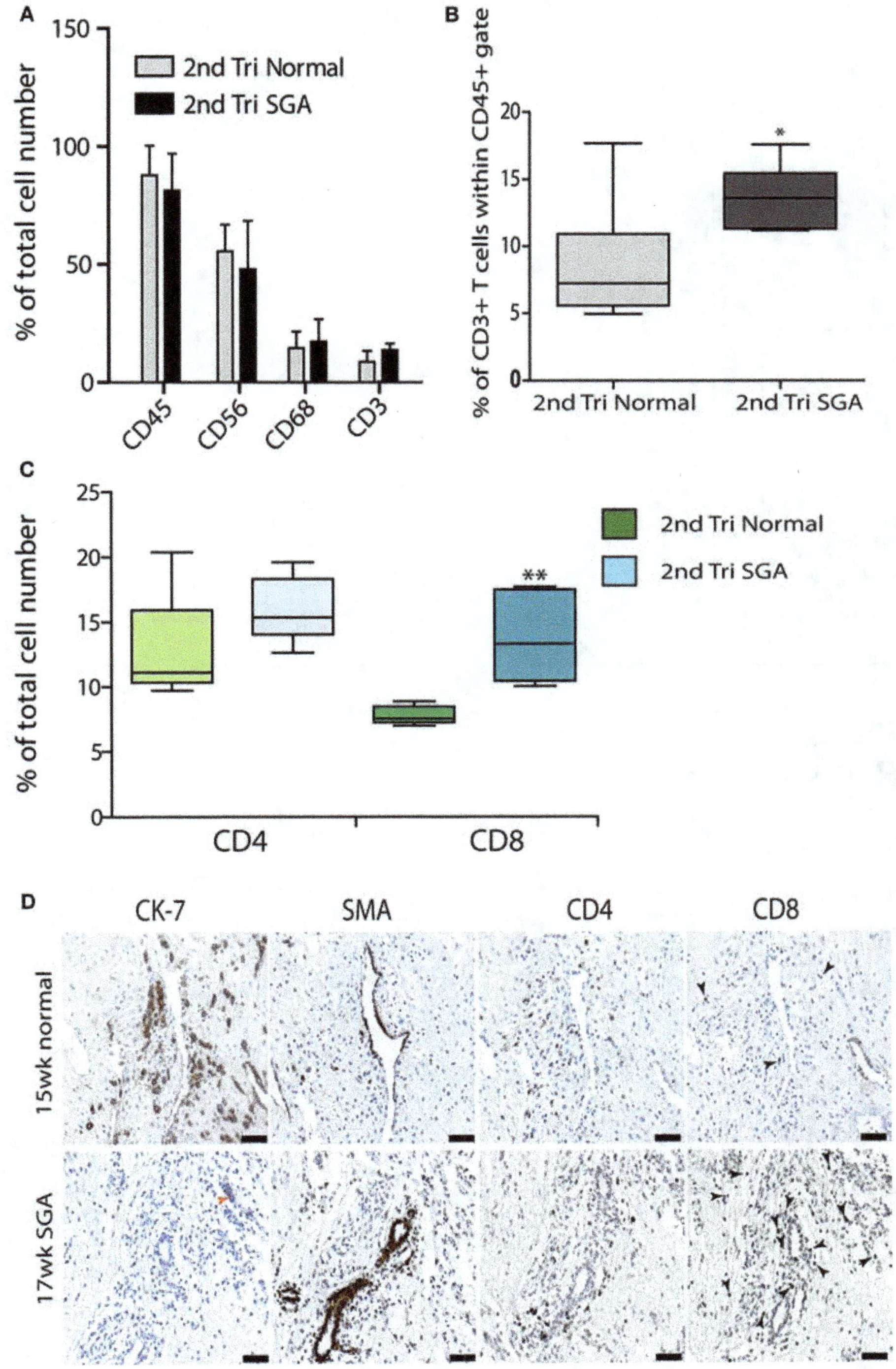

FIGURE 6 | Elevated cytotoxic $CD8^+$ T cells in 2nd trimester high Uterine artery PI and SGA decidua. Multicolored flow cytometry analysis of leukocyte subsets isolated from 2nd trimester normal or high uterine artery PI (>1.6) of decidua. Numbers of $CD45^+$ leukocytes, $CD56^{++}$ uNK, and $CD68^+$ macrophage were no different between groups **(A)**. CD3+ T cells gated within the $CD45^+$ population were doubled in the high uterine artery PI decidua **(B)**. Visiopharm Newcast image analysis system and random meander sampling was used to quantify numbers of $CD4^+$ T cells and $CD8^+$ T cells in 5% of the total tissue area of each decidual section. Percentages of the total cell number were calculated and are presented as box whisker plots in **(C)**. Representative serial sections from a 15-week normal sample (upper panel) and a 17-week high uterine artery PI SGA) stained with CK7, SMA CD4 and CD8 antibodies are shown in **(D)** (arrows identify CD8+ T cells). $^*p < 0.05$, $^{**}p < 0.01$, $n = 6$ in each group. Scale bars = 20 μM, 200x magnification.

a failure of both interstitial and endovascular invasion into the decidual myometrial junction, and high numbers of apoptotic mural and interstitial EVT. Numbers of decidual leukocytes were lower in IUGR, while mature $CD83^+$ dendritic and $CD3^+$ T cells were found in clusters in association with apoptotic EVT in the myometrial portions of these vessels. In the 2nd trimester

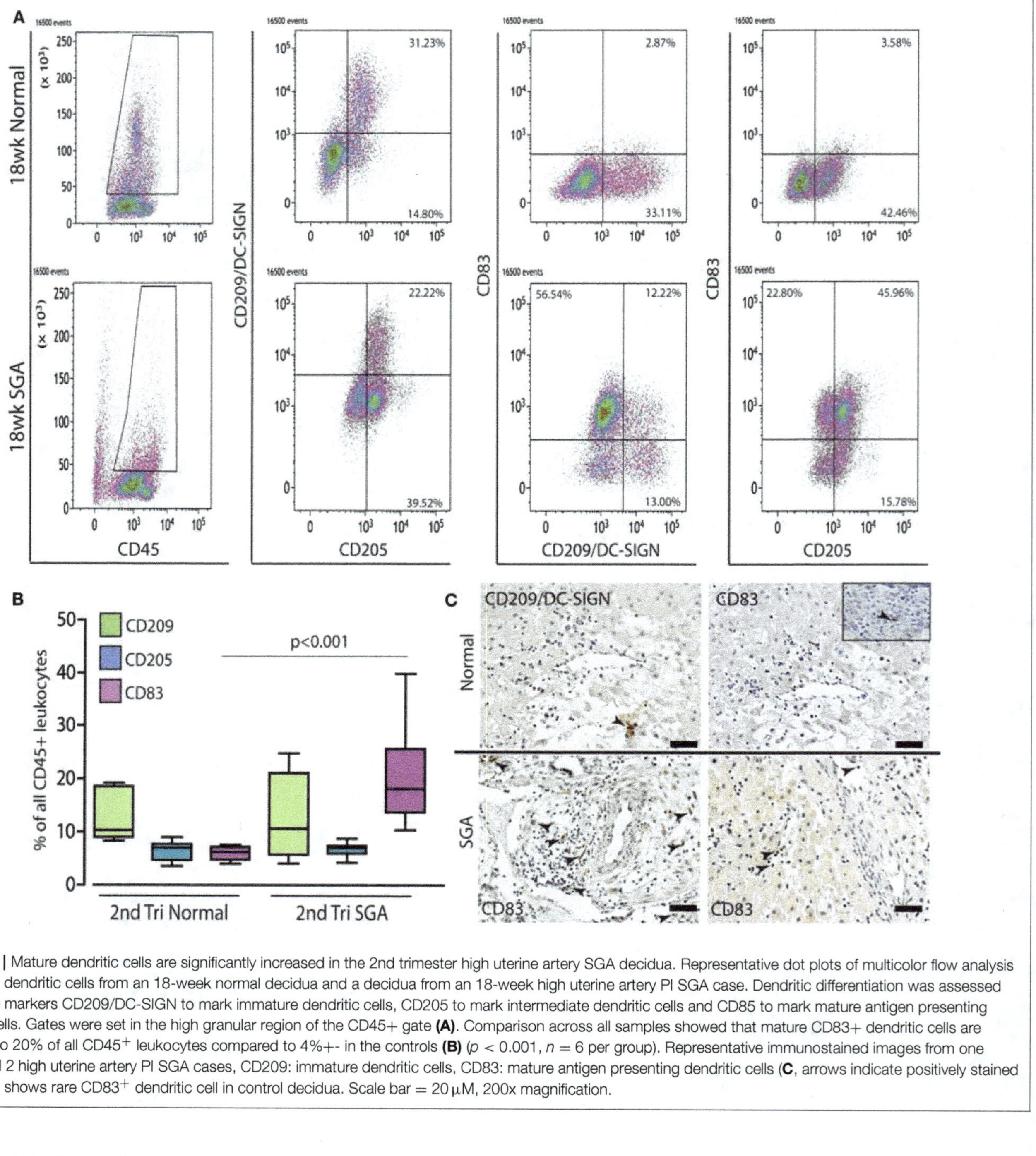

FIGURE 7 | Mature dendritic cells are significantly increased in the 2nd trimester high uterine artery SGA decidua. Representative dot plots of multicolor flow analysis of decidual dendritic cells from an 18-week normal decidua and a decidua from an 18-week high uterine artery PI SGA case. Dendritic differentiation was assessed using three markers CD209/DC-SIGN to mark immature dendritic cells, CD205 to mark intermediate dendritic cells and CD85 to mark mature antigen presenting dendritic cells. Gates were set in the high granular region of the CD45+ gate **(A)**. Comparison across all samples showed that mature CD83+ dendritic cells are increased to 20% of all CD45$^+$ leukocytes compared to 4%+- in the controls **(B)** ($p < 0.001$, $n = 6$ per group). Representative immunostained images from one control and 2 high uterine artery PI SGA cases, CD209: immature dendritic cells, CD83: mature antigen presenting dendritic cells (**C**, arrows indicate positively stained cells). Inset shows rare CD83$^+$ dendritic cell in control decidua. Scale bar = 20 μM, 200x magnification.

decidua with high uterine artery PI (>1.6) and SGA fetuses we similarly observed elevated numbers of CD8$^+$ T cells and mature CD205$^+$ CD83$^+$ dendritic cells. Most surprisingly we observed that these high uterine artery PI cases were characterized by increased numbers of lymphatic micro vessels that were packed with decidual leukocytes and a lower expression of markers of mature secretory DSC. Collectively these results provide the first direct evidence that failed progesterone mediated decidualization of the DSCs in early pregnancy leads to (1) persistence of the endometrial lymphatic vessels, (2) a failure of the DSC to recruit the leukocytes into the decidual stroma, and (3) a failure of EVT invasion and developmental maternal immune tolerance in cases of idiopathic IUGR.

Our findings regarding the lack of endovascular EVT invasion in the placental bed biopsies from idiopathic IUGR pregnancies with known abnormal uterine PI suggest that this feature is common with that of pregnancies complicated by hypertension and preeclampsia (3, 5, 15). However, there is some discrepancy regarding the complete lack of interstitial myometrial invasion that we observed in this study. Interstitial EVT were present

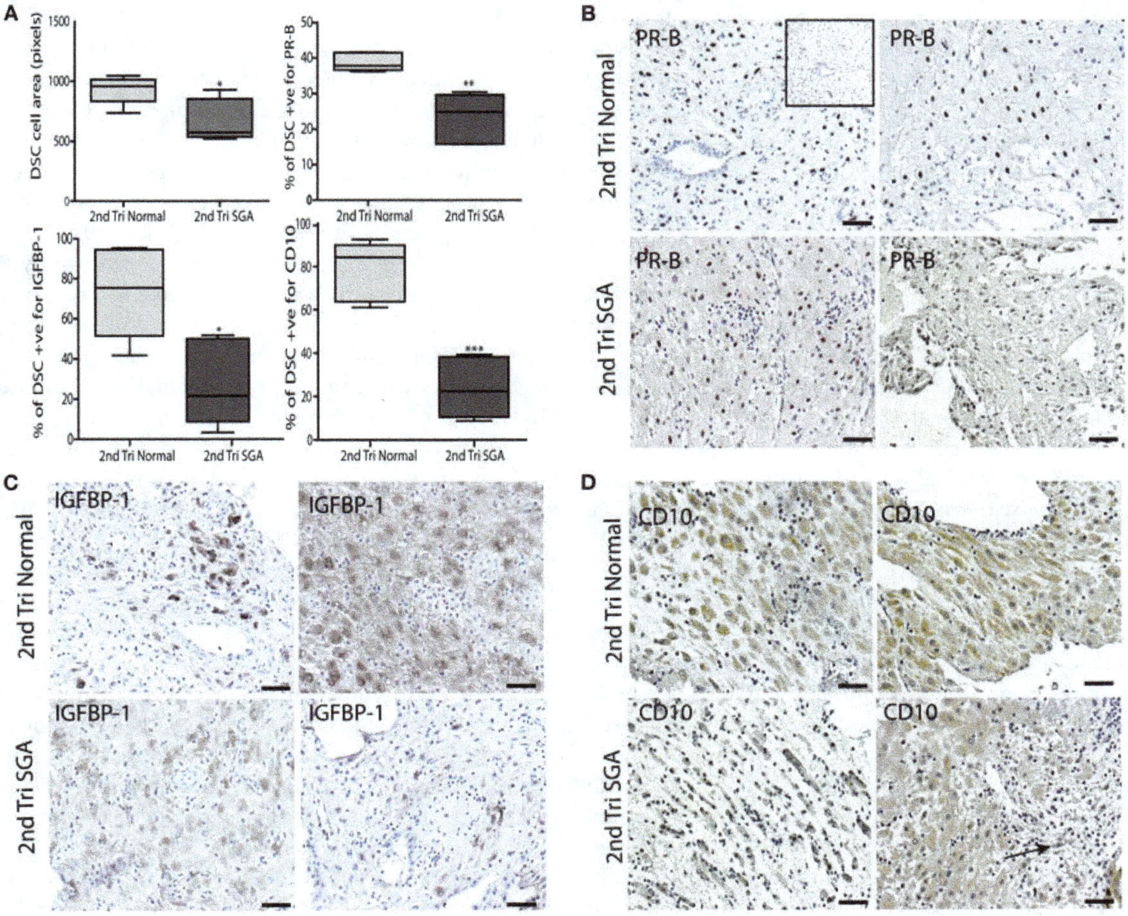

FIGURE 8 | DSC differentiation fails in the 2nd trimester high uterine artery PI SGA decidua. **(A)** DSC cell area was measured using the random ellipsoid measurement tool from the Olympus Cellsens software. Immunohistochemical image analysis was performed on serial decidual sections stained with antibodies against the decidual markers PR-B, IGFBP-1, and CD10. Visiopharm Newcast image analysis system and random meander sampling was used to quantify numbers of positively stained DSC in 5% of the total tissue area of each decidual section. Percentages of the total cell number were calculated and are presented as box whisker plots in **(A)**. Representative photographs of serial sections from 2normal 2nd trimester decidua (top panels), and 2 high uterine artery PI SGA cases (lower panels) in each case are shown stained with PR-B **(B)**, IGFBP-1**(C)** and CD10 **(D)** antibodies (arrow indicates area of increased lymphatic vessel density). $^{*}p < 0.05$, $^{**}p < 0.01$, $^{***}p < 0.0001$, $n = 6$ in each group. Inset shows no staining with the Rabbit IgG negative control. Scale bar = 50 μM, 100x magnification.

at low levels in all decidual tissues associated with the IUGR biopsies but appeared to be unable to penetrate the myometrium and many accumulated and fused at the decidual myometrial junction. There is a paucity of studies on PBBx from pure idiopathic IUGR as compared to mixed cases. In a similar study to ours, Lyall et al. contrastingly reported an increase in interstitial EVT density in association with both decidual and myometrial vessels in fetal growth restriction as compared to PE and controls (14). In their study, only 60% of patients in the growth restricted groups displayed a mean uterine artery PI >95th percentile or bilateral notching, while in our study we specifically collected idiopathic IUGR cases with confirmed elevated and abnormal uterine artery PI (>1.5), this may account for the differences between the two studies. In contrast to the pure IUGR cases, the combined IUGR and preeclamptic biopsies in the current study did demonstrate high levels of interstitial invasion into the myometrium suggesting a distinct etiology of pure IUGR. Interestingly EVT from IUGR placenta have been shown to express lower levels of the VCAM-1, alpha 2 beta 1, alpha 3 beta 1, and alpha 5 beta 1 integrin's but much higher levels of intercellular adhesion molecule 3 (ICAM3) than EVT from normal pregnancies (53). The downregulation of these integrin's is likely to negatively affect the ability of the EVT to interact with collagen, laminin and fibronectin, all major extracellular matrix components of the myometrium and decidua, and thus may underlie to inability of the EVT to penetrate the myometrium. Interestingly ICAM3 binds to DCSIGN/CD209+ immature dendritic cells that are found in the decidua, suggesting that it's over expression may lead to changes in the immunological reactions between the mother and the developing fetus and placenta.

During human pregnancy the semi-allogeneic/allogeneic fetal graft is normally accepted by the mother's immune system. Initially the contact between maternal and fetal cells is restricted to the decidua and depends on the reaction between KIR, and NKp receptors on the maternal uNK with paternally-derived non-self-human leukocyte antigens (HLA) class I and class I allotypes (54–56). In our quantitative study decidual leukocytes were shown to be lower in IUGR pregnancies but higher in preeclampsia. We suggest that this is likely to be reflective of a reported decrease in the numbers of uNK in the term IUGR decidua (41). Correlation of this data with the observed increase in the numbers of preserved or partially remodeled decidual vessels, and decreased numbers of enEVT (**Supplemental Figure 1B**) suggests that this critical interaction of EVT and uNK in early tolerance and decidual vascular transformation is compromised in IUGR.

In the myometrium maternal allo-recognition of the fetus depends on avoidance of maternal T cells recognizing and responding to fetal antigen, due to the restriction of the $CD56^+$ uNK to the decidual compartment (57). It is also known that in response to trophoblast-secreted factors, decidual $CD209^+$ dendritic cells induce differentiation of $CD4^+CD25^-$ T cells into a $CD4^+CD25^+FOXP3^+$ Treg population capable of inhibiting $CD4^+$ T lymphocyte proliferation (58). In our study we observed apoptotic TUNEL positive mural EVT near maternal leukocyte clusters of macrophage, mature $CD83^+$ antigen presenting dendritic cells and $CD3^+$ T cells. Recently depletion or malfunction of T cell populations has been associated with recurrent spontaneous abortion and incidence of preeclampsia (59, 60) and higher numbers of $CD209^+$ and $CD83^+$ DC have been reported in the preeclamptic placental bed (61). Correlation of these studies suggests that the maternal response against the trophoblast may be hostile and excessive in all of these placental pathologies. This is further supported by our quantification of decidual leukocyte populations in the second trimester with high uterine artery PI and SGA fetuses where we found a significant increase in the numbers of cytotoxic $CD8^+$ T cells and mature $CD83^+$ dendritic cells as compared to the control group. Mature CD83+ dendritic cells are capable of presenting fetal antigen to the adaptive immune cells (62). We have previously shown that in healthy 2nd trimester pregnancy the proportion of $CD3^+$ T cells doubles from 1st to 2nd second trimester from 10 to 20% of all $CD45^+$ leukocytes in the decidua and is predominated by Th2 $CD4^+$ and Th1 $CD8^+$ populations, while decidual dendritic cells are maintained in an immature status (27). In the current study the control samples similarly displayed a normal CD4:CD8 ratio (i.e., close to 2 while the high uterine artery PI SGA cases displayed a ratio of 1.21 due to the elevation in CD8+ T cells; this change in T cell ratio is indicative of altered immune function, and chronic inflammation (63). Thus, we suggest that the results in the current study support the hypothesis of activation of the maternal immune system against the fetus and placenta in these cases of maternal idiopathic IUGR. Elevation of CD8 T cells has also previously been reported in the maternal peripheral circulation in cases of IUGR (64). Furthermore, these findings suggest a contributory mechanism to the increased incidence of villitis of unknown origin (VUE), an inflammatory condition of the placenta characterized by maternal T cell infiltrates in the villous stroma in fetal growth restriction and stillbirth (65, 66). In our patient group two of eight IUGR placentas displayed signs of VUE.

The second trimester decidua with high uterine artery PI also provided an unexpected insight into the potential global decidual contribution to the utero-placental pathology of IUGR. It should however be noted that although 4 of 6 cases were shown to be 2 weeks smaller than expected for their gestational age (thus designated as SGA) we cannot conclusively say that these pregnancies, if healthy, would have progressed to IUGR rather than preeclampsia as elevated uterine artery PI has been shown to be predictive for the onset of preeclampsia (49). The most surprising finding in these cases was the persistence of significant numbers of micro-lymphatic podoplanin positive vessels in association with the decidual spiral arterioles. In the basal layer of the non-pregnant endometrium lymphatic vessels are reported to be closely associated with the spiral arterioles (67) and to regress with the onset of perivascular decidualization of the DSC in the late secretory phase such that they are rarely observed in the decidua (68–71). Higher numbers of lymphatic vessels have also been recently found in the decidua of recurrent spontaneous abortions (72), suggestive of a common defect in decidualization in these conditions. In the high uterine artery PI and SGA cases the lymphatic vessels were also packed with decidual leukocytes of uNK, macrophage and T cell lineages, while very few leukocytes were seen in the decidual stroma as is normally observed. Differentiated DSC cells secrete numerous chemokines critical to the recruitment and trafficking of these leukocyte subsets out of the lymphatics and into the stroma, where they play key role in early vascular transformation (21). This again suggested that the decidualization of the DSC was compromised in the high uterine artery PI and SGA cases. Of note, in addition to invading and transforming the uterine arteries EVT have also recently been shown to invade the walls and endothelium of veins and glands and lymphatic vessels in the decidua basalis (72–74). We also observed EVT in venous and lymphatic vessels in both control and high uterine artery PI and SGA cases (**Figure 5**).

Progesterone is known to play a key role in decidualization of the stromal cells and its effects are primarily mediated via its PR-B receptor. A recent study has shown that in human endometrial stromal cells, PR-B regulates a significantly larger transcriptome than PR-A occupying unique binding sites associated with suppression of cell cycle regulators and induction of angiogenic growth factors and chemokine expression known to be critical in DSC interactions with trophoblast and immune cells (50). In this study we have shown for the first time progesterone responsiveness is decreased in 2nd trimester high uterine artery PI SGA decidua as compared to normal PI controls. The stromal cells of these cases were much smaller and displayed abnormal cellular morphology and far fewer expressed nuclear PR-B and lower levels of the DSC markers IGFBP-1 and CD10. Moreover, PR-B and IGFBP-1 was absent in the most abnormal growth restricted cases expressing SMA in the decidua. The mechanisms underlying PR-B dysregulation are not known however defective menstrual conditioning or epigenetic modulation of PR-B expression has been proposed (75, 76). Interestingly both estrogen and progesterone levels have recently been shown to be lower in the serum of IUGR pregnancies than healthy controls (77), and a recent mouse model of stress induced IUGR has also shown that pregnant dams exhibited reduced progesterone levels and placental heme oxygenase 1 (Hmox1) expression and an increase in cytotoxic CD8+ T cells (78). We therefore conclude, in accordance with the hypothesis proposed by Pijnenborg et al. (30), that progesterone mediated decidualization is negatively affected in cases of high Uterine artery PI and SGA. Interestingly, 7 out of 8 patients in our IUGR PBBx group had either recurrent IUGR or high gravidity but low parity ($G > 3$, $P < 1$) suggestive of a recurrent problem with decidualization, implantation or maintenance of pregnancy.

In conclusion, we have shown that failure of the first step of progesterone mediated DSC decidualization has a fundamental and detrimental effect on all subsequent stages of decidual development in the second trimester. The regression of the decidual lymphatics, migration of the immune cells into the decidual stroma, maternal adaptive immune tolerance, EVT invasion and trophoblast-leukocyte mediated uterovascular transformation were all compromised. Correlation of these findings with our observations in placental bed biopsies supports the hypothesis that defective decidualization leads to the uteroplacental pathology observed in cases of IUGR.

AUTHOR CONTRIBUTIONS

CD and SL conceptualized the research program and secured the grant funding. CD, CM, SK, JK, and SL conceived and designed the placental bed biopsy study. CD, LH, RJ, and WW conceived and designed the second trimester study. CD, JW, AH, MK, and SW performed the experiments and analyzed the data. CM, WW, and JK recruited and consented patients. CD and CM wrote the manuscript. LH, CD, AH, and CM revised the manuscript. All authors read the manuscript and approved its submission.

FUNDING

The study was supported by grants to CD and SL from the Canadian Institutes of Health Research CIHR MOP-86322, CIHR MOP-82811, and FDN-143262. JW, MK, and AH were all recipients of the Richard Venn and Carol Mitchell Graduate Studentship in Women's Health Research at the Lunenfeld Tanenbaum Research Institute, Mount Sinai Hospital. CM work was supported in part by the Whitman Fellowship from Harvard Medical School, Boston, MA.

ACKNOWLEDGMENTS

The authors thank the donors, and the Research Center for Women's and Infants' Health BioBank Program of the CIHR Group in Development and Fetal Health (CIHR MGC-13299), the Lunenfeld Tanenbaum Research Institute, and the MSH/UHN Dept. of Obstetrics & Gynecology for the human specimens used in this study. We thank Ms. Annie Bang of the Flow Cytometry Facility (LTRI, Mount Sinai Hospital) for the technical support with flow cytometry and Milan Ganguly from the pathology department for performing the TUNEL staining assay.

REFERENCES

1. Benirschke K, Kaufman P, Baergen R. *Pathology of the Human Placenta*. New York, NY: Springer (2006).
2. Gerretsen G, Huisjes HJ, Elema JD. Morphological changes of the spiral arteries in the placental bed in relation to pre-eclampsia and fetal growth retardation. *Br J Obstet Gynaecol.* (1981) 88:876–81. doi: 10.1111/j.1471-0528.1981.tb02222.x
3. Khong TY, De Wolf F, Robertson WB, Brosens I. Inadequate maternal vascular response to placentation in pregnancies complicated by pre-eclampsia and by small-for-gestational age infants. *Br J Obstet Gynaecol.* (1986) 93:1049–59. doi: 10.1111/j.1471-0528.1986.tb07830.x
4. Kim YM, Chaiworapongsa T, Gomez R, Bujold E, Yoon BH, Rotmensch S, et al. Failure of physiologic transformation of the spiral arteries in the placental bed in preterm premature rupture of membranes. *Am J Obstet Gynecol.* (2002) 187:1137–42. doi: 10.1067/mob.2002.127720
5. Meekins JW, Pijnenborg R, Hanssens M, McFadyen IR, van Asshe A. A study of placental bed spiral arteries and trophoblast invasion in normal and severe pre-eclamptic pregnancies. *Br J Obstet Gynaecol.* (1994) 101:669–74. doi: 10.1111/j.1471-0528.1994.tb13182.x
6. Viero S, Chaddha V, Alkazaleh F, Simchen MJ, Malik A, Kelly E, et al. Prognostic value of placental ultrasound in pregnancies complicated by absent end-diastolic flow velocity in the umbilical arteries. *Placenta.* (2004) 25:735–41. doi: 10.1016/j.placenta.2004.03.002
7. Li N, Ghosh G, Gudmundsson S. Uterine artery Doppler in high-risk pregnancies at 23-24 gestational weeks is of value in predicting adverse outcome of pregnancy and selecting cases for more intense surveillance. *Acta Obstet Gynecol Scand.* (2014) 93:1276–81. doi: 10.1111/aogs.12488
8. Whittle W, Chaddha V, Wyatt P, Huppertz B, Kingdom J. Ultrasound detection of placental insufficiency in women with 'unexplained' abnormal maternal serum screening results. *Clin Genet.* (2006) 69:97–104. doi: 10.1111/j.1399-0004.2005.00546.x
9. McLaughlin K, Zhang J, Lye SJ, Parker JD, Kingdom JC. Phenotypes of pregnant women who subsequently develop hypertension in pregnancy. *J Am Heart Assoc.* (2018) 7:e009595. doi: 10.1161/JAHA.118.009595
10. Kadyrov M, Kingdom JC, Huppertz B. Divergent trophoblast invasion and apoptosis in placental bed spiral arteries from pregnancies complicated by maternal anemia and early-onset preeclampsia/intrauterine growth restriction. *Am J Obstet Gynecol.* (2006) 194:557–63. doi: 10.1016/j.ajog.2005.07.035
11. Lyall F. The human placental bed revisited. *Placenta.* (2002) 23:555–62. doi: 10.1053/plac.2002.0850
12. Reister F, Frank HG, Kingdom JC, Heyl W, Kaufmann P, Rath W, et al. Macrophage-induced apoptosis limits endovascular trophoblast invasion in the uterine wall of preeclamptic women. *Lab Invest.* (2001) 81:1143–52. doi: 10.1038/labinvest.3780326
13. Hustin J, Foidart JM, Lambotte R. Maternal vascular lesions in pre-eclampsia and intrauterine growth retardation: light microscopy and immunofluorescence. *Placenta. Spec No.* (1983) 4, 489–98.

14. Lyall F, Robson SC, Bulmer JN. Spiral artery remodeling and trophoblast invasion in preeclampsia and fetal growth restriction: relationship to clinical outcome. *Hypertension.* (2013) 62:1046–54. doi: 10.1161/HYPERTENSIONAHA.113.01892
15. Pijnenborg R, Anthony J, Davey DA, Rees A, Tiltman A, Vercruysse L, et al. Placental bed spiral arteries in the hypertensive disorders of pregnancy. *Br J Obstet Gynaecol.* (1991) 98:648–55. doi: 10.1111/j.1471-0528.1991.tb13450.x
16. Brosens I, Curcic A, Vejnovic T, Gargett CE, Brosens JJ, Benagiano G. The perinatal origins of major reproductive disorders in the adolescent: research avenues. *Placenta.* (2015) 36:341–4. doi: 10.1016/j.placenta.2015.01.003
17. Brosens I, Pijnenborg R, Vercruysse L, Romero R. The "Great Obstetrical Syndromes" are associated with disorders of deep placentation. *Am J Obstet Gynecol.* (2011) 204:193–201. doi: 10.1016/j.ajog.2010.08.009
18. Croy BA, van den Heuvel MJ, Borzychowski AM, Tayade C. Uterine natural killer cells: a specialized differentiation regulated by ovarian hormones. *Immunol Rev.* (2006) 214:161–85. doi: 10.1111/j.1600-065X.2006.00447.x
19. Dunk C, Smith S, Hazan A, Whittle W, Jones RL. Promotion of angiogenesis by human endometrial lymphocytes. *Immunol Invest.* (2008) 37:583–610. doi: 10.1080/08820130802191466
20. Croxatto D, Vacca P, Canegallo F, Conte R, Venturini PL, Moretta L, et al. Stromal cells from human decidua exert a strong inhibitory effect on NK cell function and dendritic cell differentiation. *PLoS ONE.* (2014) 9:e89006. doi: 10.1371/journal.pone.0089006
21. Jones RL, Hannan NJ, Kaitu'u TJ, Zhang J, Salamonsen LA. Identification of chemokines important for leukocyte recruitment to the human endometrium at the times of embryo implantation and menstruation. *J Clin Endocrinol Metab.* (2004) 89:6155–67. doi: 10.1210/jc.2004-0507
22. Kruse A, Merchant MJ, Hallmann R, Butcher EC. Evidence of specialized leukocyte-vascular homing interactions at the maternal/fetal interface. *Eur J Immunol.* (1999) 29:1116–26. doi: 10.1002/(SICI)1521-4141(199904)29:04<1116::AID-IMMU1116>3.0.CO;2-4
23. Segerer SE, Martignoni F, Bogdan A, Muller N, Kapp M, Dietl J, et al. Thrombopoietin modulates the proliferation, migration and cytokine profile of decidual cell subsets during early gestation. *Mol Hum Reprod.* (2013) 19:361–8. doi: 10.1093/molehr/gat005
24. Sojka DK, Yang L, Plougastel-Douglas B, Higuchi DA, Croy BA, Yokoyama WM. Cutting edge: local proliferation of uterine tissue-resident NK cells during decidualization in mice. *J Immunol.* (2018) 201:2551–6. doi: 10.4049/jimmunol.1800651
25. Bulmer JN, Sunderland CA. Immunohistological characterization of lymphoid cell populations in the early human placental bed. *Immunol.* (1984) 52:349–57.
26. Heikkinen J, Mottonen M, Alanen A, Lassila O. Phenotypic characterization of regulatory T cells in the human decidua. *Clin Exp Immunol.* (2004) 136:373–8. doi: 10.1111/j.1365-2249.2004.02441.x
27. Kwan M, Hazan A, Zhang J, Jones RL, Harris LK, Whittle W, et al. Dynamic changes in maternal decidual leukocyte populations from first to second trimester gestation. *Placenta.* (2014) 35:1027–34. doi: 10.1016/j.placenta.2014.09.018
28. Tilburgs T, Schonkeren D, Eikmans M, Nagtzaam NM, Datema G, Swings GM, et al. Human decidual tissue contains differentiated CD8+ effector-memory T cells with unique properties. *J Immunol.* (2010) 185:4470–7. doi: 10.4049/jimmunol.0903597
29. Craven CM, Morgan T, Ward K. Decidual spiral artery remodelling begins before cellular interaction with cytotrophoblasts. *Placenta.* (1998) 19:241–52. doi: 10.1016/S0143-4004(98)90055-8
30. Pijnenborg R, Vercruysse L, Brosens I. Deep placentation. *Best Pract Res Clin Obstet Gynaecol.* (2011) 25:273–85. doi: 10.1016/j.bpobgyn.2010.10.009
31. Smith SD, Choudhury RH, Matos P, Horn JA, Lye SJ, Dunk CE, et al. Changes in vascular extracellular matrix composition during decidual spiral arteriole remodeling in early human pregnancy. *Histol Histopathol.* (2016) 31:557–71. doi: 10.14670/HH-11-696
32. Hazan AD, Smith SD, Jones RL, Whittle W, Lye SJ, Dunk CE. Vascular-leukocyte interactions: mechanisms of human decidual spiral artery remodeling *in vitro. Am J Pathol.* (2010) 177:1017–30. doi: 10.2353/ajpath.2010.091105
33. Lash GE, Pitman H, Morgan HL, Innes BA, Agwu CN, Bulmer JN. Decidual macrophages: key regulators of vascular remodeling in human pregnancy. *J Leukoc Biol.* (2016) 100:315–25. doi: 10.1189/jlb.1A0815-351R
34. Smith SD, Dunk CE, Aplin JD, Harris LK, Jones RL. Evidence for immune cell involvement in decidual spiral arteriole remodeling in early human pregnancy. *Am J Pathol.* (2009) 174:1959–71. doi: 10.2353/ajpath.2009.080995
35. Choudhury RH, Dunk CE, Lye SJ, Harris LK, Aplin JD, Jones RL. Decidual leucocytes infiltrating human spiral arterioles are rich source of matrix metalloproteinases and degrade extracellular matrix *in vitro* and *in situ. Am J Reprod Immunol.* (2018) 81:e13054. doi: 10.1111/aji.13054
36. Harris LK, Aplin JD. Vascular remodeling and extracellular matrix breakdown in the uterine spiral arteries during pregnancy. *Reprod Sci.* (2007) 14:28–34. doi: 10.1177/1933719107309588
37. Bulmer JN, Innes BA, Levey J, Robson SC, Lash GE. The role of vascular smooth muscle cell apoptosis and migration during uterine spiral artery remodeling in normal human pregnancy. *FASEB J.* (2012) 26:2975–85. doi: 10.1096/fj.12-203679
38. Wallace AE, Cartwright JE, Begum R, Laing K, Thilaganathan B, Whitley GS. Trophoblast-induced changes in C-x-C motif chemokine 10 expression contribute to vascular smooth muscle cell dedifferentiation during spiral artery remodeling. *Arterioscler Thromb Vasc Biol.* (2013) 33:e93–101. doi: 10.1161/ATVBAHA.112.300354
39. Burton GJ, Woods AW, Jauniaux E, Kingdom JC. Rheological and physiological consequences of conversion of the maternal spiral arteries for uteroplacental blood flow during human pregnancy. *Placenta.* (2009) 30:473–82. doi: 10.1016/j.placenta.2009.02.009
40. Hanna J, Goldman-Wohl D, Hamani Y, Avraham I, Greenfield C, Natanson-Yaron S, et al. Decidual NK cells regulate key developmental processes at the human fetal-maternal interface. *Nat Med.* (2006) 12:1065–74. doi: 10.1038/nm1452
41. Williams PJ, Bulmer JN, Searle RF, Innes BA, Robson SC. Altered decidual leucocyte populations in the placental bed in pre-eclampsia and foetal growth restriction: a comparison with late normal pregnancy. *Reproduction.* (2009) 138:177–84. doi: 10.1530/REP-09-0007
42. Pollheimer J, Vondra S, Baltayeva J, Beristain AG, Knofler M. Regulation of placental extravillous trophoblasts by the maternal uterine environment. *Front Immunol.* (2018) 9:2597. doi: 10.3389/fimmu.2018.02597
43. Pijnenborg R, Dixon G, Robertson WB, Brosens I. Trophoblastic invasion of human decidua from 8 to 18 weeks of pregnancy. *Placenta.* (1980) 1:3–19. doi: 10.1016/S0143-4004(80)80012-9
44. Nair RR, Verma P, Singh K. Immune-endocrine crosstalk during pregnancy. *Gen Comp Endocrinol.* (2017) 242:18–23. doi: 10.1016/j.ygcen.2016.03.003
45. Munn DH, Shafizadeh E, Attwood JT, Bondarev I, Pashine A, Mellor AL. Inhibition of T cell proliferation by macrophage tryptophan catabolism. *J Exp Med.* (1999) 189:1363–72. doi: 10.1084/jem.189.9.1363
46. Vacca P, Cantoni C, Vitale M, Prato C, Canegallo F, Fenoglio D, et al. Crosstalk between decidual NK and CD14+ myelomonocytic cells results in induction of Tregs and immunosuppression. *Proc Natl Acad Sci USA.* (2010) 107:11918–23. doi: 10.1073/pnas.1001749107
47. Pilalis A, Souka AP, Antsaklis P, Basayiannis K, Benardis P, Haidopoulos D, et al. Screening for pre-eclampsia and small for gestational age fetuses at the 11–14 weeks scan by uterine artery Dopplers. *Acta Obstet Gynecol Scand.* (2007) 86:530–4. doi: 10.1080/00016340601155056
48. Pijnenborg R, Bland JM, Robertson WB, Brosens I. Uteroplacental arterial changes related to interstitial trophoblast migration in early human pregnancy. *Placenta.* (1983) 4:397–413. doi: 10.1016/S0143-4004(83)80043-5
49. Papageorghiou AT, Yu CK, Erasmus IE, Cuckle HS, Nicolaides KH. Assessment of risk for the development of pre-eclampsia by maternal characteristics and uterine artery Doppler. *BJOG.* (2005) 112:703–9. doi: 10.1111/j.1471-0528.2005.00519.x
50. Kaya HS, Hantak AM, Stubbs LJ, Taylor RN, Bagchi IC, Bagchi MK. Roles of progesterone receptor A and B isoforms during human endometrial decidualization. *Mol Endocrinol.* (2015) 29:882–95. doi: 10.1210/me.2014-1363
51. Bryant-Greenwood GD, Rutanen EM, Partanen S, Coelho TK, Yamamoto SY. Sequential appearance of relaxin, prolactin and IGFBP-1 during growth and differentiation of the human endometrium. *Mol Cell Endocrinol.* (1993) 95:23–9. doi: 10.1016/0303-7207(93)90025-F
52. Oliver C, Cowdrey N, Abadia-Molina AC, Olivares EG. Antigen phenotype

of cultured decidual stromal cells of human term decidua. *J Reprod Immunol.* (1999) 45:19–30. doi: 10.1016/S0165-0378(99)00041-8
53. Zygmunt M, Boving B, Wienhard J, Munstedt K, Braems G, Bohle RM, et al. Expression of cell adhesion molecules in the extravillous trophoblast is altered in IUGR. *Am J Reprod Immunol.* (1997) 38:295–301. doi: 10.1111/j.1600-0897.1997.tb00518.x
54. Marlin R, Duriez M, Berkane N, de Truchis C, Madec Y, Rey-Cuille MA, et al. Dynamic shift from CD85j/ILT-2 to NKG2D NK receptor expression pattern on human decidual NK during the first trimester of pregnancy. *PLoS ONE.* (2012) 7:e30017. doi: 10.1371/journal.pone.0030017
55. Moffett A, Chazara O, Colucci F. Maternal allo-recognition of the fetus. *Fertil Steril.* (2017) 107:1269–72. doi: 10.1016/j.fertnstert.2017.05.001
56. von Rango U. Fetal tolerance in human pregnancy–a crucial balance between acceptance and limitation of trophoblast invasion. *Immunol Lett.* (2008) 115:21–32. doi: 10.1016/j.imlet.2007.09.014
57. Bulmer JN, Lash GE. Human uterine natural killer cells: a reappraisal. *Mol Immunol.* (2005) 42:511–21. doi: 10.1016/j.molimm.2004.07.035
58. Segerer SE, Muller N, Brandt J, Kapp M, Dietl J, Reichardt HM, et al. The glycoprotein-hormones activin A and inhibin A interfere with dendritic cell maturation. *Reprod Biol Endocrinol.* (2008) 6:17. doi: 10.1186/1477-7827-6-17
59. Jung YJ, Park Y, Kim HS, Lee HJ, Kim YN, Lee J, et al. Abnormal lymphatic vessel development is associated with decreased decidual regulatory T cells in severe preeclampsia. *Am J Reprod Immunol.* (2018) 80:e12970. doi: 10.1111/aji.12970
60. Robertson SA, Care AS, Moldenhauer LM. Regulatory T cells in embryo implantation and the immune response to pregnancy. *J Clin Invest.* (2018) 128:4224–35. doi: 10.1172/JCI122182
61. Faas MM, De Vos P. Innate immune cells in the placental bed in healthy pregnancy and preeclampsia. *Placenta.* (2018) 69:125–33. doi: 10.1016/j.placenta.2018.04.012
62. Laskarin G, Kammerer U, Rukavina D, Thomson AW, Fernandez N, Blois SM. Antigen-presenting cells and materno-fetal tolerance: an emerging role for dendritic cells. *Am J Reprod Immunol.* (2007) 58:255–67. doi: 10.1111/j.1600-0897.2007.00511.x
63. McBride JA, Striker R. Imbalance in the game of T cells: what can the CD4/CD8 T-cell ratio tell us about HIV and health? *PLoS Pathog.* (2017) 13:e1006624. doi: 10.1371/journal.ppat.1006624
64. Makrydimas G, Plachouras N, Higueras MT, Thilaganathan B, Nicolaides K. Maternal peripheral blood lymphocyte subpopulations in normal and pathological pregnancies. *Fetal Diagn Ther.* (1994) 9:371–8. doi: 10.1159/000264068
65. Derricott H, Jones RL, Greenwood SL, Batra G, Evans MJ, Heazell AE. Characterizing villitis of unknown etiology and inflammation in stillbirth. *Am J Pathol.* (2016) 186:952–61. doi: 10.1016/j.ajpath.2015.12.010
66. Kovo M, Schreiber L, Ben-Haroush A, Wand S, Golan A, Bar J. Placental vascular lesion differences in pregnancy-induced hypertension and normotensive fetal growth restriction. *Am J Obstet Gynecol.* (2010) 202:e561–65. doi: 10.1016/j.ajog.2010.01.012
67. Donoghue JF, Lederman FL, Susil BJ, Rogers PA. Lymphangiogenesis of normal endometrium and endometrial adenocarcinoma. *Human Reprod.* (2007) 22:1705–13. doi: 10.1093/humrep/dem037
68. Gambino LS, Wreford NG, Bertram JF, Dockery P, Lederman F, Rogers PA. Angiogenesis occurs by vessel elongation in proliferative phase human endometrium. *Human Reprod.* (2002) 17:1199–206. doi: 10.1093/humrep/17.5.1199
69. Girling JE, Rogers PA. The endometrial lymphatic vasculature: function and dysfunction. *Rev Endocr Metab Disord.* (2012) 13:265–75. doi: 10.1007/s11154-012-9224-6
70. Plaisier M, Rodrigues S, Willems F, Koolwijk P, van Hinsbergh VW, Helmerhorst FM. Different degrees of vascularization and their relationship to the expression of vascular endothelial growth factor, placental growth factor, angiopoietins, and their receptors in first-trimester decidual tissues. *Fertil Steril.* (2007) 88:176–87. doi: 10.1016/j.fertnstert.2006.11.102
71. Volchek M, Girling JE, Lash GE, Cann L, Kumar B, Robson SC, et al. Lymphatics in the human endometrium disappear during decidualization. *Human Reprod.* (2010) 25:2455–64. doi: 10.1093/humrep/deq224
72. Windsperger K, Dekan S, Pils S, Golletz C, Kunihs V, Fiala C, et al. Extravillous trophoblast invasion of venous as well as lymphatic vessels is altered in idiopathic, recurrent, spontaneous abortions. *Human Reprod.* (2017) 32:1208–17. doi: 10.1093/humrep/dex058
73. He N, van Iperen L, de Jong D, Szuhai K, Helmerhorst FM, van der Westerlaken LA, et al. Human extravillous trophoblasts penetrate decidual veins and lymphatics before remodeling spiral arteries during early pregnancy. *PLoS ONE.* (2017) 12:e0169849. doi: 10.1371/journal.pone.0169849
74. Moser G, Weiss G, Sundl M, Gauster M, Siwetz M, Lang-Olip I, et al. Extravillous trophoblasts invade more than uterine arteries: evidence for the invasion of uterine veins. *Histochem Cell Biol.* (2017) 147:353–66. doi: 10.1007/s00418-016-1509-5
75. Brosens I, Benagiano G. Menstrual preconditioning for the prevention of major obstetrical syndromes in polycystic ovary syndrome. *Am J Obstet Gynecol.* (2015) 213:488–93. doi: 10.1016/j.ajog.2015.07.021
76. Lessey BA, Kim JJ. Endometrial receptivity in the eutopic endometrium of women with endometriosis: it is affected, and let me show you why. *Fertil Steril.* (2017) 108:19–27. doi: 10.1016/j.fertnstert.2017.05.031
77. Pecks U, Rath W, Kleine-Eggebrecht N, Maass N, Voigt F, Goecke TW, et al. Maternal serum lipid, estradiol, and progesterone levels in pregnancy, and the impact of placental and hepatic pathologies. *Geburtshilfe Frauenheilkd.* (2016) 76:799–808. doi: 10.1055/s-0042-107078
78. Solano ME, Kowal MK, O'Rourke GE, Horst AK, Modest K, Plosch T, et al. Progesterone and HMOX-1 promote fetal growth by CD8+ T cell modulation. *J Clin Invest.* (2015) 125:1726–38. doi: 10.1172/JCI68140

17

Brain Volumes and Developmental Outcome in Childhood Following Fetal Growth Restriction Leading to Very Preterm Birth

Eva Morsing[1], Mariya Malova[2], Anna Kahn[3], Jimmy Lätt[3], Isabella M. Björkman-Burtscher[3,4], Karel Maršál[5] and David Ley[1]*

[1] Department of Pediatrics, Clinical Sciences Lund, Lund University, Lund, Sweden, [2] Neonatal Intensive Care Unit, Istituto Giannina Gaslini, Genoa, Italy, [3] Department of Radiology, Clinical Sciences Lund, Lund University, Lund, Sweden, [4] Department of Medical Imaging and Physiology, Skåne University Hospital, Lund, Sweden, [5] Department of Obstetrics and Gynecology, Clinical Sciences Lund, Lund University, Lund, Sweden

***Correspondence:**
Eva Morsing
eva.morsing@med.lu.se

Background: Children born very preterm (PT) after fetal growth restriction (FGR) exhibit cognitive impairment at early school age. The relationship between neurodevelopmental impairment and attained regional brain volumes is unknown.

Methods: We studied 23 preterm children with FGR (PT-FGR), 24 matched preterm children AGA (PT-AGA), and 27 matched term AGA children (T-AGA) by measuring brain volumes with magnetic resonance imaging at early school age. Cognitive and motor functions were assessed by the Wechsler Intelligence Scales for Children and the ABC-Movement score.

Results: The mean (*SD*) full-scale IQ was 80 (17) in the PT-FGR group and 103 (12) in the PT-AGA group ($p < 0.001$). The PT-FGR group had lower mean total, gray matter, white matter, thalamic, cerebellar white matter, and hippocampal volumes as compared to the T-AGA group ($p = 0.01$, 0.04, 0.003, 0.002, 0.001, and 0.009, respectively). Brain volumes did not differ significantly between the PT groups. Reduction of hippocampal volume correlated with degree of growth restriction at birth ($r = 0.46$, $p = 0.05$). Neither the full-scale IQ nor the ABC movement score <5th percentile were related to brain volumes.

Conclusion: Brain volumes as determined by MRI at early school age were primarily associated with degree of prematurity at birth and less with FGR. Regional brain volumes did not discriminate cognitive and motor function beyond that predicted by gestational age at birth.

Keywords: brain volumes, magnetic resonance imaging, neuro-development, preterm birth, fetal growth restriction

---

Abbreviations: ADD, Attention deficit disorder; AGA, Appropriate for gestational age; ARED, Absent or reversed end-diastolic; BPD, Bronchopulmonary dysplasia; FGR, Fetal growth restriction; FIQ, Full scale IQ; GA, Gestational age; GM, Gray matter; MRI, Magnetic resonance imaging; PIQ, Performance IQ; PT, Preterm; ROP, Retinopathy of prematurity; ROI, Regions of interest; T, Term; VIQ, Verbal IQ; WM, White matter.

INTRODUCTION

Fetal growth restriction (FGR) at early GA is associated with high risk of perinatal mortality, morbidity, and long-term neurodevelopmental impairment (Torrance et al., 2010; Baschat, 2011). ARED blood flow in the umbilical artery assessed by Doppler velocimetry is associated with adverse outcome in preterm FGR (PT-FGR) fetuses (Hartung et al., 2005). No consensus on clinical management of FGR fetuses diagnosed in the second trimester (early-onset) has been achieved so far (Baschat and Odibo, 2011). Prenatal clinical management has to consider the high risk of neonatal complications associated with severe prematurity against the substantial risk of fetal death.

Previous studies, with the objective of relating impaired fetal growth to different aspects of outcome have mainly used birthweight small for GA, (SGA) as a proxy and a common denominator for FGR. As well known, this definition is imprecise and will include constitutionally small infants as well as truly growth-retarded infants. The objective of the present study is to evaluate long-term effects of FGR leading to very preterm birth (<30 GW). The patho-physiological consequences of early-onset FGR, i.e., leading to very preterm birth, are sensitively detected by fetal blood flow evaluation using Doppler ultrasound (Figueras and Gratacos, 2014).

Infants born very preterm (PT) were reported to exhibit reduction in total and regional cerebral volumes determined by MRI (Keunen et al., 2012) and the observed brain volume reduction has been shown to persist into childhood and adolescence (Reiss et al., 2004; Northam et al., 2011). In fetuses affected by late-onset growth restriction, fetal MRI showed different cortical development as compared to fetuses with normal growth (Egana-Ugrinovic et al., 2013). Subjects with late-onset FGR, as determined by birthweight small for GA and born at term age, exhibited a global reduction in brain volume as well as regional reductions in cortical surface area (Ostgard et al., 2014).

Fetal growth restriction leading to very preterm birth, i.e., early-onset FGR, has been associated with altered brain structure and lower brain volumes during the PT period and at term-equivalent age (Tolsa et al., 2004; Thompson et al., 2007). Interpretation of previous studies on FGR and brain volumes is complicated by the heterogeneity of study designs and inclusion criteria. Some authors have described reduced brain volumes in small for GA subjects born at late gestation with no information on preceding fetal blood flow examinations (Ostgard et al., 2014). Differences in age of subjects at MRI assessment also complicate comparisons of brain volumes studies, since brain growth changes with age in healthy subjects (Sussman et al., 2016).

To date, there are no controlled studies investigating the effect of FGR leading to very preterm birth on MRI-assessed regional brain volumes in children; thus, it is unclear whether the alterations in brain volumes persist into childhood. Infants with FGR and ARED flow leading to very preterm birth have an increased neonatal morbidity and an adverse cognitive outcome at school age (Brodszki et al., 2009; Morsing et al., 2011). Clinical guide-lines for management of this group of fetuses still differ between centers and countries. It is therefore essential, from a neuro-scientific as from a clinical point of view, to investigate brain development in this well-defined group of subjects. The aim of this study was to evaluate regional brain volumes and their relationship to cognitive and motor outcome at 8 years of age in children born very preterm after FGR and ARED umbilical artery blood flow.

PATIENTS AND METHODS

Population

The present work is part of a prospective case-control follow-up study of children born very preterm (<30 gestational weeks) after early-onset FGR and ARED blood flow in the umbilical artery. Doppler flow velocity signals from the umbilical artery, the middle cerebral artery, DV, umbilical veins and from both maternal uterine arteries were recorded using Philips HDI 5000 or Philips IU22 (Philips Medical Systems, Bothell, WA, United States) ultrasound systems. Abnormal DV flow was defined as absent or reverse flow during the a-wave. The Doppler velocimetry was in all cases performed in a standardized way by experienced sonographers. FHR recordings and Doppler velocimetry were performed daily. Between 1998 and 2004, 42 such live-born neonates were delivered on fetal indication at the level III perinatal center at Skane University Hospital in Lund, Sweden. Since 1998, a proactive clinical management protocol is used for management of very preterm fetuses with FGR aiming to avoid severe fetal hypoxia and deterioration of fetal condition. The protocol indicates delivery at the occurrence of reversed end-diastolic (RED) flow in the umbilical artery, and/or if there are rapidly progressing changes in the ductus venosus (DV) blood velocity waveform or pathological changes of fetal heart rate (FHR; loss of variability, late decelerations). After 26 gestational weeks, absent end-diastolic (AED) flow in the umbilical artery was indication for delivery after the full course of antenatal steroid treatment. The clinical protocol included delivery by cesarean section and neonatal active care comprising early surfactant treatment and early enteral feeding with human milk. During the same period, two control groups with birth weight AGA were identified; one group consisted of preterm infants matched for GA and sex (PT-AGA), and the other group was born at term matched for sex and age at examination (T-AGA). At the age of 7–8 years, follow-up examinations were performed. Perinatal data, prevalence of cerebral palsy, as well as neurocognitive, cardiovascular and pulmonary outcome in this cohort have been reported previously (Brodszki et al., 2009; Morsing et al., 2011, 2012, 2014).

Children from the three groups that underwent an examination with brain MRI at 8 years of age constituted the index group (PT-FGR, $n = 23$) and two control groups (PT-AGA, $n = 24$; T-AGA, $n = 27$) of the present study.

Movement ABC

Children were evaluated with The Movement Assessments Battery for Children 2nd edition (Movement ABC) consisting of eight items divided into three subtests: manual dexterity, ball skills, and static/dynamic balance. (Henderson and Barnett, 2007) High scores denote motor performance deficits. Scores below the 5th percentile indicate severe motor impairment, and scores between the 5th and 15th percentile indicate minor motor impairment.

Cognitive Tests and Behavior Questionnaire

Cognitive evaluation was performed by Wechsler scales (the Wechsler Preschool and Primary Scale of Intelligence-III and the Wechsler Intelligence Scale for Children-III, 1991 revision, British version) at 5–8 years of age (range 60–105 months). (Wechsler, 1991, 2002; Brown, 2001) Both tests consist of two IQ subscales, VIQ and PIQ, forming the full-scale IQ (FIQ). All scales have a mean of 100 points and *SD* of 15. Cognitive impairment was defined as FIQ < 70 (>2 *SD* below the normative mean).

During follow-up visit, the parents were interviewed and filled in two scoring questionnaires regarding attention-deficit disorder (ADD; Brown's ADD scales)(Brown, 2001) and behavior problems (Strengths and Difficulties Questionnaire (SDQ). Brown's ADD consists of 44 items and includes tasks examining ability to sustain attention and energy, effort to complete tasks, to regulate moods and recall learned material. A score >55 indicates risk for ADD. The SDQ is a behavioral screening questionnaire that comprises 25 items divided into subscales (prosocial, hyperactivity, emotional problems, conduct, and peer problems). A total score of 13 was considered to be borderline or high.

MRI Scanning

All children were informed about the MRI procedure beforehand and were awake during the scanning. None of the children were sedated. Ear plugs and headphones were used for hearing protection and children could watch a movie during the examination by means of projection on a screen behind the scanner and viewed through a mirror mounted to the head coil.

The MRI investigations were performed on a 3T scanner (Achieva, Philips, Best, Netherlands) with an eight channel SENSE head coil. Volumetric data were acquired using a T1 3D magnetization prepared rapid acquisition with gradient echo (MPRAGE) sequence with isotropic voxel size of 1 mm^3, allowing reconstruction in any plane, repetition time = 9 ms, echo time = 4 ms, and flip angle = 10°. Reconstruction and segmentation of the brain was performed with the FreeSurfer image analysis suite[1]. Volumetric data were acquired for total intracranial volume, GM, WM, cerebrospinal fluid, cerebellar GM and WM, and thalamus. All segmentations were subsequently reviewed and, if necessary, the automatically segmented volumes were adjusted manually using in-house MatLab (Mathworks, MA, United States) based software. In particular, the anterior border of the cerebellar WM was adjusted to consequently exclude brainstem areas. The peduncles of the cerebellum were included in the WM volumes and the vermis was included in the GM volumes.

Hippocampal segmentation was performed manually on a PACS workstation (IDS7, Sectra, Linköping, Sweden) in consensus by two radiologists blinded to perinatal data. T1 MPRAGE images were separately for both sides reformatted to an oblique coronal viewing plane perpendicular to the long axis and in parallel to the anterior and posterior limits of the hippocampus. Delineation was performed in a posterior to anterior direction with the plane showing the crus of the fornix defining the level of the most posterior aspect of the hippocampus and the plane where the temporal horn appears medially and beneath the amygdala the most anterior portion. As further boundaries of the hippocampus we used the alveus (superior), WM of the para-hippocampal gyrus (inferior), the temporal horn of the lateral ventricle (lateral), and the ambient cistern (medial). The subiculum was included in the hippocampus. Anteriorly the temporal horn of the lateral ventricle and the alveus were used to separate hippocampus from amygdala. When in doubt, an imaginary line between the ambient cistern and the middle of the temporal horn of the lateral ventricle was used. ROIs were first drawn by observer 1 according to the protocol, then observer 2, in a separate session defined visually the boundaries of the hippocampi on unmarked projections ant then checked ROIs for mismatches. All suggested changes of hippocampal delineation were discussed in consensus between the observers and then implemented.

Data Collection and Analysis

Demographic data and clinical parameters, including prenatal, perinatal, and neonatal data were collected from the obstetric and pediatric patient records. Head circumference was measured by a pediatrician at the follow-up examination. Information on socioeconomic factors was obtained from questionnaires administered to the parents while the children attended the tests. Cognitive, motor, and behavioral test results, as well as MRI data were registered. Possible associations between the volume of brain structures, clinical data and neurobehavioral test results were assessed.

Statistical analyses were performed using SPSS 23.0 statistical software (SPSS Inc, Chicago, IL, United States). Categorical variables were compared between groups by the χ^2 test. Differences in continuous variables were assessed with two-way analysis of variance (ANOVA) with *post hoc* Bonferroni correction for multiple group comparisons. *P*-values of <0.05 were considered statistically significant. Confounders were explored by linear regression analysis.

RESULTS

Perinatal Clinical Data and Postnatal Morbidity

Birth characteristics, neonatal morbidity, and rate of cerebral palsy in the three groups are presented in **Table 1**. All 23 infants of the index group had ultrasonically estimated fetal weight more than 2 *SD* below the mean of the Swedish reference population (Marsal et al., 1996). Eighteen fetuses had absent, and five had reversed end-diastolic blood flow in the umbilical

[1]http://surfer.nmr.mgh.harvard.edu

TABLE 1 | Birth characteristics, neonatal morbidity, and rate of cerebral palsy.

	PT-FGR	PT-AGA	T-AGA	Significance of difference		
	(*n* = 23)	(*n* = 24)	(*n* = 27)	PT-FGR–PT-AGA	PT-FGR – T-AGA	PT-AGA – T-AGA
Gestational age weeks, mean ± SD	26.4 ± 1.5	26.7 ± 1.6	39.4 ± 0.7	*ns*	*<0.001*	*<0.001*
ARED flow in the umbilical artery, *n* (%)	23 (100)	0	0	*<0.001*	*<0.001*	*na*
Birthweight g, median (range)	664 (395–976)	1032 (660–1790)	3550 (3000–4390)	*<0.001*	*<0.001*	*<0.001*
Birthweight deviation %, median (range)	−37 (−63 – −23)	−5 (−22 –+14)	−1 (−17 –+29)	*<0.001*	*<0.001*	*0.05*
Apgar score < 7 at 5 min *n* (%)	1 (4)	4 (17)	0	*ns*		
Cesarean section *n* (%)	23 (100)	14 (58)	0	*<0.001*		
Sex, female/male *n*	13/10	11/13	14/13	*ns*	*ns*	*ns*
Term head circumference cm, mean ± SD	34.4 ± 1.5	35.6 ± 1.0	35.5 ± 1.2	*0.02*	*0.02*	*ns*
IVH III/PVHI *n* (%)	1 (4)	2 (8)	0	*ns*		
ROP *n* (%)	4 (17)	6 (25)	0	*ns*		
NEC *n* (%)	3 (13)	0	0	*ns*		
BPD *n* (%)	16 (70)	6 (25)	0	*0.003*		
Postnatal steroid treatment *n* (%)	9 (39)	5 (21)	0	*ns*		
Septicemia *n* (%)	14 (61)	6 (25)	0	0.02		
Cerebral palsy *n* (%)	2 (9)	4 (17)	0	*ns*		

PT, preterm; T, term; AGA, appropriate for gestational age; birthweight deviation % of expected birthweight according to Swedish standard; FGR, fetal growth restriction; ARED, absent or reversed end-diastolic blood flow; ns, non-significant; IVH, Intraventricular hemorrhage; PVHI, peri-ventricular hemorrhagic infarction; ROP, retinopathy of prematurity; NEC, necrotizing enterocolitis; BPD, bronchopulmonary dysplasia.

artery. Fifteen fetuses out of 23 had signs of brain-sparing, i.e., middle cerebral artery pulsatility index >2 *SD* below the GA related mean (Mari and Deter, 1992). The mean (*SD*) GA at birth was 26.4 (1.5) weeks and all infants were small-for-GA with birthweight < mean−2 *SD* of the reference (Marsal et al., 1996).

Infants in the control groups (PT-AGA and T-AGA) had AGA birth weight. Antenatal Doppler velocimetry was not performed in the control children.

The Apgar score <7 at 5 min and sex distribution were similar in the preterm groups. Prevalence of severe intraventricular hemorrhage, ROP and necrotizing enterocolitis, as well as use of postnatal steroids was similar in the preterm groups. The PT-FGR group had higher rate of septicemia and BPD than the control PT-AGA group.

Cognitive Function, Motor Performance, and Behavior

Results of cognitive evaluation, motor performance, ADD, and behavior are shown in **Table 2**. The PT-FGR group had lower motor performance score, higher scores in attention deficit and behavior questionnaires compared to the T-AGA group. Scores from Brown's ADD and SDQ scales did not differ between the two preterm groups. PIQ and FIQ were lower in both preterm groups compared to the T-AGA group. FIQ was lower in the PT-FGR group than in the PT-AGA group.

Subjects Not Examined With MRI

The numbers of subjects evaluated for cognitive and behavioral outcome at 6–8 years of age in the background population (Morsing et al., 2011) but not examined by MRI were 11, 10, and 7 in the background PT-FGR, PT-AGA, and the T-AGA groups, respectively. Birthweight deviation and GA at birth, as well as the cognitive outcome, behavior, and motor performance did not differ between the infants examined and those not examined with MRI.

MRI Brain Volumes

The PT-FGR group had significantly lower mean total intracranial, GM and WM, thalamic, cerebellar WM and hippocampal volumes as compared to the T-AGA group (**Table 3** and **Figure 1**). The PT-AGA group had lower mean WM, thalamic and cerebellar WM volumes as compared to the T-AGA group. Brain volumes did not differ significantly between the PT-FGR and the PT-AGA groups (**Table 3** and **Figure 1**). When compared to term controls, female FGR subjects had smaller thalamic, cerebellar WM and hippocampal volumes, while males had smaller WM volumes.

Group differences were also evaluated for regional brain volumes in relation to total intracranial volume. Relative cerebellar WM volume was lower in the PT-FGR and the PT-AGA groups as compared to the T-AGA group, p = 0.016 and

TABLE 2 | Cognitive evaluation by WISC-III/WPPSI-III, motor performance by ABC-movement, attention deficit disorder and behavior by Brown's ADD and SDQ and measurements of head circumference at 5–8 years.

	PT-FGR (n = 23)	PT-AGA (n = 24)	T-AGA (n = 27)	Significance of difference		
				PT-FGR – PT-AGA	PT-FGR – T-AGA	PT-AGA – T-AGA
Parental education						
High school/university						
Mother, n (%)	9/23 (39)	12/23 (52)	14/26 (54)	*ns*	*ns*	*ns*
Father, n (%)	5/23 (22)	8/23 (35)	11/26 (42)	*ns*	*ns*	*ns*
Verbal IQ mean ± SD	85 ± 18	95 ± 14	102 ± 11	*ns*	*<0.001*	*ns*
Performance IQ mean ± SD	80 ± 16	87 ± 15	105 ± 15	*ns*	*<0.001*	*<0.001*
Full scale IQ mean ± SD	80 ± 17	90 ± 13	103 ± 12	*0.05*	*<0.001*	*0.003*
Motor performance < 5th percentile, n (%)	8 (34)	3 (12)	1 (4)	*ns*	*0.002*	*ns*
ADD combined mean ± SD	51.4 ± 10.9	48.1 ± 10.1	42.1 ± 5.6	*ns*	*0.002*	*ns*
ADD combined > 55, n (%)	8 (35)	7 (29)	1 (4)	*ns*	*0.007*	*0.019*
SDQ total, mean ± SD	9.6 ± 5.1	7.2 ± 5.9	4.4 ± 4.9	*ns*	*<0.001*	*ns*
SDQ total > 13, n (%)	6 (26)	4 (17)	1 (4)	*ns*	*0.04*	*ns*
Head circumference at MRI, cm, mean ± SD	51.7 ± 1.6	52.9 ± 1.6	54.6 ± 1.6	*ns*	*<0.001*	*0.009*

WISC, Wechsler Intelligence Scale for Children; 3rd edition. WPPSI, Wechsler Preschool and Primary Scale of Intelligence; 3rd edition. ABC-movement, Movement assessments battery for children; Brown's ADD, attention deficit disorder; SDQ, strength and difficulties questionnaire; PT, preterm; AGA, appropriate for gestational age; FGR, fetal growth restriction; MRI, magnetic resonance imaging.

0.033, respectively. Remaining regional brain volumes in relation to total intracranial volume exhibited no differences between groups.

After adjustment for GA at birth, head circumference at term age correlated positively with global as well as with regional brain volumes within the respective PT groups. Fetal brain sparing was not associated with brain volumes. Weight deviation at birth was positively correlated to all regional brain volumes, but when GA at birth and sex were taken into account, only hippocampal volume remained significantly associated ($r = 0.46$, $p = 0.05$).

The presence of neonatal risk factors with a potential impact on brain growth, such as severe intraventricular hemorrhage grade III or periventricular hemorrhagic infarction, septicemia, and necrotizing enterocolitis, was not related to brain volumes. In univariate analysis, BPD was significantly associated with decreased volumes of GM, WM and cerebellar WM, but after adjustment for GA, birth weight deviation at birth and sex only GM volumes remained associated with BPD ($r = 0.43$, $p = 0.01$). Any stage of ROP was significantly associated with decreased volumes of WM, thalamus, and cerebellar GM, but after adjustment for GA, weight deviation at birth and sex, ROP remained significantly associated with cerebellar GM ($r = 0.60$, $p = 0.02$). Postnatal steroid treatment with betamethasone did not correlate with brain volumes.

Motor performance, cognitive outcome, behavior, and ADD were not associated with differences in any of the measured brain volumes. Sex had no influence on the relationship between regional brain volumes and neurodevelopmental outcome.

DISCUSSION

In this prospective study, we examined neurodevelopmental outcome and brain growth as determined by brain MRI at early school age in children born very preterm after early-onset FGR, and in matched preterm and term AGA controls. The PT-FGR group had a higher rate of cognitive impairment than PT-AGA subjects, however, we did not observe any corresponding differences in global or regional brain volumes as determined by MRI.

All children in the PT-FGR group had ARED blood flow in the umbilical artery prior to delivery and were actively delivered before 30 gestational weeks in order to prevent further worsening of fetal distress. We have previously reported that neonatal mortality, cerebral morbidity, and rate of cerebral palsy at 2 years of age in the PT-FGR group were comparable to those of children delivered very preterm due to other indications (Brodszki et al., 2009). However, subsequent follow-up showed that cognitive impairment at early school age was more prevalent in the PT-FGR as compared to the PT-AGA group, mainly due to decreased cognitive performance in growth restricted boys (Morsing et al., 2011).

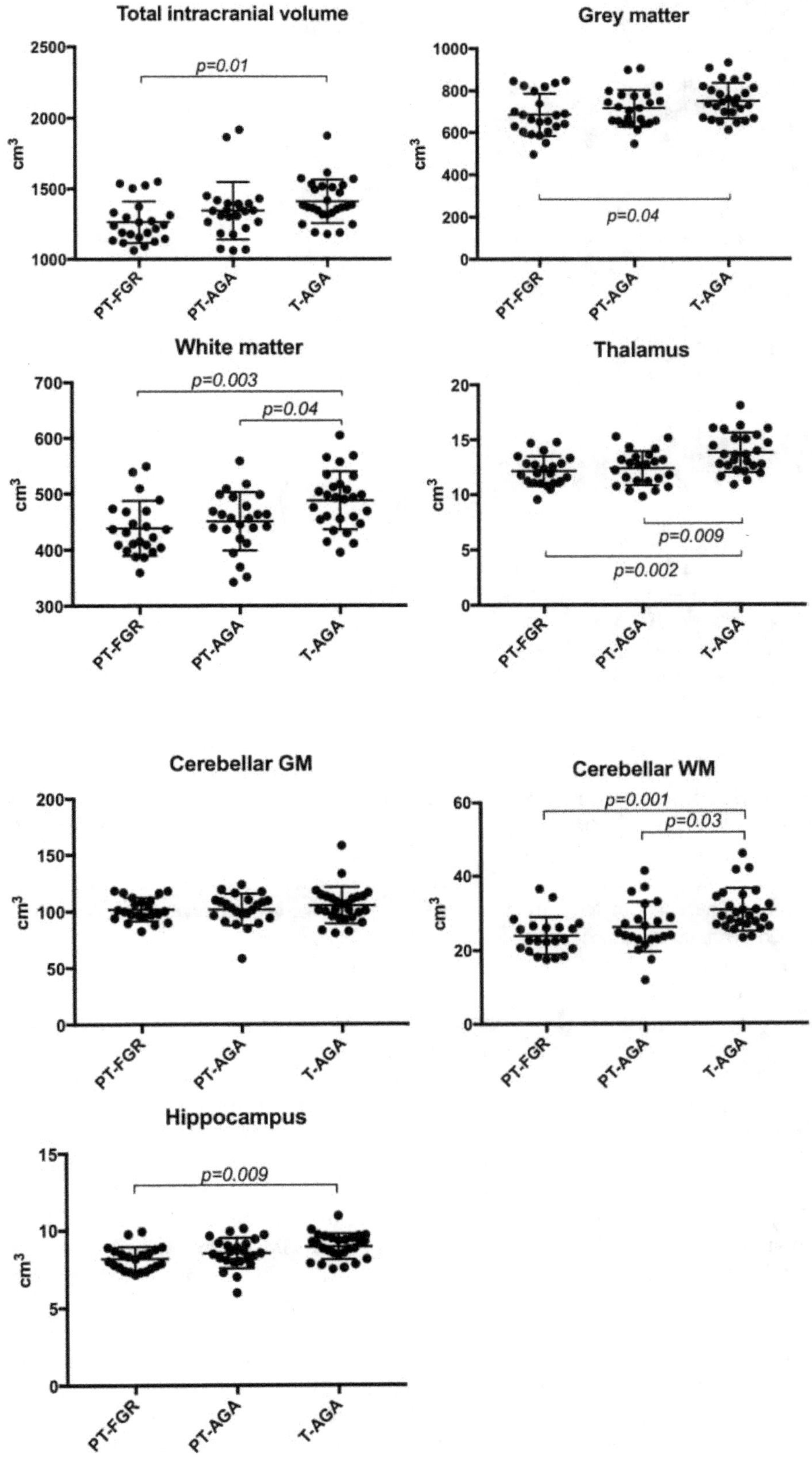

FIGURE 1 | Dot plots describing individual values of total intracranial brain volume and regional brain volumes in subjects with fetal growth restriction and very preterm birth (PT-FGR group), very preterm birth and birthweight appropriate for gestational age (PT-AGA group), and birthweight appropriate for GA at term age (T-AGA group). Horizontal lines depict group means and standard deviations. Cerebellar GM, cerebellar gray matter; Cerebellar WM, cerebellar white matter.

TABLE 3 | Brain volumes (cm^3, mean ± SD).

Brain structure	Group			Significance of difference		
cm^3	PT-FGR (*n* = 23)	PT-AGA (*n* = 24)	T-AGA (*n* = 27)	PT-FGR–PT-AGA	PT-FGR – T-AGA	PT-AGA – T-AGA
Total intracranial volume	1264 ± 147	1344 ± 203	1409 ± 153	*ns*	*0.01*	*ns*
male	1287 ± 153	1434 ± 213	1462 ± 179	*ns*	*ns*	*ns*
female	1246 ± 146	1237 ± 130	1361 ± 111	*ns*	*ns*	*ns*
Gray matter	684 ± 101	714 ± 88	750 ± 85	*ns*	*0.04*	*ns*
male	705 ± 119	747 ± 88	777 ± 102	*ns*	*ns*	*ns*
female	669 ± 87	676 ± 75	726 ± 59	*ns*	*ns*	*ns*
White matter	438 ± 49	450 ± 52	488 ± 52	*ns*	*0.003*	*0.04*
male	449 ± 52	471 ± 39	509 ± 50	*ns*	*0.02*	*ns*
female	431 ± 46	426 ± 55	468 ± 46	*ns*	*ns*	*ns*
Thalamus	12.1 ± 1.4	12.4 ± 1.5	13.8 ± 1.8	*ns*	*0.002*	*0.009*
male	12.4 ± 1.1	12.7 ± 1.8	14.1 ± 2.3	*ns*	*ns*	*ns*
female	11.9 ± 1.5	12.0 ± 1.3	13.5 ± 1.3	*ns*	*0.02*	*0.04*
Cerebellar GM	101.7 ± 10.2	101.5 ± 13.8	105.1 ± 15.9	*ns*	*ns*	*ns*
male	107.6 ± 9.7	108.9 ± 8.7	105.3 ± 21.1	*ns*	*ns*	*ns*
female	97.7 ± 8.8	93.6 ± 14.3	104.9 ± 9.7	*ns*	*ns*	*0.05*
Cerebellar WM	24.0 ± 4.9	26.0 ± 6.6	31.7 ± 9.1	*ns*	*0.001*	*0.03*
male	25.40 ± 6.4	28.3 ± 5.9	32.7 ± 10.1	*ns*	*ns*	*ns*
female	23.0 ± 3.0	23.5 ± 7.0	30.7 ± 8.2	*ns*	*0.02*	*0.03*
Hippocampus	8.2 ± 0.8	8.5 ± 1.0	8.9 ± 0.8	*ns*	*0.009*	*ns*
male	8.5 ± 0.9	8.8 ± 0.9	9.1 ± 0.9	*ns*	*ns*	*ns*
female	8.0 ± 0.6	8.3 ± 1.1	8.8 ± 0.7	*ns*	*0.04*	*ns*

ns, non-significant; GM, gray matter; WM, white matter.

Several studies have correlated adverse neurodevelopment with time of onset of growth restriction, (Baschat, 2014) severity of Doppler changes, (Schreuder et al., 2002) GA at delivery, (Baschat and Odibo, 2011), and neonatal morbidity (Yeh et al., 2004; Trittmann et al., 2013). The effect of fetal brain sparing was found to be associated with impaired cognitive outcome and to have negative effects on the brain (Scherjon et al., 2000). The majority of children in the present PT-FGR group had signs of fetal brain sparing, however, we did not find any relationship between redistribution of flow and brain volumes at early childhood.

The main result of the present study is the observation of smaller global and regional brain volumes in the preterm FGR group compared to the term AGA group, although no clear differences could be observed between the PT-FGR and PT-AGA groups. In previous studies, MRI performed at term-equivalent age (Tolsa et al., 2004) and at 12 months of age (Padilla et al., 2014) has shown reduced brain tissue volumes in infants born after FGR when compared to GA matched controls. It is important to note that subjects included in those studies had a considerably higher mean GA at birth, which, in absence of extreme prematurity, may increase the possibility of observing effects of FGR *per se*. The conflicting results might also reflect differences in pathophysiology between early-onset and late-onset FGR, and in the related clinical managements.

In our controlled study of preterm FGR subjects, hippocampal volume was positively correlated to weight deviation at birth. This is consistent with both experimental (Mallard et al., 2000) and clinical (Lodygensky et al., 2008) studies describing hippocampal vulnerability in growth restriction, possibly mediated by hypoxia and/or reduced supply of nutrients.

We observed sex-related differences in regional brain volumes in our study population. In comparison to the T-AGA reference group, female PT-FGR subjects had reduced thalamic, cerebellar, and hippocampal volumes, while male PT-FGR subjects had smaller WM volumes. These results are in accordance with literature that shows smaller WM volume at 8 years of age in preterm males (Reiss et al., 2004). Sex differences in brain morphology corresponding to those found in the present study were recently observed in a cohort of extremely preterm infants: female subjects had more abnormalities in the cerebellum and male subjects displayed delayed myelination (Skiold et al., 2014).

Among neonatal morbidities, BPD remained related to decreased GM volume after adjustment for GA and weight deviation at birth. The relationship between BPD and MRI abnormalities has been described previously. Brain abnormalities and delayed maturation in WM and thalamus were observed in MRI at term-equivalent age of PT infants with BPD. (Rose et al., 2014; Neubauer et al., 2015) In two other cohorts, BPD and exposure to postnatal dexamethasone resulted in smaller GM volume at term (Murphy et al., 2001) and in reduced total brain volume at adolescent age (Cheong et al., 2014). In our population, smaller GM volume was related to BPD but not to postnatal steroid treatment. The effect of postnatal treatment with betamethasone on brain growth has not been evaluated in

PT infants as opposed to that of dexamethasone (Cheong et al., 2014). Speculatively, betamethasone may be less harmful to the brain tissue.

Further, any stage of ROP was related to reductions in cerebellar cortex volumes and these relationships remained significant after adjustment for confounders. In a recent study, presence of ROP was associated with smaller biometric measurements and higher prevalence of brain abnormalities on term-equivalent age MRI (Naud et al., 2017). We recently reported a relationship between any stage of ROP and reduced WM and cerebellar volume at term age as determined by MRI (Sveinsdottir et al., 2018). These findings suggest that common pathways may lead to impaired neural and neurovascular development in the brain and retina.

The main strengths of the present study are its prospective design and careful matching of study groups. The study has several limitations. Fetal Doppler measurements were not performed in the control groups. However, all subjects in the control groups were AGA at birth, which suggests that fetal blood flow impairment was less probable. Further, the study and control groups were relatively small and conclusions have to be drawn with caution. Thirty per cent of the children/parents did not consent to MRI examination which further reduced the strength of the study. However, cognitive and motor performance outcomes did not differ between children who declined and those who performed the MRI assessment in our study. The latter observation is reassuring in view of the finding in a recent meta-analysis, reporting that a greater loss to follow-up was correlated to higher rates of neurodevelopmental impairment (Guillen et al., 2012).

It is still unclear to which extent FGR with hemodynamic impairment prior to very preterm birth modifies or accentuates the risks of prematurity. Contrary to other studies, our data on that the reduced brain volumes are not the most important pathophysiological factor connected to functional outcomes. Alternatively, reduced brain volumes seen at early ages, i.e., in neonates and in infancy, may normalize with age. We are the FGR group delivered very preterm did not show smaller regional brain volumes compared to those of matched PT-AGA controls. Cognitive impairment, more prevalent in the FGR group, was not related to brain volumes. One can speculate currently analyzing data from diffusion tensor imaging (DTI), performed in parallel with the MRI volumetric study. Data on WM structure may provide important additional information about the effect of FGR on brain development.

AUTHOR CONTRIBUTIONS

EM conceptualized and designed the study, coordinated and supervised the data collection, carried out the statistical analysis, drafted the initial manuscript, and reviewed and revised the manuscript. KM, DL, and IB-B, conceptualized and designed the study, designed the data collection instruments, and critically reviewed and revised the manuscript. AK, MM, and JL, collected the data, carried out the initial analyses, and reviewed and revised the manuscript. All authors approved the final manuscript as submitted and agreed to be accountable for all aspects of the work.

ACKNOWLEDGMENTS

Gunborg Mattson, physiotherapist, B.Sc., who performed the ABC-movement and Malena Åsard, psychologist, who performed the psychological tests.

REFERENCES

1. Baschat, A. A. (2011). Neurodevelopment following fetal growth restriction and its relationship with antepartum parameters of placental dysfunction. *Ultrasound Obstet. Gynecol.* 37, 501–514. doi: 10.1002/uog.9008
2. Baschat, A. A. (2014). Neurodevelopment after fetal growth restriction. *Fetal Diagn. Ther.* 36, 136–142. doi: 10.1159/000353631
3. Baschat, A. A., and Odibo, A. O. (2011). Timing of delivery in fetal growth restriction and childhood development: some uncertainties remain. *Am. J. Obstet. Gynecol.* 204, 2–3. doi: 10.1016/j.ajog.2010.10.915
4. Brodszki, J., Morsing, E., Malcus, P., Thuring, A., Ley, D., and Marsal, K. (2009). Early intervention in management of very preterm growth-restricted fetuses: 2-year outcome of infants delivered on fetal indication before 30 gestational weeks. *Ultrasound Obstet. Gynecol.* 34, 288–296. doi: 10.1002/uog.7321
5. Brown, T. E. (ed.) (2001). *Brown Attention-Deficit Disorder Scales for Children and Adolescents.* San Antonio, TX: The Psychological Corporation.
6. Cheong, J. L., Burnett, A. C., Lee, K. J., Roberts, G., Thompson, D. K., Wood, S. J., et al. (2014). Association between postnatal dexamethasone for treatment of bronchopulmonary dysplasia and brain volumes at adolescence in infants born very preterm. *J. Pediatr.* 164, 737.e1–743.e1. doi: 10.1016/j.jpeds.2013. 10.083
7. Egana-Ugrinovic, G., Sanz-Cortes, M., Figueras, F., Bargallo, N., and Gratacos, E. (2013). Differences in cortical development assessed by fetal MRI in late-onset intrauterine growth restriction. *Am. J. Obstet. Gynecol.* 209, 126.e1–128.e1. doi: 10.1016/j.ajog.2013.04.008
8. Figueras, F., and Gratacos, E. (2014). Update on the diagnosis and classification of fetal growth restriction and proposal of a stage-based management protocol. *Fetal Diagn. Ther.* 36, 86–98. doi: 10.1159/000357592
9. Guillen, U., DeMauro, S., Ma, L., Zupancic, J., Roberts, R., Schmidt, B., et al. (2012). Relationship between attrition and neurodevelopmental impairment rates in extremely preterm infants at 18 to 24 months: a systematic review. *Arch. Pediatr. Adolesc. Med.* 166, 178–184. doi: 10.1001/archpediatrics.2011.616
10. Hartung, J., Kalache, K. D., Heyna, C., Heling, K. S., Kuhlig, M., Wauer, R., et al. (2005). Outcome of 60 neonates who had ARED flow prenatally compared with a matched control group of appropriate-for-gestational age preterm neonates. *Ultrasound Obstet. Gynecol.* 25, 566–572. doi: 10.1002/uog.1906
11. Henderson, S. D., and Barnett, D. A. (eds) (2007). *Movement Assessment Battery of Children.* London: The Psychological Corporation.
12. Keunen, K., Kersbergen, K. J., Groenendaal, F., Isgum, I., de Vries, L. S., and Benders, M. J. (2012). Brain tissue volumes in preterm infants: prematurity, perinatal risk factors and neurodevelopmental outcome: a systematic review. *J. Matern. Fetal Neonatal Med.* 25(Suppl. 1), 89–100. doi: 10.3109/14767058. 2012.664343
13. Lodygensky, G. A., Seghier, M. L., Warfield, S. K., Tolsa, C. B., Sizonenko, S., Lazeyras, F., et al. (2008). Intrauterine growth restriction affects the preterm infant's hippocampus. *Pediatr. Res.* 63, 438–443. doi: 10.1203/PDR. 0b013e318165c005

14. Mallard, C., Loeliger, M., Copolov, D., and Rees, S. (2000). Reduced number of neurons in the hippocampus and the cerebellum in the postnatal guinea-pig following intrauterine growth-restriction. *Neuroscience* 100, 327–333. doi: 10.1016/S0306-4522(00)00271-2
15. Mari, G., and Deter, R. L. (1992). Middle cerebral artery flow velocity waveforms in normal and small-for-gestational-age fetuses. *Am. J. Obstet. Gynecol.* 166, 1262–1270. doi: 10.1016/S0002-9378(11)90620-6
16. Marsal, K., Persson, P. H., Larsen, T., Lilja, H., Selbing, A., and Sultan, B. (1996). Intrauterine growth curves based on ultrasonically estimated foetal weights. *Acta Paediatr.* 85, 843–848. doi: 10.1111/j.1651-2227.1996.tb14164.x
17. Morsing, E., Asard, M., Ley, D., Stjernqvist, K., and Marsal, K. (2011). Cognitive function after intrauterine growth restriction and very preterm birth. *Pediatrics* 127, e874–e882. doi: 10.1542/peds.2010-1821
18. Morsing, E., Gustafsson, P., and Brodszki, J. (2012). Lung function in children born after foetal growth restriction and very preterm birth. *Acta Paediatr.* 101, 48–54. doi: 10.1111/j.1651-2227.2011.02435.x
19. Morsing, E., Liuba, P., Fellman, V., Marsal, K., and Brodszki, J. (2014). Cardiovascular function in children born very preterm after intrauterine growth restriction with severely abnormal umbilical artery blood flow. *Eur. J. Prev. Cardiol.* 21, 1257–1266. doi: 10.1177/2047487313486044
20. Murphy, B. P., Inder, T. E., Huppi, P. S., Warfield, S., Zientara, G. P., Kikinis, R., et al. (2001). Impaired cerebral cortical gray matter growth after treatment with dexamethasone for neonatal chronic lung disease. *Pediatrics* 107, 217–221. doi: 10.1542/peds.107.2.217
21. Naud, A., Schmitt, E., Wirth, M., and Hascoet, J. M. (2017). Determinants of indices of cerebral volume in former very premature infants at term equivalent age. *PLoS One* 12:e0170797. doi: 10.1371/journal.pone.0170797
22. Neubauer, V., Junker, D., Griesmaier, E., Schocke, M., and Kiechl-Kohlendorfer, U. (2015). Bronchopulmonary dysplasia is associated with delayed structural brain maturation in preterm infants. *Neonatology* 107, 179–184. doi: 10.1159/000369199
23. Northam, G. B., Liegeois, F., Chong, W. K., Wyatt, J. S., and Baldeweg, T. (2011). Total brain white matter is a major determinant of IQ in adolescents born preterm. *Ann. Neurol.* 69, 702–711. doi: 10.1002/ana.22263
24. Ostgard, H. F., Lohaugen, G. C., Bjuland, K. J., Rimol, L. M., Brubakk, A. M., Martinussen, M., et al. (2014). Brain morphometry and cognition in young adults born small for gestational age at term. *J. Pediatr.* 165, 921.e1–927.e1. doi: 10.1016/j.jpeds.2014.07.045
25. Padilla, N., Junque, C., Figueras, F., Sanz-Cortes, M., Bargallo, N., Arranz, A., et al. (2014). Differential vulnerability of gray matter and white matter to intrauterine growth restriction in preterm infants at 12 months corrected age. *Brain Res.* 1545, 1–11. doi: 10.1016/j.brainres.2013.12.007
26. Reiss, A. L., Kesler, S. R., Vohr, B., Duncan, C. C., Katz, K. H., Pajot, S., et al. (2004). Sex differences in cerebral volumes of 8-year-olds born preterm. *J. Pediatr.* 145, 242–249. doi: 10.1016/j.jpeds.2004.04.031
27. Rose, J., Vassar, R., Cahill-Rowley, K., Stecher Guzman, X., Hintz, S. R., Stevenson, D. K., et al. (2014). Neonatal physiological correlates of near-term brain development on MRI and DTI in very-low-birth-weight preterm infants. *Neuroimage Clin.* 5, 169–177. doi: 10.1016/j.nicl.2014. 05.013
28. Scherjon, S., Briet, J., Oosting, H., and Kok, J. (2000). The discrepancy between maturation of visual-evoked potentials and cognitive outcome at five years in very preterm infants with and without hemodynamic signs of fetal brain-sparing. *Pediatrics* 105, 385–391. doi: 10.1542/peds.105.2.385
29. Schreuder, A. M., McDonnell, M., Gaffney, G., Johnson, A., and Hope, P. L. (2002). Outcome at school age following antenatal detection of absent or reversed end diastolic flow velocity in the umbilical artery. *Arch. Dis. Child. Fetal Neonatal Ed.* 86, F108–F114. doi: 10.1136/fn.86.2.F108
30. Skiold, B., Alexandrou, G., Padilla, N., Blennow, M., Vollmer, B., and Aden, U. (2014). Sex differences in outcome and associations with neonatal brain morphology in extremely preterm children. *J. Pediatr.* 164, 1012–1018. doi: 10.1016/j.jpeds.2013.12.051
31. Sussman, D., Leung, R. C., Chakravarty, M. M., Lerch, J. P., and Taylor, M. J. (2016). Developing human brain: age-related changes in cortical, subcortical, and cerebellar anatomy. *Brain Behav.* 6:e00457. doi: 10.1002/brb3.457
32. Sveinsdottir, K., Ley, D., Hovel, H., Fellman, V., Huppi, P. S., Smith, L. E. H., et al. (2018). Relation of retinopathy of prematurity to brain volumes at term equivalent age and developmental outcome at 2 years of corrected age in very preterm infants. *Neonatology* 114, 46–52. doi: 10.1159/0004 87847
33. Thompson, D. K., Warfield, S. K., Carlin, J. B., Pavlovic, M., Wang, H. X., Bear, M., et al. (2007). Perinatal risk factors altering regional brain structure in the preterm infant. *Brain* 130(Pt 3), 667–677. doi: 10.1093/brain/awl277
34. Tolsa, C. B., Zimine, S., Warfield, S. K., Freschi, M., Sancho Rossignol, A., Lazeyras, F., et al. (2004). Early alteration of structural and functional brain development in premature infants born with intrauterine growth restriction. *Pediatr. Res.* 56, 132–138. doi: 10.1203/01.pdr.0000128983.54614.7e
35. Torrance, H. L., Bloemen, M. C., Mulder, E. J., Nikkels, P. G., Derks, J. B., de Vries, L. S., et al. (2010). Predictors of outcome at 2 years of age after early intrauterine growth restriction. *Ultrasound Obstet. Gynecol.* 36, 171–177. doi: 10.1002/uog.7627
36. Trittmann, J. K., Nelin, L. D., and Klebanoff, M. A. (2013). Bronchopulmonary dysplasia and neurodevelopmental outcome in extremely preterm neonates. *Eur. J. Pediatr.* 172, 1173–1180. doi: 10.1007/s00431-013- 2016-5
37. Wechsler, D. (2002). *The Wechsler Preschool and Primary Scale of Intelligence, Third Edition (WPPSI-III).* San Antonio, TX: The Psychological Corporation. Wechsler, D. (ed.) (1991). *Wechsler Intelligence Scale for Children.* San Antonio,TX: The Psychological Corporation.
38. Yeh, T. C., Chang, J. H., Kao, H. A., Hsu, C. H., Hung, H. Y., and Peng, C. C. (2004).
39. Necrotizing enterocolitis in infants: clinical outcome and influence on growth and neurodevelopment. *J. Formos. Med. Assoc.* 103, 761–766.

18

Regulation of Placental Development and its Impact on Fetal Growth—New Insights from Mouse Models

Laura Woods [1,2], *Vicente Perez-Garcia* [1,2*] *and Myriam Hemberger* [1,2*†]

[1] *Epigenetics Programme, The Babraham Institute, Cambridge, United Kingdom,*

[2] *Centre for Trophoblast Research, University of Cambridge, Cambridge, United Kingdom*

***Correspondence:**
Vicente Perez-Garcia
vicente.perez-garcia@babraham.ac.uk
Myriam Hemberger
myriam.hemberger@babraham.ac.uk

†Present Address:
Myriam Hemberger,
Department of Biochemistry and Molecular Biology, University of Calgary, Calgary, AB, Canada

The placenta is the chief regulator of nutrient supply to the growing embryo during gestation. As such, adequate placental function is instrumental for developmental progression throughout intrauterine development. One of the most common complications during pregnancy is insufficient growth of the fetus, a problem termed intrauterine growth restriction (IUGR) that is most frequently rooted in a malfunctional placenta. Together with conventional gene targeting approaches, recent advances in screening mouse mutants for placental defects, combined with the ability to rapidly induce mutations *in vitro* and *in vivo* by CRISPR-Cas9 technology, has provided new insights into the contribution of the genome to normal placental development. Most importantly, these data have demonstrated that far more genes are required for normal placentation than previously appreciated. Here, we provide a summary of common types of placental defects in established mouse mutants, which will help us gain a better understanding of the genes impacting on human placentation. Based on a recent mouse mutant screen, we then provide examples on how these data can be mined to identify novel molecular hubs that may be critical for placental development. Given the close association between placental defects and abnormal cardiovascular and brain development, these functional nodes may also shed light onto the etiology of birth defects that co-occur with placental malformations. Taken together, recent insights into the regulation of mouse placental development have opened up new avenues for research that will promote the study of human pregnancy conditions, notably those based on defects in placentation that underlie the most common pregnancy pathologies such as IUGR and pre-eclampsia.

Keywords: placenta, trophoblast, mouse models, IUGR, fetal growth restriction, DMDD

INTRODUCTION

Intrauterine growth restriction (IUGR; also referred to as fetal growth restriction, FGR) is a common pregnancy complication, affecting around 3–8% of pregnancies worldwide (1–3). IUGR overlaps but is distinct from the more general condition known as small for gestational age (SGA), which is most commonly defined as weight below the 10th percentile for the gestational age. Whilst SGA babies are small but may be physiologically normal, IUGR is a pathological condition defined as the failure of a fetus to attain its full genetic growth potential. IUGR is a leading cause of stillbirth, prematurity, cerebral palsy and perinatal mortality (4–6). In the most severe cases, IUGR can lead to embryonic lethality and miscarriage during pregnancy. IUGR babies may have to be delivered prematurely, and therefore IUGR is also an indirect cause of preterm birth (7). Moreover, IUGR increases an infants' lifelong risk of adverse health outcomes including long-term poor neurological development, poor postnatal growth, and other childhood conditions, including serious and long-lasting immune deficiencies. Even well beyond infancy and childhood, IUGR is associated with a significant increase in the risk of cardiovascular disease, diabetes mellitus and hyperinsulinemia (8–10). Despite the distinction between IUGR and SGA, it is noteworthy that SGA infants are also affected by increased perinatal morbidity and mortality similar to IUGR, including neurodevelopmental disorders, stillbirth, and lifelong risk of adverse health outcomes (11).

IUGR is a complex and multifactorial disorder with a wide spectrum of potential causes. Some of these originate in specific genetic defects or congenital abnormalities in the embryo itself, or are a consequence of intrauterine infections. However, the majority of IUGR cases are caused by a failure of the placenta (10). The placenta is the extra-embryonic organ that only persists for the duration of pregnancy but that is absolutely essential for all intrauterine development. It has a number of essential functions such as anchoring the conceptus to the uterine wall, producing hormones to sustain pregnancy, inducing an immune-privileged environment and—as the perhaps most widely appreciated role—providing the embryo with sufficient amounts of nutrients and oxygen. Because of the pivotal role of the placenta in the etiology of IUGR, we here provide a brief overview of placental development, focussing for the most part on the mouse as the genetically most tractable model system to study early developmental processes at the molecular level. Specifically, we concentrate on fetal-specific effects of gene mutations. Interactions between placental trophoblast cells and maternal immune cells are also known to have an influence on growth trajectories of the fetus, but this aspect is outside the scope of this review and has been summarized elsewhere (12). Following this, we discuss novel insights into genetic causes of placental dysmorphologies. We will focus on recent findings that highlight the highly under-estimated number of genes contributing to placental development, and offer first approaches on how these may serve to identify novel molecular hubs that may be of key importance for placentation. These advances in the field harbor the prospect of enabling a better appreciation of the various causes of IUGR at the molecular and genetic level, which may lead to improved disease sub-classification, refined diagnosis and potentially to improved treatment options in the future.

BRIEF OVERVIEW OF PLACENTAL DEVELOPMENT

Tracing back in developmental time, the first definitive emergence of future placental cells occurs at the blastocyst stage with the formation of the trophectoderm. The trophectoderm forms the outer shell of the blastocyst, which is set aside from cells of the inner cell mass that will generate the embryo proper. Trophectoderm-derived cells ultimately give rise to all trophoblast cell types of the future placenta. Trophoblast cells make up the majority and defining aspects of the placenta. However, the most important exception to this placental cell provenance is the fetal placental vasculature. Endothelial cells of the fetal placental vasculature descend from cells of the extra-embryonic mesoderm that form the allantois and umbilical cord (13). These extra-embryonic mesodermal cells emerge slightly later in development at gastrulation, but ultimately have their cell lineage origin in the inner cell mass and epiblast. Thus, the placenta is a composite organ of two distinct cell lineages that arise from the fertilized embryo and that are established in early development, (1) the trophoblast lineage as the first lineage to differentiate that exclusively gives rise to placental trophoblast cell types, and (2) the extra-embryonic mesoderm that originates from cells of the inner cell mass and forms the fetal placental vasculature (**Figure 1A**).

Apart from these fetal-derived cell types, a vital aspect of placental development is the maternal uterine tissue into which the blastocyst is embedded upon implantation. The cells of the uterine lining, the so-called endometrium, undergo a specialized decidualization reaction upon implantation that is instrumental to support normal placentation and hence embryonic growth and survival (14). Indeed, the decidua will form part of the mature placenta. These principal tissue contributions are broadly similar between murine and human placentas. It is because of this complex and unique composition, combining fetal and maternal parts and thus amalgamating cells with different genetic constitution in a single organ, that often makes it difficult to discern where precisely the putative causes of a placental malformation may reside.

Placentation in the Mouse

Mouse models have been instrumental for advancing our knowledge of the impact of extra-embryonic development on pregnancy outcome and tracing the cell lineage origins of particular defects. For this reason, it is important to appreciate the progression of extra-embryonic development in the mouse, in comparison to that in humans. Following on from blastocyst formation, the trophectoderm cells surrounding the murine blastocoel cavity will soon cease to proliferate and enter endoreduplicative cell cycles, forming early (primary) trophoblast giant cells (TGCs). These TGCs help the embryo penetrate the uterine epithelium and implant into the endometrium, a process that takes place from developmental day (E) 4.5 onwards. Following implantation, polar trophectoderm cells overlying the inner cell mass continue to proliferate in response to a fibroblast growth factor 4 (FGF4) signal emanating from the epiblast (15). The arising column of diploid trophoblast cells forms the extra-embryonic ectoderm (ExE), a tightly packed epithelial tissue that retains stem cell potency (**Figure 1A**). Cells at the proximal tip of the ExE, farthest away from the epiblast, will further differentiate into the ectoplacental cone (EPC) that sits like a cap on top of the ExE. The cells at the margins of the EPC differentiate into secondary TGCs. It is these secondary TGCs in particular that acquire invasive characteristics, penetrating deeply into the endometrial stroma and making contact with

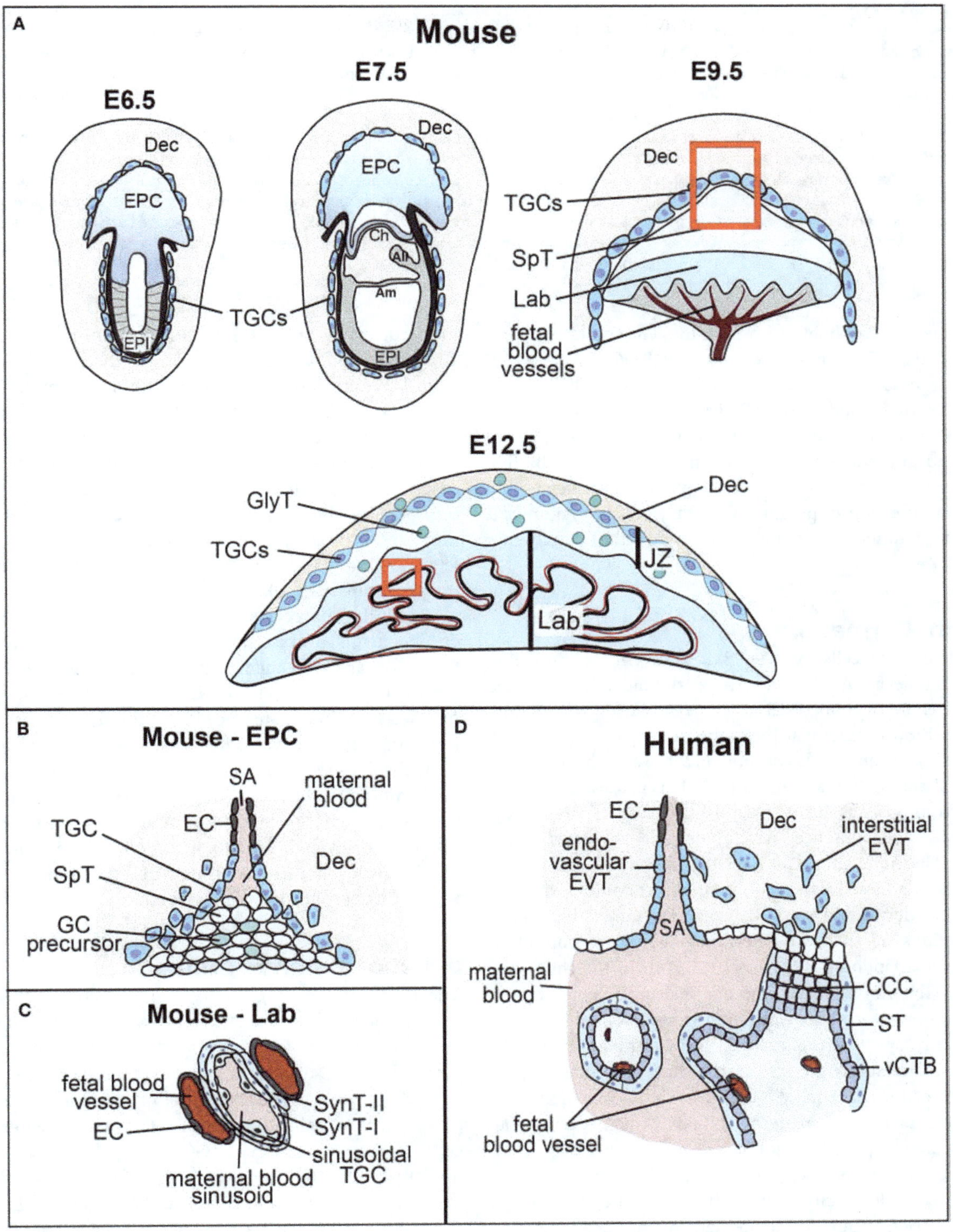

FIGURE 1 | Overview of mouse placental development and similarities to human placenta. **(A)** Following implantation, the blastocyst's mural trophectoderm differentiates into trophoblast giant cells (TGCs), while trophectodermal cells that overlie the inner cell mass form the extra-embryonic ectoderm (ExE) and the ectoplacental cone (EPC). The future embryo originates from the blastocyst's inner cell mass that differentiates into the epiblast (EPI). The conceptus is embedded into the maternal decidua (Dec) which differentiates from the uterine endometrium. With gastrulation, the chorion (Ch) consisting of a trophoblast and an extra-embryonic mesodermal cell layer, the amnion (Am) and the allantois (All) are formed. Cells at the margins of the of the EPC differentiate into invasive, secondary TGCs, that remodel the maternal vasculature [highlighted by the inset, see **(B)**]. The allantois grows out and attaches to the chorion (chorio-allantoic fusion) around E8.5, a critical process for developmental progression. At E9.5, allantoic blood vessels start to invaginate into the chorionic ectoderm to initiate formation of the placental labyrinth (Lab). Trophoblast cells overlying this layer differentiate into future spongiotrophoblast (SpT) and glycogen cells (GCs). The mature mouse placenta is established

(Continued)

FIGURE 1 | around mid-gestation (~E10.5) and continues to grow in size and complexity. It consists of three main layers: the labyrinth (Lab), the junctional zone (JZ) made up of SpT, GCs and TGCs, and the maternal decidua (Dec). The labyrinth is the main site of nutrient and gas exchange [highlighted by the inset, see **(C)**]. Black bar indicates thickness of the labyrinth zone. **(B)** Magnified view of the tip of the EPC where invasive TGCs remodel maternal spiral arteries (SA) by eroding their smooth muscle lining and displacing their endothelial cell (EC) layer. **(C)** Close-up view of the interhaemal barrier, consisting (from maternal to fetal side) of a discontinuous layer of sinusoidal TGCs, two layers of syncytiotrophoblast (SynT-I and -II), and the endothelial cell layer of the fetal blood vessels. **(D)** Despite significant morphological differences, comparison with the human placenta reveals structural and/or functional similarities. Human placental villi are made up of a mesenchymal core that contains the fetal blood vessels, a layer of villous cytotrophoblast (vCTB) and one overlying layer of syncytiotrophoblast (ST) that is directly exposed to maternal blood. Thus, the haemochorial organization and the exchange barrier are similarly organized between mouse and human placentas. vCTBs are perhaps most analogous to the chorionic ectoderm in mice. In anchoring villi, cytotrophoblast cells form cytotrophoblast cell columns (CCCs) that invade into the maternal decidua (Dec). Cells at the base of the CCCs proliferate, pushing cells along the column where they progressively differentiate into invasive extravillous trophoblast (EVT). Trophoblast invasion occurs along two routes, interstitially into the decidual stroma, and along an endovascular route to replace the endothelial cell (EC) lining of maternal spiral arteries (SA). This spiral artery remodeling process is instrumental for healthy pregnancy progression, and is equally shared with the mouse where these processes occur between ~E7.5 and E10.5 as shown.

maternal arteries. Trophoblast invasion by TGCs peaks between ~E7.5 and E9.5. This process entails that TGCs erode away the smooth muscle layer and displace the endothelial cell lining of maternal blood vessels (**Figure 1B**). As a consequence, maternal blood is funneled into the placenta in trophoblast-lined conduits and in the absence of vaso-constrictive control by the mother (16). These vascular remodeling processes are key to the successful progression of pregnancy, as they lay the anatomical foundations for the functional capacity of the developing placenta.

Labyrinth Formation

With gastrulation, cells of the ExE differentiate into the chorionic ectoderm. At the same time, the allantois develops from extra-embryonic mesoderm at the posterior end of the embryo, positioned exactly at the embryonic—extra-embryonic boundary. The allantois grows out and toward the chorion, ultimately attaching to it at around E8.5. This process of chorio-allantoic fusion is absolutely essential for further pregnancy progression. In its absence, development is abrogated soon afterwards. Chorio-allantoic fusion establishes a scenario where extra-embryonic mesodermal cells are in direct contact with the chorionic ectoderm, and start to invaginate into it in finger-like projections at sites pre-determined by expression of a particular transcription factor, *Gcm1* (17, 18). In the chorionic trophoblast, these invaginating mesodermal protrusions trigger a differentiation process in which individual trophoblast cells fuse to form syncytiotrophoblast. Syncytiotrophoblast cells ultimately will establish the transport surface, or "interhaemal membrane," of the placenta (**Figure 1C**). They form the blood sinusoids through which maternal blood (brought in by the trophoblast-lined spiral arteries and canals) percolates, and across which nutrients and oxygen must be transported to reach the fetal blood circulation. In the mouse, the entire exchange barrier, from the maternal to the fetal side, is made up of a total of three continuous cell layers, two layers of syncytiotrophoblast (SynT-I and SynT-II, respectively) and the extra-embryonic mesoderm-derived fetal endothelial cells (19). Sinusoidal TGCs that are likely of chorionic trophoblast origin are also present at the maternal side, apposed to the SynT-I layer, but they only form a fenestrated, discontinuous layer that does not constitute a complete barrier (**Figure 1C**). These intricate developmental steps start to occur from around mid-gestation in the mouse (E9.5–10.5) and lead to the formation of the so-called labyrinth. With labyrinth formation, the mature mouse placenta is being established. The labyrinth continues to grow for the next days by continued branching morphogenesis leading to further elongation and refinement of these inter-digitated vascular spaces. This architecture achieves a large surface area for transport in which maternal and fetal blood circulations come into close contact but never mix. Moreover, maternal and fetal blood flow in a counter-current direction, thus optimizing transport capacity (20).

As can be appreciated from these complicated and intricate developmental processes, defects and deficiencies in labyrinth formation are a frequent cause of developmental failure and growth deficits, respectively. Up until mid-gestation, the yolk sac meets the nutritional needs of the early embryo. However, from around E10 onwards the transport capacity of the placenta is an absolute requirement to ensure embryo survival. Indeed, this requirement to switch from yolk sac nutrition to placental nutrient supply, tied to the necessity for chorio-allantoic fusion and labyrinth formation to occur successfully, creates a developmental bottleneck around mid-gestation in the mouse when a large proportion of mutants die.

Junctional Zone Formation

The junctional zone (JZ) is positioned between the labyrinth and the maternal decidua. Together with the labyrinth, it forms the other major layer of the fetal part of the mature mouse placenta. The JZ originates mainly from cells of the core of the EPC, as judged by gene expression of prominent markers, such as *Tpbpa*. It contains three main cell types: spongiotrophoblast cells (SpT), glycogen cells (GCs) and a layer of TGCs that directly border the decidua (21). GCs often associate with maternal blood canals and sinuses. From about E12.5 onwards, they invade into the decidua where they become associated with maternal blood spaces. Because of their glycogen content and location, GCs are believed to serve as an energy store that can provide additional nutrition to the placenta and/or embryo. Apart from that, the JZ constitutes the main endocrine compartment of the placenta. It produces vast amounts of hormones, growth factors and cytokines that are important for the normal progression of pregnancy, acting on both the maternal and fetal physiology (22, 23).

The Human Placenta

Although mammalian placentas are functionally convergent, placental morphology is remarkably different between species. Mouse and human placentas share in common a haemochorial type of placentation, meaning that fetal trophoblast cells are directly bathed in maternal blood. In both species trophoblast is invasive and penetrates deeply into the endometrium, in humans even farther reaching into the muscular layer of the myometrium. Cellular morphology and overlapping gene expression patterns have helped identify analogous cell types in mouse and human placentas, although a direct comparison is not always clear-cut. The structure analogous to the murine labyrinth are the placental villi in the human placenta. As in the mouse, the cells exposed to the maternal blood are syncytial in nature, however, in humans there is only one layer of syncytiotrophoblast (**Figure 1D**). Immediately underlying the syncytiotrophoblast is a layer of villous cytotrophoblast cells (vCTBs) that continuously fuse into the syncytium and replenish it. These cells may be analogous to chorionic ectoderm cells in the early mouse placenta, but whether such a cell population persists into later murine gestation remains unknown. The core of the villus is made up of mesenchymal cells, fetal blood vessels, and a macrophage cell type known as Hofbauer cells. The blood vessels come close to the vCTB layer at presumptive sites of nutrient transfer, which hence in humans has to cross at least one syncytiotrophoblast layer, one cytotrophoblast layer and the fetal endothelial cells (19).

While there is appreciable morphological and functional similarity between the mouse labyrinth and the human placental villous structure, the equivalent to the JZ is harder to make out. Conceivably, such a relationship exists with the cytotrophoblast cell columns (CCCs). These columns grow out at certain points from the villi and anchor the placenta to the uterine wall. They consist of tightly packed cytotrophoblast cells that are highly proliferative at the base of the CCC, thereby contributing to the growth of the column. At their distal tips, extravillous cytotrophoblast (EVT) cells leave the context of the column and invade deeply into the uterine stroma. As in the mouse, this process of trophoblast invasion is instrumental to remodel maternal spiral arteries into large, trophoblast-lined canals that bring blood into the placenta (24). From the base of the column to the tip, cytotrophoblast cells undergo a well-documented epithelial-mesenchymal transition that coincides with acquiring invasive characteristics (25, 26). Like TGCs, EVT cells are also becoming polyploid and/or aneuploid, but not to the same extent as in the mouse where the genome content of TGCs can gain an equivalent of up to 1000N. In many regards, this morphological layout is somewhat similar to the ExE-EPC structure in the early mouse conceptus. It translates less obviously into the JZ structure of the mature mouse placenta, although by cellular descent these cells will be related to their earlier ExE/EPC progenitors.

PLACENTAL STRUCTURES LINKED TO EMBRYONIC GROWTH

Despite this mixed picture of structural and functional similarities and discrepancies between mouse and human placentas, the mouse model has been instrumental for gaining insights into molecular pathways that direct early trophoblast cell fate decisions as well as for identifying genes that affect placental development. For this reason, we focus below on key examples of what we have learnt from mouse mutants over recent years.

Maternal Spiral Arteries and Blood Canals

Trophoblast invasion and the remodeling of maternal spiral arteries are perhaps the most widely accepted processes associated with the patho-etiology of IUGR. A large number of genes have been linked to conferring invasive characteristics to mouse and human trophoblast, thereby endowing this cell type with the capacity to target and remodel maternal spiral arteries deep within the maternal decidua. Disruption of this process impairs placental blood flow and is a major cause of IUGR and pre-eclampsia (27). Pre-eclampsia is a pregnancy complication characterized by high blood pressure, proteinuria, and often fetal growth restriction. Both disorders share common risk factors and outcomes, however they are distinct conditions, i.e. not all cases of IUGR are also complicated by pre-eclampsia, and *vice versa*. In the mouse, invasive TGCs originate from the margins of the EPC. Their vital role in remodeling the maternal vasculature has been demonstrated in cell type-specific ablation experiments that took advantage of the regulatory elements of the *Tpbpa* gene to drive Cre recombinase expression. *Tpbpa* is a key marker gene of the precursors of invasive TGCs located within the core of the EPC. Ablation of *Tpbpa*-positive cells by conditional activation of a *Diphteria* toxin gene results in trophoblast invasion deficiencies and consequently in defective remodeling of maternal spiral arteries (28). Mature placentas from such mice exhibit a small JZ with reduced SpT, GC and TGC numbers, and the conceptuses die around E11.5. A comparable placental phenotype is observed upon deletion of the serine peptidase *Htra1*, which targets a similar cell population and partially ablates *Tpbpa*-positive EPC cells (29). These data show that in mouse, as in humans, trophoblast invasion and the vascular remodeling process mediated by these invading cells are pivotal determinants of fetal growth and survival.

In addition to these proof-of-concept phenotypes in the mouse, strong evidence suggests that the diameter of maternal blood canals is regulated by the NOTCH signaling pathway. Deletion of the transmembrane receptor *Notch2* in trophoblast causes developmental delay due to impaired invasion of maternal spiral arteries and a reduced size of maternal blood canals and -sinuses at the entry point into the placenta (30, 31). The importance of NOTCH signaling has also been demonstrated in the human placenta. In the first trimester placenta, NOTCH1 is expressed exclusively by progenitors of invasive EVTs (32), suggesting a role in spiral artery remodeling. In term placentas the NOTCH1,−2,−4 receptors, and the NOTCH pathway ligand JAGGED2 are expressed in the brush border of the syncytiotrophoblast layer, with NOTCH1 and NOTCH4 also marking vascular endothelial cells. Expression of these NOTCH family components is disrupted in placentas affected by IUGR and pregnancy-induced hypertension (33).

Junctional Zone Defects

Numerous mouse models with JZ defects exhibit an IUGR phenotype (**Figure 2**, **Supplementary Table 1**). A small JZ is associated with impaired production of the large family of prolactin-like hormones. However, deletion of the gene encoding prolactin (*Prl*) alone does not cause overt JZ defects (34), potentially implying functional redundancy with the other 22 prolactin-like genes present in the mouse genome (35). Alternatively, the abnormal expression of prolactin family hormones that is observed in many mutants with JZ defects may represent a readout rather than a cause of abnormal JZ size. In any case, fetal growth is affected by the size of the developing JZ. Apparently, this effect is indeed linked to the JZ and not the placenta as a whole, as fetal growth is impaired in mouse models which exhibit differences in the JZ but not the labyrinth (36, 37). JZ defects cause an altered endocrine environment in the placenta locally, but also have systemic effects on both fetus and mother. Such dysmorphologies may therefore affect fetal growth due to deregulation of the control of placental growth and structure, or by controlling the allocation of maternal resources, for example by altering maternal insulin resistance (38).

A major component of the JZ are GCs. Their ability to store and release large amounts of glycogen suggests they play a role in supplying glycogen as an energy source to the growing conceptus. For example, the volume of the JZ, the proportion of GCs it contains, and their total glycogen content is reduced when pregnant females are subjected to chronic or acute dietary restriction (39–41). Imprinted genes, i.e. the small collection of genes that are expressed in a parent-of-origin dependent manner, are a chief regulator of JZ development and maternal resource allocation. Disruption of imprinted gene expression in the placenta can be associated with both, fetal growth restriction or overgrowth in mice and humans. Prominent examples in humans are Beckwith-Wiedemann syndrome which is associated with fetal overgrowth, and Silver-Russell syndrome characterized by growth restriction. Both syndromes are caused by imprinting errors on chromosome 11p15, notably a paternal and maternal duplication of the imprinting control region, respectively. In the mouse, imprinting defects are commonly associated with JZ defects affecting the size of this compartment and hence the number of SpT and GCs (42). For instance, increasing the gene dosage of the imprinted gene *Phlda2* (encoding a pleckstrin homology domain protein) by a single copy dramatically reduces the size of the JZ and the amount of stored glycogen by between 25 and 35% (43). The remaining GCs fail to migrate into the decidua in late

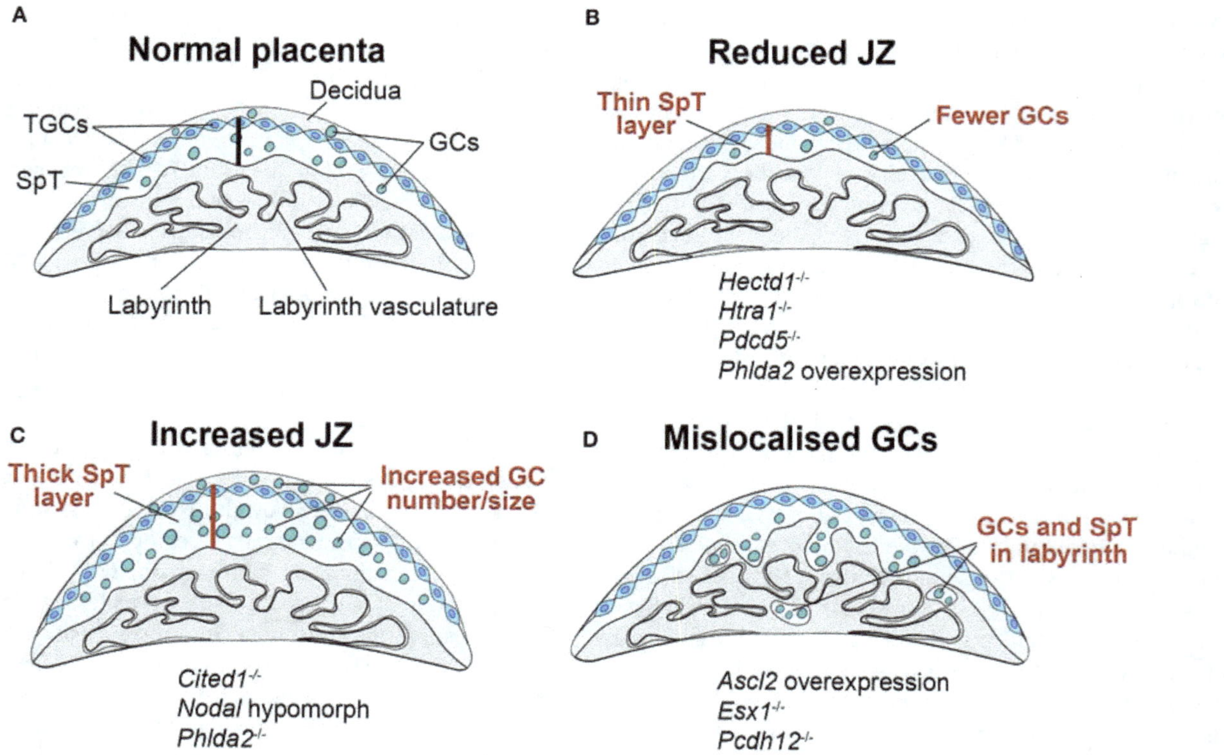

FIGURE 2 | Schematic representation of JZ defects that can be associated with IUGR. **(A)** The junctional zone (JZ) is composed of three cell types: spongiotrophoblast cells (SpT), glycogen cells (GCs) and trophoblast giant cells (TGCs). The JZ provides energetic (glycogen), hormonal and physical support to ensure correct placentation and pregnancy progression. **(B–D)** Recurring JZ phenotypes entail **(B)** a reduced thickness of the JZ layer (indicated by the red bar) with fewer SpT and/or GCs, **(C)** an increased size of the JZ with more SpT and/or GCs and **(D)** a mislocalisation of GCs and SpT in the labyrinth. All of these phenotypes can be associated with IUGR, highlighting that JZ size alone is not indicative of placental efficiency, but that other parameters such as effect on cellular function, and precise cell localisation in relation to blood vessels and blood conduits, is important. Examples of mouse mutants or overexpression models in which these dysmorphologies are observed are given (fetal genotype is shown).

gestation but persist in the JZ. Instead, *Tpbpa*-positive SpT cells and GCs become progressively mislocalized in the labyrinth compartment. Partial loss-of-function of another imprinted gene, *Ascl2,* which regulates *Phlda2* expression, similarly leads to depletion of SpT and ablation of GCs, and fetal growth restriction (44).

The common co-occurrence of a growth-retarded fetus with reduced GC numbers and less total glycogen content suggests that IUGR could be linked to the scarcity of glycogen in these placentas (**Figure 2B**). However, overabundance of glycogen is also associated with reduced fetal growth (**Figures 2C,D**). This is observed in the *Phlda2* knockout, which is associated with expansion of the junctional zone resulting in an over-accumulation of placental glycogen to 3x its normal levels, and leads to fetal growth restriction (45). Similarly, overexpression of *Ascl2* or knockout of *H19*, a maternally expressed non-coding RNA, leads to increased placental glycogen stores and reduced fetal growth (46, 47). An increase in GC numbers and glycogen content can also be associated with GC mislocalisation. This is the case in the *Ascl2* overexpression model or also in knockouts of the cell adhesion molecule *Pcdh12* or the homeobox gene *Esx1*, where GCs are ectopically located in the labyrinth (47–49). Hence, GC mislocalisation is emerging as a common feature of several gene manipulations that cause JZ defects associated with fetal growth restriction (**Figure 2D**). Although it may appear counter-intuitive that increased placental glycogen stores restrict fetal and placental growth, it may be that in such cases GCs are unable to supply their stored glycogen to the conceptus. This could be due to the inability of GCs to migrate into the decidua and access the maternal blood supply, or failure to break down and release stored glycogen, resulting in its over-accumulation. These deficits in turn may be caused by cell intrinsic defects in glycogen release, or altered hormonal control of glycogen metabolism, potentially due to defects in hormone production by the JZ. Taken together, these findings suggest that accumulation and storage of glycogen, and its subsequent release, are distinct and delicately balanced processes. Failure of GCs to either store adequate quantities of glycogen or to degrade and supply it as an energy source is detrimental to fetal and placental growth and development.

Although the human placenta does not contain specialized GCs akin to those found in the mouse, EVT cells located distally in the basal plate have the ability to store and metabolize large quantities of glycogen (19). The human placenta accumulates glycogen mainly in the first trimester, which then declines toward term, potentially contributing to the increased fetal and/or placental growth at this time (50, 51). Several studies have investigated glycogen content and metabolism in placentas complicated by IUGR, however as of yet no differences have been found in glycogen deposition (52, 53), or the expression and activity of enzymes involved in glycogen synthesis (54). The role of placental glycogen in normal human pregnancy and in pregnancy disorders is relatively understudied, however a recent review highlighted the association between altered glycogen deposition and metabolism in pathological pregnancy, including pre-eclampsia with IUGR, and diabetes (55). The strong association between altered placental glycogen stores and IUGR in the mouse prompts further research into understanding the role of placental glycogen in healthy and pathological pregnancies.

Labyrinth Defects

The role of the labyrinth as the site of nutrient exchange strongly implicates this placental layer in the pathogenesis of IUGR. Any defect in the labyrinth which alters its ability to mediate the transfer of nutrients and oxygen to the fetus may impact on fetal growth. Such defects lead to an imbalance between the metabolic demands of the fetus and the ability of the placenta to meet that need. Indeed, in a recent systematic screen of embryonic lethal or sub-viable mouse mutants that are frequently associated with IUGR prior to death, labyrinth defects stood out as a prominent site of placental failure (56). Many other reports of individual gene knockouts support the direct link between placental labyrinth development and fetal growth and viability (**Figure 3, Supplementary Table 1**) (57).

Small Labyrinth Size

The size of the labyrinth compartment is an important determinant of its capacity to nourish the fetus. A small labyrinth has a reduced transport surface area, thereby limiting the nutrients available to the fetal circulation and hence restricting the extent of fetal growth (**Figure 3B**). A small labyrinth can be the result of a labyrinth-restricted failure to expand this particular compartment, or because of an overall reduced placental size. For example, deletion of the translation initiation factor *Eif2s1* causes endoplasmic reticulum stress in the placenta and specifically reduces the size of the labyrinth layer, resulting in growth restriction of the fetus (2). These scenarios can sometimes be difficult to distinguish, as the labyrinth forms a substantial fraction of the placenta, and hence labyrinth-to-JZ ratios are often used as a measure of disruptions in the relative proportion of labyrinth size. Labyrinth growth is regulated by genes encoding key growth factor pathway components, including the receptors for fibroblast growth factor (*Fgfr2*), leukemia inhibitory factor (*Lifr*), epidermal growth factor (*Egfr*) and hepatocyte growth factor (*Met*) (58). *Met* (also known as *c-Met*), for example, is involved in the proliferation of labyrinth trophoblast progenitors, and its deletion leads to reduced labyrinth size and cellularity, and poor development of the vascular branching structure (59). The *Fgfr2-IgIII*, and *Egfr* mutants are embryonic lethal at midgestation due to disrupted labyrinth and JZ development (60–63), whilst the *Lifr* mutant displays perinatal lethality with poor organization of the labyrinth and spongiotrophoblast (64).

The insulin-like growth factor (IGF) axis is another important regulator of placental growth and development, and the placenta itself is a major source of IGF2 during pregnancy (65). Deletion of the imprinted, placenta-specific *Igf2 P0* transcript significantly reduces labyrinth thickness and surface area (66, 67), causing fetal growth restriction. Human IUGR pregnancies are characterized by altered IGF signaling, with low levels of IGF1 in umbilical cord blood and increased IGFBP1 and IGFBP2 (68–70). Human *IGF1* mutations are associated with severe IUGR (71–73), suggesting the conserved importance of the IGF

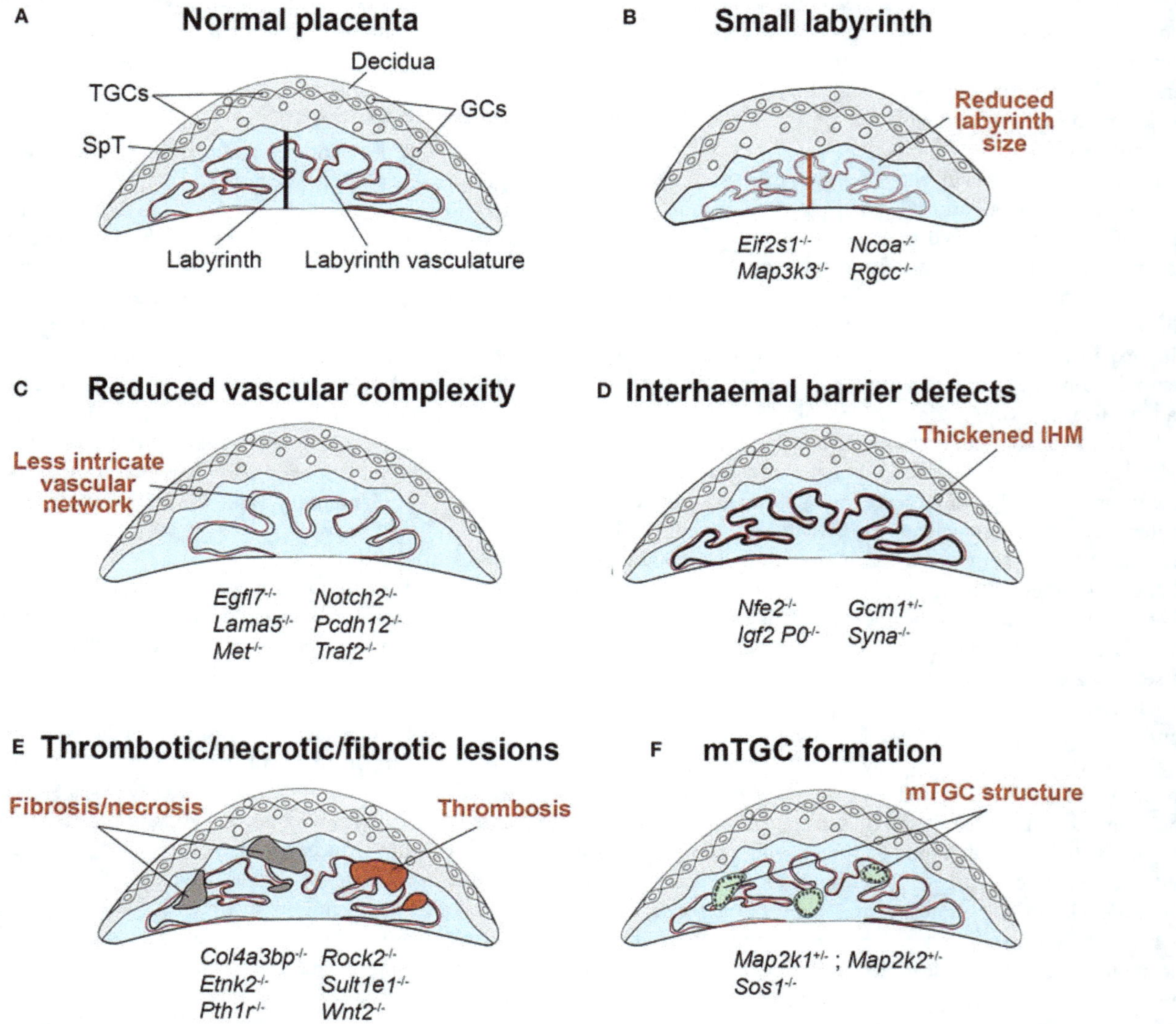

FIGURE 3 | Schematic representation of labyrinth defects associated with IUGR. **(A)** Within a normal placenta, the labyrinth is the largest layer and is the site of all nutrient and gas exchange between the maternal and fetal blood circulations (black bar indicates thickness of the labyrinth layer). As such, failure in the establishment of this intricately organized layer is a direct cause of IUGR, or in more severe cases of intrauterine lethality. Defects in the development of the labyrinth often originate from defective or insufficient invagination of allantoic blood vessels into the chorionic ectoderm (see **Figure 1**, E9.5) and the subsequent branching morphogenesis that has to occur to form this exchange surface. **(B)** Such defects can lead to a small labyrinth layer (indicated by the red bar, often coupled with an overall reduced size of the placenta) or **(C)** a reduced complexity of the vascular organization within the labyrinth, in which there are fewer, disorganized and/or inappropriately dilated fetal blood vessels and maternal conduits. Principally, these structural defects lead to a reduction of the surface area available for transport, which hence cause placental insufficiency. **(D)** Impaired nutrient transfer may also occur because of a thickened or dysfunctional interhaemal barrier (IHM). **(E)** The transport surface may be diminished due to overt lesions in the labyrinth layer, that frequently entail thrombotic or necrotic patches or the accumulation of fibrotic tissue. **(F)** An unusual trophoblast differentiation defect is observed in some mouse mutants with the formation of multinucleate trophoblast giant cells (mTGCs). These mTGCs likely have their origin in inappropriate fusion and syncytialisation of labyrinth trophoblast cells, disrupting the intricate labyrinthine architecture. Examples of mouse mutants or overexpression models in which these dysmorphologies are observed are given (fetal genotype is shown).

axis in placental development and fetal growth in mice and humans. The signaling cascades activated by the aforementioned growth factors and their receptors ultimately converge on the MAPK signaling cascade. Therefore, unsurprisingly, mutations in several MAPK pathway components also lead to varying degrees of labyrinth expansion deficits. As such, mutants of SOS1, GAB1, GRB2, RAF1, MEK1 (*Map2k1*), MEKK3 (*Map3k3*), and p38a (*Mapk14*) are characterized by a small labyrinth layer (**Supplementary Table 1**) (57, 74).

A small placental labyrinth is also a common feature of maternal undernutrition and diabetic mouse models leading to IUGR, showing that maternal exposure to external factors can affect labyrinth proliferation and expansion (39, 40, 75).

Vascular Organization

The intricately branched network of fetal blood vessels in the labyrinth develops initially by vasculogenesis, when angioblasts that are specified in the allantois extend into the chorion to form the fetal labyrinth vasculature. As outlined above, failure in chorio-allantoic fusion prevents any such vascular development and is associated with mid-gestational lethality in the mouse. A key factor required for the specification of invagination points into the chorionic ectoderm is the transcription factor *Gcm1*. Homozygous *Gcm1* mutants develop normally until E9.5 but are growth restricted and die at E10.5 due to failing branching morphogenesis of the labyrinth. Instead, the chorion remains a flat layer in these mutants (17). Apart from complete failure of vessel invagination, milder forms of chorion folding defects and insufficient vessel invagination can also be observed in many other mutants (**Figure 3C, Supplementary Table 1**). Development of the chorio-allantoic vasculature is in part regulated by the TGF-β pathway, and *Tgfb*, *Alk1*, and *Alk5* null mutants all show labyrinth vascularisation defects (76, 77). Additionally, mutations in the WNT and BMP family components *Wnt2*, *Rspo3*, *Bmp4* and *Smad1* display abnormalities such as a small or absent allantois and failure of chorio-allantoic fusion, as well as defects in formation of the labyrinth vasculature, including failure of fetal vessels to invaginate into the chorion, and the inappropriate formation of large edematous maternal blood spaces (77). The PPAR signaling pathway also plays a role, as *Pparg* null trophoblast cells fail to undrego terminal syncytium formation, which disrupts the integrity of the vascular exchange interface and restricts growth of the fetus (78, 79). Members of the PPAR family, as well as *GCM1* and its antagonist *NFE2* have been implicated in human IUGR placentas (80–82), demonstrating that abnormal differentiation of the villous trophoblast, especially of the syncytiotrophoblast layer, also contributes to placental insufficiency and IUGR in humans.

From mid-gestation onwards, the fetal vessels undergo extensive branching by angiogenesis, which contributes to placental expansion to meet the increasing needs of the growing fetus. These processes are regulated by members of the vascular endothelial growth factor (VEGF), placental growth factor (PGF), FGF, WNT, and the TGF-β and BMP families (83). Disruption of such key angiogenic pathways in the placenta has significant impact on placental vascularisation and is causally associated with IUGR in mouse and human pregnancies (84). Commonly, placentas exhibiting such vascularisation defects show a reduction in the number of fetal and/or maternal blood spaces, or an abnormal lumen diameter (85–88). For example, mouse mutants with deletion of *Rgcc*, a VEGF-inducible angiogenic inhibitor (89), develop a small placenta with fewer and wider fetal capillaries. Poorly vascularised $Rgcc^{-/-}$ placentas show decreased expression of *Vegf2* and *Pgf*, and embryos are growth restricted from E16.5 onwards (87).

The VEGF and PGF families constitute some of the prime regulators of angiogenesis in the labyrinth. Deletion of *Vegf* or overexpression of *Pgf* leads to severe labyrinth vascularisation defects, causing IUGR and embryonic death due to placental insufficiency (90–92). Similarly, ablation of the VEGF receptor *Vegfr1* (*Flt1*) in the mouse causes vasculogenesis and angiogenesis problems, resulting embryonic lethality (93). Overexpression of the soluble isoform of the human VEGF receptor, sFLT1, in mouse embryos induces pre-eclampsia like symptoms in pregnant dams, including IUGR, hypertension, and proteinuria, which can be ameliorated by PGF induction suggesting that PGF works antagonistically with sFLT1 to regulate placental angiogenesis (94). Dysregulated expression of sFLT1, PGF, and other angiogenic factors has been observed in human pregnancies complicated by IUGR and early onset pre-eclampsia complicated by IUGR (95–97). Indeed, determination of the sFLT1:PGF ratio, in combination with ultrasound findings, shows promise as a test of pre-eclampsia risk in the clinic, with an elevated ratio as an indicator of disease risk in pregnant women before the clinical onset of symptoms (98, 99).

Interhemal Barrier Defects

In addition to reduced labyrinth size, placental transfer insufficiency can also be caused by defects in the exchange barrier itself (**Figure 3D**). This may entail a mis-regulated expression of particular transporter molecules, or an increased thickness of the interhaemal membrane (IHM), thus hampering transport efficiency. These defects may occur in isolation or as compounding factor of small labyrinth size or reduced vascular complexity.

The IHM is a selectively permeable trilaminar barrier whose surface area increases throughout gestation as the labyrinth expands and becomes more intricately branched. The IHM also becomes significantly thinner between E12.5 and E16.5 of pregnancy, thereby reducing the distance over which substances must diffuse between the maternal and fetal blood supplies. This increases the theoretical diffusion capacity of the placenta, and in conjunction with expansion and branching of the labyrinth maximizes materno-fetal exchange (100, 101). Therefore, an increased thickness of the IHM can impede the efficiency of nutrient transfer to the fetus (**Figure 3D**). Disrupted morphology and thickness of the IHM is evident in the *Igf2 P0* knockout and in Syncytin A (*Syna*)-ablated mice, both of which display fetal growth impairment followed by embryonic lethality (67, 102). Manipulation of *Gcm1* expression to levels both below or above normal, by heterozygous *Gcm1* deletion or upregulation due to deletion of its antagonist p45NF-E2 (*Nfe2*), respectively, increases the thickness of the IHM (86, 103). Although fetal growth in $Gcm1^{+/-}$ conceptuses is not affected, wild-type females carrying $Gcm1^{+/-}$ conceptuses develop late gestational hypertension similar to what is seen in pre-eclampsia patients. Human placentas from IUGR pregnancies express reduced levels of *NFE2*, leading to upregulation of *GCM1* and excessive development of the syncytium (82), suggesting that similar molecular pathways operate in the establishment of the human placental IHM and may contribute to IUGR when disrupted.

In addition to IHM thickness, nutrient supply deficits may also be caused by mis-expression of specific transporter proteins. The *Igf2 P0* knockout affects in particular the system A amino acid transport system. Embryos overexpressing human *sFlt1*, which as mentioned earlier is implicated in early-onset pre-eclampsia with IUGR, develop a small labyrinth with reduced expression of the glucose diffusion channel *Connexin26* (*Cx26*). In contrast to their decreased expression of *Cx26*, *sFlt1* overexpressing embryos increase fatty acid and cholesterol transport by upregulation of *Cd36* and *Abca1* expression, respectively (104). Similarly, mice subjected to dietary restriction during pregnancy increase system A amino acid transporter activity leading to increased fetal amino acid accumulation (39). Amino acid and fatty acid/cholesterol uptake is increased in placentas with reduced ability to transport glucose, which may represent an attempt to compensate for an insufficient glucose supply. In fact, one study found that in normal pregnancies, the smallest placentas in a litter are more efficient in their nutrient transfer capacity to promote adequate fetal growth (105). Thus, up to a certain extent, small placentas may be able to compensate for reduced labyrinth size by increasing transport efficiency, but as labyrinth defects become more severe such compensatory mechanisms are insufficient to support normal embryonic growth.

Vascular Lesions

Additionally, defects in the integrity of the labyrinth can lead to the formation of edematous regions and thrombosis, generating infarcts which may impair fetal growth by disrupting the flow of fetal and maternal blood (**Figure 3E**). Mouse strains and mutants affected by placental thrombosis and infarction often show reduced fetal growth (106–109). Similar defects are a common feature of placentas from human pregnancies complicated by IUGR (110, 111). Likewise, failing development and impaired perfusion of the labyrinth can lead to tissue fibrosis and necrosis, thus limiting the available healthy labyrinth tissue for nutrient and gas exchange (**Figure 3E**) (112–114). For example, *Traf2*$^{-/-}$ (a regulator of NF-kappa-B and JNK) and *Col4a3bp*$^{-/-}$ (a collagen binding protein) placentas exhibit regions of fibrosis and necrosis within the vascularised labyrinth compartment, and deletion of the parathyroid hormone receptor *Pth1r* causes disruption of the labyrinth vasculature due to the presence of spongiotrophoblast inclusions and abnormal accumulation of maternal blood in the labyrinth (56).

Additionally, several mouse mutants with deletion of MAPK pathway components, including *Map2k1*, *Map2k2*, and the Ras guanine nucleotide exchange factor *Sos1*, display an unusual defect characterized by the formation of large multinucleate structures in the labyrinth (**Figure 3F**) (115, 116). These are referred to as multinucleate TGCs (mTGCs) in the literature but are unlikely to be true TGCs and may instead be a result of aberrant fusion of SynT-I and SynT-II, as they display characteristics of both layers (116). Mutants exhibiting mTGC formation also show reduced embryo growth (117) suggesting their presence may impede placental nutrient transfer due to severe disruption of the labyrinth branching structure and interruption of the vascular network.

As already alluded to, the placental defects described do not necessarily occur in isolation, as labyrinth growth, villous branching, and angiogenesis are interlinked. For example, a labyrinth with a simple branching structure is likely also small, with a reduced network of fetal capillaries. A placenta with failure in SynT differentiation or placental vascularisation may be both small, and have a thickened IHM due to defects in formation of the syncytium or fetal capillaries (67, 86, 102, 103). Defects in labyrinth morphogenesis and integrity are likely to also be affected by the presence of vascular thrombosis and infarction (106, 107).

Moreover, defects in labyrinth formation often co-occur with abnormal development of the JZ, suggesting that development of the two layers is interlinked. For example, deletion of *Ascl2* reduces the size of the JZ layer with an absence of GCs, in addition to severe defects in labyrinth morphogenesis and vascularisation (44). Maternal dietary restriction during pregnancy initially reduces the volume and glycogen content of the JZ with no effect on labyrinth size at E16, however by E19 the labyrinth compartment is significantly reduced in these placentas (39). These observations raise the possibility that hormone secretion by the JZ influences labyrinth morphogenesis, and JZ glycogen stores may be utilized during late gestation to fuel expansion of the labyrinth. In fact, the glycogen content of the JZ decreases in late gestation as GCs are lysed, coinciding with expansion of the labyrinth compartment at this time (100, 118). If so, this may contribute to abnormal development of the labyrinth in placentas with JZ defects (119, 120).

ENDOMETRIAL CAUSES OF IUGR

Development of the placenta is dependent upon successful implantation of the blastocyst into the uterine wall, followed by decidualization of the surrounding uterine stroma. This is necessary to facilitate a controlled trophoblast invasion into and remodeling of the stromal compartment, key pillars for subsequent placental development. Implantation and decidualization are regulated by a series of highly orchestrated and synchronized interactions between a competent blastocyst and the receptive endometrium. In the mouse, implantation occurs on the evening of day 4 of pregnancy when the blastocyst becomes attached to the receptive endometrium and starts to embed itself into the uterine wall. Implantation of the embryo is a prerequisite for pregnancy progression without which development cannot occur (121–123). Disruption of implantation and decidualisation, or a delay in its timing can create a ripple effect through pregnancy, leading to poor placentation and abnormal growth and development of the embryo (124). Maternal deletion of the cytosolic phospholipase A2 (*Pla2g4a*), prostaglandin synthase 2 (*Ptgs2*), or lysophosphatidic acid receptor 3 (*Lpar3*), factors involved in the prostaglandin synthesis pathway, or of the homeobox gene *Msx1*, causes implantation to be deferred beyond the normal window (125–127). This leads to a spectrum of complications ranging from mild to severe growth restriction through to embryonic demise, which may be secondary to developmental abnormalities of the placenta. A similar outcome was observed when blastocysts developed to E4 were allowed to implant in an E5 uterus (125). This pathological deferred implantation is distinct from embryonic diapause when a blastocyst is retained dormant in the uterus for an extended period before resuming implantation (128). Thus, defects in implantation can have a knock-on effect on development of the placenta, with ramifications for fetal growth and development. Human studies suggest that deferred implantation may be a factor in pregnancies affected by growth restriction. Late implantation occurring >12 days after ovulation in human pregnancy is associated with early pregnancy loss (129). Additionally, pregnancies with a longer interval between ovulation and implantation have a smaller first trimester crown-rump length than those that implant earlier (130), which has been shown to be a predictor of low birth weight and IUGR (131–133).

Implantation stimulates uterine stromal cells to proliferate and differentiate in response to progesterone. Decidualized uterine stromal cells acquire a unique secretory phenotype, which facilitates deep trophoblast invasion and remodeling of the maternal uterine stroma to form the maternal portion of the placenta, the decidua. Inhibiting formation of the decidua by deletion of key genes such as progesterone receptor (*Pgr*), *Bmp2* or *Hoxa11* abrogates the maintenance of pregnancy (134–137), and impaired growth of decidual tissue limits the size of the placenta. As such, defects which attenuate the decidualization response lead to the development of a small placenta with limited capacity to nourish the fetus, such as in mice with uterine-specific deletion of the TGF-β family receptor *Bmpr2* (138). Decidualization and formation of the decidua is dependent on the action of progesterone in an estrogen-primed uterus. Uterine stromal cells in the receptive endometrium express high levels of *Pgr* and its co-receptors including *Stat3*, which renders them competent to undergo decidualisation. Mice with deletion of *Pgr* or *Stat3* in the uterus are infertile as their progesterone resistance leads to complete failure of decidualization (135, 139). In recent studies into placental development with advanced maternal age in mice, it was shown that PGR and pSTAT3 levels are reduced in the uterine stroma of aged females, thus decreasing the ability of the endometrium to respond to progesterone (140, 141). This causes a blunted and delayed decidualization response with reduced proliferation and differentiation of uterine stromal cells, thus retarding the development of the decidua by up to 2 days in aged pregnancies. Such maternal-age related defects in the decidua impact on development of the trophoblast compartment, such that placentas from aged pregnancies often exhibit a small, malformed labyrinth and increased numbers of TGCs due to abnormal and skewed trophoblast differentiation. This is likely the result of dysregulation of the reciprocal signaling between the abnormal decidua and the trophoblast compartments. Other studies have similarly shown that defective decidualization has a knock-on effect on development of the trophoblast. Decidualization defects stemming from the maternal uterus can lead to reduced thickness of the labyrinth and SpT layers, with defects in GC differentiation and localisation (142–144), and increased differentiation into the TGC lineage (138, 143–146). These defects are likely to have a significant impact on placental function and fetal growth. Most strikingly, transfer of embryos from aged females into a young uterine environment rescues the placentation defects as well as embryonic growth and development, thus unequivocally attributing the effect to the mother and not the fetus (141). This is as of yet an understudied area in human pregnancy. Whilst abnormal decidualization with advanced maternal age has not yet been shown in humans, older women are at increased risk of pregnancy complications including fetal growth restriction and pre-eclampsia. The findings in the mouse suggest that this may be a result of defective decidualization due to endometrial dysfunction.

Abnormal decidualization can be associated with shallow invasion and inadequate transformation of the maternal vasculature, which is thought to be a causative factor and defining feature of obstetric complications such as pre-eclampsia and fetal growth restriction. In the mouse, deletion of the PI3K antagonist *Pten* in the decidua causes the development of an abnormally thick decidual compartment, due to decreased levels of apoptosis. The persistence of a thick decidual layer impedes trophoblast invasion and delays the remodeling of maternal blood vessels. This presumably limits the maternal blood supply to the placenta in early gestation, thus restricting fetal growth (142). Expression of a dominant negative form of the gap junction protein connexin-43 (*Gja1*) increases the expression of angiogenic factors *Flt1* and *Vegfa*, thus altering decidual angiogenesis. As a consequence, maternal blood spaces are disorganized and abnormally dilated, thus decreasing the surface area available for exchange (147). Conversely, deletion of the TGF-β family receptor *Bmpr2* in the uterus impairs decidual angiogenesis, resulting in a hypo-vascularised, under-perfused decidua with a poor capacity to nourish the fetus. This leads to reduced fetal growth and a miscarriage-like phenotype with progressive hemorrhaging of the placenta (138). These examples highlight the maternal impact on placentation and fetal growth as a consequence.

NEW INSIGHTS INTO MOLECULAR PATHWAYS CONTRIBUTING TO PLACENTAL DEVELOPMENT

Based on all the genetic and histopathological evidence summarized in the examples outlined above, it is clear that the placenta plays a pivotal role in the etiology of IUGR. With this in mind, the insights from a recent consortium study termed "Deciphering the Mechanisms of Developmental Disorders" (DMDD) is of key importance (148). This initiative aimed at systematically examining the impact of embryonic lethal or sub-viable gene mutations on embryonic and placental development in the mouse. It revealed that the placenta is far more frequently affected in these mutants than previously thought. Indeed, almost 70% of the mutant mouse lines examined that do not produce viable offspring at weaning exhibit a placental phenotype, a number that far exceeds the ~10% placentation defects estimated on the basis of published data deposited in the Mouse Genome Informatics (MGI) database (56). Even though this study was conducted on mutants that do not produce viable offspring at the expected Mendelian ratios post-weaning, the vast majority of these mutants is also affected by IUGR prior to demise. Thus, these insights are highly valuable as it is conceivable that hypomorphic mutations in such genes may contribute to the spectrum of IUGR pathologies in viable offspring.

The key realization that most embryonic lethal or subviable mouse mutations will also suffer from placentation defects is of great impact. With some ~5000 genes causing embryonic lethality, and an estimated two-thirds of these being associated with placental defects, there are literally hundreds if not thousands of genes that remain unknown for their role in placental development. At least in some instances, these placentation defects will be causative of the developmental retardation and embryonic lethal phenotype. Even with the relatively limited number of genes analyzed as part of DMDD, it was possible to determine functional gene "hubs," i.e., clusters of physically or functionally interacting factors that very likely play pivotal roles in normal placentation. One example highlighted in that study was the Polycomb group gene *L3mbtl2*. Further mining of the DMDD database also reveals, for instance, the glycosylphosphatidylinositol (GPI)-anchor biosynthesis pathway as an important player in formation of the early labyrinth. Thus, efforts to identify embryonic lethal and subviable mutants are of immense value to identify novel genes, and functional protein complexes, that are important for normal placental development and hence also likely involved in the etiology of IUGR.

Data Mining Approaches

Apart from providing a first systematic survey of placental pathologies in embryonic lethal mouse mutants, another key advantage afforded by the DMDD study is the parallel analysis of both embryo and placenta for all mutant lines, allowing statistical co-association analyses of phenotype correlations. This analysis revealed a strong link between placental defects and heart, brain, and vascular abnormalities. These co-associations are not entirely unexpected, as a "heart-placenta axis" that describes an inter-dependence in the development of both organ systems has previously been suggested (78). However, this concept has so far been based on the analysis of very few, select genes only. The clear-cut nature of these developmental correlations in an entirely unbiased survey was hence compelling. They may indeed prove of great benefit for hypothesis-generating approaches to identify novel candidates for functional analysis in placental development. Thus, gene mutations that affect embryonic viability as well as heart, brain, or vascular development should enrich for factors that are also involved in normal placentation.

Underpinning the validity of this rationale on the above example of the GPI-anchor biosynthesis pathway, mutations in human *DPM1* and *PGAP2*, two pivotal genes implicated in placentation failure in the mouse, cause congenital disorders in which severe neurological dysmorphologies are a common feature (149, 150). Similarly, mutations in human *PIGL*, another placental regulator and GPI anchor synthesis protein identified by the DMDD study, are linked to a general developmental delay causing congenital heart disease, ocular colobomas, ichthyosiform dermatosis, mental retardation, ear anomalies and epilepsy (CHIME) syndrome (151). The fact that deletion of these genes in the mouse induces a severe trophoblast phenotype suggests an essential role of the GPI pathway in regulating early placentation linked to heart and neural development in the fetus.

Following this line of thought, we here screened the MGI database for the mammalian phenotype term "embryonic growth retardation" (MP: 0003984). This revealed 505 gene mutations, of which 54.7% (276) are also known to exhibit placental abnormalities (**Figure 4A**). Intriguingly, the remaining 229 lines in which a placental phenotype remains unknown show a significant prevalence of cardiovascular system phenotypes (51.1%), brain development defects (33.2%), or both (21.4 %) (**Figure 4B**). Therefore, it is tempting to speculate that at least some of these gene mutations will also display placentation defects.

To take this analysis even further we screened the genes associated with cardiovascular and/or brain phenotypes for expression in embryonic (ESCs) and trophoblast (TSCs) stem cells. In doing so we uncovered several genes that cluster into functional networks with an enriched expression in the trophoblast compartment compared to ESCs, thus suggesting a likely role in placentation (**Figure 4C**). One such node, identified within the cardiovascular phenotype gene collection, centers around a hydroxyacyl-CoA dehydrogenase complex (*Hadha*) gene. *Hadha* encodes the alpha subunit of the mitochondrial trifunctional protein complex involved in the mitochondrial beta-oxidation of fatty acids. The gene, as well as its known interactors, shows increased expression in TSCs compared to ESCs, reinforcing the notion of the likely functionality of this complex in trophoblast differentiation. Along similar lines, the *Coq7* gene encoding the enzyme demethoxyubiquinone monooxygenase was identified in the overlap between search terms "embryonic growth retardation" and "abnormal brain morphology." COQ7 is essential for ubiquinone biosynthesis. Ubiquinone acts as a cofactor during several redox processes like mitochondrial respiration. *Coq7*-deficient mice are embryonic lethal during mid-gestation with impaired neurogenesis and mitochondrial defects (152, 153). Although placental defects have not been described to date, *Coq7* is highly expressed in TSCs and placental trophoblast. Recently, a mutation of *COQ7* has been reported in a pregnancy complicated by oligohydramniosis, fetal lung hypoplasia, and growth retardation (154).

Finally, the joint overlap between search terms embryonic growth retardation, abnormal brain morphology and heart morphology reveals a number of genes that are highly expressed in TSCs, for example the muscle segment homeobox 2 (*Msx2*) transcription factor. *Msx1/2*-deficient mice show severe defects in cardiovascular and brain development and are growth-retarded (155). Our data would suggest that this mutant is likely to also exhibit defects in placental development. In fact, recent reports demonstrated that MSX2 is expressed in the human placenta and may regulate human trophoblast invasion (156). Another tangible example is the Hippo pathway component centered around *Lats2* (**Figure 4C**), that is known for its function in establishing cell polarity in the early embryo and the acquisition of trophoblast cell fate (15, 157). The phosphorylation state of YAP1 in particular is known as the broker between "inner" and "outer" cells in the morula-stage embryo, with unphosphorylated nuclear Yap1 being essential to induce trophoblast identity. The cytoskeletal protein Ezrin (*Ezr*) is a core hallmark of microvilli in epithelial cells and is strongly expressed in trophectoderm and its derivatives.

These various examples highlight the value of mining available large-scale datasets to identify novel candidate factors

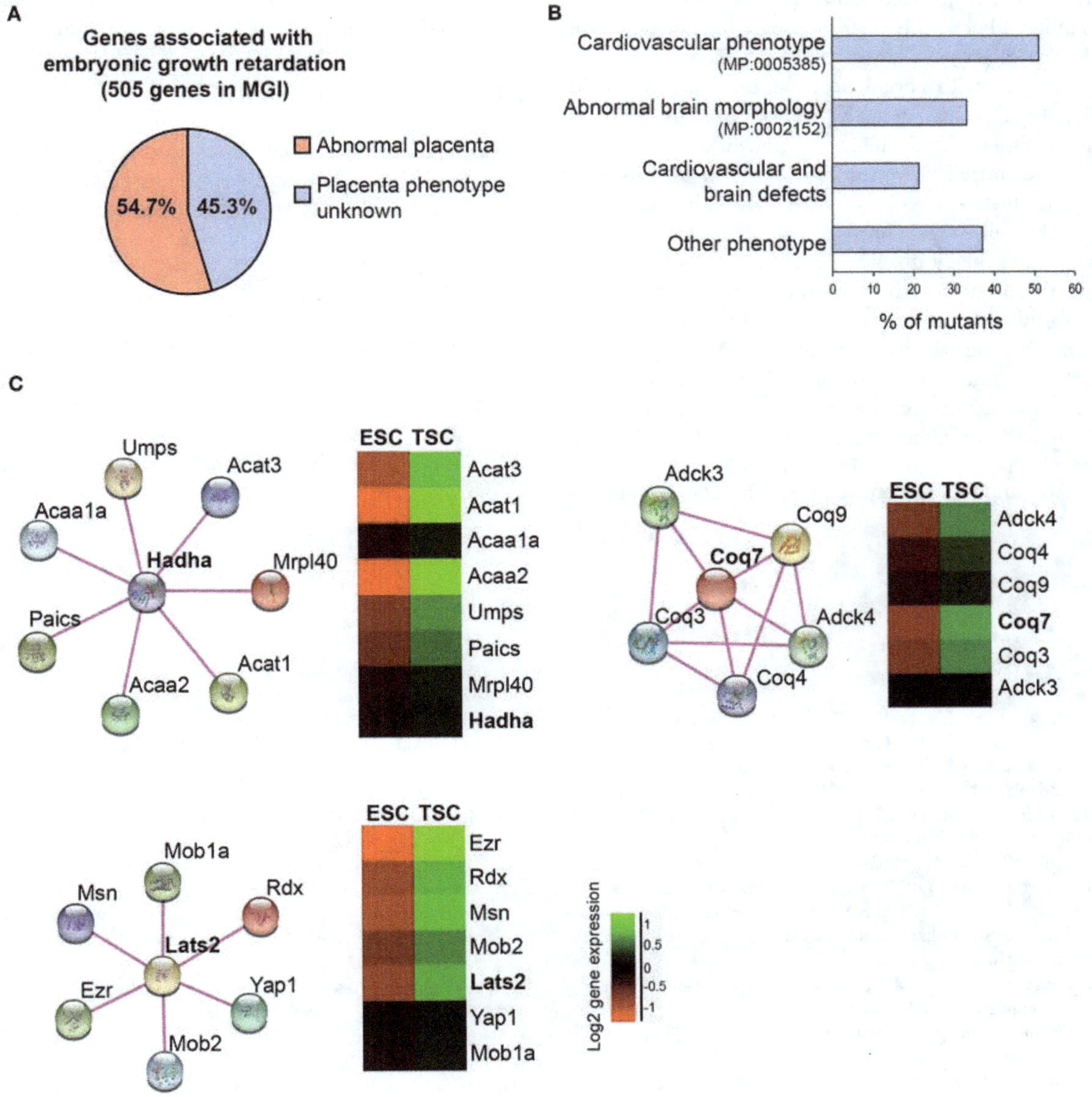

FIGURE 4 | Data mining approaches to identify molecular networks of potential importance in placental development. **(A)** Pie chart of genes extracted from the Mouse Genome Informatics database (www.informatics.jax.org) that are associated with embryonic growth retardation (MP: 0003984; 505 genes in total) and that are either scored as having an abnormal placenta (MP:0002086 or MP:0004264) or an unknown placental phenotype. **(B)** Breakdown of the proportion of mutants with unknown placental phenotype that also exhibit defects in heart and/or brain development. Since placental defects are often co-associated with cardiovascular and brain abnormalities (56), this selection will enrich for genes that have a function in the placenta. **(C)** Molecular network analysis using String (https://string-db.org/) to identify physical and/or functional gene interactions for selected examples, and expression levels of the identified complex components in trophoblast stem cells (TSCs) compared to embryonic stem cells (ESCs). The network components are enriched in the trophoblast compartment, arguing for a potential function in placental development.

and pathways that may be required for normal placentation. Once identified, these putative placental hubs require in-depth phenotypic and functional screening to confirm their involvement in extra-embryonic development. Nevertheless, they may prove powerful to accelerate the much-needed efforts in gaining a broader understanding of the collection of genes involved in placental biology both in healthy and pathological conditions.

CONCLUSIONS AND OUTLOOK

Perhaps the most striking outcome of the recent DMDD mouse phenotyping screen is the realization of the extent to which the number of genes contributing to placental development has been underestimated. The above examples provide a starting point on how these new and extensive datasets can be mined in the future with the aim of identifying novel molecular networks that may have key functions during placentation. Even within the small set of genes highlighted here, it is clear that some have already been linked to human placentation and/or developmental problems. These links inspire with confidence that the combination of mouse phenotyping data, gene expression profiles, physical, and/or functional protein interaction networks and human disease links are indeed powerful approaches to identify such functional gene clusters. Arguably, rather than individual genes, the functionality of larger protein complexes and/or gene networks is more likely to be conserved between species, making this approach more powerful and more promising for translational studies. Once confirmed for an involvement in the etiology of placental defects, it is conceivable that such genes may become part of mutation screening panels for refined diagnosis and may constitute targets for drug development to improve our understanding and potential treatment options of IUGR in the future. Overall, the depth and molecular detail of the analysis of recent mouse mutants has opened up many new avenues for research aimed at understanding the molecular basis of normal placentation and of placental pathologies in humans.

AUTHOR CONTRIBUTIONS

LW, VP-G, and MH contributed to the conceptualisation and writing of the manuscript. MH assembled **Figure 1**, LW **Figures 2, 3**, and VP-G **Figure 4** and **Supplementary Table 1.**

ACKNOWLEDGMENTS

This work was supported by the Biotechnology and Biological Sciences Research Council (BBSRC), and by a Ph.D. studentship from the Medical Research Council (MRC) to LW. VP-G is recipient of a Next Generation Fellowship from the Centre for Trophoblast Research, University of Cambridge, UK.

REFERENCES

1. Militello M, Pappalardo EM, Ermito S, Dinatale A, Cavaliere A, Carrara S. Obstetric management of IUGR. *J Prenat Med.* (2009) 3:6–9.
2. Yung HW, Hemberger M, Watson ED, Senner CE, Jones CP, Kaufman RJ, et al. Endoplasmic reticulum stress disrupts placental morphogenesis: implications for human intrauterine growth restriction. *J. Pathol.* (2012) 228:554–64. doi: 10.1002/path.4068
3. Vijayaselvi R, Cherian AG. Risk assessment of intrauterine growth restriction. *Curr Med Issues* (2017) 15:262–6. doi: 10.4103/cmi.cmi_76_17
4. Gardosi J, Madurasinghe V, Williams M, Malik A, Francis A. Maternal and fetal risk factors for stillbirth: population based study. *BMJ* (2013) 346:f108. doi: 10.1136/bmj.f108
5. von Beckerath AK, Kollmann M, Rotky-Fast C, Karpf E, Lang U, Klaritsch P. Perinatal complications and long-term neurodevelopmental outcome of infants with intrauterine growth restriction. *Am J Obstet Gynecol.* (2013) 208:130.e1–6. doi: 10.1016/j.ajog.2012.11.014
6. Blair EM, Nelson KB. Fetal growth restriction and risk of cerebral palsy in singletons born after at least 35 weeks' gestation. *Am J Obstet Gynecol.* (2015) 212:520.e1–7. doi: 10.1016/j.ajog.2014.10.1103
7. Hui L, Challis D. Diagnosis and management of fetal growth restriction: the role of fetal therapy. *Best Pract Res Clin Obstet Gynaecol.* (2008) 22:139–58. doi: 10.1016/j.bpobgyn.2007.06.004
8. Barker DJ, Osmond C, Golding J, Kuh D, Wadsworth ME. Growth in utero, blood pressure in childhood and adult life, and mortality from cardiovascular disease. *BMJ* (1989) 298:564–7. doi: 10.1136/bmj.298.6673.564
9. Barker DJ. The fetal and infant origins of disease. *Eur J Clin Invest.* (1995) 25:457–63. doi: 10.1111/j.1365-2362.1995.tb01730.x
10. Sharma D, Shastri S, Sharma P. Intrauterine growth restriction: antenatal and postnatal aspects. *Clin Med Insights Pediatr.* (2016) 10:67–83. doi: 10.4137/CMPed.S40070
11. Sharma D, Farahbakhsh N, Shastri S, Sharma P. Intrauterine growth restriction - part 2. *J Matern Fetal Neonatal Med.* (2016) 29:4037–48. doi: 10.3109/14767058.2016.1154525
12. Erlebacher A. Immunology of the maternal-fetal interface. *Annu Rev Immunol.* (2013) 31:387–411. doi: 10.1146/annurev-immunol-032712-100003
13. Rossant J, Cross JC. Placental development: lessons from mouse mutants. *Nat Rev Genet.* (2001) 2:538–48. doi: 10.1038/35080570
14. Ramathal CY, Bagchi IC, Taylor RN, Bagchi MK. Endometrial decidualization: of mice and men. *Semin Reprod Med.* (2010) 28:17–26. doi: 10.1055/s-0029-1242989
15. Latos PA, Hemberger M. From the stem of the placental tree: trophoblast stem cells and their progeny. *Development* (2016) 143:3650–60. doi: 10.1242/dev.133462
16. Hemberger M. Health during pregnancy and beyond: fetal trophoblast cells as chief co-ordinators of intrauterine growth and reproductive success. *Ann Med.* (2012) 44:325–37. doi: 10.3109/07853890.2012.663930
17. Anson-Cartwright L, Dawson K, Holmyard D, Fisher SJ, Lazzarini RA, Cross JC. The glial cells missing-1 protein is essential for branching morphogenesis in the chorioallantoic placenta. *Nat Genet.* (2000) 25:311–4. doi: 10.1038/77076
18. Simmons DG, Natale DR, Begay V, Hughes M, Leutz A, Cross JC. Early patterning of the chorion leads to the trilaminar trophoblast cell structure in the placental labyrinth. *Development* (2008) 135:2083–91. doi: 10.1242/dev.020099
19. Georgiades P, Ferguson-Smith AC, Burton GJ. Comparative developmental anatomy of the murine and human definitive placentae. *Placenta* (2002) 23:3–19. doi: 10.1053/plac.2001.0738
20. Adamson SL, Lu Y, Whiteley KJ, Holmyard D, Hemberger M, Pfarrer C, et al. Interactions between trophoblast cells and the maternal and fetal circulation in the mouse placenta. *Dev Biol.* (2002) 250:358–73. doi: 10.1006/dbio.2002.0773
21. Simmons DG, Fortier AL, Cross JC. Diverse subtypes and developmental origins of trophoblast giant cells in the mouse placenta. *Dev Biol.* (2007) 304:567–78. doi: 10.1016/j.ydbio.2007.01.009
22. Ain R, Canham LN, Soares MJ. Gestation stage-dependent intrauterine trophoblast cell invasion in the rat and mouse: novel endocrine phenotype and regulation. *Dev Biol.* (2003) 260:176–90. doi: 10.1016/S0012-1606(03)00210-0
23. Soares MJ. The prolactin and growth hormone families: pregnancy-specific hormones/cytokines at the maternal-fetal interface. *Reprod Biol Endocrinol.* (2004) 2:51. doi: 10.1186/1477-7827-2-51
24. Pijnenborg R, Vercruysse L, Brosens I. Deep placentation. *Best Pract Res Clin Obstet Gynaecol.* (2011) 25:273–85. doi: 10.1016/j.bpobgyn.2010.10.009
25. DaSilva-Arnold S, James JL, Al-Khan A, Zamudio S, Illsley NP. Differentiation of first trimester cytotrophoblast to extravillous trophoblast involves an epithelial-mesenchymal transition. *Placenta* (2015) 36:1412–8. doi: 10.1016/j.placenta.2015.10.013

26. Davies JE, Pollheimer J, Yong HE, Kokkinos MI, Kalionis B, Knofler M, et al. Epithelial-mesenchymal transition during extravillous trophoblast differentiation. *Cell Adh Migr.* (2016) 10:310–21. doi: 10.1080/19336918.2016.1170258
27. Brosens I, Pijnenborg R, Vercruysse L, Romero R. The "Great Obstetrical Syndromes" are associated with disorders of deep placentation. *Am J Obstet Gynecol.* (2011) 204:193–201. doi: 10.1016/j.ajog.2010.08.009
28. Hu D, Cross JC. Ablation of Tpbpa-positive trophoblast precursors leads to defects in maternal spiral artery remodeling in the mouse placenta. *Dev Biol.* (2011) 358:231–9. doi: 10.1016/j.ydbio.2011.07.036
29. Hasan MZ, Ikawati M, Tocharus J, Kawaichi M, Oka C. Abnormal development of placenta in HtrA1-deficient mice. *Dev Biol.* (2015) 397:89–102. doi: 10.1016/j.ydbio.2014.10.015
30. Hamada Y, Hiroe T, Suzuki Y, Oda M, Tsujimoto Y, Coleman JR, et al. Notch2 is required for formation of the placental circulatory system, but not for cell-type specification in the developing mouse placenta. *Differentiation* (2007) 75:268–78. doi: 10.1111/j.1432-0436.2006.00137.x
31. Hunkapiller NM, Gasperowicz M, Kapidzic M, Plaks V, Maltepe E, Kitajewski J, et al. A role for Notch signaling in trophoblast endovascular invasion and in the pathogenesis of pre-eclampsia. *Development* (2011) 138:2987–98. doi: 10.1242/dev.066589
32. Haider S, Meinhardt G, Saleh L, Fiala C, Pollheimer J, Knofler M. Notch1 controls development of the extravillous trophoblast lineage in the human placenta. *Proc Natl Acad Sci USA.* (2016) 113:E7710–9. doi: 10.1073/pnas.1612335113
33. Sahin Z, Acar N, Ozbey O, Ustunel I, Demir R. Distribution of Notch family proteins in intrauterine growth restriction and hypertension complicated human term placentas. *Acta Histochem.* (2011) 113:270–6. doi: 10.1016/j.acthis.2009.10.006
34. Horseman ND, Zhao W, Montecino-Rodriguez E, Tanaka M, Nakashima K, Engle SJ, et al. Defective mammopoiesis, but normal hematopoiesis, in mice with a targeted disruption of the prolactin gene. *EMBO J.* (1997) 16:6926–35. doi: 10.1093/emboj/16.23.6926
35. Simmons DG, Rawn S, Davies A, Hughes M, Cross JC. Spatial and temporal expression of the 23 murine Prolactin/Placental Lactogen-related genes is not associated with their position in the locus. *BMC Genomics* (2008) 9:352. doi: 10.1186/1471-2164-9-352
36. Salas M, John R, Saxena A, Barton S, Frank D, Fitzpatrick G, et al. Placental growth retardation due to loss of imprinting of Phlda2. *Mech Dev.* (2004) 121:1199–210. doi: 10.1016/j.mod.2004.05.017
37. Tunster SJ, Van de. Pette M, John RM. Impact of genetic background on placental glycogen storage in mice. *Placenta* (2012) 33:124–7. doi: 10.1016/j.placenta.2011.11.011
38. Fowden AL, Moore T. Maternal-fetal resource allocation: co-operation and conflict. *Placenta* (2012) 33(Suppl 2):e11–15. doi: 10.1016/j.placenta.2012.05.002
39. Coan PM, Vaughan OR, Sekita Y, Finn SL, Burton GJ, Constancia M, et al. Adaptations in placental phenotype support fetal growth during undernutrition of pregnant mice. *J Physiol.* (2010) 588:527–38. doi: 10.1113/jphysiol.2009.181214
40. Sferruzzi-Perri AN, Vaughan OR, Coan PM, Suciu MC, Darbyshire R, Constancia M, et al. Placental-specific Igf2 deficiency alters developmental adaptations to undernutrition in mice. *Endocrinology* (2011) 152:3202–12. doi: 10.1210/en.2011-0240
41. Gonzalez PN, Gasperowicz M, Barbeito-Andres J, Klenin N, Cross JC, Hallgrimsson B. Chronic protein restriction in mice impacts placental function and maternal body weight before fetal growth. *PLoS ONE* (2016) 11:e0152227. doi: 10.1371/journal.pone.0152227
42. Lefebvre L. The placental imprintome and imprinted gene function in the trophoblast glycogen cell lineage. *Reprod Biomed Online* (2012) 25:44–57. doi: 10.1016/j.rbmo.2012.03.019
43. Tunster SJ, Tycko B, John RM. The imprinted Phlda2 gene regulates extraembryonic energy stores. *Mol Cell Biol.* (2010) 30:295–306. doi: 10.1128/MCB.00662-09
44. Oh-McGinnis R, Bogutz AB, Lefebvre L. Partial loss of Ascl2 function affects all three layers of the mature placenta and causes intrauterine growth restriction. *Dev Biol.* (2011) 351:277–86. doi: 10.1016/j.ydbio.2011.01.008
45. Tunster SJ, Creeth HDJ, John RM. The imprinted Phlda2 gene modulates a major endocrine compartment of the placenta to regulate placental demands for maternal resources. *Dev Biol.* (2016) 409:251–60. doi: 10.1016/j.ydbio.2015.10.015
46. Esquiliano DR, Guo W, Liang L, Dikkes P, Lopez MF. Placental glycogen stores are increased in mice with H19 null mutations but not in those with insulin or IGF type 1 receptor mutations. *Placenta* (2009) 30:693–9. doi: 10.1016/j.placenta.2009.05.004
47. Tunster SJ, McNamara GI, Creeth HDJ, John RM. Increased dosage of the imprinted Ascl2 gene restrains two key endocrine lineages of the mouse placenta. *Dev Biol.* (2016) 418:55–65. doi: 10.1016/j.ydbio.2016.08.014
48. Li Y, Behringer RR. Esx1 is an X-chromosome-imprinted regulator of placental development and fetal growth. *Nat Genet.* (1998) 20:309–11. doi: 10.1038/3129
49. Rampon C, Bouillot S, Climescu-Haulica A, Prandini MH, Cand F, Vandenbrouck Y, et al. Protocadherin 12 deficiency alters morphogenesis and transcriptional profile of the placenta. *Physiol Genomics* (2008) 34:193–204. doi: 10.1152/physiolgenomics.00220.2007
50. Shafrir E, Barash V. Placental glycogen metabolism in diabetic pregnancy. *Isr J Med Sci.* (1991) 27:449–61.
51. Hahn D, Blaschitz A, Korgun ET, Lang I, Desoye G, Skofitsch G, et al. From maternal glucose to fetal glycogen: expression of key regulators in the human placenta. *Mol Hum Reprod.* (2001) 7:1173–8. doi: 10.1093/molehr/7.12.1173
52. Yung HW, Calabrese S, Hynx D, Hemmings BA, Cetin I, Charnock-Jones DS, et al. Evidence of placental translation inhibition and endoplasmic reticulum stress in the etiology of human intrauterine growth restriction. *Am J Pathol.* (2008) 173:451–62. doi: 10.2353/ajpath.2008.071193
53. Gheorman V, Gheorman L, Ivanus C, Pana RC, Goganau AM, Patrascu A. Comparative study of placenta acute fetal distress and diabetes associated with pregnancy. *Rom J Morphol Embryol.* (2013) 54:505–11.
54. Laviola L, Perrini S, Belsanti G, Natalicchio A, Montrone C, Leonardini A, et al. Intrauterine growth restriction in humans is associated with abnormalities in placental insulin-like growth factor signaling. *Endocrinology* (2005) 146:1498–505. doi: 10.1210/en.2004-1332
55. Akison LK, Nitert MD, Clifton VL, Moritz KM, Simmons DG. Review: alterations in placental glycogen deposition in complicated pregnancies: current preclinical and clinical evidence. *Placenta* (2017) 54:52–8. doi: 10.1016/j.placenta.2017.01.114
56. Perez-Garcia V, Fineberg E, Wilson R, Murray A, Mazzeo CI, Tudor C, et al. Placentation defects are highly prevalent in embryonic lethal mouse mutants. *Nature* (2018) 555:463–8. doi: 10.1038/nature26002
57. Watson ED, Cross JC. Development of structures and transport functions in the mouse placenta. *Physiology* (2005) 20:180–93. doi: 10.1152/physiol.00001.2005
58. El-Hashash AH, Warburton D, Kimber SJ. Genes and signals regulating murine trophoblast cell development. *Mech Dev.* (2010) 127:1–20. doi: 10.1016/j.mod.2009.09.004
59. Ueno M, Lee LK, Chhabra A, Kim YJ, Sasidharan R, Van Handel B, et al. c-Met-dependent multipotent labyrinth trophoblast progenitors establish placental exchange interface. *Dev Cell* (2013) 27:373–86. doi: 10.1016/j.devcel.2013.10.019
60. Sibilia M, Wagner EF. Strain-dependent epithelial defects in mice lacking the EGF receptor. *Science* (1995) 269:234–8. doi: 10.1126/science.7618085
61. Arman E, Haffner-Krausz R, Chen Y, Heath JK, Lonai P. Targeted disruption of fibroblast growth factor (FGF) receptor 2 suggests a role for FGF signaling in pregastrulation mammalian development. *Proc Natl Acad Sci USA.* (1998) 95:5082–7. doi: 10.1073/pnas.95.9.5082
62. Sibilia M, Steinbach JP, Stingl L, Aguzzi A, Wagner EF. A strain-independent postnatal neurodegeneration in mice lacking the EGF receptor. *EMBO J.* (1998) 17:719–31. doi: 10.1093/emboj/17.3.719
63. Xu X, Weinstein M, Li C, Naski M, Cohen RI, Ornitz DM, et al. Fibroblast growth factor receptor 2 (FGFR2)-mediated reciprocal regulation loop between FGF8 and FGF10 is essential for limb induction. *Development* (1998) 125:753–65.
64. Ware CB, Horowitz MC, Renshaw BR, Hunt JS, Liggitt D, Koblar SA, et al. Targeted disruption of the low-affinity leukemia inhibitory factor receptor gene causes placental, skeletal, neural and metabolic defects and results in perinatal death. *Development* (1995) 121:1283–99.

65. Sferruzzi-Perri AN, Owens JA, Pringle KG, Roberts CT. The neglected role of insulin-like growth factors in the maternal circulation regulating fetal growth. *J Physiol.* (2011) 589:7–20. doi: 10.1113/jphysiol.2010.198622
66. Constância M, Hemberger M, Hughes J, Dean W, Ferguson-Smith A, Fundele R, et al. Placental-specific IGF-II is a major modulator of placental and fetal growth. *Nature* (2002) 417:945–8. doi: 10.1038/nature00819
67. Sibley CP, Coan PM, Ferguson-Smith AC, Dean W, Hughes J, Smith P, et al. Placental-specific insulin-like growth factor 2 (Igf2) regulates the diffusional exchange characteristics of the mouse placenta. *Proc Natl Acad Sci USA.* (2004) 101:8204–8. doi: 10.1073/pnas.0402508101
68. Street ME, Seghini P, Fieni S, Ziveri MA, Volta C, Martorana D, et al. Changes in interleukin-6 and IGF system and their relationships in placenta and cord blood in newborns with fetal growth restriction compared with controls. *Eur J Endocrinol.* (2006) 155:567–74. doi: 10.1530/eje.1.02251
69. Gupta MB. The role and regulation of IGFBP-1 phosphorylation in fetal growth restriction. *J Cell Commun Signal.* (2015) 9:111–23. doi: 10.1007/s12079-015-0266-x
70. Tzschoppe A, Riedel C, von Kries R, Struwe E, Rascher W, Dorr HG, et al. Differential effects of low birthweight and intrauterine growth restriction on umbilical cord blood insulin-like growth factor concentrations. *Clin Endocrinol.* (2015) 83:739–45. doi: 10.1111/cen.12844
71. Woods KA, Camacho-Hubner C, Barter D, Clark AJ, Savage MO. Insulin-like growth factor I gene deletion causing intrauterine growth retardation and severe short stature. *Acta Paediatr Suppl.* (1997) 423:39–45. doi: 10.1111/j.1651-2227.1997.tb18367.x
72. Bonapace G, Concolino D, Formicola S, Strisciuglio P. A novel mutation in a patient with insulin-like growth factor 1 (IGF1) deficiency. *J Med Genet.* (2003) 40:913–7. doi: 10.1136/jmg.40.12.913
73. Netchine I, Azzi S, Houang M, Seurin D, Perin L, Ricort JM, et al. Partial primary deficiency of insulin-like growth factor (IGF)-I activity associated with IGF1 mutation demonstrates its critical role in growth and brain development. *J Clin Endocrinol Metab.* (2009) 94:3913–21. doi: 10.1210/jc.2009-0452
74. Hemberger M, Cross JC. Genes governing placental development. *Trends Endocrinol Metab.* (2001) 12:162–8. doi: 10.1016/S1043-2760(01)00375-7
75. Salbaum JM, Kruger C, Zhang X, Delahaye NA, Pavlinkova G, Burk DH, et al. Altered gene expression and spongiotrophoblast differentiation in placenta from a mouse model of diabetes in pregnancy. *Diabetologia* (2011) 54:1909–20. doi: 10.1007/s00125-011-2132-6
76. Hong KH, Seki T, Oh SP. Activin receptor-like kinase 1 is essential for placental vascular development in mice. *Lab Invest.* (2007) 87:670–9. doi: 10.1038/labinvest.3700560
77. Arora R, Papaioannou VE. The murine allantois: a model system for the study of blood vessel formation. *Blood* (2012) 120:2562–72. doi: 10.1182/blood-2012-03-390070
78. Barak Y, Nelson MC, Ong ES, Jones YZ, Ruiz-Lozano P, Chien KR, et al. PPAR gamma is required for placental, cardiac, and adipose tissue development. *Mol Cell* (1999) 4:585–95. doi: 10.1016/S1097-2765(00)80209-9
79. Parast MM, Yu H, Ciric A, Salata MW, Davis V, Milstone DS. PPARgamma regulates trophoblast proliferation and promotes labyrinthine trilineage differentiation. *PLoS ONE* (2009) 4:e8055. doi: 10.1371/journal.pone.0008055
80. Baczyk D, Drewlo S, Proctor L, Dunk C, Lye S, Kingdom J. Glial cell missing-1 transcription factor is required for the differentiation of the human trophoblast. *Cell Death Differ.* (2009) 16:719–27. doi: 10.1038/cdd.2009.1
81. Holdsworth-Carson SJ, Lim R, Mitton A, Whitehead C, Rice GE, Permezel M, et al. Peroxisome proliferator-activated receptors are altered in pathologies of the human placenta: gestational diabetes mellitus, intrauterine growth restriction and preeclampsia. *Placenta* (2010) 31:222–9. doi: 10.1016/j.placenta.2009.12.009
82. Kohli S, Hoffmann J, Lochmann F, Markmeyer P, Huebner H, Fahlbusch FB, et al. p45 NF-E2 regulates syncytiotrophoblast differentiation by post-translational GCM1 modifications in human intrauterine growth restriction. *Cell Death Dis.* (2017) 8:e2730. doi: 10.1038/cddis.2017.127
83. Chen DB, Zheng J. Regulation of placental angiogenesis. *Microcirculation* (2014) 21:15–25. doi: 10.1111/micc.12093
84. Barut F, Barut A, Gun BD, Kandemir NO, Harma MI, Harma M, et al. Intrauterine growth restriction and placental angiogenesis. *Diagn Pathol.* (2010) 5:24. doi: 10.1186/1746-1596-5-24
85. Rodriguez TA, Sparrow DB, Scott AN, Withington SL, Preis JI, Michalicek J, et al. Cited1 is required in trophoblasts for placental development and for embryo growth and survival. *Mol Cell Biol.* (2004) 24:228–44. doi: 10.1128/MCB.24.1.228-244.2004
86. Kashif M, Hellwig A, Kolleker A, Shahzad K, Wang H, Lang S, et al. p45NF-E2 represses Gcm1 in trophoblast cells to regulate syncytium formation, placental vascularization and embryonic growth. *Development* (2011) 138:2235–47. doi: 10.1242/dev.059105
87. Cui XB, Guo X, Chen SY. Response gene to complement 32 deficiency causes impaired placental angiogenesis in mice. *Cardiovasc Res.* (2013) 99:632–9. doi: 10.1093/cvr/cvt121
88. Lacko LA, Hurtado R, Hinds S, Poulos MG, Butler JM, Stuhlmann H. Altered feto-placental vascularization, feto-placental malperfusion and fetal growth restriction in mice with Egfl7 loss of function. *Development* (2017) 144:2469–79. doi: 10.1242/dev.147025
89. An X, Jin Y, Guo H, Foo SY, Cully BL, Wu J, et al. Response gene to complement 32, a novel hypoxia-regulated angiogenic inhibitor. *Circulation* (2009) 120:617–27. doi: 10.1161/CIRCULATIONAHA.108.841502
90. Carmeliet P, Ferreira V, Breier G, Pollefeyt S, Kieckens L, Gertsenstein M, et al. Abnormal blood vessel development and lethality in embryos lacking a single VEGF allele. *Nature* (1996) 380:435–9. doi: 10.1038/380435a0
91. Ferrara N, Carver-Moore K, Chen H, Dowd M, Lu L, O'Shea KS, et al. Heterozygous embryonic lethality induced by targeted inactivation of the VEGF gene. *Nature* (1996) 380:439–42. doi: 10.1038/380439a0
92. Kang MC, Park SJ, Kim HJ, Lee J, Yu DH, Bae KB, et al. Gestational loss and growth restriction by angiogenic defects in placental growth factor transgenic mice. *Arterioscler Thromb Vasc Biol.* (2014) 34:2276–82. doi: 10.1161/ATVBAHA.114.303693
93. Fong G-H, Rossant J, Gertsenstein M, Breitman ML. Role of the Flt-1 receptor tyrosine kinase in regulating the assembly of vascular endothelium. *Nature* (1995) 376:66–70. doi: 10.1038/376066a0
94. Kumasawa K, Ikawa M, Kidoya H, Hasuwa H, Saito-Fujita T, Morioka Y, et al. Pravastatin induces placental growth factor (PGF) and ameliorates preeclampsia in a mouse model. *Proc Natl Acad Sci USA.* (2011) 108:1451–5. doi: 10.1073/pnas.1011293108
95. Nevo O, Many A, Xu J, Kingdom J, Piccoli E, Zamudio S, et al. Placental expression of soluble fms-like tyrosine kinase 1 is increased in singletons and twin pregnancies with intrauterine growth restriction. *J Clin Endocrinol Metab.* (2008) 93:285–92. doi: 10.1210/jc.2007-1042
96. Kwiatkowski S, Dolegowska B, Kwiatkowska E, Rzepka R, Torbe A, Bednarek-Jedrzejek M. A common profile of disordered angiogenic factor production and the exacerbation of inflammation in early preeclampsia, late preeclampsia, and intrauterine growth restriction. *PLoS ONE* (2016) 11:e0165060. doi: 10.1371/journal.pone.0165060
97. Chang YS, Chen CN, Jeng SF, Su YN, Chen CY, Chou HC, et al. The sFlt-1/PlGF ratio as a predictor for poor pregnancy and neonatal outcomes. *Pediatr Neonatol.* (2017) 58:529–33. doi: 10.1016/j.pedneo.2016.10.005
98. Chelli D, Hamdi A, Saoudi S, Jenayah AA, Zagre A, Jguerim H, et al. Clinical assessment of soluble FMS-like tyrosine kinase-1/placental growth factor ratio for the diagnostic and the prognosis of preeclampsia in the second trimester. *Clin Lab.* (2016) 62:1927–32. doi: 10.7754/Clin.Lab.2016.151004
99. Chau K, Hennessy A, Makris A. Placental growth factor and pre-eclampsia. *J Hum Hypertens.* (2017) 31:782–6. doi: 10.1038/jhh.2017.61
100. Coan PM, Ferguson-Smith AC, Burton GJ. Developmental dynamics of the definitive mouse placenta assessed by stereology. *Biol Reprod.* (2004) 70:1806–13. doi: 10.1095/biolreprod.103.024166
101. Burton GJ, Fowden AL, Thornburg KL. Placental origins of chronic disease. *Physiol Rev.* (2016) 96:1509–65. doi: 10.1152/physrev.00029.2015
102. Dupressoir A, Vernochet C, Bawa O, Harper F, Pierron G, Opolon P, et al. Syncytin-A knockout mice demonstrate the critical role in placentation of a fusogenic, endogenous retrovirus-derived, envelope gene. *Proc Natl Acad Sci USA.* (2009) 106:12127–32. doi: 10.1073/pnas.0902925106
103. Bainbridge SA, Minhas A, Whiteley KJ, Qu D, Sled JG, Kingdom JC, et al. Effects of reduced Gcm1 expression on trophoblast morphology,

fetoplacental vascularity, and pregnancy outcomes in mice. *Hypertension* (2012) 59:732–9. doi: 10.1161/HYPERTENSIONAHA.111.183939
104. Kuhnel E, Kleff V, Stojanovska V, Kaiser S, Waldschutz R, Herse F, et al. Placental-specific overexpression of sFlt-1 alters trophoblast differentiation and nutrient transporter expression in an iugr mouse model. *J Cell Biochem.* (2017) 118:1316–29. doi: 10.1002/jcb.25789
105. Coan PM, Angiolini E, Sandovici I, Burton GJ, Constancia M, Fowden AL. Adaptations in placental nutrient transfer capacity to meet fetal growth demands depend on placental size in mice. *J Physiol.* (2008) 586:4567–76. doi: 10.1113/jphysiol.2008.156133
106. Thumkeo D, Keel J, Ishizaki T, Hirose M, Nonomura K, Oshima H, et al. Targeted disruption of the mouse rho-associated kinase 2 gene results in intrauterine growth retardation and fetal death. *Mol Cell Biol.* (2003) 23:5043–55. doi: 10.1128/MCB.23.14.5043-5055.2003
107. Tong MH, Jiang H, Liu P, Lawson JA, Brass LF, Song WC. Spontaneous fetal loss caused by placental thrombosis in estrogen sulfotransferase-deficient mice. *Nat Med.* (2005) 11:153–9. doi: 10.1038/nm1184
108. Tian Y, Jackson P, Gunter C, Wang J, Rock CO, Jackowski S. Placental thrombosis and spontaneous fetal death in mice deficient in ethanolamine kinase 2. *J Biol Chem.* (2006) 281:28438–49. doi: 10.1074/jbc.M605861200
109. McKelvey KJ, Yenson VM, Ashton AW, Morris JM, McCracken SA. Embryonic/fetal mortality and intrauterine growth restriction is not exclusive to the CBA/J sub-strain in the CBA x DBA model. *Sci Rep.* (2016) 6:35138. doi: 10.1038/srep35138
110. Vedmedovska N, Rezeberga D, Teibe U, Melderis I, Donders GG. Placental pathology in fetal growth restriction. *Eur J Obstet Gynecol Reprod Biol.* (2011) 155:36–40. doi: 10.1016/j.ejogrb.2010.11.017
111. Biswas S, Adhikari A, Chattopadhyay JC, Ghosh SK. Histological changes of placentas associated with intra-uterine growth restriction of fetuses: a case control study. *Nepal Med Coll J.* (2012) 14:18–24.
112. Witlin AG, Li ZY, Wimalawansa SJ, Grady JJ, Grafe MR, Yallampalli C. Placental and fetal growth and development in late rat gestation is dependent on adrenomedullin. *Biol Reprod.* (2002) 67:1025–31. doi: 10.1095/biolreprod.101.002196
113. Suh CH, Cho NK, Lee CK, Lee CH, Kim DH, Kim JH, et al. Perfluorooctanoic acid-induced inhibition of placental prolactin-family hormone and fetal growth retardation in mice. *Mol Cell Endocrinol.* (2011) 337:7–15. doi: 10.1016/j.mce.2011.01.009
114. Lee CK, Kang SG, Lee JT, Lee SW, Kim JH, Kim DH, et al. Effects of perfluorooctane sulfuric acid on placental PRL-family hormone production and fetal growth retardation in mice. *Mol Cell Endocrinol.* (2015) 401:165–72. doi: 10.1016/j.mce.2014.10.026
115. Qian X, Esteban L, Vass WC, Upadhyaya C, Papageorge AG, Yienger K, et al. The Sos1 and Sos2 Ras-specific exchange factors: differences in placental expression and signaling properties. *EMBO J.* (2000) 19:642–54. doi: 10.1093/emboj/19.4.642
116. Nadeau V, Charron J. Essential role of the ERK/MAPK pathway in blood-placental barrier formation. *Development* (2014) 141:2825–37. doi: 10.1242/dev.107409
117. Parekh V, McEwen A, Barbour V, Takahashi Y, Rehg JE, Jane SM, et al. Defective extraembryonic angiogenesis in mice lacking LBP-1a, a member of the grainyhead family of transcription factors. *Mol Cell Biol.* (2004) 24:7113–29. doi: 10.1128/MCB.24.16.7113-7129.2004
118. Coan PM, Conroy N, Burton GJ, Ferguson-Smith AC. Origin and characteristics of glycogen cells in the developing murine placenta. *Dev Dyn.* (2006) 235:3280–94. doi: 10.1002/dvdy.20981
119. Sarkar AA, Nuwayhid SJ, Maynard T, Ghandchi F, Hill JT, Lamantia AS, et al. Hectd1 is required for development of the junctional zone of the placenta. *Dev Biol.* (2014) 392:368–80. doi: 10.1016/j.ydbio.2014.05.007
120. Singh VP, Alex JL, Lakshmi BJ, Sailasree SP, Raj TA, Kumar S. Role of mouse Wdr13 in placental growth; a genetic evidence for lifetime body weight determination by placenta during development. *Sci Rep.* (2015) 5:13371. doi: 10.1038/srep13371
121. Stewart CL, Kaspar P, Brunet LJ, Bhatt H, Gadi I, Kontgen F, et al. Blastocyst implantation depends on maternal expression of leukaemia inhibitory factor. *Nature* (1992) 359:76–9. doi: 10.1038/359076a0
122. Kurihara I, Lee DK, Petit FG, Jeong J, Lee K, Lydon JP, et al. COUP-TFII mediates progesterone regulation of uterine implantation by controlling ER activity. *PLoS Genet.* (2007) 3:e102. doi: 10.1371/journal.pgen.0030102
123. Monsivais D, Clementi C, Peng J, Titus MM, Barrish JP, Creighton CJ, et al. Uterine ALK3 is essential during the window of implantation. *Proc Natl Acad Sci USA.* (2016) 113:E387–95. doi: 10.1073/pnas.1523758113
124. Wang H, Dey SK. Roadmap to embryo implantation: clues from mouse models. *Nat Rev Genet.* (2006) 7:185–99. doi: 10.1038/nrg1808
125. Song H, Lim H, Paria BC, Matsumoto H, Swift LL, Morrow J, et al. Cytosolic phospholipase A2alpha is crucial [correction of A2alpha deficiency is crucial] for 'on-time' embryo implantation that directs subsequent development. *Development* (2002) 129:2879–89.
126. Ye X, Hama K, Contos JJ, Anliker B, Inoue A, Skinner MK, et al. LPA3-mediated lysophosphatidic acid signalling in embryo implantation and spacing. *Nature* (2005) 435:104–8. doi: 10.1038/nature03505
127. Daikoku T, Cha J, Sun X, Tranguch S, Xie H, Fujita T, et al. Conditional deletion of Msx homeobox genes in the uterus inhibits blastocyst implantation by altering uterine receptivity. *Dev Cell* (2011) 21:1014–25. doi: 10.1016/j.devcel.2011.09.010
128. Cha J, Dey SK. Cadence of procreation: orchestrating embryo-uterine interactions. *Semin Cell Dev Biol.* (2014) 34:56–64. doi: 10.1016/j.semcdb.2014.05.005
129. Macklon NS, Geraedts JP, Fauser BC. Conception to ongoing pregnancy: the 'black box' of early pregnancy loss. *Hum Reprod Update* (2002) 8:333–43. doi: 10.1093/humupd/8.4.333
130. Mahendru AA, Daemen A, Everett TR, Wilkinson IB, McEniery CM, Abdallah Y, et al. Impact of ovulation and implantation timing on first-trimester crown-rump length and gestational age. *Ultrasound Obstet Gynecol.* (2012) 40:630–5. doi: 10.1002/uog.12277
131. Smith GC, Smith MF, McNay MB, Fleming JE. First-trimester growth and the risk of low birth weight. *N Engl J Med.* (1998) 339:1817–22. doi: 10.1056/NEJM199812173392504
132. Bukowski R, Smith GC, Malone FD, Ball RH, Nyberg DA, Comstock CH, et al. Fetal growth in early pregnancy and risk of delivering low birth weight infant: prospective cohort study. *BMJ* (2007) 334:836. doi: 10.1136/bmj.39129.637917.AE
133. Mook-Kanamori DO, Steegers EA, Eilers PH, Raat H, Hofman A, Jaddoe VW. Risk factors and outcomes associated with first-trimester fetal growth restriction. *JAMA* (2010) 303:527–34. doi: 10.1001/jama.2010.78
134. Hsieh-Li HM, Witte DP, Weinstein M, Branford W, Li H, Small K, et al. Hoxa 11 structure, extensive antisense transcription, and function in male and female fertility. *Development* (1995) 121:1373–85.
135. Lydon JP, DeMayo FJ, Funk CR, Mani SK, Hughes AR, Montgomery CAJr, et al. Mice lacking progesterone receptor exhibit pleiotropic reproductive abnormalities. *Genes Dev.* (1995) 9:2266–78. doi: 10.1101/gad.9.18.2266
136. Lee KY, Jeong JW, Wang J, Ma L, Martin JF, Tsai SY, et al. Bmp2 is critical for the murine uterine decidual response. *Mol Cell Biol.* (2007) 27:5468–78. doi: 10.1128/MCB.00342-07
137. Li Q, Kannan A, Wang W, Demayo FJ, Taylor RN, Bagchi MK, et al. Bone morphogenetic protein 2 functions via a conserved signaling pathway involving Wnt4 to regulate uterine decidualization in the mouse and the human. *J Biol Chem.* (2007) 282:31725–32. doi: 10.1074/jbc.M704723200
138. Nagashima T, Li Q, Clementi C, Lydon JP, DeMayo FJ, Matzuk MM. BMPR2 is required for postimplantation uterine function and pregnancy maintenance. *J Clin Invest.* (2013) 123:2539–50. doi: 10.1172/JCI65710
139. Pawar S, Starosvetsky E, Orvis GD, Behringer RR, Bagchi IC, Bagchi MK. STAT3 regulates uterine epithelial remodeling and epithelial-stromal crosstalk during implantation. *Mol Endocrinol.* (2013) 27:1996–2012. doi: 10.1210/me.2013-1206
140. Li MQ, Yao MN, Yan JQ, Li ZL, Gu XW, Lin S, et al. The decline of pregnancy rate and abnormal uterine responsiveness of steroid hormones in aging mice. *Reprod Biol.* (2017) 17:305–11. doi: 10.1016/j.repbio.2017.09.001
141. Woods L, Perez-Garcia V, Kieckbusch J, Wang X, DeMayo F, Colucci F, et al. Decidualisation and placentation defects are a major cause of age-related reproductive decline. *Nat Commun.* (2017) 8:352. doi: 10.1038/s41467-017-00308-x
142. Lague MN, Detmar J, Paquet M, Boyer A, Richards JS, Adamson SL, et al. Decidual PTEN expression is required for trophoblast invasion

in the mouse. *Am J Physiol Endocrinol Metab.* (2010) 299:E936–46. doi: 10.1152/ajpendo.00255.2010

143. Plaks V, Rinkenberger J, Dai J, Flannery M, Sund M, Kanasaki K, et al. Matrix metalloproteinase-9 deficiency phenocopies features of preeclampsia and intrauterine growth restriction. *Proc Natl Acad Sci USA.* (2013) 110:11109–14. doi: 10.1073/pnas.1309561110
144. Peng B, Zhu H, Ma L, Wang YL, Klausen C, Leung PC. AP-1 transcription factors c-FOS and c-JUN mediate GnRH-induced cadherin-11 expression and trophoblast cell invasion. *Endocrinology* (2015) 156:2269–77. doi: 10.1210/en.2014-1871
145. Park CB, DeMayo FJ, Lydon JP, Dufort D. NODAL in the uterus is necessary for proper placental development and maintenance of pregnancy. *Biol Reprod.* (2012) 86:194. doi: 10.1095/biolreprod.111.098277
146. Peng J, Monsivais D, You R, Zhong H, Pangas SA, Matzuk MM, et al. Uterine activin receptor-like 1081 kinase 5 is crucial for blastocyst implantation and placental development. *Proc Natl Acad Sci USA.* (2015)112:E5098–107. doi: 10.1073/pnas.1514498112
147. Winterhager E, Gellhaus A, Blois SM, Hill LA, Barr KJ, Kidder GM. Decidual angiogenesis and placental orientation are altered in mice heterozygous for a dominant loss-of-function Gja1 (connexin43) mutation. *Biol Reprod.* (2013) 89:111. doi: 10.1095/biolreprod.113.111690
148. Mohun T, Adams DJ, Baldock R, Bhattacharya S, Copp AJ, Hemberger M, et al. Deciphering the Mechanisms of Developmental Disorders (DMDD): a new programme for phenotyping embryonic lethal mice. *Dis Model Mech.* (2013) 6:562–6. doi: 10.1242/dmm.011957
149. Kim S, Westphal V, Srikrishna G, Mehta DP, Peterson S, Filiano J, et al. Dolichol phosphate mannose synthase (DPM1) mutations define congenital disorder of glycosylation Ie (CDG-Ie). *J Clin Invest.* (2000) 105:191–8. doi: 10.1172/JCI7302
150. Krawitz PM, Murakami Y, Riess A, Hietala M, Kruger U, Zhu N, et al. PGAP2 mutations, affecting the GPI-anchor-synthesis pathway, cause hyperphosphatasia with mental retardation syndrome. *Am J Hum Genet.* (2013) 92:584–9. doi: 10.1016/j.ajhg.2013.03.011
151. Ng BG, Hackmann K, Jones MA, Eroshkin AM, He P, Wiliams R, et al. Mutations in the glycosylphosphatidylinositol gene PIGL cause CHIME syndrome. *Am J Hum Genet.* (2012) 90:685–8. doi: 10.1016/j.ajhg.2012.02.010
152. Levavasseur F, Miyadera H, Sirois J, Tremblay ML, Kita K, Shoubridge E, et al. Ubiquinone is necessary for mouse embryonic development but is not essential for mitochondrial respiration. *J Biol Chem.* (2001) 276:46160–4. doi: 10.1074/jbc.M108980200
153. Nakai D, Yuasa S, Takahashi M, Shimizu T, Asaumi S, Isono K, et al. Mouse homologue of coq7/clk-1, longevity gene in *Caenorhabditis elegans*, is essential for coenzyme Q synthesis, maintenance of mitochondrial integrity, and neurogenesis. *Biochem Biophys Res Commun.* (2001) 289:463–71. doi: 10.1006/bbrc.2001.5977
154. Freyer C, Stranneheim H, Naess K, Mourier A, Felser A, Maffezzini C, et al. Rescue of primary ubiquinone deficiency due to a novel COQ7 defect using 2,4-dihydroxybensoic acid. *J Med Genet.* (2015) 52:779–83. doi: 10.1136/jmedgenet-2015-102986
155. Ishii M, Han J, Yen HY, Sucov HM, Chai Y, Maxson REJr. Combined deficiencies of Msx1 and Msx2 cause impaired patterning and survival of the cranial neural crest. *Development* (2005) 132:4937–50. doi: 10.1242/dev.02072
156. Liang H, Zhang Q, Lu J, Yang G, Tian N, Wang X, et al. MSX2 Induces Trophoblast Invasion in Human Placenta. *PLoS ONE* (2016) 11:e0153656. doi: 10.1371/journal.pone.0153656
157. Ajduk A, Zernicka-Goetz M. Polarity and cell division orientation in the cleavage embryo: from worm to human. *Mol Hum Reprod.* (2016) 22:691–703. doi: 10.1093/molehr/gav068

19

The Possible Role of Placental Morphometry in the Detection of Fetal Growth Restriction

Nastaran Salavati[1], Maddy Smies[2], Wessel Ganzevoort[2], Adrian K. Charles[3], Jan Jaap Erwich[1], Torsten Plösch[1] and Sanne J. Gordijn[1]*

[1] Department of Obstetrics and Gynecology, University Medical Center Groningen, University of Groningen, Groningen, Netherlands, [2] Department of Obstetrics and Gynecology, Amsterdam University Medical Centers, University of Amsterdam, Amsterdam, Netherlands, [3] Department of Anatomical Pathology, Sidra Medicine, Doha, Qatar

***Correspondence:**
Nastaran Salavati
n.salavati@umcg.nl

Fetal growth restriction (FGR) is often the result of placental insufficiency and is characterized by insufficient transplacental transport of nutrients and oxygen. The main underlying entities of placental insufficiency, the pathophysiologic mechanism, can broadly be divided into impairments in blood flow and exchange capacity over the syncytiovascular membranes of the fetal placenta villi. Fetal growth restriction is not synonymous with small for gestational age and techniques to distinguish between both are needed. Placental insufficiency has significant associations with adverse pregnancy outcomes (perinatal mortality and morbidity). Even in apparently healthy survivors, altered fetal programming may lead to long-term neurodevelopmental and metabolic effects. Although the concept of fetal growth restriction is well appreciated in contemporary obstetrics, the appropriate detection of FGR remains an issue in clinical practice. Several approaches have aimed to improve detection, e.g., uniform definition of FGR, use of Doppler ultrasound profiles and use of growth trajectories by ultrasound fetal biometry. However, the role of placental morphometry (placental dimensions/shape and weight) deserves further exploration. This review article covers the clinical relevance of placental morphometry during pregnancy and at birth to help recognize fetuses who are growth restricted. The assessment has wide intra- and interindividual variability with various consequences. Previous studies have shown that a small placental surface area and low placental weight are associated with a slower growth of the fetus. Parameters such as placental surface area, placental volume and placental weight in relation to birth weight can help to identify FGR. In the future, a model including sophisticated antenatal placental morphometry may prove to be a clinically useful method for screening or diagnosing growth restricted fetuses, in order to provide optimal monitoring.

Keywords: FGR, IUGR, SGA, fetal growth restriction, intra uterine growth restriction, small for gestational age, placenta morphometry, birth weight

BACKGROUND

The diagnosis of fetal growth restriction (FGR) has for long mainly be based on birth weight below a reference cut-off, most commonly the 10th percentile (p10) (Beune et al., 2018). Birth weight (BW) or estimated fetal weight (EFW) below p10 indicates that the BW or EFW is within the lowest 10% of BW compared to the reference population. This is in essence not FGR but small for gestational age (SGA). There are some important diagnostic issues with this misnomer. First, about 75% of fetuses who are SGA (and therefore many who are FGR) remain unrecognized until they are born and the diagnosis is made on the baby scale, postnatally (Monier et al., 2017; Beune et al., 2018), meaning some are severely compromised, exposed to potential long term sequelae, or even stillborn. Second, fetuses who are too small according to the intra uterine reference chart may be physiologically small and appropriate grown according to their individual growth potential (based upon their genetic and epigenetic inheritance at conception), and therefore not at risk from diseases related to FGR, but are exposed to unnecessary investigations for FGR. Third, many cases of growth restriction remain unacknowledged, when a baby or fetus is too small according to its *individual* growth potential, but not necessarily too small in the *population* based reference chart. Thus FGR overlaps with, but is not synonymous to, SGA (Zhang et al., 2010) ("SGA-FGR confusion"), as two overlapping distribution curves. It is self-evident that the incidence of growth restricted fetuses increases as EFW or BW percentiles decreases (Vasak et al., 2015). Yet, there is not a single cut-off above which all babies have grown appropriately, or below which none have grown appropriately for their individual biological growth potential. If SGA is used as the proxy for FGR in clinical practice, healthy SGA fetuses and neonates without FGR are prone to unnecessary monitoring intervention strategies and FGR fetuses and neonates who are FGR but not SGA remain unrecognized ("masked" FGR). Furthermore, if SGA is used as proxy for FGR in research, the study population is diluted by healthy small fetuses and newborns, hampering adequate association studies. It is estimated that in the SGA group, 60% were growth restricted, and 40% were constitutionally small (**Figure 1**) (Figueras and Gratacos, 2017). In this study, "constitutionally small" was defined as fetuses with moderately low BW (>3rd percentile) and normal placental function on both the fetal (normal cerebroplacental ratio) and maternal (normal uterine Doppler) sides. Severe growth restriction or evidence of placental dysfunction was defined as "growth restricted" (Figueras and Gratacos, 2017).

This study implies the relevance of appropriate, possibly easy to obtain, and cheap diagnostic tools to detect only those fetuses who are growth restricted because these are the fetuses who have an increased risk of adverse short- and long-term outcomes when not delivered in time (Jaddoe et al., 2014; Meher et al., 2015; Miller et al., 2016).

The causes of FGR can be divided into pre-utero-placental (e.g., maternal anemia, hypoxia, malnourishment), utero-placental (e.g., poor implantation, pre-eclampsia) and fetal conditions (e.g., fetal infection, some maldevelopments), and

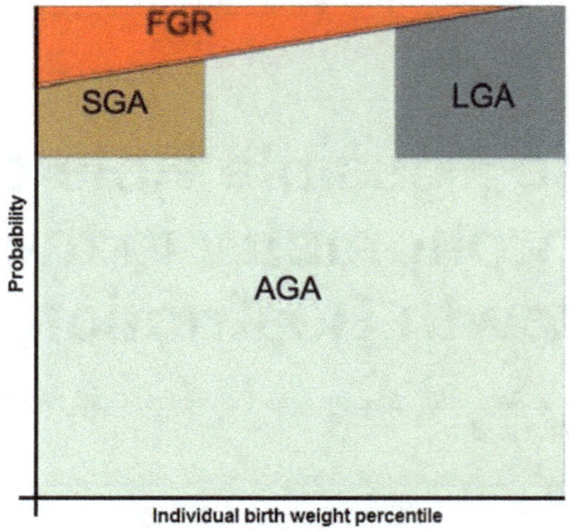

FIGURE 1 | Schematic representation of the possible distribution of FGR within the total population consisting of SGA, AGA, and LGA fetuses at a certain gestational age. Another gestational age-period or population will most likely have a different distribution. FGR, fetal growth restriction; SGA, small for gestational age; AGA, appropriate for gestational age; LGA, large for gestational age [reproduced with permission from (Gordijn et al., 2018)].

conditions like twin to twin transfusion. The utero-placental group appears the largest (ACOG Practice Bulletin no. 134: Fetal Growth Restriction, 2013), and the main focus to date has been on histopathological changes such as maternal malperfusion, villitis and more recently terminal villous hypoplasia. However, recently more focus has been made on examining the role of the gross examination of the placenta, with weight, shape, cord insertion. With better identification of the factors that are associated or causative for FGR, the baby who may or may not be small can still be identified as at risk for sequelae of FGR, based upon the severity of the changes. The issue is complex as the relationship is not straightforward, and several opposing forces are occurring. The placenta is not inert and does not grow purely as its genes dictate, but it appears to respond to the demands of the fetus and also the supply from the mother, appearing to adapt and compensate. It does this on a local level controlling blood flow through the stem villi with the arterial muscle, and globally, causing the increased placental resistance that in turn is identified by the Doppler studies. Furthermore, the fetus does the same with its redistribution of the blood, to the brain, at the cost of the liver glycogen and fatty tissue stores. There may also be a tradeoff on how much of the overall nutrient going to the conceptus is used for the placenta (to maximize uptake) or to the fetus, but usually the birth weight to placenta weight-ratio (BWP-ratio) increases in conditions with FGR. In addition, there are also well established differences between male and female fetuses.

Ideally for every fetus, all the relevant factors are assessed to give a rational approach to answer the question whether the fetus has reached its full growth percentile, based on the assessment of significant evidence of less than optimal maternal factors, uteroplacental factors including gross and histopathological placental examination, and fetal factors.

Abbreviations: AGA, appropriate for gestational age; BW, birth weight; CPR, cerebroplacental ratio; EFW, estimated fetal weight; FGR, fetal growth restriction; GA, gestational age; GV, growth velocity; HC, head circumference; LGA, large for gestational age; MRI, Magnetic Resonance Imaging; PAPP-A, pregnancy-associated plasma protein A; PI, pulsatility index; PIGF, placenta growth factor; PT, placental thickness; PV, placental volume; PW, placental weight; PQ, placenta quotient (=PV/gestational age); sFLIT1, soluble fms-like tyrosine kinase 1; SGA, small for gestational age; UmA, umbilical artery; UtA, uterine artery.

In this literature review we focus of the gross examination of the placenta and we aim to give an overview on the possible use of *placental morphometry* in recognizing fetuses and neonates with growth restriction, independent of their weight.

Diagnosis of Fetal Growth Restriction

The most common pathophysiologic mechanism of FGR is placental insufficiency, with multiple underlying maternal, fetal and placental causes, resulting in insufficient nutrition and oxygen supply to the fetus (ACOG Practice Bulletin no. 134: Fetal Growth Restriction, 2013). As mentioned above, the diagnostic process is complicated by the "SGA-FGR confusion." Placental insufficiency, placing fetuses at increased risk of hypoxia and malnourishment related morbidity, as well as stillbirth, is not restricted to those fetuses who are growth restricted and small, but also to those within normal weight ranges. The "masked" FGR fetuses in the subgroup of appropriate for gestational age (AGA) or even large for gestational age (LGA) fetuses, also experience placental insufficiency [assessed by umbilical artery pulsatility index (PI), middle cerebral artery PI, cerebroplacental ratio] (Morales Roselló et al., 2012). They show a slower growth trajectory during pregnancy, and are prone to the same risks. In addition, these fetuses have a further doubling of stillbirth risk compared to those fetuses with detected FGR, because no interventions to modify that risk are installed (Lindqvist and Molin, 2005; Gardosi et al., 2013). Clinically, these fetuses can only be recognized with sequential ultrasound measurements that show a decline in weight centiles, which is not routinely applied in general midwifery and obstetric practice. FGR, particularly early onset, is associated with histopathological changes through later onset may be histologically unremarkable (Mifsud and Sebire, 2014).

The major challenge of FGR is the diagnostic standard. In 2016 an international Delphi procedure among 56 experts on FGR was established to come to a consensus definition for both early ($<$32 weeks of gestation) and late FGR ($\geq$32 weeks of gestation) (Gordijn et al., 2016). In this definition not only size parameters of the fetus but also parameters of placental function, either alone or in combination, are included and have been used widely since publication. The clinical applicability of these definitions in predicting adverse outcomes is yet to be assessed.

The Role of Placental Size in Fetal Growth

Normal growth of the fetus is mainly dependent on normal placental function, with normal placental morphometry (size and shape) and normal structure. Impairments in placental development, including reduced placental size, or altered placental nutrient transport capability contribute to placental dysfunction (Zhang et al., 2015). Placental dysfunction attributable to structural fetal or genetic fetal defects share similar pathophysiologic pathways but are characterized by a different set of pathophysiologic features and are not included in this review. These factors contributing to placental dysfunction, as well as changes in the placental transport system, result in FGR.

To illustrate, it is known that transporter activity of system A amino acid uptake is reduced in placentas from FGR fetuses with abnormal umbilical artery Dopplers, and that it is also related to the severity of FGR (Glazier et al., 1997). The capability of the placenta to maintain sufficient nutrient supply is commonly described as "placental efficiency" and is described to be reflected by BWPW-ratio (Wilson and Ford, 2001). The increased risk of stillbirth may reflect less "placental reserve" with a high BWPW-ratio, where the fetus is running higher risk of stillbirth and yet maximizing its albeit constrained weight and growth. In animal studies, positive correlations were found between BWPW-ratio and placental uptake of nutrient transport system A amino acid uptake, indicating that nutrient transfer per gram placenta must have increased compared to low or normal BWPW-ratio (Hayward et al., 2016). However, in human studies these effects are less conclusive regarding the system A transporter. A low BWPW-ratio describes fetuses with a relatively large placenta (higher placental weight) compared to the birth weight, whereby the nutrient transfer is reduced per gram placenta.

Antenatal Measurement of Placental Function

Prenatal screening for FGR in general obstetrical populations involves identifying risk factors for impaired fetal growth. When the fetus is identified to be at risk for FGR, sequential assessment of fetal size, either by anatomical reference points or by sequential ultrasound is executed. Actual fetal size reflects past placental function until that point in time, whereby "real time" placental function can be assessed *in vivo* by measurement of vascular resistance Doppler flows in the mother (uterine artery) or in the fetus (umbilical artery and middle cerebral artery) (Alfirevic et al., 2010). Doppler flow measurements enable the non-invasive detection of signs of placental insufficiency and fetal hemodynamic changes that occur during oxygen deprivation. During the course of normal, healthy, pregnancies, umbilical artery resistance decreases gradually throughout gestation, and increases with placental insufficiency (Unterscheider et al., 2013). Ghosh et al. suggested in their study on pregnancies complicated by suspected FGR fetuses that abnormal Doppler patterns of the uterine arteries could identify a fetus at increased risk, even in the presence of normal umbilical artery Doppler flow (Ghosh and Gudmundsson, 2009). Regarding fetal biometry, abdominal circumference is smaller in FGR fetuses due to depletion of abdominal adipose tissue as well as smaller liver size, because of reduced glycogen storage. As solitary parameter in the detection of FGR, measurement of the abdominal circumference is the most sensitive (Nardozza et al., 2017). In case of placental insufficiency and decreased oxygen and nutrients supply, the fetus redistributes the blood to the brain, at the costs of the liver glycogen and fatty issue stores, resulting in normal fetal brain growth and decline of growth of the abdominal circumference.

Measurement of Serum Biomarkers

Biochemical biomarkers that reflect placental function and adverse pregnancy outcomes, including FGR, are increasingly subject of research. A systematic review conducted in 2013, assessed 53 studies investigating biomarkers that could potentially have a role in screening for FGR. They concluded that none of the 37 different biomarkers were sufficiently accurate to function as a predictor of FGR (Conde-Agudelo et al., 2013). However, different definitions of FGR were used in the evaluated studies in which the vast majority; 47 of the 53 studies, used SGA as a proxy for FGR. Gaccioli and colleagues, investigated whether an EFW below the 10th percentile in combinations with an elevated sFLIT1: PIGF ratio (at 36 weeks of gestation) was predictive for adverse pregnancy outcomes. They showed that this combination was strongly predictive for delivering a SGA infant (birth weight < 10th centile) plus perinatal morbidity and/or preeclampsia (Gaccioli et al., 2018a). In a subsequent study, elevated FLIT1:PIGF ratio was combined with low abdominal circumference growth velocity (ACGV), and a composite measure generated by, the earlier mentioned, Delphi procedure (Gordijn et al., 2016), described as indicators of FGR (Gaccioli et al., 2018b). They found that at a gestational age of 28 as well as 36 weeks, the positive predictive value of ultrasonic screening for the delivery of a SGA infant with complications was doubled when it was combined with biochemical markers compared to the ultrasonic screening method alone. The relation with placental morphometry has not been examined in these studies.

CLINICAL RELEVANCE OF ANTENATAL AND POSTNATAL ASSESSMENT OF PLACENTAL MORPHOMETRY

In current clinical practice, placental morphometry is only routinely investigated and described at pathological examination, after delivery. In general, placentas are only routinely investigated in case of some adverse pregnancy outcomes. However, examination of placental morphometry, both in the antenatal and postnatal phase, can possibly disclose information for the detection of fetal growth restriction.

Antenatal Assessment of Placental Morphometry

Evaluation of the placenta during pregnancy is usually only performed to assess the location of the placenta or to diagnose placental adhesion disorders (e.g., *placenta praevia*, *placenta increta*, *placenta bilobata*). Antenatal assessment of placental morphometry, alone or in relation to fetal size, is not routinely performed but may improve the identification of fetuses at risk for adverse outcomes caused by placental insufficiency. The theoretical advantage of antenatal assessment compared to postnatal assessment of placenta morphometry is obvious; relevant information from antenatal assessment does not only apply to the newborn or future pregnancies, but could also be of vital importance in the current pregnancy. It can allow the clinician to tailor monitoring- and intervention strategies to reduce the risk of adverse outcomes.

Unfortunately, literature regarding the clinical relevance of antenatal assessment of placental morphometry is still scarce. In this paragraph, we will summarize the existing literature on placental morphometry assessment during pregnancy with both ultrasound and MRI.

Antenatal Assessment of Placental Morphometry With Ultrasound

Measurements of placental diameter and thickness, using two-dimensional ultrasound, have been used as indicator of high-risk pregnancies and correlates with birth weight (Afrakhteh et al., 2013). Several studies have investigated these ultrasound measures in relation to SGA (birth weight < p10), and showed that placental diameter and thickness are lower in SGA fetuses (Habib, 2002; Afrakhteh et al., 2013; Mathai et al., 2013; Schwartz et al., 2014). In addition, Schwartz and colleagues had the aim to combine early, direct ultrasound assessment of the placenta with other markers of placental development, such as mean of the uterine artery Doppler PI, to identify pregnancies delivering SGA infants (Schwartz et al., 2014). Placental volume, placental quotient (PQ = placental volume/gestational age), and mean placental diameter were significantly smaller in fetuses in the SGA group, compared to the AGA group. This indicates that a smaller placental mass is associated with SGA (Heinonen et al., 2001; Chisholm and Folkins, 2016).

On the other hand, the placental morphology index [defined by mean placental diameter divided by placental quotient (PQ)] was significantly higher in the SGA group, demonstrating a closer association between slower fetal growth and a relatively wide and flat placenta, rather than a relatively thick placenta (Schwartz et al., 2014).

Studies that used FGR as outcome variable (**Table 1**) showed that abnormal placental shape (placental thickness > 4 cm or >50% of placental length) were predictive for experiencing FGR (Viero et al., 2004; Toal et al., 2007, 2008). In addition, Proctor et al. showed that FGR was associated with small placental size (linear placental length <10 cm), in a group of women with low first trimester PAPP-A (≤0.30 multiples of median) (Proctor et al., 2009).

In order to assess placental morphometry during pregnancy with ultrasound, sonographic reliability of placental measurements has to be adequate. In this regard, a couple of limitations have to be addressed. First, there are no existing, *in vivo*, ultrasound reference charts of normal placental size. Although Higgins et al. described that the estimated placental biometry and volume during pregnancy are correlated with their measurements at postnatal assessment, they are not equal (Higgins et al., 2016). *In vivo* measurements, performed within 7 days before delivery, of placental length and width, and 3D placental volume measurements were smaller compared to *ex vivo* measurements (Higgins et al., 2016). Placental depth and 2D placental volume measurements were found to be larger compared to their *ex vivo* correlates. These differences are probably caused by the collapse of intervillous space due to loss of maternal blood flow after birth and less stretching of the placenta due to the loss of intrauterine pressure from amniotic fluid and the baby volumes after birth. Azpurua et al. described that placental weight could be accurately predicted by 2D ultrasound with volumetric calculation (Azpurua et al., 2010). Second, intra- and inter-observer variability play a much bigger role with *in-vivo* sonographic measurements than *ex-vivo*, real life measurements (Higgins et al., 2016). Higgins et al. investigated the intra- and inter-observer variability between observations

TABLE 1 | Literature overview of antenatal placental morphometry assessment with ultrasound in relation to FGR (markers).

Author, year, country	Study type and population	FGR definition	Determinant(s)	Outcome	Results
Viero et al., 2004, Canada	Prospective 60 SP with ARED flow velocities in UmA.	EFW <p10 and - Elevated HC/AC - Amniotic fluid index (AFI) <10 cm	PL, PT, cord insertion Small/thick placenta: max PT > 4 cm, in absence of uterine contraction OR >50% of PL	Pregnancies with ARED in UmA.	Ultrasound was accurate in identifying lateral or marginal cords (sensitivity 86%, PPV 71%; $p < 0.0001$) Ultrasound examination of the placenta and its maternal blood supply may contribute to the perinatal management of pregnancies with high risk of perinatal morbidity/mortality.
Toal et al., 2007, Canada	Prospective 212 high risk* SP	EFW <p10 delivered at <34 wks and - Ultrasound examinations demonstrating reduced fetal growth - AFI <10 cm - ARED in UmA	Abnormal placental shape: PT > 4 cm or >50% of PL. Abnormal placental cord insertion. Placental texture. GA: 18–23 wks	FGR	The odds of the development of FGR were sign. less in women with all normal test results. Combining those women with two ($n = 21$) of three ($n = 3$) abnormal test results together predicted 14 of 19 severe FGR.
Toal et al., 2008, Canada	Prospective 60 high risk* SP with abnormal UtA Doppler flow at GA 19–23 weeks	EFW <p10 delivered at <34 wks and -Ultrasound examinations demonstrating reduced fetal growth - AFI < 10 cm - Abnormal UmA Doppler waveforms	Abnormal placental shape (PT/PL ratio of >0.5 or PT of >4 cm)	FGR	Women with abnormal placental shape had higher odds of FGR (odds, 4.7; 95% CI, [1.6–14.1]). Combined abnormal UtA Doppler flow and placental dysmorphologic condition before fetal viability identifies a subset of women who are at risk for adverse outcomes.
Proctor et al., 2009, Canada	Prospective 90 SP with first trimester PAPP-A ≤ 0.30 multiples of median.	EFW <p10 with UmA PI >p95 or ARED in UmA, and - Serial fetal biometry demonstrating growth failure. - AFI < 5 cm	Placental size (linear placental length). GA: 18–24 wks	FGR, preterm delivery before 32 weeks, stillbirth	FGR was sign. associated with small placental size (linear placental length <10 cm), in group of women with low PAPP-A.

**defined as "significant medical and/or obstetric risk factors for hypertensive disease/placental insufficiency."*
AC, abdominal circumference; AFI, amniotic fluid index; ARED, absent or reversed end diastolic; EFW, estimated fetal weight; FGR, fetal growth restriction; GA, gestational age; HC, head circumference; PAPP-A, pregnancy-associated plasma protein A; PL, placental length; PPV, positive predictive value; PT, placental thickness; SP, singleton pregnancies; UmA, umbilical artery; UtA, uterine artery; wks, weeks.

for placental measurements length, width, depth and volume performed by 2D ultrasound. The variability in measurements (intra- and inter-) was suboptimal with no intraclass correlation coefficient >0.75 (Higgins et al., 2016). More recently, a new technique was established for estimating placental volume from 3D ultrasound scans through an semi-automated technique (Looney et al., 2018). In this study, placental volume of 2,393 pregnancies was assessed by three operators on the one hand, and this semi-automated tool on the other hand. The clinical utility of placental volume was tested by looking at prediction of SGA at term. Results showed good similarity between the operators and the tool, and almost identical clinical results for the prediction of SGA (Looney et al., 2018).

Antenatal Assessment of Placental Morphometry With Magnetic Resonance Imaging

Magnetic resonance imaging (MRI) is an established, safe method of imaging during second and third trimester of pregnancy, but currently mainly used for fetal imaging (Wang et al., 2012a,b; Bulas and Egloff, 2013). The advantages of MRI compared to ultrasound, are the more accurate measurements of anatomical volume and the higher soft tissue contrast, and thus it has specific strengths in detecting abnormal placental morphometry. Furthermore, it has a larger field of view and, other than ultrasound, it is not dependent on its ability to penetrate tissue.

Reference values of placental volume by MRI measurements throughout gestation of healthy pregnancies, although in relatively small sample size, have been studied and are available now (Duncan et al., 2001; Langhoff et al., 2017; León et al., 2018). Current research on placental imaging is much more focused on the more advanced techniques of functional MRI (fMRI), rather than assessment of placental morphometry with conventional MRI. These fMRI techniques, and their implications for diagnosing FGR, are not in the scope of this review but are described in the reviews of Avni et al. (2015) and Siauve et al. (2015).

Although current research focuses more on the possibilities of fMRI, five studies specifically investigated the placenta morphometry measurements with MRI in relation to FGR, or markers of FGR (**Table 2**). The study of Derwig et al. was the only one that used SGA as outcome rather than FGR, and showed that small placental volume is predictive for delivering a SGA-neonates, which is in line with the findings from other (ultrasound) studies and could be a physiological phenomenon (Derwig et al., 2011). They also described that small placental volume was significantly associated with higher PI of the uterine artery, a marker of FGR. Increased uterine artery PI is thought to reflect defective trophoblast invasion, which could result in reduced placental growth (Arakaki et al., 2015).

Three studies (Damodaram et al., 2010; Ohgiya et al., 2016; Andescavage et al., 2017) investigated placental morphometry measurements in a FGR population compared to healthy controls. Although different definitions of FGR have been used (see **Table 2**), they all showed significantly reduced placental volume in the FGR population compared to the healthy pregnant population. Furthermore, Damodaram et al. showed that the placental volume remained significantly smaller throughout gestation in the FGR group, and that a lower placental volume was also associated with the severity of the FGR (detailed information on the severity subgroups can be found in **Table 2**) (Damodaram et al., 2010). Finally, Andescavage et al. described that the placental volume was significantly lower in a subgroup of the FGR-population with abnormal umbilical artery Doppler (Andescavage et al., 2017). Higher mean placental thickness, lower macroscopic placental surface area and increase in max placental thickness/placental volume (PT/PV) ratio, were placental morphometry parameters that were significantly associated with FGR (Damodaram et al., 2010; Ohgiya et al., 2016).

Further substantiation of the relevance of the max PT/PV ratio was shown by the significant correlation found between a higher max PT/PV ratio and the severity of the FGR, and the association with fetal and early neonatal morbidity in case of an increase of the max PT/PV ratio above the 95th percentile for gestation (Damodaram et al., 2010).

The last and most recent study of Dahdouh et al. had a slightly different study design. In this study placenta morphometry, although in combination with placental textural features computed on 3D MRI images, were used in two machine learning frameworks to predict FGR and BW for both healthy and FGR fetuses (Dahdouh et al., 2018). This semi-automated framework was able to detect FGR-fetuses with a diagnostic accuracy of 86%, sensitivity of 86% and a specificity of 87%. In line with the other four studies, placental volume was one of the most important features for identification of FGR. Although this study had a small sample size ($n = 80$), these results are promising, outperforming the current standard clinical tools for diagnosing FGR. Although MRI is increasingly used during pregnancy, especially at advanced gestation or in obese women (Millischer et al., 2013), availability is limited and costs are high. Therefore, current clinical use of MRI in the assessment of placental morphometry is very limited.

Postnatal Assessment of Placental Morphometry

After birth, standard placental measures are placental disk shape, diameter, surface area, disk thickness, weight, location of umbilical cord insertion site relative to the edge of the placental disk, and placental weight in relation to birth weight (Khong et al., 2016). It is advised to use placental weight trimmed of extraplacental membranes and umbilical cord (Khong et al., 2016). Inconsistencies in preparation of the placenta before weighing remains in different studies. Therefore, it is important to check whether trimmed or untrimmed placental weights are used, as for direct comparisons between absolute placental weights, values should be standardized to trimmed placental weight (Leary et al., 2003).

There is increasing evidence that features of placental gross morphology are linked biologically to the functional capacity of the placenta (Burton et al., 2016), but it has received little clinical interest. The reason for this is the timing of investigation of the placenta: pregnancy conditions have either developed or not, and intra-uterine problems already have taken place before

TABLE 2 | Literature overview of antenatal placental morphometry assessment with MRI in relation to FGR (markers).

Author, year, country	Study type and population	FGR definition	Determinant(s)	Outcome	Results
Damodaram et al., 2010, United Kingdom	Prospective 48 SP **A:** 20 FGR fetuses (1) $n = 3$, (2) $n = 3$, (3) $n = 10$, (4) $n = 1$, (5) $n = 3$ **B**: 28 controls	EFW <p5 and (1) PI UmA >p95 (2) PI UmA>p95 and PI MCA <p5 (3) AEDF in UmA (4) REDF in UmA (5) Absent or reversed "a" wave in DV and/or pulsatility in UV	PV, max PT, PT/PV ratio GA: 20–38 wks	Morphometry determinants in relation to: - Group A vs. B - Severity of FGR - Fetal and neonatal mortality	Sign. increase in max PT/PV ratio in group A Sign. correlation: max PT/PV ratio –severity FGR, PV–EFW, PV–severity of FGR Association: increase in max PT/PV ratio >p95–fetal and early neonatal mortality PV remained sign. smaller in group A
Dahdouh et al., 2018, United States of America	Prospective 49 SP **A:** 43 FGR fetuses **B:** 46 controls	EFW <p10 and - Abnormal Doppler of fetal vessels - Asymmetric growth with lagging AC	PV, PT, PL icw textural features used in machine learning frameworks GA: 18–39 wks	Identification of the FGR pregnancies	The proposed machine-learning based method using shape features identified FGR pregnancies with 86% accuracy, 77% precision and 86% recall.
Ohgiya et al., 2016, Japan	Prospective 50 SP **A:** 25 FGR fetuses **B:** 25 controls	No definition given	PT, PSA, PV GA: 19–38 wks	Morphometry determinants in group A vs. B	Sign. lower mean PSA and PV in group A compared to group B. Sign. higher mean PT in group A compared to group B.
Andescavage et al., 2017, United States of America	Prospective 114 SP **A:** 35 FGR fetuses **B:** 79 controls	EFW < p10 and - UmA PI >p95 or CPR<1 - AC lagged HC > 1 week	PV GA: 18–40 wks	Morphometry determinant in relation to: - group A vs. B - UmA Doppler, UtA Doppler, MCA Doppler, CPR	Sign. lower mean PV in group A vs. B Sign. lower mean PV in subgroup of group A with abnormal UmA Doppler. no association between: PV–UtA Doppler, PV–MCA Doppler, PV–CPR
Derwig et al., 2011, United Kingdom	Prospective 83 SP	Not applicable	PV GA: 24 - 29 wks	Morphometry determinant in relation to UtA Doppler and BW-centile	Median PV was sign decreased in pregnancies delivering a SGA-neonate (<p10) PV is sign related to the degree of uterine perfusion reflected in the PI of the UtA.

AC, abdominal circumference; CPR, cerebroplacental ratio; DV, ductus venosus; EFW, estimated fetal weight; FGR, fetal growth restriction; GA, gestational age; HC, head circumference; icw, in combination with; MCA, middle cerebral artery; PI, pulsatility index; PL, placental length; PSA, macroscopic placental surface area; PT, placental thickness; PV, placental volume; sign, significantly; SP, singleton pregnancies; UtA, uterine artery; UmA, umbilical artery; UV, umbilical vein; wks, weeks.

the possibility to investigate the placenta. However, postnatal morphology studies of the placenta give the opportunity to help in finding the neonate who suffered undetected growth restriction and should be monitored more closely during postnatal care. It is thus important to focus on the possible clinical relevance of placental morphometry in retrospectively diagnosing impaired growth.

Postnatal Placental Morphometry in Relation to Ultrasound Markers of Fetal Growth Restriction

It has been shown that utero-placental blood flow and fetal growth can be related to the gross morphometry of the placenta (Salavati et al., 2016). Small placental area and low placental weight were associated with, respectively, higher uterine and higher umbilical artery PI. Both placental area and weight were associated with a slower fetal ACGV (Salavati et al., 2016). The circularity of the placenta was associated with the uterine artery, but not the umbilical artery, flow velocity waveform. These results show that size and shape of the placenta are depending on the vascular function of the placenta from both the maternal and fetal side. Although some studies have focused on the relationship between ultrasound measurements (e.g., fetal biometry, Doppler flow velocity waveforms) and adverse pregnancy outcome (Ghosh and Gudmundsson, 2009; Sovio et al., 2015), more literature on the relationship with postnatal placental morphometry is lacking.

Birth weight to placenta weight-ratio in relation to ultrasound markers

Research showed that not only the size and weight of the placenta, but also the weight of the placenta in relation to birth weight was associated with both umbilical and uterine artery PI (Salavati et al., 2018). Specifically, high BWPW-ratio was associated with both higher umbilical artery PI (26 weeks of gestation) and higher uterine artery PI (20 weeks of gestation), two markers of decreased placental function. Low BWPW-ratio was not associated with either umbilical or uterine artery PI, however it was with maternal and neonatal morbidity (Salavati et al., 2018). Decreased placental function may sound contradictory, since placentas in the group of high BWPW-ratio can also be seen as very efficient. It might be plausible that the relatively small placentas in the group of high BWPW-ratio work at their maximum function capability for that volume, and that the birth weight actually could have been higher with higher placental volume. With this said, we would expect high BWPW-ratio to be related to adverse postnatal outcome related to starvation caused by too relatively small placentas, which was not shown by recent research (Salavati et al., 2018). This might be the result of intervention bias: those cases with high umbilical and uterine artery PI might have experienced an earlier induction of labor, resulting in lower neonatal morbidity (Gibson et al., 2014). Another explanation might be the role of placental surface area. Those placentas in the group of low BWPW-ratio might be thicker but have a small macroscopic placental surface area, resulting in a less efficiently exchange process of oxygen, nutrients, and fetal waste products. In the group of high BWPW-ratio the reverse might be true; within this group the placentas might have a large macroscopic placental surface area, but are really thin, explaining the lower placental weight.

Postnatal Placental Morphometry in Relation to Birth Weight and Fetal Growth Restriction

Various studies have looked at the relationship between postnatal placental morphometry and birth weight. These studies showed that low birth weight was associated with lower placental weight and volume, and a smaller placental area (Balihallimath et al., 2013; Kowsalya et al., 2013). Balihallimath et al. studied the relationship of placenta morphometry more specifically in different birth weight groups, classified by gender (Balihallimath et al., 2013). In the groups with birth weight less than 3,000 g, the surface area of the placenta was smaller in male babies compared to female babies. When birth weight exceeded 3,000 g, the surface area was larger in male babies (Balihallimath et al., 2013). In addition, it has been described that male babies have a higher birth weight compared to female babies, but have the same placental weight (increased BWPW-ratio) (Eriksson et al., 2010; Macdonald et al., 2014). Male babies also have a higher perinatal mortality (Drevenstedt et al., 2008), rather than more efficient they may also be just the fetus that runs the risk of increased mortality to maximize growth. We think the placenta has a functional reserve to cope with extra demands, which explains why many stillbirths have pre-existing injury (Gardosi et al., 2013).

Although a small placenta suggests reduced reserve, the association between low birth weight and low placental weight and size, could potentially be physiological (small baby, small placenta) therefore statements regarding the association between placental morphometry and pathological, low or high, birth weight, require an investigation of proportionality, of the relationship of placental morphometry with BWPW-ratio. Also the site of the umbilical cord insertion has been linked to birth weight (Yampolsky et al., 2009; Haeussner et al., 2013; Kowsalya et al., 2013). Kowsalya et al. indicated that the cord insertion was more often eccentric or marginal in the group of infants with low birth weight (Kowsalya et al., 2013). Yampolsky et al. pointed out that this central insertion influences placental efficiency positively (Yampolsky et al., 2009). Conflicting results were published by Haeussner et al. who reported that the location of the cord insertion in relation to the edge of the placental disk did not correlate with birth weight, and eccentric cord insertion did not necessarily compromise efficiency of the normal human placenta (Haeussner et al., 2013). Furthermore, they reported that parameters regarding the form of the placenta (e.g., diameter, thickness, roundness, eccentricity of the cord insertion) correlate with both birth weight and placental weight (Haeussner et al., 2013).

It has been proposed that FGR and morphologic changes of the placenta, are caused by impaired placental perfusion, due to reduced placental vascular bed in chronic fetal hypoxia, which causes oxidative stress of the fetal vasculature (Kingdom and Kaufmann, 1997; Kuzmina et al., 2005). Junaid et al. investigated micro and microvasculature of placentas from normal and FGR pregnancies, and observed hyposvascularity in the peripheral lobules of placentas from FGR pregnancies (Junaid et al., 2014).

TABLE 3 | Literature overview of postnatal placental morphometry assessment in relation to FGR (markers).

Author, year, country	Study type and population	FGR definition	Determinant(s)	Outcome	Results
Egbor et al., 2006 United Kingdom	Prospective **A:** 17 FGR **B:** 16 PE-FGR **C:** 16 controls	- Clinical evidence of suboptimal growth - Ultra sonographic evidence of deviation from appropriate growth percentile - BW <p10	PV, PW	FGR	FGR was associated with a significant reduction in PV and PW
Mayhew et al., 2007, United Kingdom	Prospective **A:** 5 FGR **B:** 5 PE-FGR **C:** 9 controls	- Deficient fetal growth on ultrasound scans - IBR <p10	PSA	Morphometry determinant in the different groups	FGR (with or without PE) was associated with a reduced PSA
Almasry and Elfayomy, 2012, Saudi Arabia	Case-control **A:** 50 FGR **B:** 25 controls	EFW<p10 icw two criteria: - Abnormal UmA Doppler - Oligohydramnios; AFI<5 - Asymmetric growth; HC/AC ratio	PD, PW, "placenta co-efficient" (PW/BW).	FGR	Significant reduction in PD and PW in FGR group as compared with controls. Placental coefficient greater in FGR group.

AC, abdominal circumference; BW, birth weight; EFW, estimated fetal weight; FGR, fetal growth restriction; HC, head circumference; IBR, individualized birth weight ratio (is calculated using factors including fetal gender, GA, parity, ethnic origin and maternal age, height and booking weight); icw, in combination with; PE, preeclampsia; PD, placental diameter; PSA, macroscopic placental surface area; PV, placental volume; PW, placental weight; UmA, umbilical artery.

Another aspect that may result in altered morphometry, is the fact that FGR related hypoxia influences angiogenesis via various growth factor receptors (Mayhew et al., 2004). Three studies were found that investigated the relationship between postnatal placental morphometry and FGR (Egbor et al., 2006; Mayhew et al., 2007; Almasry and Elfayomy, 2012) (**Table 3**).

These three studies classified FGR based on deficient fetal growth on ultrasound scans and EFW less than 10th centile. They found that FGR was associated with changes in placental morphometry such as decreased surface areas, decreased placental diameter, and decreased placental volume and placental weight (Egbor et al., 2006; Mayhew et al., 2007; Almasry and Elfayomy, 2012).

FUTURE PERSPECTIVES

As described, various studies have focused on the relationship between placental morphometry and fetal growth and birth weight. Unfortunately, only limited research has been performed focusing on associations between placental morphometry and FGR. The often seen "SGA-FGR confusion" in FGR studies will lead to weaker associations with any effective screening test, including placental morphometry imaging. Although cheap and easy to obtain, the postnatal placenta will only aid the diagnosis of FGR in retrospect. This could result in altered management by less monitoring in healthy SGA and more monitoring in FGR, regardless of birth weight. Although we expect that aspects of placental morphometry can play a role in the diagnostic process of FGR, mainly postnatally, additional components, as part of a multiparameter model, might need to be taken into account with the aspects of placental morphometry. A small placenta, or abnormally flat or thick placenta may prompt review for assessment of the baby and the histology of the placenta to see if other findings to suggest maternal malperfusion or other pathology is present.

Further use of placenta morphometry in the diagnostic process of FGR can be explored by for example BWPW-ratio in relation to abdominal circumference growth velocity (ACGV), macroscopic placental surface area (and placental volume) and placenta serum biomarkers. As suggested in a recent paper about screening for fetal growth restriction (Gaccioli et al., 2018a), it is expected that future screening tests for FGR will include several measurements, which are obtained from both imaging procedures and measurements of biomarkers. For the development of such a model it is essential that every single parameter is measured and scaled in the association with FGR, in order to generate consistent associations. Regarding imaging procedures, research has shown that placental imaging through MRI might be of clinical use in predicting FGR. Nowadays, MRI is already in use for fetal imaging, so possibly placental imaging can be used in the near future.

CONCLUSIONS

It is of great importance that clinically useful, and easy to perform, methods will be generated in order to improve the antenatal and postnatal screening for, and diagnosis of, fetuses with FGR who have increased risk on adverse pregnancy outcomes. In this literature review we intended to give an overview on the clinical relevance of placenta morphometry in the detection of FGR. In current clinical practice, antenatal placental imaging is difficult, and the placenta is not routinely examined after birth, nor in a standardized way, despite the possible value in several parameters of impaired growth of the fetus. Future research can focus on the relationship between placental morphometry, FGR and its complications, to improve screening for FGR, and to determine the biological pathways that can be linked to placental dysfunction, in a group of optimally phenotyped cases of FGR. With this, placental morphometry might be implemented in clinical practice, possibly as part of a multiparameter model.

AUTHOR CONTRIBUTIONS

All authors made substantial contributions to the conception of this review and the critical appraisal of the literature summarized herein. NS and MS generated the initial draft of the manuscript, and this was critically revised by SG, WG, AC, TP, and JE. All authors approved the final version and submission of the article.

REFERENCES

1. ACOG Practice Bulletin no. 134: Fetal Growth Restriction (2013). *Obstet. Gynecol.* 121, 1122–1133. doi: 10.1097/01.AOG.0000429658.85846.f9
2. Afrakhteh, M., Moeini, A., Taheri, M. S., and Haghighatkhah, H. R. (2013). Correlation between placental thickness in the second and third trimester and fetal weight. *Rev. Bras. Ginecol. Obstet.* 35, 317–322. doi: 10.1590/S0100-72032013000700006
3. Alfirevic, Z., Stampalija, T., and Gyte, G. M. (2010). Fetal and umbilical Doppler ultrasound in high-risk pregnancies. *Cochr. Database Syst. Rev.* CD007529. doi: 10.1002/14651858.CD007529.pub2
4. Almasry, S. M., and Elfayomy, A. K. (2012). Morphometric analysis of terminal villi and gross morphological changes in the placentae of term idiopathic intrauterine growth restriction. *Tissue Cell* 44, 214–219. doi: 10.1016/j.tice.2012.03.006
5. Andescavage, N., duPlessis, A., Metzler, M., Bulas, D., Vezina, G., Jacobs, M., et al. (2017). *In vivo* assessment of placental and brain volumes in growth-restricted fetuses with and without fetal Doppler changes using quantitative 3D MRI. *J. Perinatol.* 37, 1278–1284. doi: 10.1038/jp.2017.129
6. Arakaki, T., Hasegawa, J., Nakamura, M., Hamada, S., Muramoto, M., Takita, H., et al. (2015). Prediction of early- and late-onset pregnancy-induced hypertension using placental volume on three-dimensional ultrasound and uterine artery Doppler. *Ultrasound Obstet. Gynecol.* 45, 539–543. doi: 10.1002/uog.14633
7. Avni, R., Neeman, M., and Garbow, J. R. (2015). Functional MRI of the placenta–from rodents to humans. *Placenta* 36, 615–622. doi: 10.1016/j.placenta.2015.04.003
8. Azpurua, H., Funai, E. F., Coraluzzi, L. M., Doherty, L. F., Sasson, I. E., Kliman, M., et al. (2010). Determination of placental weight using two-dimensional sonography and volumetric mathematic modeling. *Am. J. Perinatol.* 27, 151–155. doi: 10.1055/s-0029-1234034
9. Balihallimath, R. L., Shirol, V. S., Gan, A. M., Tyagi, N. K., and Bandankar, M. R. (2013). Placental morphometry determines the birth weight. *J. Clin. Diagn. Res.* 7, 2428–2431. doi: 10.7860/JCDR/2013/7478.3564
10. Beune, I. M., Pels, A., Gordijn, S. J., and Ganzevoort, W. (2018). Definitions of fetal growth restriction in existing literature over time. *Ultrasound Obstet. Gynecol.* doi: 10.1002/uog.19189. [Epub ahead of print].
11. Bulas, D., and Egloff, A. (2013). Benefits and risks of MRI in pregnancy. *Semin. Perinatol.* 37, 301–304. doi: 10.1053/j.semperi.2013.06.005
12. Burton, G. J., Fowden, A. L., and Thornburg, K. L. (2016). Placental origins of chronic disease. *Physiol. Rev.* 96, 1509–1565. doi: 10.1152/physrev.00029.2015
13. Chisholm, K. M., and Folkins, A. K. (2016). Placental and clinical characteristics of term small-for-gestational-age neonates: a case-control study. *Pediatr. Dev. Pathol.* 19, 37–46. doi: 10.2350/15-04-1621-OA.1
14. Conde-Agudelo, A., Papageorghiou, A. T., Kennedy, S. H., and Villar, J. (2013). Novel biomarkers for predicting intrauterine growth restriction: a systematic review and meta-analysis. *BJOG* 120, 681–694. doi: 10.1111/1471-0528.12172
15. Dahdouh, S., Andescavage, N., Yewale, S., Yarish, A., Lanham, D., Bulas, D., et al. (2018). *In vivo* placental MRI shape and textural features predict fetal growth restriction and postnatal outcome. *J. Magn. Reson. Imaging* 47, 449–458. doi: 10.1002/jmri.25806
16. Damodaram, M., Story, L., Eixarch, E., Patel, A., McGuinness, A., Allsop, J., et al. (2010). Placental MRI in intrauterine fetal growth restriction. *Placenta* 31, 491–498. doi: 10.1016/j.placenta.2010.03.001
17. Derwig, I. E., Akolekar, R., Zelaya, F. O., Gowland, P. A., Barker, G. J., and Nicolaides, K. H. (2011). Association of placental volume measured by MRI and birth weight percentile. *J. Magn. Reson. Imaging* 34, 1125–1130. doi: 10.1002/jmri.22794
18. Drevenstedt, G. L., Crimmins, E. M., Vasunilashorn, S., and Finch, C. E. (2008). The rise and fall of excess male infant mortality. *Proc. Natl. Acad. Sci. U.S.A.* 105, 5016–5021. doi: 10.1073/pnas.08002 21105
19. Duncan, K. R., Sahota, D. S., Gowland, P. A., Moore, R., Chang, A., Baker, P. N., et al. (2001). Multilevel modeling of fetal and placental growth using echo-planar magnetic resonance imaging. *J. Soc. Gynecol. Investig.* 8, 285–290. doi: 10.1177/107155760100800505
20. Egbor, M., Ansari, T., Morris, N., Green, C. J., and Sibbons, P. D. (2006). Pre-eclampsia and fetal growth restriction: how morphometrically different is the placenta? *Placenta* 27, 727–734. doi: 10.1016/j.placenta.2005.06.002
21. Eriksson, J. G., Kajantie, E., Osmond, C., Thornburg, K., and Barker, D. J. P. (2010). Boys live dangerously in the womb. *Am. J. Hum. Biol.* 22, 330–335. doi: 10.1002/ajhb.20995
22. Figueras, F., and Gratacos, E. (2017). An integrated approach to fetal growth restriction. *Best Pract. Res. Clin. Obstet. Gynaecol.* 38, 48–58. doi: 10.1016/j.bpobgyn.2016.10.006
23. Gaccioli, F., Aye, I. L. M. H., Sovio, U., Charnock-Jones, D. S., and Smith, G. C. S. (2018a). Screening for fetal growth restriction using fetal biometry combined with maternal biomarkers. *Am. J. Obstet. Gynecol.* 218, S725–S737. doi: 10.1016/j.ajog.2017.12.002
24. Gaccioli, F., Sovio, U., Cook, E., Hund, M., Charnock-Jones, D. S., and Smith, G. C. S. (2018b). Screening for fetal growth restriction using ultrasound and the sFLT1/PlGF ratio in nulliparous women: a prospective cohort study. *Lancet Child Adolesc. Health* 2, 569–581. doi: 10.1016/S2352-4642(18) 30129-9
25. Gardosi, J., Madurasinghe, V., Williams, M., Malik, A., and Francis, A. (2013). Maternal and fetal risk factors for stillbirth: population based study. *BMJ* 346:f108. doi: 10.1136/bmj.f108
26. Ghosh, G., and Gudmundsson, S. (2009). Uterine and umbilical artery Doppler are comparable in predicting perinatal outcome of growth-restricted fetuses. *BJOG An Int. J. Obstet. Gynaecol.* 116, 424–430. doi: 10.1111/j.1471-0528.2008.02057.x
27. Gibson, K. S., Waters, T. P., and Bailit, J. L. (2014). Maternal and neonatal outcomes in electively induced low-risk term pregnancies. *Am. J. Obstet. Gynecol.* 211, 249.e1–249.e16. doi: 10.1016/j.ajog.2014.03.016
28. Glazier, J. D., Cetin, I., Perugino, G., Ronzoni, S., Grey, A. M., Mahendran, D., et al. (1997). Association between the activity of the system a amino acid transporter in the microvillous plasma membrane of the human placenta and severity of fetal compromise in intrauterine growth restriction. *Pediatr. Res.* 42, 514–519. doi: 10.1203/00006450-19971000 0-00016
29. Gordijn, S. J., Beune, I. M., and Ganzevoort, W. (2018). Building consensus and standards in fetal growth restriction studies. *Best Pract. Res. Clin. Obstet. Gynaecol.* 49, 117–126. doi: 10.1016/j.bpobgyn.2018.02.002
30. Gordijn, S. J., Beune, I. M., Thilaganathan, B., Papageorghiou, A.,

Baschat, A. A., Baker, P. N., et al. (2016). Consensus definition of fetal growth restriction: a Delphi procedure. *Ultrasound Obstet. Gynecol.* 48, 333–339. doi: 10.1002/uog.15884

31. Habib, F. A. (2002). Prediction of low birth weight infants from ultrasound measurement of placental diameter and placental thickness. *Ann. Saudi Med.* 22, 312–314. doi: 10.5144/0256-4947.2002.312
32. Haeussner, E., Schmitz, C., von Koch, F., and Frank, H.-G. (2013). Birth weight correlates with size but not shape of the normal human placenta. *Placenta* 34, 574–582. doi: 10.1016/j.placenta.2013.04.011
33. Hayward, C. E., Lean, S., Sibley, C. P., Jones, R. L., Wareing, M., Greenwood, S. L., et al. (2016). Placental adaptation: what can we learn from birthweight:placental weight ratio? *Front. Physiol.* 7:28. doi: 10.3389/fphys.2016.00028
34. Heinonen, S., Taipale, P., and Saarikoski, S. (2001). Weights of placentae from small-for-gestational age infants revisited. *Placenta* 22, 399–404. doi: 10.1053/plac.2001.0630
35. Higgins, L. E., Simcox, L., Sibley, C. P., Heazell, A. E. P., and Johnstone, E. D. (2016). Third trimester placental volume and biometry measurement: a method-development study. *Placenta* 42, 51–58. doi: 10.1016/j.placenta.2016.04.010
36. Jaddoe, V. W. V., de Jonge, L. L., Hofman, A., Franco, O. H., Steegers, E. A. P., and Gaillard, R. (2014). First trimester fetal growth restriction and cardiovascular risk factors in school age children: population based cohort study. *BMJ* 348:g14. doi: 10.1136/bmj.g14
37. Junaid, T. O., Brownbill, P., Chalmers, N., Johnstone, E. D., and Aplin, J. D. (2014). Fetoplacental vascular alterations associated with fetal growth restriction. *Placenta* 35, 808–815. doi: 10.1016/j.placenta.2014.07.013
38. Khong, T. Y., Mooney, E. E., Ariel, I., Balmus, N. C. M., Boyd, T. K., Brundler, M.-A., et al. (2016). Sampling and definitions of placental lesions: amsterdam placental workshop group consensus statement. *Arch. Pathol. Lab. Med.* 140, 698–713. doi: 10.5858/arpa.2015-0225-CC
39. Kingdom, J. C., and Kaufmann, P. (1997). Oxygen and placental villous development: origins of fetal hypoxia. *Placenta* 18, 613–21; discussion 623–626. doi: 10.1016/S0143-4004(97)90000-X
40. Kowsalya, V., Vijayakumar, R., Valli, G., Bharath, K. P., Srikumar, R., Kishor Kumar, C., et al. (2013). Morphometry examination of placenta in birth weight of full-term newborns in Puducherry, India. *Pakistan J. Biol. Sci.* 16, 895–897.
41. Kuzmina, I. Y., Hubina-Vakulik, G. I., and Burton, G. J. (2005). Placental morphometry and Doppler flow velocimetry in cases of chronic human fetal hypoxia. *Eur. J. Obstet. Gynecol. Reprod. Biol.* 120, 139–145. doi: 10.1016/j.ejogrb.2004.09.001
42. Langhoff, L., Grønbeck, L., von Huth, S., Axelsson, A., Jørgensen, C., Thomsen, C., et al. (2017). Placental growth during normal pregnancy-a magnetic resonance imaging study. *Gynecol. Obstet. Invest.* 82, 462–467. doi: 10.1159/000452661
43. Leary, S. D., Godfrey, K. M., Greenaway, L. J., Davill, V. A., and Fall, C. H. D. (2003). Contribution of the umbilical cord and membranes to untrimmed placental weight. *Placenta* 24, 276–278. doi: 10.1053/plac.2002.0888
44. León, R. L., Li, K. T., and Brown, B. P. (2018). A retrospective segmentation analysis of placental volume by magnetic resonance imaging from first trimester to term gestation. *Pediatr. Radiol.* 48, 1936–1944. doi: 10.1007/s00247-018-4213-x
45. Lindqvist, P. G., and Molin, J. (2005). Does antenatal identification of small-for-gestational age fetuses significantly improve their outcome? *Ultrasound Obstet. Gynecol.* 25, 258–264. doi: 10.1002/uog.1806
46. Looney, P., Stevenson, G. N., Nicolaides, K. H., Plasencia, W., Molloholli, M., Natsis, S., et al. (2018). Fully automated, real-time 3D ultrasound segmentation to estimate first trimester placental volume using deep learning. *JCI insight* 3:e120178. doi: 10.1172/jci.insight.120178
47. Macdonald, E. M., Koval, J. J., Natale, R., Regnault, T., and Campbell, M. K. (2014). Population-based placental weight ratio distributions. *Int. J. Pediatr.* 2014:291846. doi: 10.1155/2014/291846
48. Mathai, B. M., Singla, S. C., Nittala, P. P., Chakravarti, R. J., and Toppo, J. N. (2013). Placental thickness: its correlation with ultrasonographic gestational age in normal and intrauterine growth-retarded pregnancies in the late second and third trimester. *J. Obstet. Gynecol. India* 63, 230–233. doi: 10.1007/s13224-012-0316-8
49. Mayhew, T., Charnock-Jones, D., and Kaufmann, P. (2004). Aspects of human fetoplacental vasculogenesis and angiogenesis. iii. changes in complicated pregnancies. *Placenta* 25, 127–139. doi: 10.1016/j.placenta.2003.10.010
50. Mayhew, T. M., Manwani, R., Ohadike, C., Wijesekara, J., and Baker, P. N. (2007). The placenta in pre-eclampsia and intrauterine growth restriction: studies on exchange surface areas, diffusion distances and villous membrane diffusive conductances. *Placenta* 28, 233–238. doi: 10.1016/j.placenta.2006.02.011
51. Meher, S., Hernandez-Andrade, E., Basheer, S. N., and Lees, C. (2015). Impact of cerebral redistribution on neurodevelopmental outcome in small-for-gestational-age or growth-restricted babies: a systematic review. *Ultrasound Obstet. Gynecol.* 46, 398–404. doi: 10.1002/uog.14818
52. Mifsud, W., and Sebire, N. J. (2014). Placental pathology in early-onset and late-onset fetal growth restriction. *Fetal Diagn. Ther.* 36, 117–128. doi: 10.1159/000359969
53. Miller, S. L., Huppi, P. S., and Mallard, C. (2016). The consequences of fetal growth restriction on brain structure and neurodevelopmental outcome. *J. Physiol.* 594, 807–823. doi: 10.1113/JP271402
54. Millischer, A. E., Sonigo, P., Ville, Y., Brunelle, F., Boddaert, N., and Salomon, L. J. (2013). Standardized fetal anatomical examination using magnetic resonance imaging: a feasibility study. *Ultrasound Obstet. Gynecol.* 42, 553–559. doi: 10.1002/uog.12415
55. Monier, I., Ancel, P.-Y., Ego, A., Jarreau, P.-H., Lebeaux, C., Kaminski, M., et al. (2017). Fetal and neonatal outcomes of preterm infants born before 32 weeks of gestation according to antenatal vs postnatal assessments of restricted growth. *Am. J. Obstet. Gynecol.* 216, 516.e1–516.e10. doi: 10.1016/j.ajog.2017.02.001
56. Morales Roselló, J., Hervás Marín, D., Fillol Crespo, M., and Perales Marín, A. (2012). Doppler changes in the vertebral, middle cerebral, and umbilical arteries in fetuses delivered after 34 weeks: relationship to severity of growth restriction. *Prenat. Diagn.* 32, 960–967. doi: 10.1002/pd.3941
57. Nardozza, L. M. M., Caetano, A. C. R., Zamarian, A. C. P., Mazzola, J. B., Silva, C. P., Marçal, V. M. G., et al. (2017). Fetal growth restriction: current knowledge. *Arch. Gynecol. Obstet.* 295, 1061–1077. doi: 10.1007/s00404-017-4341-9
58. Ohgiya, Y., Nobusawa, H., Seino, N., Miyagami, O., Yagi, N., Hiroto, S., et al. (2016). MR imaging of fetuses to evaluate placental insufficiency. *Magn. Reson. Med. Sci.* 15, 212–219. doi: 10.2463/mrms.mp.2015-0051
59. Proctor, L. K., Toal, M., Keating, S., Chitayat, D., Okun, N., Windrim, R. C., et al. (2009). Placental size and the prediction of severe early-onset intrauterine growth restriction in women with low pregnancy-associated plasma protein-A. *Ultrasound Obstet. Gynecol.* 34, 274–282. doi: 10.1002/uog.7308
60. Salavati, N., Gordijn, S. J., Sovio, U., Zill-E-Huma, R., Gebril, A., Charnock-Jones, D. S., et al. (2018). Birth weight to placenta weight ratio and its relationship to ultrasonic measurements, maternal and neonatal morbidity: a prospective cohort study of nulliparous women. *Placenta* 63, 45–52. doi: 10.1016/j.placenta.2017.11.008
61. Salavati, N., Sovio, U., Mayo, R. P., Charnock-Jones, D. S., and Smith, G. C. S. (2016). The relationship between human placental morphometry and ultrasonic measurements of utero-placental blood flow and fetal growth. *Placenta* 38, 41–48. doi: 10.1016/j.placenta.2015.12.003
62. Schwartz, N., Sammel, M. D., Leite, R., and Parry, S. (2014). First-trimester placental ultrasound and maternal serum markers as predictors of small- for-gestational-age infants. *Am. J. Obstet. Gynecol.* 211, 253.e1–253.e8. doi: 10.1016/j.ajog.2014.02.033
63. Siauve, N., Chalouhi, G. E., Deloison, B., Alison, M., Clement, O., Ville, Y., et al. (2015). Functional imaging of the human placenta with magnetic resonance. *Am. J. Obstet. Gynecol.* 213, S103–S114. doi: 10.1016/j.ajog.2015.06.045
64. Sovio, U., White, I. R., Dacey, A., Pasupathy, D., and Smith, G. C. S. (2015). Screening for fetal growth restriction with universal third trimester ultrasonography in nulliparous women in the Pregnancy Outcome Prediction (POP) study: a prospective cohort study. *Lancet* 386, 2089–2097. doi: 10.1016/S0140-6736(15)00131-2
65. Toal, M., Chan, C., Fallah, S., Alkazaleh, F., Chaddha, V., Windrim, R. C., et al. (2007). Usefulness of a placental profile in high-risk pregnancies. *Am. J. Obstet. Gynecol.* 196, 363.e1–363.e7. doi: 10.1016/j.ajog.2006. 10.897
66. Toal, M., Keating, S., Machin, G., Dodd, J., Adamson, S. L., Windrim, R. C., et al. (2008). Determinants of adverse perinatal outcome in high-risk women with abnormal uterine artery Doppler images. *Am. J. Obstet. Gynecol.* 198, 330. e1–330.e7. doi: 10.1016/j.ajog.2007.09.031
67. Unterscheider, J., Daly, S., Geary, M. P., Kennelly, M. M., McAuliffe, F. M., O'Donoghue, K., et al. (2013). Optimizing the definition of intrauterine growth restriction: the multicenter prospective PORTO Study. *Am. J. Obstet. Gynecol.* 208, 290.e1–290.e6. doi: 10.1016/j.ajog.2013.02.007

68. Vasak, B., Koenen, S. V., Koster, M. P. H., Hukkelhoven, C. W. P. M., Franx, A., Hanson, M. A., et al. (2015). Human fetal growth is constrained below optimal for perinatal survival. *Ultrasound Obstet. Gynecol.* 45, 162–167. doi: 10.1002/uog.14644
69. Viero, S., Chaddha, V., Alkazaleh, F., Simchen, M. J., Malik, A., Kelly, E., et al. (2004). Prognostic value of placental ultrasound in pregnancies complicated by absent end-diastolic flow velocity in the umbilical arteries. *Placenta* 25, 735–741. doi: 10.1016/j.placenta.2004.03.002
70. Wang, P. I., Chong, S. T., Kielar, A. Z., Kelly, A. M., Knoepp, U. D., Mazza,
71. M. B., et al. (2012a). Imaging of pregnant and lactating patients: part 1, evidence-based review and recommendations. *Am. J. Roentgenol.* 198, 778–784. doi: 10.2214/AJR.11.7405
72. Wang, P. I., Chong, S. T., Kielar, A. Z., Kelly, A. M., Knoepp, U. D., Mazza, M. B., et al. (2012b). Imaging of pregnant and lactating patients: part 2, evidence-based review and recommendations. *Am. J. Roentgenol.* 198, 785–792. doi: 10.2214/AJR.11.8223
73. Wilson, M. E., and Ford, S. P. (2001). Comparative aspects of placental efficiency. *Reprod. Suppl.* 58, 223–232.
74. Yampolsky, M., Salafia, C. M., Shlakhter, O., Haas, D., Eucker, B., and Thorp, J. (2009). Centrality of the umbilical cord insertion in a human placenta influences the placental efficiency. *Placenta* 30, 1058–1064. doi: 10.1016/j.placenta.2009.10.001
75. Zhang, J., Merialdi, M., Platt, L. D., and Kramer, M. S. (2010). Defining normal and abnormal fetal growth: promises and challenges. *Am. J. Obstet. Gynecol.* 202, 522–528. doi: 10.1016/j.ajog.2009.10.889
76. Zhang, S., Regnault, T., Barker, P., Botting, K., McMillen, I., McMillan, C., et al. (2015). Placental adaptations in growth restriction. *Nutrients* 7, 360–389. doi: 10.3390/nu7010360

Permissions

All chapters in this book were first published by Frontiers; hereby published with permission under the Creative Commons Attribution License or equivalent. Every chapter published in this book has been scrutinized by our experts. Their significance has been extensively debated. The topics covered herein carry significant findings which will fuel the growth of the discipline. They may even be implemented as practical applications or may be referred to as a beginning point for another development.

The contributors of this book come from diverse backgrounds, making this book a truly international effort. This book will bring forth new frontiers with its revolutionizing research information and detailed analysis of the nascent developments around the world.

We would like to thank all the contributing authors for lending their expertise to make the book truly unique. They have played a crucial role in the development of this book. Without their invaluable contributions this book wouldn't have been possible. They have made vital efforts to compile up to date information on the varied aspects of this subject to make this book a valuable addition to the collection of many professionals and students.

This book was conceptualized with the vision of imparting up-to-date information and advanced data in this field. To ensure the same, a matchless editorial board was set up. Every individual on the board went through rigorous rounds of assessment to prove their worth. After which they invested a large part of their time researching and compiling the most relevant data for our readers.

The editorial board has been involved in producing this book since its inception. They have spent rigorous hours researching and exploring the diverse topics which have resulted in the successful publishing of this book. They have passed on their knowledge of decades through this book. To expedite this challenging task, the publisher supported the team at every step. A small team of assistant editors was also appointed to further simplify the editing procedure and attain best results for the readers.

Apart from the editorial board, the designing team has also invested a significant amount of their time in understanding the subject and creating the most relevant covers. They scrutinized every image to scout for the most suitable representation of the subject and create an appropriate cover for the book.

The publishing team has been an ardent support to the editorial, designing and production team. Their endless efforts to recruit the best for this project, has resulted in the accomplishment of this book. They are a veteran in the field of academics and their pool of knowledge is as vast as their experience in printing. Their expertise and guidance has proved useful at every step. Their uncompromising quality standards have made this book an exceptional effort. Their encouragement from time to time has been an inspiration for everyone.

The publisher and the editorial board hope that this book will prove to be a valuable piece of knowledge for researchers, students, practitioners and scholars across the globe.

All chapters in this book were first published by Frontiers; hereby published with permission under the Creative Commons Attribution License or equivalent. Every chapter published in this book has been scrutinized by our experts. Their significance has been extensively debated. The topics covered herein carry significant findings which will fuel the growth of the discipline. They may even be implemented as practical applications or may be referred to as a beginning point for another development.

The contributors of this book come from diverse backgrounds, making this book a truly international effort. This book will bring forth new frontiers with its revolutionizing research information and detailed analysis of the nascent developments around the world.

List of Contributors

Marius Schmidt, Manfred Rauh, Rainer Wachtveitl, Nada Cordasic, Wolfgang Rascher, Carlos Menendez-Castro, Andrea Hartner and Fabian B. Fahlbusch
Department of Pediatrics and Adolescent Medicine, Friedrich-Alexander University Erlangen-Nuremberg, Erlangen, Germany

Matthias C. Schmid
Institute of Medical Biometry, Informatics and Epidemiology, Faculty of Medicine, Rheinische Friedrich-Wilhelms-University, Bonn, Germany

Hanna Huebner and Matthias Ruebner
Department of Gynaecology and Obstetrics/ Comprehensive Cancer Center Erlangen-EMN, Friedrich-Alexander University Erlangen-Nuremberg, Erlangen, Germany

Olivier Baud
Division of Neonatology and Pediatric Intensive Care, Department of Women-Children-Teenagers, University Hospitals Geneva, Geneva, Switzerland
Inserm U1141, Sorbonne, Paris Diderot University, Paris, France

Nadia Berkane
Division of Obstetrics and Gynecology, Department of Women-Children-Teenagers, University Hospitals Geneva, Geneva, Switzerland

Tamara Yawno, Graham Jenkin and Suzanne L. Miller
The Ritchie Centre, Hudson Institute of Medical Research, Monash University, Clayton, VIC, Australia
Department of Obstetrics and Gynaecology, Monash University, Clayton, VIC, Australia

Amy E. Sutherland, Yen Pham and Margie Castillo-Melendez
The Ritchie Centre, Hudson Institute of Medical Research, Monash University, Clayton, VIC, Australia

Kristin Thiele, Alexandra Maximiliane Hierweger, Julia Isabel Amambay Riquelme, María Emilia Solano and Petra Clara Arck
Division of Experimental Feto-Maternal Medicine, Department of Obstetrics and Fetal Medicine, University Medical Center Hamburg-Eppendorf, Hamburg, Germany

John P. Lydon
Department of Molecular and Cellular Biology, Baylor College of Medicine, Houston, TX, United States

Johanna Seitz, Diana Maria Morales-Prieto, Rodolfo R. Favaro and Udo Rudolf Markert
Placenta Lab, Department of Obstetrics, Jena University Hospital, Jena, Germany

Henning Schneider
Institute of Biochemistry and Molecular Medicine, University of Bern, Bern, Switzerland
Department of Obstetrics and Gynecology, Inselspital, Bern University Hospital, University of Bern, Bern, Switzerland

Brigitte Vollmer
Clinical and Experimental Sciences, Faculty of Medicine, University of Southampton, Southampton, United Kingdom
Paediatric and Neonatal Neurology, Southampton Children's Hospital, University Hospital Southampton NHS Foundation Trust, Southampton, United Kingdom

Beth J. Allison, Hannah Youn, Courtney A. McDonald, Margie Castillo-Melendez, Yen Pham, Amy E. Sutherland, Graham Jenkin, Graeme R. Polglase and Suzanne L. Miller
The Ritchie Centre, Hudson Institute of Medical Research, Clayton, VIC, Australia
Department of Obstetrics and Gynaecology and Paediatrics, Monash University, Clayton, VIC, Australia

Atul Malhotra
The Ritchie Centre, Hudson Institute of Medical Research, Clayton, VIC, Australia
Monash Newborn, Monash Medical Centre, Clayton, VIC, Australia

Bobbi Fleiss
School of Health and Biomedical Sciences, RMIT University, Bundoora, VIC, Australia
NeuroDiderot, INSERM, Université Paris Diderot, Sorbonne Paris Cité, Paris, France
Centre for the Developing Brain, School of Biomedical Engineering and Imaging Sciences, King's College London, St Thomas' Hospital, London, United Kingdom

Flora Wong
The Ritchie Centre, Hudson Institute of Medical Research, Clayton, VIC, Australia
Department of Paediatrics, Monash University, Clayton, VIC, Australia
Monash Newborn, Monash Children's Hospital, Clayton, VIC, Australia

Caroline J. Edmonds
School of Psychology, University of East London, London, United Kingdom

Fiona Brownfoot
Translational Obstetrics Group, Department of Obstetrics and Gynaecology, Mercy Hospital for Women, University of Melbourne, Heidelberg, VIC, Australia

Isabelle K. Shearer, David W. Walker and Mary Tolcos
School of Health and Biomedical Sciences, RMIT University, Bundoora, VIC, Australia

Olivier Baud
NeuroDiderot, INSERM, Université Paris Diderot, Sorbonne Paris Cité, Paris, France
Division of Neonatal Intensive Care, University Hospitals of Geneva, Children's Hospital, University of Geneva, Geneva, Switzerland

Pierre Gressens
NeuroDiderot, INSERM, Université Paris Diderot, Sorbonne Paris Cité, Paris, France
Centre for the Developing Brain, School of Biomedical Engineering and Imaging Sciences, King's College London, St Thomas' Hospital, London, United Kingdom

Marjon E. Feenstra, Torsten Plösch, Jelmer R. Prins, Sicco A. Scherjon and Sanne J. Gordijn
Department of Obstetrics and Gynecology, University Medical Center Groningen, University of Groningen, Groningen, Netherlands

Mirthe H. Schoots, Albertus Timmer and Harry van Goor
Department of Pathology and Medical Biology, University Medical Center Groningen, University of Groningen, Groningen, Netherlands

Immaculate M. Langmia
Experimental and Clinical Research Center, A Joint Cooperation Between the Max-Delbrueck Center for Molecular Medicine and the Charité Universitätsmedizin Berlin, Berlin, Germany
Berlin Institute of Health (BIH), Berlin, Germany
Alexander von Humboldt Foundation, Bonn, Germany

Till Schütte
Berlin Institute of Health (BIH), Berlin, Germany
DZHK (German Centre for Cardiovascular Research), Partner Site Berlin, Berlin, Germany
Center for Cardiovascular Research, Institute of Pharmacology, Charité -Universitätsmedizin Berlin, Berlin, Germany

Kristin Kräker and Nadine Haase
Experimental and Clinical Research Center, A Joint Cooperation Between the Max-Delbrueck Center for Molecular Medicine and the Charité Universitätsmedizin Berlin, Berlin, Germany
Berlin Institute of Health (BIH), Berlin, Germany
Charité–Universitätsmedizin Berlin, Corporate member of Freie Universität Berlin, Berlin Institute of Health, Humboldt-Universität zu Berlin, Berlin, Germany
Max-Delbrueck Center for Molecular Medicine in the Helmholtz Association, Berlin, Germany
DZHK (German Centre for Cardiovascular Research), Partner Site Berlin, Berlin, Germany

Sara E. Weiss
Experimental and Clinical Research Center, A Joint Cooperation Between the Max-Delbrueck Center for Molecular Medicine and the Charité Universitätsmedizin Berlin, Berlin, Germany
Berlin Institute of Health (BIH), Berlin, Germany
Charité–Universitätsmedizin Berlin, Corporate member of Freie Universität Berlin, Berlin Institute of Health, Humboldt-Universität zu Berlin, Berlin, Germany

Florian Herse
Experimental and Clinical Research Center, A Joint Cooperation Between the Max-Delbrueck Center for Molecular Medicine and the Charité Universitätsmedizin Berlin, Berlin, Germany
Berlin Institute of Health (BIH), Berlin, Germany
Max-Delbrueck Center for Molecular Medicine in the Helmholtz Association, Berlin, Germany

Ralf Dechend
Experimental and Clinical Research Center, A Joint Cooperation Between the Max-Delbrueck Center for Molecular Medicine and the Charité Universitätsmedizin Berlin, Berlin, Germany
Berlin Institute of Health (BIH), Berlin, Germany
Charité–Universitätsmedizin Berlin, Corporate member of Freie Universität Berlin, Berlin Institute of Health, Humboldt-Universität zu Berlin, Berlin, Germany
DZHK (German Centre for Cardiovascular Research), Partner Site Berlin, Berlin, Germany
HELIOS-Klinikum, Berlin, Germany

Yohan van de Looij
Division of Child Development and Growth, Department of Pediatrics, School of Medicine, University of Geneva, Geneva, Switzerland
Laboratory for Functional and Metabolic Imaging, Ecole Polytechnique Fédérale de Lausanne, Lausanne, Switzerland

Kim E. Boers
Haaglanden Medical Centre, The Hague, Netherlands

Camille Larpin, Eduardo F. Sanches, Audrey Toulotte and Stéphane V. Sizonenko
Division of Child Development and Growth, Department of Pediatrics, School of Medicine, University of Geneva, Geneva, Switzerland

Jan-Harry Cabungcal and Kim Q. Do
Department of Psychiatry, Centre for Psychiatric Neuroscience, Lausanne University Hospital, Lausanne, Switzerland

Atul Malhotra
Monash Newborn, Monash Children's Hospital, Melbourne, VIC, Australia
The Ritchie Centre, Hudson Institute of Medical Research, Melbourne, VIC, Australia
Department of Paediatrics, Monash University, Melbourne, VIC, Australia

Beth J. Allison, Margie Castillo-Melendez, Graham Jenkin, Graeme R. Polglase and Suzanne L. Miller
The Ritchie Centre, Hudson Institute of Medical Research, Melbourne, VIC, Australia
Department of Obstetrics and Gynaecology, Monash University, Melbourne, VIC, Australia

Linda van Wyk
Departments of Obstetrics, Leiden University Medical Centre, Leiden, Netherlands
Department of Obstetrics, University Medical Centre Groningen, Groningen, Netherlands

Aleid G. van Wassenaer-Leemhuis and Joris A. M. van der Post
Academic Medical Centre, Amsterdam, Netherlands

Henk A. Bremer
Reinier de Graaf Hospital, Delft, Netherlands

Friso M. C. Delemarre
Elkerliek Hospital, Helmond, Netherlands

Sanne J. Gordijn and Sicco A. Scherjon
Department of Obstetrics, University Medical Centre Groningen, Groningen, Netherlands

Kitty W. M. Bloemenkamp and Jan M. M. van Lith
Departments of Obstetrics, Leiden University Medical Centre, Leiden, Netherlands

Frans J. M. E. Roumen
Atrium Medical Centre, Heerlen, Netherlands

Martina Porath
Maxima Medical Centre, Veldhoven, Netherlands

Ben W. J. Mol
Department of Obstetrics, Monash University Medical Centre, Clayton, VIC, Australia

Saskia le Cessie
Department of Clinical Epidimiology, Leiden University Medical Centre, Leiden, Netherlands

Christina E. Hayward, Kirsty R. McIntyre, Colin P. Sibley, Susan L. Greenwood and Mark R. Dilworth
Maternal and Fetal Health Research Centre, Division of Developmental Biology and Medicine, Faculty of Biology, Medicine and Health, School of Medical Sciences, University of Manchester, Manchester, United Kingdom
Manchester Academic Health Science Centre, St. Mary's Hospital, Manchester University NHS Foundation Trust, Manchester, United Kingdom

Julia Hartkopf and Franziska Schleger
Institute for Diabetes Research and Metabolic Diseases of the Helmholtz Center Munich at the University of Tuebingen, Tuebingen, Germany
German Center for Diabetes Research (DZD e.V.), Tuebingen, Germany
fMEG Center, University of Tuebingen, Tuebingen, Germany

Jana Keune
Department of Neurology, Klinikum Bayreuth GmbH, Bayreuth, Germany

Cornelia Wiechers
Department of Neonatology, University of Tuebingen, Tuebingen, Germany

Jan Pauluschke-Froehlich and Sara Brucker
Department of Women's Health, University of Tuebingen, Tuebingen, Germany

Magdalene Weiss and Isabelle Kiefer-Schmidt
fMEG Center, University of Tuebingen, Tuebingen, Germany
Department of Women's Health, University of Tuebingen, Tuebingen, Germany

Annette Conzelmann
Department of Child and Adolescent Psychiatry, Psychosomatics and Psychotherapy, University of Tuebingen, Tuebingen, Germany

Lynda K. Harris
Division of Pharmacy and Optometry, University of Manchester, Manchester, United Kingdom
Faculty of Biology Medicine and Health, Maternal and Fetal Health Research Centre, University of Manchester, Manchester, United Kingdom
Academic Health Science Centre, St Mary's Hospital, Manchester,United Kingdom

Hubert Preissl
Institute for Diabetes Research and Metabolic Diseases of the Helmholtz Center Munich at the University of Tuebingen, Tuebingen, Germany
German Center for Diabetes Research (DZD e.V.), Tuebingen, Germany
fMEG Center, University of Tuebingen, Tuebingen, Germany
Department of Internal Medicine, Division of Endocrinology, Diabetology, Angiology, Nephrology and Clinical Chemistry, University of Tuebingen, Tuebingen, Germany

Caroline Dunk, Melissa Kwan, Aleah Hazan, Sierra Walker and Julie K. Wright
Research Centre for Women's and Infants' Health, Lunenfeld Tanenbaum Research Institute, Mount Sinai Hospital, Sinai Health System, Toronto, ON, Canada

Rebecca Lee Jones
Faculty of Biology Medicine and Health, Maternal and Fetal Health Research Centre, University of Manchester, Manchester, United Kingdom
Academic Health Science Centre, St Mary's Hospital, Manchester, United Kingdom

Sarah Keating, Wendy Whittle and Cynthia Maxwell
Department of Obstetrics and Gynaecology, Faculty of Medicine, University of Toronto, Toronto, ON, Canada

John C. P. Kingdom
Research Centre for Women's and Infants' Health, Lunenfeld Tanenbaum Research Institute, Mount Sinai Hospital, Sinai Health System, Toronto, ON, Canada
Department of Obstetrics and Gynaecology, Faculty of Medicine, University of Toronto, Toronto, ON, Canada

Stephen J. Lye
Research Centre for Women's and Infants' Health, Lunenfeld Tanenbaum Research Institute, Mount Sinai Hospital, Sinai Health System, Toronto, ON, Canada
Department of Obstetrics and Gynaecology, Faculty of Medicine, University of Toronto, Toronto, ON, Canada
Department of Physiology, Faculty of Medicine, University of Toronto, Toronto, ON, Canada

Eva Morsing and David Ley
Department of Pediatrics, Clinical Sciences Lund, Lund University, Lund, Sweden

Mariya Malova
Neonatal Intensive Care Unit, Istituto Giannina Gaslini, Genoa, Italy

Anna Kahn and Jimmy Lätt
Department of Radiology, Clinical Sciences Lund, Lund University, Lund, Sweden

Isabella M. Björkman-Burtscher
Department of Radiology, Clinical Sciences Lund, Lund University, Lund, Sweden
Department of Medical Imaging and Physiology, Skåne University Hospital, Lund, Sweden

Karel Maršál
Department of Obstetrics and Gynecology, Clinical Sciences Lund, Lund University, Lund, Sweden

Laura Woods, Vicente Perez-Garcia and Myriam Hemberger
Epigenetics Programme, The Babraham Institute, Cambridge, United Kingdom
Centre for Trophoblast Research, University of Cambridge, Cambridge, United Kingdom

Nastaran Salavati, Jan Jaap Erwich, Torsten Plösch and Sanne J. Gordijn
Department of Obstetrics and Gynecology, University Medical Center Groningen, University of Groningen, Groningen, Netherlands

Maddy Smies and Wessel Ganzevoort
Department of Obstetrics and Gynecology, Amsterdam University Medical Centers, University of Amsterdam, Amsterdam, Netherlands

Adrian K. Charles
Department of Anatomical Pathology, Sidra Medicine, Doha, Qatar

Index

www.ingramcontent.com/pod-product-compliance
Lightning Source LLC
LaVergne TN
LVHW080926210926
848485LV00004B/735